Series Editors: Stephen Wagg, Leeds Beckett University, UK, and David Andrews, University of Maryland, USA.

The Global Culture and Sport series aims to contribute to and advance the debate about sport and globalization by engaging with various aspects of sport culture as a vehicle for critically excavating the tensions between the global and the local, transformation and tradition and sameness and difference. With studies ranging from snowboarding bodies, the globalization of rugby and the Olympics, to sport and migration, issues of racism and gender, and sport in the Arab world, this series showcases the range of exciting, pioneering research being developed in the field of sport sociology.

David L. Andrews
Holly Thorpe • Joshua I. Newman
Editors

Sport and Physical Culture in Global Pandemic Times

COVID Assemblages

palgrave
macmillan

Editors
David L. Andrews
Physical Cultural Studies Research Group
Department of Kinesiology
University of Maryland
College Park, MD, USA

Holly Thorpe
School of Health
University of Waikato
Hamilton, New Zealand

Joshua I. Newman
College of Education
Florida State University
Tallahassee, FL, USA

ISSN 2662-3404 ISSN 2662-3412 (electronic)
Global Culture and Sport Series
ISBN 978-3-031-14386-1 ISBN 978-3-031-14387-8 (eBook)
https://doi.org/10.1007/978-3-031-14387-8

Cover illustration: electravk

This Palgrave Macmillan imprint is published by the registered company Springer Nature Switzerland AG.
The registered company address is: Gewerbestrasse 11, 6330 Cham, Switzerland

Contents

1 **Introduction: Assembling COVID/COVID Assemblages** 1
Holly Thorpe, Joshua I. Newman, and David L. Andrews

2 **The Political Physics of an Unkicked Ball: On Diffractive No-Bodies and Pandemic Non-Matter in Footballing China** 37
Hanhan Xue and Joshua I. Newman

3 **Sporting Coronapolitics: Politics, Ideology and U.S. Nationalism in Pandemic Times** 65
Anthony J. Weems

4 **Lockdown Cartographies: Active Bodies, Public Spaces and Pandemic Atmospheres in Italy** 91
Nicola De Martini Ugolotti, Antonio Donato, and Leonardo Tonelli

5 **Women Sport and Fitness Professionals in Pandemic Times: Feminist Ethics, Digital Connection and Becoming Community** 117
Holly Thorpe, Allison Jeffrey, and Nida Ahmad

6 **Meeting the Physical Online: Thinking with Agential Realism About Digitally Entangled Becoming in the Time of Corona** 145
Kathrine Liedtke Thorndahl, Lasse Nørgaard Frandsen, and Sine Agergaard

7 **Dreaming of "Level Free": Lockdown and the Cultural Politics of Surfing during the COVID-19 Pandemic in South Africa** 165
Glen Thompson

8 **Proximity to Precarity: Confronting the COVID-19 Pandemic as Graduate Apprentices in Physical Cultural Studies** 191
Eric A. Stone, Anna Posbergh, and Brandon Wallace

9 **Black Bodies and Green Spaces: Remembering the Eminence of Nature During a Pandemic** 213
Jennifer D. Roberts, Shadi Omidvar Tehrani, and Gregory N. Bratman

10 **Experimenting with Research Creation During a Pandemic: Making Time Capsules with Girls in Sport** 241
Adele Pavlidis, Simone Fullagar, Erin Nichols, Deborah Lupton, Kirsty Forsdike, and Holly Thorpe

11 **Access & Crisis: Disrupting Ableist Definitions of Physical Activity & Culture** 269
Sara H. Olsen, Stephanie J. Cork, Mollie M. Greenberg, and Erica Gavel

12 **A Community of Athletic Pariahs?: Guilt, Shame, and Social Control in the COVID-19 Pandemic** 295
Eileen Narcotta-Welp and Elizabeth S. Cavalier

13 **On the Subject of Race and Sport: Covid-19, Zoom, and the Necessity of Antiracist Dialogic Pedagogy** 321
Ronald L. Mower

14 **Sport-for-Development and Peace and COVID-19: Technologies, the Body, and Virtual Forms of Programming** 347
Mitchell McSweeney and Lyndsay Hayhurst

15 **Reorienting the Cartography of Coaching to Pandemic Times** 373
Jordan Maclean

16 **Virat over Virus, Cricket over Covid: IPL during a Global Pandemic** 395
Kailash Koushik and M. M. Padmakumar

17 **From Football Nation to COVID 19-Land: Cultural Pedagogies and Political Protests during Syndemic Times in Brazil** 419
Jorge Knijnik and Luiz Guilherme Burlamaqui

18 **Parenting in Pandemic Times: Notes on the Emotional Geography of Youth Sport Culture** 445
Ryan King-White and Michael D. Giardina

19 **Te Mana Whakahaere: COVID-19 And Resetting Sport in Aotearoa New Zealand** 471
Jeremy Hapeta, Farah Palmer, Rochelle Stewart-Withers, and Haydn Morgan

20 **The Uptake of Modern Monetary Theory (MMT) and the COVID-19 Pandemic: Implications for Sport and Physical Culture** 495
Andrew M. Hammond

21 **Furlough, Food Banks and Vaccine Hesitancy: Sport in Britain During the COVID-19 Pandemic** 517
Jon Dart

22 **COVID-19, the Anthropocene, and the Need for Post-Sport** 545
Samuel M. Clevenger, Oliver J. C. Rick, and Jacob J. Bustad

23 **A Syndemics Approach to NCAA Collegiate Sport Participation During COVID-19** 569
Caitlin Vitosky Clarke, Kaitlin Pericak, Brynn C. Adamson, and Kassidy Mahoney

24 **On the Politics and Embodiments of Longing: Snapshots from a Digital Photo Diary Study of Australians' Movement Experiences During Lockdown** 597
Marianne Clark

25 **Playing Through a Pandemic: Football Bodies, Racialized Violence, and Institutionalized Care** 623
Tracie Canada

26 **Mapping the Geographies of Combat Sport during COVID-19: Dana White, Trumpism, and the Landscapes of the UFC** 645
Ted Butryn, Matthew A. Masucci, and jay a. johnson

27 **Corona Games: The Tokyo 2020 Olympics, Celebration Capitalism, and COVID-19** 667
Jules Boykoff

28 **"You realise you tick a lot of boxes": Exploring the Impact of COVID-19 on the Rehabilitating Body Through a Bourdieusian Lens** 691
Joanna Blackwell, Hannah Henderson, Adam Evans, and Jacquelyn Allen-Collinson

29 Paradoxical Effects of the Health Crisis within the Esports Industry: How French Esports Organizations Illuminate the Perceived Revenue Growth Façade 715
Nicolas Besombes and Seth E. Jenny

30 Disaster Football: Billionaire Owners, Shock Therapy, and the Exploitation of the COVID-19 Pandemic in European Football 743
Adam Beissel and David L. Andrews

31 Interview(s) with the Vampire: Research Opportunism During a Global Catastrophe 771
Michael Atkinson

Index 797

Notes on Contributors

Brynn C. Adamson is an Assistant Professor in the Department of Health Sciences at the University of Colorado Colorado Springs. Her research focuses on disability and the medicalization of exercise. Specifically, she identifies ways that medical exercise promotion paradigms contribute to guilt, shame, stigma and compulsory able-bodiedness. She works to develop and deliver peer-led group exercise programs for populations that experience chronic disease and disability and which utilize a critical framework for understanding the role of exercise among these groups. Additionally, she implements disability training among community-based recreation facilities in order to reduce ableism and increase accessibility of physical activity.

Sine Agergaard holds a Ph.D. in ethnography and social anthropology from Aarhus University, Denmark, supplemented with courses on the anthropology of the body from Brunel University. Since 2004, Sine has worked in the field of sports sciences; in 2018, securing a position as professor with specific responsibilities in humanistic and social sports sciences at Aalborg University, where she is now head of the Sports and Social Issues research group. Sine's research engages critically with policies and programs for the inclusion of underserved groups in sporting communities. Sine is manager of the International Network for Research in Sport and Migration Issues.

Nida Ahmad is an independent researcher. Her research focuses on Muslim women's experiences of sport and social media.

Jacquelyn Allen-Collinson is Professor Emerita in Sociology and Physical Cultures, in the School of Sport and Exercise Science, at the University of Lincoln, UK. She is a qualitative sociologist with current research interests focusing on investigating the lived experience of various sporting and physical cultures, together with the sociology of endurance, the senses, weather and 'weather work', and identity. She continues to address the challenges of combining sociology with existential-phenomenological perspectives. Jacquelyn was formerly Director of the Health Advancement Team (HART) at Lincoln.

David L. Andrews is Professor of Physical Cultural Studies in the Department of Kinesiology at the University of Maryland, College Park. His research contextualizes sport and physical culture in relation to the intersecting cultural, political, economic, and technological forces shaping contemporary society.

Michael Atkinson is Professor of Physical Cultural Studies in the Faculty of Kinesiology at the University of Toronto, and cross-appointed with the Dalla Lana School of Public Health. His research and teaching interests pertain to the study of pain, violence, and suffering. Michael's current projects include ethnographic research on invisible disabilities in post-sport movement cultures, storytelling work with male athletes who have suffered intimate partner violence, and arts-based research with people suffering from insomnia. He is past Editor of the Sociology of Sport Journal, and current Co-Editor of Qualitative Research in Sport, Exercise and Health.

Adam Beissel is an Associate Professor of Sport Leadership & Management at Miami University (OH—USA). Adam's scholarship interrogates the geopolitical economy of sport. His primary research interests include: the Economics of Sport Mega-Events; Geopolitics of Sport; Sport Stadiums and Urban Development; Social and Economic (in)justice in College Sport; Sports Labor Markets and Global Athletic Migration; and Sport Globalization. Adam is currently working on two research projects critically examining the political economy of the 2023

FIFA Women's World Cup in Australia and New Zealand and the 2026 FIFA Men's World Cup joint hosted by Canada, Mexico, and the United States.

Nicolas Besombes is an Associate Professor at the Sports Faculty of the Université Paris Cité. His research is focused on sports' digital practices and more specifically on competitive gaming and esports. Through a transdisciplinary approach at the crossroads of the sociology of sport and the game studies, his research topics are related to esports and physicality, esports and public policies, esports and health, and esports and diversity. In parallel, he also is a Board Member of the *Esports Research Network*, Founding Member of the *French Speaking Association for Esports Research and Studies*, Editorial Board Member of the *International Journal of Esports* and the *Journal of Electronic Gaming and Esports*. He is the former Vice President of *France Esports*, the French national esports association, and has advised the Olympic Movement and many sports stakeholders on their esports strategies. Twitter: @NicoBesombes

Joanna Blackwell is a Research Associate and Mildred Blaxter Fellow in the College of Social Science at the University of Lincoln, UK. Jo's research interests focus on the lived experience of health, illness, and physical activity, with sociological exploration a frequent feature of her research. She completed a dual PhD with the School of Sport and Exercise Science at the University of Lincoln, UK, and the Department of Nutrition, Exercise, and Sport at the University of Copenhagen, Denmark, with her thesis entitled 'Socio-cultural influences on exercise and health along the cardiac patient journey: A Bourdieusian perspective'.

Jules Boykoff is the author of five books on the Olympic Games, most recently, *The 1936 Berlin Olympics: Race, Power, and Sportswashing* (Common Ground, 2022), *NOlympians: Inside the Fight Against Capitalist Mega-Sports in Los Angeles, Tokyo, and Beyond* (Fernwood, 2020) and *Power Games: A Political History of the Olympics* (Verso, 2016). His writing on the Olympics has appeared in places like the *New York Times*, the *Los Angeles Times*, the *Guardian*, the *Washington Post*, and the *Nation*. He teaches political science at Pacific University in Oregon. On Twitter: @JulesBoykoff

Gregory N. Bratman is Assistant Professor of Nature, Health, and Recreation, and the director of the Environment and Well-Being Lab in the School of Environmental and Forest Sciences at the University of Washington. His work takes place at the nexus of psychology, public health and ecology, and is focused on investigating the ways in which natural environments impact human well-being. He also develops proposals to integrate these effects into ecosystem service studies and to support ways in which this science can be put into practice to address health inequities that are disproportionately experienced by underserved and socially disadvantaged communities.

Luiz Guilherme Burlamaqui holds a PhD in Social History at Universidade de São Paulo (USP/Brazil). He is currently an Assistant Professor at Instituto Federal de Brasília (Brazil). He has recently published *A dança das cadeiras: a eleição de João Havelange à presidência da FIFA* (Editora Intermeios) and *A Blond Pelé: Cold War Politics and João Havelange election to FIFA* (De Gruyter, 2023).

Jacob J. Bustad (Ph.D.) is Associate Professor in the Department of Kinesiology at Towson University. His primary research and teaching interests are in the fields of sport management, physical cultural studies, the sociology of sport and urban studies. His research has been published in international journals such as *Cities*, *Qualitative Research in Sport, Exercise and Health*, *International Journal of Sport Communication*, and *The International Journal of the History of Sport.*

Ted Butryn is a Professor of Sport Sociology and Sport Psychology in the Department of Kinesiology at San José State University. He received his Ph.D. in Cultural Studies and Sport Studies from the University of Tennessee. His research agenda is positioned at the nexus of critical sport sociology and sport psychology. His work on issues related to athlete activism, whiteness and race in sport, cyborg athletes, and doping has appeared in a range of journals including the *Sociology of Sport Journal*, *The Sport Psychologist*, and *Qualitative Research in Sport, Exercise and Health.*

Tracie Canada is a cultural anthropologist with research and teaching interests in race, sport, kinship, care, and the performing body. Her ethnographic work about American football foregrounds issues of anti-Black racism, racial capitalism, labor exploitation, and structural violence. She is particularly interested in highlighting what football, and its Black players, can tell us about power dynamics in the contemporary United States. Canada is currently an assistant professor of cultural anthropology at Duke University and is working on a book project about the lived experiences of Black college football players.

Elizabeth S. Cavalier is a Professor of Sociology and Human Development at Georgia Gwinnett College in Lawrenceville, GA. Her research focuses on sexuality, gender, and sport, with a specific focus on women's soccer. She has published about the interplay between sports and politics, roller derby, racialized mascots, and gay men in sport. She received her Ph.D. from Georgia State University in 2009, and lives in Atlanta, Georgia with her wife, son, and crazy dogs.

Marianne Clark is an Assistant Professor in the School of Kinesiology at Acadia University, Canada and an adjunct fellow with the Vitalities Lab, University of New South Wales, Sydney. Her research examines the socio-political and embodied dimensions of human movement practices and the intersections between digital and physical cultures. She is also interested people's sensory, embodied engagements with digital technologies in everyday life. Her research has been published in *New Media & Society*, *Sociology of Sport Journal*, *Qualitative Research in Sport, Exercise and Health* and she is the co-author of *The Face Mask in Covid Times: A Sociomaterial Analysis* (De Gruyter), and *New Materialisms, Sport and Fitness: A Lively Entanglement* (Palgrave Macmillan).

Caitlin Vitosky Clarke is teaching assistant professor of kinesiology and community health at the University of Illinois Urbana-Champaign. Trained in UIUC's Cultural Interpretive and Science Studies group, her primary research agenda focuses on examining the use of physical activity interventions as a solution for mental health. She considers how researchers conceptualize their research participants, the disorders, and the relationship between the variables. She is interested in the production of knowledge in this area and social perceptions of people with mental illness. Collectively, her work uses a biosocial approach to exercise science for mental health and holistic college athlete health.

Samuel M. Clevenger is Assistant Professor in the Department of Kinesiology at Towson University. His research interests center on the history of sport and physical culture, with particular interests in the historical intersections of capitalism, Western colonialism, and the construction of physical cultural spaces. His research has been published in such international journals as *Rethinking History*, *Sport in Society*, *Sport, Education and Society*, and *The International Journal of the History of Sport*. In collaboration with Dr. Oliver Rick, he also co-produces the *Somatic Podcast* project.

Stephanie J. Cork (She/They), BAH, MA, PhD currently works at Ontario Tech University (formerly UOIT) as the Manager of Student Accessibility Services. She received her PhD in Kinesiology (Physical Cultural Studies) from the School of Public Health at the University of Maryland, College Park. Stephanie completed her Bachelor's (Honours) and Master's in Sociology at Queen's University in Kingston, Ontario, Canada. Her research focuses on Justice, Equity, Diversity and Inclusion (JEDI) with a focus on accessibility. Stephanie is extremely dedicated to integrating her service, teaching and research, working on large scale projects such as the Including Disability, Global Disability Summit and companion Journal. ORCID 0000-0001-6189-0324

Jon Dart is a Senior Lecturer in the Carnegie School of Sport at Leeds Beckett University. His teaching and research interests are focused on the intersection of sport, politics and protest. He has published in a range of academic journals on the political economy of sport and social media, sports fandom, and sports politics and policy in the Middle East, specifically the Palestine/Israel conflict. His most recent book is an edited collection, with Stephen Wagg, titled *Sport, Protest and Globalisation: Stopping Play*.

Nicola De Martini Ugolotti is Senior Lecturer in Sport and Physical Culture at Bournemouth University (UK) and member of Associazione

Frantz Fanon (Italy). His research follows two related strands. The first focuses on leisure and physical cultural practices as lenses to explore the reciprocal constitution of bodies, spaces, and power in contexts of (forced) migration and uneven urban transformations. The second interrogates the physical culture—environment nexus in times of planetary upheaval. Nicola has co-edited the book "Leisure and Forced Migration: Lives Lived in Asylum Systems" (with Jayne Caudwell, 2021) and has published in journals/books across leisure, urban and migration studies, sociology of sport and cultural geography.

Antonio Donato holds a PhD in Pedagogical Sciences at the University of Padua, Italy. He is currently Research fellow at the Department for Life Quality Studies—University of Bologna, Italy. His research focuses on body pedagogies in institutional and social/ecological contexts, mainly in the areas of Physical Cultural Studies (PCS) end Education Studies. He is co-editor of the book "Le pieghe del corpo" (2019, Mimesis—with Eduardo Galak and Leonardo Tonelli). He is a member of Associazione Leib, Italy.

Adam Evans is Associate Professor in the sociology of sport at the Department of Nutrition, Exercise and Sport (NEXS) at the University of Copenhagen, Denmark. He currently directs the 'Sport, Health and Implementation' research group at the same institution. He is currently Editor in Chief for the European Journal for Sport and Society, and a 'member at large' of the Qualitative Research in Sport and Exercise network. His work focuses upon sport development at both the local and European levels, and understanding the lived experiences of sport, exercise and physical activity amongst marginalised groups.

Kirsty Forsdike is a Senior Lecturer in Management in La Trobe Business School, a Researcher in the Centre of Sport and Social Impact, and Chair of La Trobe Violence against Women Network, at La Trobe University. Her research examines organisational responses to and prevention of violence against women, particularly sport organisations response to women's safety and their wellbeing in community sport. She specialises in qualitative research methodology and multidisciplinary mixed-method evaluations.

Lasse Nørgaard Frandsen holds a master's degree in sports science from Aalborg University, Denmark. During his studies, Lasse focused on (problematic) practices of talent identification and development in European football academies in Uganda. Using a posthumanist perspective informed by Barad's performative ethico-onto-epistemology, Lasse sought to think, re-think, and write critically and differently about these practices in order to expose the exploitative nature of European involvement in talent development in Africa. While Lasse imagined he would be pursuing a career in academia, he now finds himself the head coach of a Norwegian sports club, asking himself questions about Barad and badminton.

Simone Fullagar is an interdisciplinary sociologist who has published widely on gender equity in sport, mental health, active communities and social well-being. With an interest in social and organisational change her work contributes to thinking differently about inequalities. Simone is Professor and Chair of the Sport and Gender Equity research hub at Griffith University. She has received funding from the Australian Research Council and other sources to conduct (post)qualitative research into leisure, sport and health related areas. She is a Fellow of the Academy of Social Sciences, UK.

Erica Gavel is a Paralympian, and PhD Candidate at Ontario Tech University in the Faculty of Science studying "environmental physiology and Paralympic performance". Erica completed a Master of Science at the University of Toronto and was awarded the "Own the Podium—Dr. Gord Sleivert Young Investigator Award" for her research. Erica is a member of the Canadian Paralympic Committee Athletes' Council, the International Wheelchair Basketball Federation Athlete Commission, and the International Paralympic Committee Sport Science and Research Working Group.

Michael D. Giardina is Professor of Physical Culture and Qualitative Inquiry in the Department of Sport Management at Florida State University, USA. He is the author or editor of more than 25 books, including *The SAGE Handbook of Qualitative Research (6/e)* (with Norman K. Denzin, Yvonna S. Lincoln, and Gaile S. Cannella; SAGE, 2023) and

Collaborative Futures in Qualitative Inquiry: Research in a Pandemic (with Norman K. Denzin; Routledge, 2021). He is the Co-Editor of *Qualitative Inquiry*, Co-Editor of *Cultural Studies/Critical Methodologies*, Co-Editor of *International Review of Qualitative Research*, Co-editor of three book series on qualitative inquiry for Routledge, and Director of the International Congress of Qualitative Inquiry (ICQI). He can followed on Twitter @mdgiardinaFSU

Mollie M. Greenberg, M.A., is the senior lecturer of sociology in the Department of Social Inquiry. She received her B.A. in both sociology and women and gender studies from Smith College, her M.A. in sociology from the University of Maryland, and will soon receive her Ph.D., in sociology from the University of Maryland. Her areas of expertise include stigma, deviance and disability. Her work focuses on how perceptions of social status and stigma affect marginalized groups, with an emphasis on people with physical disabilities. Greenberg is currently working on a project examining how origin and type of disability affect perception of people with physical disabilities.

Andrew M. Hammond is an independent scholar based in Staffordshire in the UK. Dr. Hammond is primarily interested in political economies of health, sport, and education. His work has been featured in the *Sociology of Sport Journal* and *Sport, Education and Society*. He has held academic posts at the University of Essex (UK) and the University of British Columbia in Vancouver, Canada.

Jeremy Hapeta (Ngāti Raukawa) is a Senior Lecturer of Māori Physical Education and co-Director of Te Koronga at the University of Otago. Formerly a fully registered Teacher, he taught in primary, intermediate and high schools, before leaving New Zealand to play and coach rugby professionally in Japan, Italy and France. Post-playing and coaching careers, he returned to New Zealand to embark on an academic career. His research interests include critical and Kaupapa Māori theories. He is currently working on a Royal Society, Marsden funded, project to do with Indigenous (Māori) perspectives of Sport for Development (SFD).

Lyndsay Hayhurst is a York Research Chair (Tier II) in Sport, Gender, Development and Digital Participatory Research, an Associate Professor in the School of Kinesiology and Health Science at York University in Toronto, Canada. Her research focuses on sport for development and peace; bicycles and gendered mobilities; gender-based violence prevention; and corporate social responsibility. She has conducted research with a range of sport and development-focused organizations. Her current research—funded by SSHRC and CFI—examines the role of the bicycle, as a possible catalyst for achieving gender equality objectives in relation to the UN Sustainable Development Goals.

Hannah Henderson is Associate Professor in the School of Sport and Exercise Science, at the University of Lincoln, UK. She is also director of the Health Advancement Research Team (HART) at Lincoln. Hannah's research interests focus on physical activity and community health. She is particularly interested in the design, delivery, and evaluation of complex, health promoting interventions and people-centred initiatives delivered in community settings.

Allison Jeffrey Ph.D. is an Assistant Professor in Community Studies, Sport and Physical Activity Leadership at Cape Breton University, Nova Scotia, Canada. She engages various theoretical approaches in attempts towards broadening understandings of embodied experiences in a range of movement cultures. Her research interests include posthumanism, feminist new materialisms and post-structuralism.

Seth E. Jenny PhD, is an Assistant Professor within the Department of Exercise Science and Athletic Training at Slippery Rock University of Pennsylvania (SRU), performance advisor to *KovaaK 2.0* FPS aim trainer, Board Member of the *Esports Research Network*, Deputy Editor of the *International Journal of Esports*, and Associate Editor of the *Journal of Electronic Gaming and Esports*. Dr. Jenny teaches esports courses in SRU's undergraduate Esports Minor and serves as the faculty advisor to SRU's Esports Team. He has provided 100+ professional presentations and has published 50+ peer-reviewed academic journal articles. *Website*: SethJenny.com *Twitter*: @DrSethJenny

jay a. johnson is a professor in the Faculty of Kinesiology and Recreation Management at the University of Manitoba. His current research explores the impact(s) of climatic change on our physical experiences and the interfaces with the environment and climate change. He is investigating how Indigenous and non-Indigenous youth experience the built environment and outdoor adventure/land-based education; community-based research examining the function of the bicycle, culture and community in activ(ism); child labor issues; bullying; sport doping; the use of marijuana and CBD by professional athletes; the Ultimate Fighting Championship (UFC) and the pandemic; and the cultural intersections of gender, masculinity, race, ethnicity, sexuality and homophobia in team hazing/initiation rituals. He has published extensively on hazing, co-editing *Making the Team: Inside the World of Sport Initiations and Hazing* with Dr. Margery Holman.

Ryan King-White is currently Associate Professor of Sport Management in the Department of Kinesiology at Towson University. He has edited a book Sport in the Neoliberal University: Profit, Politics and Pedagogy and more than 20 peer-reviewed journal articles and book chapters. His articles have been awarded as the article of the year in the Sociology of Sport Journal as well as an article designated For the Sociology of Sport spotlight article meant to define a key theoretical issue in the field. He is a NASSS Research Fellow in recognition for his contributions to the sociology of sport.

Jorge Knijnik is an Associate Professor in the School of Education at Western Sydney University (Australia). He holds a PhD in Social Psychology by Universidade de São Paulo (Brazil). Dr Knijnik's most recent books are: *Tales of South American football: passion, revolution and glory* (Fair Play Publishing); *Historias Australianas: Cultura, Educação e Esporte do outro lado do mundo* (Fontoura); *Women's Football in Latin America: Social Challenges and Historical Perspectives* (Palgrave Macmillan) and *The World Cup Chronicles: 31 days that rocked Brazil* (Fair Play Publishing). He is a board member of Women in Football Australia and of the Brazilian *Torcidas Organizadas* Association (ANATORG). Twitter @JorgeKni

Kailash Koushik is an assistant professor of media studies at the Department of Media Studies, CHRIST University, Bangalore, India. He completed his PhD from Florida State University, prior to which he was in Manipal Institute of Communication and London School of Economics for his postgraduate education. His research interests include Critical political economy of media & communication, Media labor, Sports and media, Marxist theory, and Qualitative methods for communication research.

Deborah Lupton is SHARP Professor in the Faculty of Arts, Design & Architecture, University of New South Wales (UNSW) Sydney, Australia. Her research is interdisciplinary, spanning sociology, media studies and cultural studies. She is located in the Centre for Social Research in Health and the Social Policy Research Centre, leading both the Vitalities Lab and the UNSW Node of the Australian Research Council Centre of Excellence for Automated Decision-Making and Society.

Jordan Maclean is a research assistant in the Institute for Social Marketing and Health, University of Stirling, UK. His research interests include sport and public health using socio-material and post-structuralist lenses. He is currently working on two projects related to children and young people's responses to high in fat, sugar or salt brand advertising and an independent statutory review of Northern Ireland's licensing system. He previously worked on the Limiting Virus Transmission during a Sporting Mega Event project.

Kassidy Mahoney holds a BA as a triple major in History, Political Science, and Sociology from the University of Illinois Urbana-Champaign. She wrote an honors thesis in History exploring prostitution in the United States during the Great War and an honors thesis in Political Science on political theory, focusing on neoliberalism and clinical labor. Kassidy received the Martha Barrett Scholarship in American History, the Robert H. Bierma Scholarship for Superior Academic Merit in History, and the Robert W. Johannsen Scholarship for Promising Senior Honors Thesis Research. Kassidy is a second-degree black belt and an international karate athlete on Team USA.

Matthew A. Masucci is Professor in the Department of Kinesiology at San José State University and currently serves as the Associate Dean in the College of Health and Human Sciences. His research is interdisciplinary and interrogates sport and physical activity through the lenses of cultural studies, philosophy, and critical sport studies. Current collaborative research projects include critical, historical, and political analysis of Mixed Martial Arts (MMA) and the Ultimate Fighting Championship (UFC), discourse surrounding the use of marijuana and CBD by professional athletes, and a multi-dimensional investigation of a local social movement called the San José Bike Party.

Mitchell McSweeney is a Assistant Professor of Sport Management in the School of Kinesiology at the University of Minnesota. His research agenda focuses on social entrepreneurship, innovation, sport for development and peace (SDP), and livelihoods, and he often utilizes postcolonial theory, institutional theory, and diaspora to critically investigate these areas. His publications have appeared in *Sociology of Sport Journal, International Review for the Sociology of Sport*, and *Sport Management Review*. His research has been funded by the Social Sciences and Humanities Research Council of Canada and the North American Society for Sport Management.

Haydn Morgan is a Lecturer in Sport Management at the University of Bath, United Kingdom. His research explores the connection between participation in sport and the enhancement of social inclusion within marginalized populations. More specifically, his research seeks to examine how engagement with sport and physical activity may facilitate access into education, employment, and training; develop citizen qualities; or enable young people to accumulate and enhance various forms of capital.

Ronald L. Mower is Lecturer in the Physical Cultural Studies program at the University of Maryland, Department of Kinesiology, School of Public Health, and creator of the Action Assemblage for Justice, Equity, and Peace (AAJEP). His research and teaching are generally focused around critical examinations of social injustice within sport, physical culture and society; more specifically, the contextually contingent, conjunctural, and intersectional processes of material and discursive racialization.

An avowed antiracism educator, Ron seeks to develop students' capacities for collaborative dialogue and critical self-awareness leading to empathetic action and equitable social change.

Eileen Narcotta-Welp is an Associate Professor in the Department of Exercise and Sport Science at the University of Wisconsin—La Crosse. In 2016, she earned her Ph.D. in Health and Sport Studies from the University of Iowa. As a feminist cultural studies scholar, Narcotta-Welp's research interests include intersections of race, class, gender, and sexuality in regards to high performance women's sport in both the U.S. and transnational contexts. Her work appears in the *Journal of Sport History*, *Sport in Society, and Soccer and Society* as well as in multiple edited book collections.

Joshua I. Newman is a Professor of media and cultural studies in the Department of Sport Management and Associate Dean for Research in the College of Education at Florida State University. His research focuses on social inequalities, cultural politics, and political economics and ecologies of sport and physical activity.

Erin Nichols is a PhD candidate in the Department of Tourism, Sport, and Hotel Management at Griffith University. Her research focuses on embodiment, feminist theory and the mediation of sportswomen, with a specific focus on contact and combat sports. She is also interested in visual and participatory methodologies in exploring these movement practices as well as the mobility of these physical cultures.

Sara H. Olsen, PhD, MS, MPH co-founded Crossroads Adaptive Athletic Alliance, a nonprofit designed to increase inclusive fitness for all people with disabilities. Working with people with disabilities in fitness opened Sara's eyes to all the social and environmental barriers to participation. As a result, her PhD focused on the lived experiences of disabled people. She currently works as a Disability Rights Program Specialist supporting investigation and litigation efforts against States that may have violated the ADA. ORCID 0000-0001-6054-2248

M. M. Padmakumar is an avid researcher and follower of sports, and a teacher of English, Media Studies, and Cultural Studies for 16 years now.

His PhD dissertation explored the link between sports and nationalism within Indian popular cinema, studying the intersecting strains of religion, caste, class, gender and colonialism. His research and teaching interests include ecological discourses, cultural studies, critical media studies, peace and conflict studies. Currently he is the Head of the Department of Media Studies at CHRIST University, Bangalore.

Farah Palmer (Waikato; Ngāti Maniapoto) is the Associate Dean Māori for the Massey University Business School and Senior Lecturer for the School of Management, Massey University. She is also a Sport New Zealand Board Member, Deputy Chair of NZ Rugby and Chair of the NZ Māori Rugby Board. Her research interests are primarily informed by critical, Kaupapa Māori and feminist theories. She is currently working on a Royal Society, Marsden funded, project to do with Indigenous (Māori) perspectives of Sport for Development (SFD).

Adele Pavlidis is an interdisciplinary sociologist whose work traverses sport, leisure and mental health. She is interested in concepts, theories and methods that disrupt notions of linearity and fixity. Her 2013 doctorate was focused on the affective dynamics of power in roller derby and since then she has continued to explore gendered power relations in sporting contexts. She was an Australian Research Council DECRA Fellow (2018 to 2021) and is now a Senior Lecturer at Griffith University.

Kaitlin Pericak is an Assistant Professor of Sociology at North Carolina Wesleyan University. Dr. Pericak earned her Ph.D. in Sociology at the University of Miami with specializations in medical sociology and race, ethnic relations, and immigration. Her research uses the case of sport to examine health and illness, the body, and organizations. Her published work appears in *Sociological Focus* and *Journal of the Advanced Practitioner in Oncology*

Anna Posbergh is a recent PhD graduate from the University of Maryland-College Park in the Department of Kinesiology and is an incoming postdoctoral fellow at the University of Minnesota for the Tucker Center for Research on Girls & Women in Sport. Her research focuses on gender, sport policy, safeguarding, and the body, and she has been published in the Sociology of Sport Journal, Qualitative Research in

Sport, Exercise and Health, and International Review for the Sociology of Sport.

Oliver J. C. Rick is currently Assistant Professor in the Department of Sport Management and Recreation at Springfield College. He graduated with a Ph.D. and a Master's degree in Kinesiology specializing in Physical Cultural Studies. Since graduating from the University of Maryland with his doctoral degree he has developed a research agenda that has three main strands: critical analyses of sports media and communication, globalization processes in sport, and urban physical activity cultures.

Jennifer D. Roberts is a tenured Associate Professor in the Department of Kinesiology, School of Public Health at the University of Maryland College Park (UMD). Dr. Roberts is also the Founder and Director of the Public Health Outcomes and Effects of the Built Environment (PHOEBE) Laboratory as well as the Co-Founder and Co-Director of NatureRx@UMD, an initiative that emphasizes the natural environmental benefits interspersed throughout and around the UMD campus. Her scholarship focuses on the impact of built, social, and natural environments, including the institutional and structural inequities of these environments, on the public health outcomes of marginalized communities. More specifically, much of her research has explored the dynamic relationship between environmental, social, and cultural determinants of physical activity and using empirical evidence of this relationship to infer complex health outcome patterns and disparities as well as instigate a powerful shift that recognizes, breaks, and transforms these conditions and determinants of health.

Rochelle Stewart-Withers (Te Ati Awa) is Head of programme for the Institute of Development Studies at Massey University, in Palmerston North, New Zealand. She is an indigenous scholar whose research critically explores the potential of sport as a means for improving economic and social outcomes in developing countries, especially at the community and household level. She is particularly interested in how sport is used as an entry point into communities when looking to address gender and indigenous social and economic disparities, as well as how athletes and communities see sport to be a livelihood option.

Eric A. Stone is a Doctoral candidate in the department of Kinesiology with a concentration in Physical Cultural Studies at the University of Maryland in College Park. His research focuses on understanding the emergence and coalescence of private/non-profit sport programming in disadvantaged communities in Baltimore. He has written on discourses of pain and injury, the exclusionary nature of historical and contemporary greenspace, contemporary discussions of race, sport, and protest, and the role of surveillance in youth sport programs in Baltimore.

Shadi Omidvar Tehrani is a Ph.D. student in the Community Research and Action Program in the Department of Human and Organizational Development at Vanderbilt University. Shadi has a master's degree *in Urban Designing from the Iran University of Science and Technology. Her research is focused on* the Global Development of Applied Community Studies, Public Health Outcomes, and Effects of the Built Environment, and Harnessing Emerging Transit Solutions for Underserved Communities. Currently, Shadi is involved with urban planning, public health, and community psychology research.

Glen Thompson (PhD, Stellenbosch University) is an independent researcher based in Cape Town, South Africa. He is a southern Africanist scholar working on the socio-cultural and political history of surfing and the beach. He has recently published in Hough-Snee and Eastman's *The Critical Surf Studies Reader* (2017) and lisahunter's *Surfing, Sex, Genders and Sexualities* (2018) and has articles in the *Journal of African Cultural Studies*, *Journal of Natal and Zulu History*, *Radical History Review* and *The International Journal of the History of Sport*. He is currently completing a book on South African surfing culture during the apartheid years.

Kathrine Liedtke Thorndahl graduated with a master's degree in sports science, English literature, and cultural studies from Aalborg University, Denmark, in 2015. Since 2016, Kathrine has been enrolled as a Ph.D. student with the graduate program for problem-based learning (PBL) in health science education at Aalborg University, working on a project that aims to think with agential realism to explore how such a perspective might affect possibilities for thinking differently about the assumptions undergirding conceptualizations of problem-based pedagogies, and, inspired by an agential realist ethico-onto-epistemology, to fabulate—to imagine, that is, what a socially just problem-based pedagogy-to-come might look like.

Holly Thorpe (she/her) is a Professor in the Sociology of Sport and Physical Culture at the University of Waikato, Aotearoa, New Zealand. Her research focuses on sport, physical culture and gender, and she continues to seek new innovations in social theory, qualitative methods, and representational styles to better understand the complexities of moving bodies and sporting cultures.

Leonardo Tonelli has a degree in Physical Education with a Specialization in Science and Techniques of Preventive and Adapted Physical Activity from the University of Bologna, Italy, and a Master in Public Health from the Federal University of Rio Grande do Sul (UFRGS), Brazil. He is currently a high school Physical Education teacher in Bologna, Italy. He is co-editor of the book "Le pieghe del corpo" (2019, Mimesis—with Eduardo Galak and Antonio Donato) and a member of Associazione Leib, Italy.

Brandon Wallace is a Doctoral Candidate in the Physical Cultural Studies program in the Department of Kinesiology at the University of Maryland. Broadly, his work examines sport as a vehicle for understanding how hierarchies of race, class, and gender are produced and contested in popular culture, while driven by an optimism that sport can serve as a powerful conduit of social justice. Brandon's past research analyzed the cultural politics of athletic apparel, as well as the representations of Black bodies, spaces, and culture in sports media. His current research examines the Know Your Rights Camp led by Colin Kaepernick to explore the transformative possibilities of community-based sporting activism initiatives. Brandon's work has been published in various academic books, as well as in academic journals such as *Media, Culture, and Society; Communication and Sport*; *Journal of Sport and Social Issues*, and *International Journal of the History of Sport*.

Anthony J. Weems (Ph.D., Texas A&M University) is an assistant professor of recreation and sport management at Florida International University where his research explores the social and political functions of sport. More narrowly, his work focuses on racism, ethno-nationalism, and the politics of domination. He is a founding member of The Sporting Justice Collective and serves on the leadership team for Anti Racist Soccer Club. Both initiatives bring together scholars, athletes, and activists for anti-racist movement in and through sport.

Hanhan Xue is an Assistant Professor of Sport Management at Florida State University. Her research and teaching focuses on the field of management of international business for professional sport organizations, particularly in the Chinese market, as well as e-sports.

List of Figures

Fig. 9.1	Buffalo, New York Urban Renewal. (Source: Puma, Mike. Developing: Bringing Black an Olmsted Parkway, Buffalo Spree, April 1, 2015)	225
Fig. 9.2	USA COVID-19 Rates by Race and Ethnicity	226
Fig. 9.3	Washington, DC COVID-19 Rates by Race and Ethnicity	227
Fig. 10.1	Fragments of Adele's creative rendering of a COVID time capsule	252
Fig. 10.2	Simone's Padlet	253
Fig. 10.3	A soccer player's time capsule	255
Fig. 10.4	A hockey time capsule	257
Fig. 10.5	fragment of Zarlee's hockey time capsule creative renderings	260
Fig. 15.1	Idle goalposts. (Figure 15.1 was taken by Jordan in August 2020 when lockdown restrictions on sport were easing in Scotland)	375
Fig. 17.1	Map on spacial inequality and COVID. (Source Rocha et al. (2021))	422
Fig. 29.1	Number of worldwide esports competitions per year between 1998 and 2021 per Esports Earnings (2022)	717
Fig. 29.2	Esports ecosystem at a glance	719
Fig. 29.3	Respondents' main esports activities	727
Fig. 29.4	Estimated percentage loss or gain in revenues per respondent	728
Fig. 29.5	Total prize money distributed in esports per year between 1998 and 2021 per Esports Earnings (2022)	734

List of Tables

Table 16.1	Categorization of BCCI presidents	399
Table 16.2	Income received by BCCI through sale of broadcast rights	401
Table 19.1	Summary of Results	482
Table 29.1	Estimated amount of lost or gained revenue per respondent	730
Table 29.2	Estimated percentage of lost revenue for each respondent based on the number of FTEs	732

1

Introduction: Assembling COVID/COVID Assemblages

Holly Thorpe, Joshua I. Newman, and David L. Andrews

The COVID-19 pandemic has brought about immeasurable loss. To date, the millennium's first global virological catastrophe has resulted in a death toll estimated to be between 6 and 24 million people (Johns Hopkins Coronavirus Resource Center, 2022; World Health Organization, 2022). Entire families, communities, cities, and nations have been permanently damaged by the spread and effects of the SARS-CoV-2 virus and its variants. Beyond the loss of human life, significant swathes of humanity have also experienced a profound interruption of the prevailing social order, and associated cultural formations and

H. Thorpe (✉)
School of Health, University of Waikato, Hamilton, New Zealand
e-mail: holly.thorpe@waikato.ac.nz

J. I. Newman
College of Education, Florida State University, Tallahassee, FL, USA

D. L. Andrews
Physical Cultural Studies Research Group, Department of Kinesiology, University of Maryland, College Park, MD, USA

D. L. Andrews et al. (eds.), *Sport and Physical Culture in Global Pandemic Times*, Global Culture and Sport Series, https://doi.org/10.1007/978-3-031-14387-8_1

practices. During the pandemic, established conventions of speaking, moving, connecting, cohabitating, and relationally and ecologically existing have been called into question, redefined, and/or eliminated.

COVID-19 has also fecundated *new forms of life* and laid bare *new ways of living*. It has brought to life chaos, precarity, and uncertainty for many people around the world. The pandemic has generated—by necessity or otherwise—new systems of control, new biological and immunological paradigms, and new rationalities for the human condition. It has given rise to new industry, new immunological science, new health and psychological modalities. These rationalities of life have generated discovery, articulation, and control. That which was once seen exceptional has become normalized as entire cities have been shuttered, as children have been abducted by the state and cordoned off from their parents, as health care facilities have been locked down and turned away critically-ill patients, and as governments have redefined the role of the state in preserving (or taking away) human life.

Days and months—and what has become years—have passed since January 2, 2020, the date that the World Health Organization first activated its incident management system in response to a sharp rise in "cases of pneumonia with an unknown etiology emanating from Wuhan, China" (World Health Organization, 2020, para 1). In the weeks that followed that WHO action, the world watched as the city of Wuhan went into lockdown (January 23, 2020), hospitals were instantaneously erected across the central Chinese city to accommodate the mass influx of patients, and the life that filled streets of a once bustling major metropolis vanished. While the local government in Wuhan and the central government in Beijing were eventually able to get the local spread of COVID-19 under control, inevitably, the COVID-19 pandemic spread across the globe.

By March 2020, major cities across Europe, Asia, Africa, North America, South America, and across the Pacific were experiencing major outbreaks of the COVID-19 pandemic (for a visualization of the pandemic's spread, see "Time Lapse Global Spread of COVID-19," 2022). This rapid expansion of the virus infected the bodies and body politics of national populations from China and India to Brazil and Peru, to the United States and Mexico, to the United Kingdom and Russia, to Iran and Zambia, and every nation therebetween. As the virus spread, its effects incited a wide range of political and cultural responses from government officials, to public health officials, to national publics. In many contexts, governments took aggressive measures to contain the spread of the virus. For example, following the initial wave of infections in Wuhan, the Chinese central government instituted a nation-wide system of controls including: mandatory lockdowns in cities with even minimal new cases, swift surveillance and utilization of social tracking technologies (tracking where citizens go and if they might be exposed to new cases), quarantine and social-distancing measures, mandatory face masks and school closures, and other strategies intended to limit the movement of the human population and the spread of the virus therein. China also moved quickly to close its borders to foreign travellers, restricting entry into the Peoples' Republic as early as April 2020. Some admixture of similar controls were put in place in many other national contexts, including New Zealand, Japan, and South Korea.

By contrast, many other national governments took an unstructured or 'hands off' approach to containing the spread of the virus. After a brief period of lockdown beginning in late March 2020, officials in the United Kingdom soon began to publicly downplay the severity of the pandemic for fear of its potentially dire consequences for the national economy. Indeed, as early as August 2020, through Chancellor Rishi Sunak's ill-timed "Eat Out to Help Out" scheme, citizens were actively encouraged to socialize outside the home. Furthermore, such was the apparent governmental antipathy toward actively managing the crisis, that when faced with the unavoidable prospect of a second national lockdown in October 2020 following a dramatic spike in COVID-19 infection rates, Prime Minister Boris Johnson allegedly stated to his Downing Street aides that he "would rather see the 'bodies pile high in their thousands' than approve a third lockdown" (Ellyatt, 2021, para 1). In Sweden, the government took a *laissez faire* approach to managing the pandemic, as citizens were encouraged to 'go on with their lives largely as before,' indulging in nightlife, visiting elderly relatives, and participating in mass gatherings. Government officials stated that a large enough portion of the Swedish population would gain immunity to COVID-19, making the diseases' spread less consequential (Jonsdottir, 2021).

In the United States—which has to date recorded the greatest number of COVID-related deaths—then-President Donald Trump persistently and publicly antagonized his own medical and public health officials, by questioning the effectiveness of masks, of lockdowns and of social distancing, of vaccines, all-the-while proffering a series of scientifically unproven treatments for the COVID-19 virus. In these and other contexts, political officials often cited the slowing of the economy, and the need to get 'back to normal', as major justifications for avoiding any significant actions against limiting human movement or contact during the pandemic.

As the pandemic spread and political actors around the world took (in) action, two defining aspects of the human condition—*life* and *human movement*—were seemingly put at odds with one another. Leaders across the political spectrum enacted a range of technologies, policies, and direct actions intended to manage the spread of the COVID-19 virus. For those nation-states prioritizing the *preservation of human life*, a range of technologies and controls—including mandatory lockdowns, mask requirements, travel restrictions, and containment of public gatherings, were instituted in the name of keeping the population alive. In more draconian contexts, and often as correspondent to surges in positive cases and/or COVID-related deaths, local and national governments enlisted a broad set of repressive practices including policing the streets to enforce quarantines and lockdowns, deploying national guards to quell any resistance of protests movements, and developing integrated surveillance systems to monitor and limit population movement in the name of public safety and security (see Bergamo, Italy c. March 2020 or Shanghai, China c. April 2022).

Conversely, in settings where government leaders, public health officials, and virologists sought to manage the pandemic by *promoting the freedom of human movement*, state action was often framed as antithetical to human life. In contexts such as the United States, Sweden, the United Kingdom, Brazil, and elsewhere, public discourses and state *praxis* cohered around a prevailing ideology of a human's right to move freely, to encounter and interject the transmissible self onto the community, and to allow for the human corpus to move and speak and secrete un-monitored and un-regulated. In the state of Florida within the US, for example, the governor Ron DeSantis and state Surgeon General Joseph A. Ladapo vigilantly decried the use of measures such as vaccination, mask requirements, and social distancing—enacting laws that punished local government and school officials seeking to require or expand quarantine and masking efforts, publicly admonishing school children for wearing masks at mass gatherings, and censuring university researchers and public health officials from reporting evidence of the negative effects and death toll of the pandemic.

In the spaces between draconian statism and viral liberalism, many of the old ways of organizing and experiencing life remained. For example, the benefits of scientific breakthroughs such as COVID-19 vaccines have been unevenly distributed across the global population. As vaccines were made available to the public in late 2020 and into 2021, many Western nations hoarded the supply of the Pfizer, Moderna, AstraZeneca, and Johnson & Johnson vaccines. Consequently, while vaccination rates in Europe and North America surged in early 2021, so too did the infection and death rates in those parts of the world where the vaccine was made unavailable. By confluence of commercial interests, vaccine geopolitics, and scientific stratification, the distributive politics of life-sustaining technologies revealed that the new virus had largely revealed long established geopolitically-contingent framings and formations of human existence.

This stratification of life (and death) during the pandemic was, of course, formed well in advance of the Wuhan outbreak. Through a prefabricated network of biomedical patents, proprietary rights, and pharmaceutical distribution channels, the science of life and life itself was organized in ways that gifted access to some and denied access to others. In 2021 the EU, United States, and other nations refused to support a proposal by over 100 nations to waive patents on vaccines and COVID related technologies. At the same time, leading pharmaceutical companies refused to openly share their technology with the World Health Organisation to enable developing countries to make their own vaccines and save lives.

While the transmission of the virus, and lack of transmission of the technologies needed to save lives therefrom, brings into sharp relief the state of biological and scientific imbalance and interconnectivity during pandemic times, it also allows us to trace the compositional dimensions of the global pandemic. The COVID-19 pandemic has brought about new ideas, new structurations, and new understandings of what it means to be alive: to live. It has also formed new, contested, and negotiated narratives and framings about the healthy body, the healthy body politic, and the role of the state and its scientific apparatuses in preserving life. It has asked questions such as: how does the state allow for the will of its people while maintaining life? What is the role of science in making and sustaining life? What is the role of the responsible citizen in preserving the lives of self and citizenry?

Many of these questions return us to the issues of life, death, and association. The novel coronavirus connected the world—pathogenetically linking the human population. It also created disassociation, *vis a vis* quarantines, travel bans, scientific propriety, xenophobia, lockdowns, and a new global biopolitics. Against and within the dualisms of association and disassociation, life and death, community and immunity, fast and slow, locking down and opening up, we are reminded that life is relational. The relationships of body, virus, immunity, discourse, are all entangled within and constitutive of a broader *life assemblage*. Our focus in this book is specifically on the COVID-19 pandemic as experienced in, lived through, embodied within, interjected onto, and formed within, sport and physical culture assemblages. Following Salman Khan (2022), we wonder: how can the COVID-19 pandemic be conceptualized as an assemblage that is organized through an interplay between a set of heterogeneous, human and more-than-human elements? How can we understand the situatedness, entangled-ness, and productive associativeness of human and more-than-human agents as they moved about, into, and out of sporting and physical cultural fields? In what ways did those movements make, and in what ways were they made by, the pandemic?

Assembling Sport-COVID

The authors in this book take inspiration from a range of theoretical perspectives to help make sense of the social, cultural, material, economic, and political complexities of pandemic in their local, national, and international communities. As well as engaging with individual chapters, we also offer a theoretical apparatus to encourage the reading of chapters-contexts-sports through each other. In conceptualizing, proposing, and compiling this anthology, we re-turned—back, forward, over and over—with feminist materialisms and assemblage theory to examine the contextual nature of the material-discursive expressions of sport in pandemic times. In so doing, we considered how practicing, coaching, researching, writing, teaching, and intervening in sport during the pandemic encourages us to build upon what we have learned over the past five decades in the sociology of sport and physical cultural studies, while also responding to the rapidly changing world around us.

Our diffractive approach to editing, writing and reading this book extends the emergent body of scholarship on the sociology of COVID (Lupton, 2022; Lupton & Willis, 2021; Matthewman & Huppatz, 2020) and the impact of COVID on sport, physical activity, and leisure (Evans et al., 2020; Fullagar & Pavlidis, 2020; Grix et al., 2020; King, 2021; Majumdar & Nahab, 2020; Pedersen et al., 2020; Rowe, 2020; Thibaut et al., 2021). Building upon this important work, we theoretically, methodologically, and representationally explore COVID-sport assemblages as a dynamic and diverse "ad hoc grouping" (Bennett, 2005) of interpenetrating affecting elements encompassing material and expressive forms, human and non-human, animate and inanimate matter: "humans and nonhumans; animals, vegetables, and minerals; nature, culture, and technology" (Bennett, 2005, p. 445). Empirically exploring the dynamic and diverse COVID assemblage, and its complex relationship with equally dynamic and diverse sport/physical culture assemblages, this anthology thus reveals the contingency of sport in pandemic times in multiple different ways: cultural, social, historical, economic, political, technological, and spatial. Here we signpost some of the theoretical "lines of flight" (Deleuze & Guattari, 1987) for reading this book, and for reimagining the future of sport beyond pandemic times.

Moving Bodily Boundaries

In responding to the significant social and personal disruptions prompted by the COVID-19 pandemic, some scholars have turned to new materialisms to "reimagine humanist objectives through a posthumanist accounting of the complex, enduring relations between people, ecologies, and nonhuman actors" (Clevenger et al., 2020, p. 561; Bozalek & Hölscher, 2021; Bozalek et al., 2020; Bozalek & Hölscher, 2021; Lupton & Willis, 2021; Sikka, 2021). In particular, feminist materialist scholars have examined the gendered and embodied affects of COVID-19, prompting reimaginings of the more-than-human condition within and beyond the pandemic (Bozalek et al., 2020; Braidotti, 2020). In so doing, some explain how the pandemic is prompting new ways of thinking about and knowing bodies. For example, drawing upon feminist and queer scholarship, as well as critical fat and disability studies, Lupton (2022) states the "Covid crisis has itself queered human embodiment" (p. 151). Writing in her book *COVID Societies*, Lupton (2022) explains "ideas about the integrity of bodily boundaries and the types of bodies that are more permeable and open to the world have changed" (p. 112). Indeed, the porosity of bodies—the edges and boundaries of bodies—have been brought to the fore, and "notions about intimacy have been overturned, as fears not only of touching others' potentially contagious bodies but of sharing the same air" (p. 112). These risks, vulnerabilities, and intimacies come to the fore in thinking about sporting and moving bodies. As Newman and Thorpe (2021) wrote early in the pandemic, COVID-19 has forced us to reconsider "the relatedness of the body—to other bodies, to vulnerable bodies, to the population as a whole, to particulate matter, to the state and its medical-industrial-complexes. We have been forced to reimagine how bodies move, how movement is relative, how we breathe, and where we can stand or walk or travel or live" (p. 129).

As various chapters in this anthology reveal, the pandemic radically altered when, how and with whom we move. In so doing, it also prompted new reflections and ways of knowing the importance of sport in our society and movement in our everyday lives (Clark & Lupton, 2021;

Clevenger et al., 2020; Fullagar & Pavlidis, 2020; Jeffrey et al., 2022; Wheaton, 2022). Recognising the importance of physical activity for health and well-being during the early months of the COVID-19 pandemic, the World Health Organization and many governments encouraged populations to remain physically active, offering various sets of guidelines and recommendations (Chen et al., 2020; Sallis & Pratt, 2020; WHO, 2020). However, while exercise was often encouraged, and in many places considered an 'essential activity', options for engagement were increasingly constrained. Organized sports and commercial fitness centres were closed and many countries also closed parks, beaches and other indoor and outdoor recreational facilities, with such closures felt unevenly (Duncan et al., 2020; Tupekci, 2020). Important forms of incidental activity (accumulated through daily work, shopping and care routines) were also dramatically diminished during lockdowns and periods of state and self-imposed isolation (Drake et al., 2020). Put simply, the arrival of COVID-19 meant that most people stopped moving in their usual ways (Thorpe et al., 2021).

As a result, our relationships with bodies (our own and those of others) and the spaces and places around us were dramatically altered. For devoted athletes, exercisers and gym-goers, digital spaces became paramount, as a plethora of free offerings (synchronous and asynchronous) emerged from fitness juggernauts such as Nike, Strava, Peloton and Les Mills, as well as smaller boutique studios and individual instructors (Jeffrey et al., 2022). New leisure and fitness pursuits were also created in the home–backyards, balconies and garages–and in available and allowable public spaces (Clark & Lupton, 2021). Sidewalks and roads were soon taken over by runners and families and children on bikes, scooters and skateboards. In many countries, daily walks and connection with nature (i.e., parks, waterways, beaches, forests) became imperative elements of new daily routines. With the rhythms and routines of physical activity significantly disrupted, many people created alternative movement practices, while others opted for less active lifestyles during periods of quarantine (Garmin, 2020; Sallis & Pratt, 2020). Whereas some worried about adding the 'COVID pounds' due to new eating practices and lack of physical activity, others developed new fitness obsessions. In these varied ways, COVID-19 was an 'arrhythmic experience' (Lefebvre, 2004), stopping and (re)starting our regular sporting and fitness practices (Glenney & O'Connor, 2022). For many, the biopsychosocial body responded (i.e., sleep disturbances; increases in anxiety, depression and other mental health conditions; many women experienced changes in the menstrual cycle; weight loss and gain) to such disruptions to the rhythms to daily life (Thorpe et al., 2023).

Throughout the past two years, governments and health organizations have administered familiar and revised information about the benefits and risks of sporting and fitness engagements. WHO and other health organizations advocated the benefits of exercise for minimising the physical effects of COVID-19 and mental health impacts of social isolation, and yet sport and fitness simultaneouly came to occupy an ever more contradictory space in popular and medical discourse (Koren, 2020). Previously framed as 'good' for our health, sport and physical activity suddenly held new 'risks'. In the early stages, heightened anxieties about viral-laden breath, and moving bodies and their secretions, meant exercise in public spaces was associated with the potential for risk and contagion (Freeman & Eykelbosh, 2020). Suddenly breath and breathing mattered differently, the boundaries of the body were thrust into a new light (Allen, 2020; Thorpe et al., 2021). For example, during the early stages of the pandemic, running and cycling bodies were said to pose additional risk because aerosols were more widely dispersed through people's noses and mouths as they exercised (Scanlan, 2020; Thoelen, 2020). As well as the traces of breath, sweat and spit also raised new bioethical questions as to the lingerings of sporting bodies (Newman et al., 2016). Similar debates continued to rage among exercising communities as to the risks of participating outdoors (i.e., surfing, walking, swimming), as well as the benefits and challenges of wearing a mask while exercising.

More recently, with new waves (re)emerging and fears of long COVID-19 circulating, the discourse around exercise continues to shift, with increased messaging about the importance of rest and not returning too soon to strenuous exercise after infection. Sport, health and fitness 'influencers' share their experiences and advice on an array of social platforms, often with very little medical or scientific evidence to support claims that become widespread among particular communities. In New Zealand, for example, beautiful, young, activewear clad 'mumfluencers' have been identified as proliferating dangerous messaging about vaccines and mandates, and proffering alternative 'healthy' and 'wellness' lifestyles, that fuelled one of the country's most significant and sustained violent protests on parliamentary grounds in recent history (Johnston, 2022). Around the world, sport and fitness programmes are being designed to specifically support those struggling with the debilitating effects of COVID-19 to various health systems. Understandings of risk and the boundaries of moving bodies—as they are policed, regulated and navigated—are highly contextual with different countries, regions, sports, communities and individuals reading different sources of knowledge (i.e., public health information, sporting policies, social media, personal experience) through each other. In pandemic and beyond, our individual and collective actions—to move or not to move, where and with whom—have become ever more political, ethical and deeply personal.

Affective Contagion

Another important thread weaving through our individual and collective experiences, and the chapters in this book, are the emotional and affective respondings to COVID-19. According to Lupton (2022), "Intra-acting with humans, the virus has generated intense affective forces of fear, anxiety, dread and loneliness" (p. 138). Similarly, Braidotti (2020) described the "psychic landscape" (p. 1) during pandemic as one of conflicted emotions:

> The underlying mood during this pandemic is affective. It involves complex and internally contradictory alternation of emotions—that mark what I have called the posthuman convergence (Braidotti 2013, 2019). An intense sense of suffering alternating with hope, fear unfolding alongside resilience, boredom merging into vulnerability. (p. 1)

As the pandemic continues without the possibility of a conclusive end in sight, affective respondings of frustration, despair and fatigue continue to refract from and through bodies—on screens, in sports field, at the stadium, on the street, and in the classroom. And yet there must be hope. Writing on the power of 'collective exhaustion' as a more-than-human condition, Braidotti (2020) prompts us to consider the potential of this affective and 'psychic landscape' to contribute towards affirmative ethics in which we not only come to know the human condition differently, but imagine intervening, acting in small and large ways, to build towards posthuman, post-pandemic futures in which human and nonhuman justice must be sought (Jeffrey et al., 2022).

Others have taken up such ideas with a focus on gender, affect and a rethinking of feminist politics. For example, writing early in the pandemic, Fullagar and Pavlidis (2020) explored the affective, embodied and gendered experiences generated by the COVID-19 disruption, explaining "the disruptive biocultural force of the coronavirus highlights the value of more-than-human perspectives for examining the gendered effects and affects on our everyday lives and leisure practices" (p. 152). Drawing upon feminist new materialisms, they embark on a process of writing through the "complexity of embodied affects (fear, loss, hope)", and in so doing, highlight the challenges to "humanist notions of 'agency' posed by these shifting timespace relations of home confinement, restricted movement and altered work-leisure routines" (p. 152). Continuing, they acknowledge the limitations of humanist notions of 'agency' for understanding "what the coronavirus 'does' as a gendered phenomenon" (p. 152). Reimagining the affective and agential potential of more-than-human actants encourages new ways of thinking about politics in pandemic times and beyond.

Sport SpaceTimeMattering

Engaging Barad's concepts of spacetimemattering and re-turning also encourages more dynamic and nonlinear understandings of the relationships between sport-movement-bodies during the pandemic. Barad (2010) writes, "past, present and future, [are] not in a relation of linear unfolding, but threaded through one another in a nonlinear enfolding of spacetimemattering, a topology that defies any suggestion of a smooth manifold" (p. 244; see Brice, 2021; Simpkins, 2017). Although not writing specifically about the pandemic, Barad's (2010) conceptualizing of spacetimemattering encourages new ways of thinking about the "relationship of continuity and discontinuity", the "joins and disjoins", with time and space "out of joint. Dispersed. Diffracted" (Barad, 2010, p. 244). Such an ethico-ontological shift in knowing sport, encourages us to rethink how we know pandemic sport within and across local, national and international contexts. In so doing, we might come to reimagine our past, present, and future sporting, healthy, active selves as not limited to before-during-after COVID-19, but rather as refracting across spacetime, and always in relation with human and nonhuman matter. What do our COVID-19 bodies (with, without, not yet, recovered, still suffering) remember from the past? What do they long and desire for in the future? How are our COVID-19 bodies entangled with past-present-future versions of ourselves, intra-acting with other bodies across a range of spaces (i.e., home, work, the street, the gym, the field of play, social media)? What are the 'hauntings' of our own and others bodies—pre/post COVID—that linger in the sporting spaces we re-turn to, differently? (Thorpe, Jeffrey & Fullagar, 2023).

Engaging with feminist materialisms and assemblage theory, the structure of this book enables new possibilities for tracing the multiple and more-than-human relations and practices through which sporting bodies and risk are co-implicated in particular ways during times of disruption, dis/continuity, and disjointedness. Reading chapters through each other thus prompts new ways of thinking about spacetimematter during and beyond the pandemic. Many chapters, for example, are country specific and located within particular governmental and organizational policy responses to mitigating risk within and across moments and stretches of time. The language within and across chapters differs, from the violence of the 'jab' to effervescence of 'bubbles' (Pavlidis & Rowe, 2021), to the militarism of 'shielding' and 'shuttering', the metaphors are country-specific in many cases, and yet as we read the nation-specific responses through each other, the similarities and differences emerge. In some countries, scientific knowledge played a key role in shaping governmental response, in others science became highly politicized and polarising. As time passed, and vaccines became (more or less) hegemonic—mandated differently across time and space—counter knowledge (i.e., antivaccine and mandate-related conspiracy theories) gained momentum, evoking anger and violence, dividing communities. Human bodies, as they intra-act with each other in sport and movement contexts, and with the virus, and the variety in human, community, organizational and governmental responses, reveal much about how the pandemic has impacted us all, but certainly not in the same ways. Importantly, however, the pandemic is not beyond previous ways of knowing, but rather calls forth a re-turning, over and over again, past, present and future ways of knowing the power and politics of sport, amidst shifting understandings of risk, the value of human life and the ever more desperate need for profit and productivity as signs of 'success' in neoliberal pandemic times.

Vital and Viral Matter

Amongst all of this, the matter of moving bodies—i.e., masks, balls, goal posts, gloves—also came to matter in new ways. Writing in *Vibrant Matter*, Bennett (2010) explores the vital materialities that flow in and through objects. In what she calls 'thing-power', objects or 'inanimate things' are agentic, they "speak to us", affect and move us, with a "curious ability… to animate, to act, to produce effects dramatic and subtle" (Bennett, 2004, p. 351). Taking up such ideas and exploring the agential activation of 'everyday objects' during COVID-19, Sikka (2021) explores the face mask and toilet roll as agentic, "nodal technologies within the assemblages of objects (human and non), relations, institutions, and structures" (p. 12) (also Lupton et al., 2021). For many involved in sport and fitness practices, the socio-material intra-actions with objects of health (i.e., sanitizer, vaccines), sport (i.e., bibs, cones, goals) and fitness (i.e., mats, weights, gloves) prompted new affective relations, sensory experiences, embodied routines and strange new intimacies with sporting human and nonhuman matter (Thorpe et al., 2022). Such objects, while seemingly mundane, 'do' something in that they prompt new haptic encounters of touch and contact in and through our own and others moving bodies. What are the sporting objects that have come to matter differently in and through the pandemic? What do these objects 'do' in shifting our affective, embodied and relational experiences with our own and others sporting bodies? How is sporting matter 'sticky' with affect, abjection, disgust, fear, pleasure and joy? Indeed, how are sporting pleasures, the relational affective respondings of pride and shame, felt differently through and beyond COVID-19?

In Braidotti's (2020) discussion of the "posthuman condition" (p. 1) and the pandemic, she described the limitations of approaches that focus solely on human agency and encouraged the inclusion of non-human forces (including viral formations) to be considered as agentic. Taking up similar ideas in *COVID Societies*, Lupton (2022) writes, "Like other microorganisms, viruses are our companion species, living with and co-evolving with humans as well as sometimes having mortal effects on our bodies" (p. 137). In pandemic sport, what and who are our companion species? Beyond the virus itself, how might other nonhuman actants impact sport-body-assemblages? How might we think of our own and others pets, sporting objects (i.e., running shoes, medicine ball, weights, bike), the wind, sun, tides, storms, dirt and trees, birds in the sky, as agentic in reimagining sport in and beyond the pandemic?

Importantly, acknowledging the agentic capacities of the more-than-human world have much longer histories. Some of the chapters in this book re-turn with ancient and contemporary Indigenous and First Nations philosophies, ways of knowing and learning with nonhuman creatures, objects and forces (see, in particular, Chap. 19 by Jeremy Hapeta and colleagues). Such ways of relating, caring with and for more-than-human communities hold enormous potential for understanding and readdressing the "imbalances of human–nonhuman assemblages, and the violence and crises they create for human and planetary well- being" (Lupton, 2022, p. 126; Smith, 2017; Smith et al., 2021; Todd, 2016). As Indigenous sports, environmental and health scholars have argued, the time to reimagine sporting past-present-futures is long overdue (Hokowhitu, 2021). The human and more-than-human trauma of sport–as an assemblage of intersecting racist, nationalist, homophobic and sexist, ableist, anthropocentric and capitalist vectors–is intergenerational, and despite signs of change, we must not let sport 'off the hook' just because it offers fleeting signs of hope through its compromising "normality" in what are desperate times.

Writing early in the pandemic, Clevenger et al. (2020) turned towards new materialisms to ask searching and novel questions about sport beyond anthropocentrism, prompting us to use the brief 'hiatus' to reflect, challenge and demand alternatives to *uber-sport*, particularly the "corporatization, commercialization, spectacularization, and celebritization" of traditional sports events as they exist in twenty-first-century consumer, neoliberal capitalism (Andrews, 2019, p. 10). Rather than using this moment to demand change, however, many athletes, coaches, organizations and audiences hankered for a 'return' to sport as they knew and loved it prior to the pandemic. In one sense, the pandemic offered us a gift–an opportunity to stop, rethink, re-turn, overturn sport as we've come to accept, desire or despise it. Yet this moment seems to have passed, the hiatus quickly gone with an urgency to return to life as 'normal', economies churning again, and with it, the NFL, Super Bowl, Olympic Games, and FIFA World Cups returned, with all the imbalances, violence and crises they continue to impose on human and planetary wellbeing.

In and beyond sport, COVID-19 is multiply agentic—as virus, as dominant and competing discourses around risk, health and profit, as bodies interacting under new and old ethical, moral, political and economic imperatives. As well as the physical objects in sport and fitness, other nonhuman agents (i.e., the weather, trees, virus/es, policies, money, medals) intra-act with human bodies—individual and in the collective form as in teams, organizations and fans—to produce more-than-human sporting futures. As we discuss below, however, the COVID-sport assemblage has brought bodies together-apart in new ways, communities have fractured and come back together, repeating familiar structures of injustice and inequity, as well as prompting subtle and significant shifts in relations of power operating on and through more-than-human actants.

Connection and Convergence

COVID-19 has radically shifted modes of connection and communication, as well as ways of knowing, doing and becoming sporting communities. Digital technologies became increasingly popular as workplaces, classrooms, and other everyday social settings grasped at new methods of operation, communication and connection. Facing extended periods of social and physical isolation, many workplaces, as well as educational and sporting facilities, were prompted to adapt. Similarly, sports teams and physical cultural communities engaged an array of social media and digital technologies to continue to move together. Beyond considerations of operational capacities, some of these sporting, artistic, workplace and educational communities were also concerned with the question of cultivating a sense of intimacy (or togetherness) through their online interactions (Gallagar et al., 2020). Cultivating connection through screens and online platforms (e.g. Zoom, WhatsApp, Clubhouse) quickly became commonplace as families, friends, colleagues, teammates and communities sought out new ways of coming together during a time of great challenge. As Watson et al. (2021) describe, "the literature on digitally mediated intimacies and affects points to the significant opportunity for digital media to be used for expressions of affection, friendship, familial ties, emotional connection and concern for others" (p. 138). Also writing during the pandemic, Koch and Miles (2020) reveal the many opportunities for welcoming relative strangers into a closer intimacy (defined as connection) through digital environments, and Matthews et al. (2021) explore the "embodied interpersonal interaction[s]" of remote presence enabled in complex new ways by digital technologies (p. 199). Drawing upon feminist materialisms, Clark and Lupton (2021) explored Australian adults use of digital technologies to support their home-based fitness practices during extended periods of social isolation. In so doing, they revealed the sociomaterialities and affective dimensions promoted through 'pandemic fitness assemblages' of bodies, technologies, objects and home spaces.

As revealed in some of the chapters of this book, moving learning, training and research to online environments radically shifted the social dynamics and ways of connecting with others. It is also important to consider how such new digital technologies (i.e., Zwift, Peloton, Rouvy) and training methods are changing the gendered, affective and bodily relations within sporting participation (Thorpe, Jeffrey, Fullagar & Ahmad, 2022). While such changes may have felt necessary to enable ongoing participation in difficult times, they are far from unproblematic. For example, Zwift required competitors to publicly enter their weight, prompting new anxieties among some athletes in these digital environments (Schwenker, 2021). Research on sporting and fitness communities, and new forms of connection and care, as well as emergent forms of regulation, policing, politics and activisms, would do well to consider "digital platforms and communities finding contingent ways of responding to the global coronavirus pandemic" (Margolies & Strub, 2021, p. 12).

Importantly, our understandings of sport-pandemic-assemblages must include the broader entanglements with systemic racism and sexism, ongoing and resurgent transphobia, war and conflict, environmental crisis (i.e., flooding, fire, sea level rise), as well as natural and human-made disasters. Many of the chapters in this book work at the intersections of the pandemic with other significant social, cultural, political and environmental injustices. Many bodies marginalized before COVID-19 have experienced pandemic convergence, with inequalities being exacerbated alongside the ongoing effects of colonialism and neoliberalism. Such injustices are seen all too potently in the demographics of those killed by, and suffering the ongoing debilitating effects of, COVID as it intersects with poverty and inequitable social structures. Access to medical and financial support, to outdoor and recreational facilities, and to sport, have privileged some bodies (particularly able-bodied, wealthy, white men) over others. We can only hope that writing-thinking-moving-teaching-acting-reading this book encourages a rethinking of the biopolitics, ecopolitics, and corporeal politics of sport in and beyond pandemic times.

Re-Turning the Sociology of Sport in Pandemic Times

While the primary contribution of this anthology is that it offers a comprehensive and innovative examination of the impact of COVID-19 on sport in local and global contexts, it also explores how the pandemic has affected (and continues to affect) the international community of sociology of sport and physical cultural studies scholars. Underpinned by the necessity of doing research (and editing anthologies) differently following the upheavals caused by the pandemic (Adamson et al., 2022), this project began with a call to the full diversity of critical scholars of sport/physical culture with the hope of bringing into association important research projects and reflections that, once assembled, illuminate the diverse ways in which COVID-19 is impacting on our current and future imaginings of sport and physical culture. Authors were invited to consider: What are the generative articulations between COVID-19 and our objects of study? What are the impacts of COVID-19 on the people within our field, and the politics and practices of our work within this potentially transformative moment? What are the new noticings, reflections, imaginings that COVID-19 is prompting within our field? With the call for chapters garnering a wave of interest from scholars around the world, the editorial team then worked with care to ensure the voices in the anthology represent the diversity of the field, in terms of geography (authors are writing from and about the pandemic in Aotearoa New Zealand, Australia, Brazil, Canada, China, Denmark, India, Italy, South Africa, UK, and the USA), as well as identities and career stages (including postgraduates, early careers, and established researchers). As Braidotti (2020) explains, COVID-19 evokes an affirmative ethics of "we-who-are-not-one-and-the-same-but-are-in-this-convergence-together." The fields of sociology of sport and physical cultural studies are diverse, and COVID-19 both accentuates our differences, but also brings us together in our observations and reflections on the new articulations of sport and physical culture in local, national, and global contexts. In this anthology we show how the pandemic is compelling many to forge new assemblages that help us understand the effects of COVID, and how these emergent human and nonhuman relations open new possibilities for intellectual practice and the academic fields in which we operate. As such, COVID-19 provides an important opportunity to rethink the political, pedagogical, and paradigmatic approaches/innovations that are required to respond to the significantly altered conditions of our lives: as academics, activists, educators, researchers, and sporting and social beings.

At its most fundamental level, however, the primary aim of this anthology is to make a definitive and comprehensive contribution to the understandably expanding body of research related to sport/physical culture and the COVID-19 global pandemic. To that end, we—editors and authors—individually and collectively examine the generative complexities simultaneously linking, and shaping, the sport/physical culture and COVID assemblages within the current conjuncture. This was achieved by developing a project incorporating a collection of multi-faceted readings of the complex interconnections through which the sport/physical culture and COVID assemblages have, and continue to be, formatively enmeshed. In doing so, the anthology is framed by an ontological understanding prefigured on relationality, liminality, and perpetual becoming. Broadly speaking, the objectives of the anthology are three-fold:

1. To empirically elucidate the complex interconnectivity linking sport/physical culture and various other assemblages, within different spatial, sporting, and societal settings.
2. To highlight the global/local inadequacies and/or injustices of the established sporting/physical cultural order exposed by the multiple and multiplying effects of the COVID-19 pandemic
3. To point to the possibilities of, in Ien Ang's (2021) terms, transitioning to better sporting/physical cultural formations out of the possibilities/opportunities/necessities resultant from the COVID-19 crisis.

Our authors take up and engage these issues in a range of ways. Some chapters are more empirical, others more theoretical, many provide important contextual detail about the specifics of governmental responses in their own countries, and how sports organizations and communities have responded to such radical disruptions to social life. In this way, each chapter is an important contribution in and of itself. We acknowledge that doing research from 'within the ruins' of pandemic life was (and continues to be) difficult. New logistical challenges and ethical tensions emerge, and the context has continued to shift and change, thus making the 'doings' of empirical, theoretically-nuanced, passion-driven sociological research difficult. For most of our authors, personal and professional lives have undergone radical disruption—working from home, teaching online, managing risk and illness, and caring for self and others—and thus we are grateful for their commitment to this anthology, and for the passion they continue to bring to the field, even amidst conditions of uncertainty, disruption and 'collective exhaustion' (Braidotti, 2020).

For many, the pandemic has pushed people to ask new questions about what they do and why. Some are turning away from their careers, or choosing to work differently, prioritising other aspects of their personal and professional lives that feel more meaningful, more urgent. The pandemic has also prompted us to rethink the boundaries within our discipline, the familiar, well-worn categories in which we have learned—through the structuring of our graduate courses, edited books, conference programs etc.—to 'do' critical sport studies. The pandemic has caused such radical disruption to our social, political, cultural and economic structures more broadly, and to sport and physical culture more specifically, but there seems to be a strong tendency for many to yearn for the familiar ways of doing life, to the patterns and rhythms of pre-pandemic life, even if many such patterns are deeply entangled with overly rationalized neoliberal and capitalist ways of working and living. Yet, what have we learned from this disruption, this temporary pause, the grief and trauma, of it all? Rather than returning to our pre-pandemic patterns, might this be an opportunity to revisit some of our deeply embodied assumptions about the structuring of daily life, the doing of sport and sport-related research, and the being of sport scholars? Might we take this moment to rethink the boundaries that have become engrained in our ways of writing, thinking, acting as critical sport scholars? In doing so, how might we—as a community of scholars—reimagine future post-pandemic politics, activisms and pedagogies of our field?

In this anthology, we embraced the opportunity to sit with these tensions, and to consider new lines of flight for our field. As editors, we recognize that we have played a role in crafting some of these boundaries to date; from the selection of topics and the invitation of authors, to the organization of chapters, in a range of pre-pandemic anthologies. Herein, we offer an alternative, a call for a rethinking of the boundaries of doing and (un)knowing sport sociology and physical cultural studies. Thus, rather than organizing the 30 chapters neatly (though artificially) into editor-outlined, logically structured, and nicely balanced sections (that risk reinforcing familiar bounded ways of knowing in our field), we have organized the chapters alphabetically Z-A from the first authors last name, both in an attempt to disrupt the tyranny of alphabetism (Noah, 2011), and perhaps more pointedly, to challenge readers to engage with, and think through, how the contents of this project inform and hopefully extend their own, unique intellectual projects. Hence, within and through this anthology we are encouraging more diffractive ways of reading within and across its constituent chapters, with the hope that doing so sparks new considerations and conversations: "reading insights through one another in attending to and responding to the details and specificities of relations of difference and how they matter" (Barad, 2003, p. 811). Reading chapters through each other in this way may prompt some tensions. It is a subtle reorganizing of power, putting the onus on the reader to carve their own path, their own lines of flight, through the book. For some, such shifting power relations may be uncomfortable. If/when such tensions emerge, we encourage you to sit with the discomfort a little longer. What happens when reading outside our comfort zones, beyond our familiar territories and contexts? Diffractively reading chapters through each other, we hope, will unsettle and reignite the field of sport sociology and physical cultural studies. What can we (re)learn from and through pandemic times? How might we come to know differently what we do, with whom, and for what purposes, in our post-pandemic sport sociology community? What has the pandemic taught us, if anything? Is this the moment to lean back to our familiar pre-pandemic grooves, our disciplinary ruts, as un/comfortable as they may be, or is this an opportunity to sit with the tensions, to reflect, and to consider new ways forward?

The (un)structuring of this anthology is our small attempt to encourage a rethinking of the many ways that we (re)produce the boundaries within and around the sociology of sport and physical cultural studies. Below we present some possible ways of reading the anthology, some chapters that we believe might be brought together into productive dialogue. This schema was adopted from Nelson et al.'s (1992) introduction to the seminal Cultural Studies anthology (Grossberg et al., 1992). As with the aforementioned, we deduced that a conventional table of contents, however sectionalized, could never begin to capture the "multiple investments and interventions and the many alternative ways" that the chapters comprising this anthology could be grouped together (Nelson et al., 1992, p. 17). In this vein, we have adopted a more open and suggestive approach, incorporating chapters divided into multiple thematized sections as determined by the editors. Each of the chapters in this project could be multiply thematized–the dividing lines between major and minor emphases being "far from precise" (Nelson et al., 1992, p. 17)–consequently, we offer the following as our attempt to thematically map the contents of the book. As such, we readily acknowledge the subjective nature of this (and indeed any other) editorial practice in performing the following 'agential cuts' (Barad, 2007), through which the boundaries of, and within, this assemblant project become momentarily stabilized and potentially affecting:

I. **Affect**
   5. Thorpe, Jeffrey, & Ahmad: *Women Sport and Fitness Professionals in Pandemic Times*
   7. Thompson: *Dreaming of "Level Free"*
   8. Stone, Posbergh, & Wallace: *Proximity to Precarity*
   24. Clark: *On the politics and embodiments of longing*

II. **Bodies**
   4. Ugolotti, Donato, & Tonelli: *Lockdown Cartographies*
   6. Thorndahl, Frandsen, & Agergaard: *Meeting the Physical Online*
   11. Olsen, Cork, Greenberg, & Gavel: *Access & Crisis*
   14. McSweeney & Hayhurst: *Sport-for-development and peace and COVID-19*
   28. Blackwell, Henderson, Evans, & Allen-Collinson: *"You realise you tick a lot of boxes"*

III. **Disability, Illness, and Rehabilitation**
   11. Olsen, Cork, Greenberg, & Gavel: *Access & Crisis*
   12. Narcotta-Welp & Cavalier: *A Community of Athletic Pariahs?*
   28. Blackwell, Henderson, Evans, & Allen-Collinson: *"You realise you tick a lot of boxes"*

IV. **Embodied Performance**
   5. Thorpe, Jeffrey, & Ahmad: *Women Sport and Fitness Professionals in Pandemic Times*
   7. Thompson: *Dreaming of "Level Free"*
   10. Pavlidis, Fullagar, Nichols, Lupton, Forsdike, & Thorpe: *Experimenting with research creation during a pandemic*
   24. Clark: *On the politics and embodiments of longing*
   25. Canada: *Playing through a Pandemic*

V. **Gender and Feminist Understandings**
   5. Thorpe, Jeffrey, & Ahmad: *Women Sport and Fitness Professionals in Pandemic Times*
   10. Pavlidis, Fullagar, Nichols, Lupton, Forsdike, & Thorpe: *Experimenting with research creation during a pandemic*

18. King-White & Giardina: *Parenting in pandemic times*
25. Canada: *Playing through a Pandemic*

VI. **Injustices and Activisms**
2. Xue & Newman: *The Political Physics of an Unkicked Ball*
3. Weems: *Sporting Coronapolitics*
9. Roberts, Tehrani, & Bratman: *Black Bodies and Green Spaces*
13. Mower: *On the Subject of Race and Sport*
17. Knijnik & Burlamaqui: *From football nation to coronavirus-land*
21. Dart: *Furlough, Food Banks and Vaccine Hesitancy*
23. Clarke, Pericak, Adamson, & Mahoney: *A Syndemics Approach to NCAA Collegiate Sport Participation During COVID-19*
25. Canada: *Playing through a Pandemic*

VII. **Labor and Precarity**
8. Stone, Posbergh, & Wallace: *Proximity to Precarity*
12. Narcotta-Welp & Cavalier: *A Community of Athletic Pariahs?*
14. McSweeney & Hayhurst: *Sport-for-development and peace and COVID-19*
21. Dart: *Furlough, Food Banks and Vaccine Hesitancy*
23. Clarke, Pericak, Adamson, & Mahoney: *A Syndemics Approach to NCAA Collegiate Sport Participation During COVID-19*
25. Canada: *Playing through a Pandemic*

VIII. **The Agency of Matter**
2. Xue & Newman: *The Political Physics of an Unkicked Ball*
5. Thorpe, Jeffrey, & Ahmad: *Women Sport and Fitness Professionals in Pandemic Times*
10. Pavlidis, Fullagar, Nichols, Lupton, Forsdike, & Thorpe: *Experimenting with research creation during a pandemic*
15. Maclean: *Reorienting the cartography of coaching to pandemic times*
24. Clark: *On the politics and embodiments of longing*

IX. **Methods**
2. Xue & Newman: *The Political Physics of an Unkicked Ball*
4. Ugolotti, Donato, & Tonelli: *Lockdown Cartographies*

10. Pavlidis, Fullagar, Nichols, Lupton, Forsdike, & Thorpe: *Experimenting with research creation during a pandemic*
19. Hapeta, Palmer, Stewart-Withers, & Morgan: *Te Mana Whakahaere*
24. Clark: *On the politics and embodiments of longing*
31. Atkinson: *Interview(s) with the Vampire*

X. **Nationalism**

3. Weems: *Sporting Coronapolitics*
12. Narcotta-Welp & Cavalier: *A Community of Athletic Pariahs?*
16. Koushik & Padmakumar: *Virat over Virus, Cricket over Covid*
17. Knijnik & Burlamaqui: *From football nation to coronavirus-land*
18. King-White & Giardina: *Parenting in pandemic times*
21. Dart: *Furlough, Food Banks and Vaccine Hesitancy*
26. Butryn, Masucci, & Johnson: *Mapping the geographies of combat sport during COVID-19*
27. Boykoff: *Corona Games*
30. Beissel & Andrews: *Disaster Football*

XI. **Materialisms**

2. Xue & Newman: *The Political Physics of an Unkicked Ball*
5. Thorpe, Jeffrey, & Ahmad: *Women Sport and Fitness Professionals in Pandemic Times*
6. Thorndahl, Frandsen, & Agergaard: *Meeting the Physical Online*
10. Pavlidis, Fullagar, Nichols, Lupton, Forsdike, & Thorpe: *Experimenting with research creation during a pandemic*
14. McSweeney & Hayhurst: *Sport-for-development and peace and COVID-19*
15. Maclean: *Reorienting the cartography of coaching to pandemic times*
22. Clevenger, Rick, & Bustad: *COVID-19, the Anthropocene, and the Need for Post-Sport*

XII. **Organization of Sport**

2. Xue & Newman: *The Political Physics of an Unkicked Ball*

16. Koushik & Padmakumar: *Virat over Virus, Cricket over Covid*
19. Hapeta, Palmer, Stewart-Withers, & Morgan: *Te Mana Whakahaere*
20. Hammond: *The Uptake of Modern Monetary Theory (MMT)*
21. Dart: *Furlough, Food Banks and Vaccine Hesitancy*
22. Clevenger, Rick, & Bustad: *COVID-19, the Anthropocene, and the Need for Post-Sport*
23. Clarke, Pericak, Adamson, & Mahoney: *A Syndemics Approach to NCAA Collegiate Sport Participation During COVID-19*
25. Canada: *Playing through a Pandemic*
29. Besombes & Jenny: *Paradoxical Effects of the Health Crisis within the Esports Industry*
30. Beissel & Andrews: *Disaster Football*

XIII. **Pedagogies**

8. Stone, Posbergh, & Wallace: *Proximity to Precarity*
13. Mower: *On the Subject of Race and Sport*
15. Maclean: *Reorienting the cartography of coaching to pandemic times*
17. Knijnik & Burlamaqui: *From football nation to coronavirus-land*
31. Atkinson: *Interview(s) with the Vampire*

XIV. **People**

5. Thorpe, Jeffrey, & Ahmad: *Women Sport and Fitness Professionals in Pandemic Times*
6. Thorndahl, Frandsen, & Agergaard: *Meeting the Physical Online*
8. Stone, Posbergh, & Wallace: *Proximity to Precarity*
13. Mower: *On the Subject of Race and Sport*
15. Maclean: *Reorienting the cartography of coaching to pandemic times*
18. King-White & Giardina: *Parenting in pandemic times*
22. Clevenger, Rick, & Bustad: *COVID-19, the Anthropocene, and the Need for Post-Sport*

23. Clarke, Pericak, Adamson, & Mahoney: *A Syndemics Approach to NCAA Collegiate Sport Participation During COVID-19*

XV. **Physical Activity and Health**

9. Roberts: *Black Bodies and Green Spaces*
11. Olsen, Cork, Greenberg, & Gavel: *Access & Crisis*
16. Koushik & Padmakumar: *Virat over Virus, Cricket over Covid*
18. King-White & Giardina: *Parenting in pandemic times*
23. Clarke, Pericak, Adamson, & Mahoney: *A Syndemics Approach to NCAA Collegiate Sport Participation During COVID-19*
24. Clark: *On the politics and embodiments of longing*
28. Blackwell, Henderson, Evans, & Allen-Collinson: *"You realise you tick a lot of boxes"*
29. Besombes & Jenny: *Paradoxical Effects of the Health Crisis within the Esports Industry*

XVI. **(Post)Pandemic Futures**

19. Hapeta, Palmer, Stewart-Withers, & Morgan: *Te Mana Whakahaere*
20. Hammond: *The Uptake of Modern Monetary Theory (MMT)*
22. Clevenger, Rick, & Bustad: *COVID-19, the Anthropocene, and the Need for Post-Sport*
30. Beissel & Andrews: *Disaster Football*
31. Atkinson: *Interview(s) with the Vampire*

XVII. **Private/Public Spaces**

4. Ugolotti, Donato, & Tonelli: *Lockdown Cartographies*
7. Thompson: *Dreaming of "Level Free"*
9. Roberts: *Black Bodies and Green Spaces*
20. Hammond: *The Uptake of Modern Monetary Theory (MMT)*
24. Clark: *On the politics and embodiments of longing*
26. Butryn, Masucci, & Johnson: *Mapping the geographies of combat sport during COVID-19*
27. Boykoff: *Corona Games*

XVIII. **Race, Ethnicity, and Indigeneity**

9. Roberts: *Black Bodies and Green Spaces*

13. Mower: *On the Subject of Race and Sport*
16. Koushik & Padmakumar: *Virat over Virus, Cricket over Covid*
19. Hapeta, Palmer, Stewart-Withers, & Morgan: *Te Mana Whakahaere*
23. Clarke, Pericak, Adamson, & Mahoney: *A Syndemics Approach to NCAA Collegiate Sport Participation During COVID-19*
25. Canada: *Playing through a Pandemic*
26. Butryn, Masucci, & Johnson: *Mapping the geographies of combat sport during COVID-19*

XIX. **Social Class**

9. Roberts: *Black Bodies and Green Spaces*
17. Knijnik & Burlamaqui: *From football nation to coronavirus-land*
18. King-White & Giardina: *Parenting in pandemic times*
21. Dart: *Furlough, Food Banks and Vaccine Hesitancy*

XX. **Sporting Politics**

2. Xue & Newman: *The Political Physics of an Unkicked Ball*
3. Weems: *Sporting Coronapolitics*
7. Thompson: *Dreaming of "Level Free"*
12. Narcotta-Welp & Cavalier: *A Community of Athletic Pariahs?*
16. Koushik & Padmakumar: *Virat over Virus, Cricket over Covid*
26. Butryn, Masucci, & Johnson: *Mapping the geographies of combat sport during COVID-19*
30. Beissel & Andrews: *Disaster Football*

XXI. **Technologies**

5. Thorpe, Jeffrey, & Ahmad: *Women Sport and Fitness Professionals in Pandemic Times*
6. Thorndahl, Frandsen, & Agergaard: *Meeting the Physical Online*
14. McSweeney & Hayhurst: *Sport-for-development and peace and COVID-19*
24. Clark: *On the politics and embodiments of longing*
29. Besombes & Jenny: *Paradoxical Effects of the Health Crisis within the Esports Industry*

XXII. **Youth**

6. Thorndahl, Frandsen, & Agergaard: *Meeting the Physical Online*
10. Pavlidis, Fullagar, Nichols, Lupton, Forsdike, & Thorpe: *Experimenting with research creation during a pandemic*
15. Maclean: *Reorienting the cartography of coaching to pandemic times*
18. King-White & Giardina: *Parenting in pandemic times*

It needs to be stressed that rather than being any way definitive, these thematic sections are mere suggestions for the way this project could be diffractively read; the ways of reading through the chapters are multiple, and we challenge readers to reflect upon their own lines of flight, and to consider what emerges when they breach some of the familiar boundaries of our field, and our own ways of knowing and doing sport sociology and physical cultural studies. Thus, we encourage readers to curate and annotate their own diffractive reading processes. What chapters might you bring into productive tension as you read between national, sporting, theoretical, methodological, political and embodied perspectives and ways of knowing during pandemic times? By challenging the reader to become more active in the manner in which research is engaged, we hope this anthology provokes new conversations about the politics, practices and pedagogies of a post-pandemic sociology of sport and physical cultural studies. We hope it prompts new possibilities for reimagining the boundaries around what we know and do, in the classroom, in our books and journals, conferences, and in gyms and on playing fields too.

References

Adamson, B., Adamson, M., Clarke, C., Richardson, E., & Sydnor, S. (2022). Social justice through sport and exercise studies: A manifesto. *Journal of Sport & Social Issues*. https://doi.org/10.1177/01937235221099150

Allen, I. K. (2020). Thinking with a feminist political ecology of air-and-breathing-bodies. *Body & Society, 26*(2), 79–105.

Andrews, D. L. (2019). *Making sport great again: The Uber-sport assemblage, neoliberalism, and the trump conjuncture*. Palgrave Pivot.
Ang, I. (2021). Beyond the crisis: Transitioning to a better world? *Cultural Studies, 35*(2–3), 598–615.
Barad, K. (2003). Posthumanist performativity: Toward an understanding of how matter comes to matter. *Signs: Journal of Women in Culture and Society, 28*(3), 801–831.
Barad, K. (2010). Quantum entanglements and hauntological relations of inheritance: Dis/continuities, SpaceTime enfoldings, and justice-to-come. *Derrida Today, 3*(2), 240–268.
Barad, K. M. (2007). *Meeting the universe halfway: Quantum physics and the entanglement of matter and meaning*. Duke University Press.
Bennett, J. (2004). The force of things: Steps toward an ecology of matter. *Political Theory, 32*(3), 347–372.
Bennett, J. (2005). The agency of assemblages and the North American blackout. *Public Culture, 17*(3), 445–465.
Bennett, J. (2010). *Vibrant matter*. Duke University Press.
Bozalek, V., & Hölscher, D. (2021). Higher education hauntologies and spacetimemattering: Response-ability and non-innocence in times of pandemic. In V. Bozalek, M. Zembylas, S. Motala, & D. Holscher (Eds.), *Higher education hauntologies: Living with ghosts for a justice-to-come* (pp. 171–186). Routledge.
Bozalek, V., Newfield, D., Romano, N., Carette, L., Naidu, K., Mitchell, V., & Noble, A. (2020). Touching matters: Affective entanglements in coronatime. *Qualitative Inquiry, 27*, 1–9. https://doi.org/10.1177/1077800420960167
Braidotti, R. (2020). "We" are in this together, but we are not one and the same. *Journal of Bioethical Inquiry, 17*(4), 465–469.
Brice, J. (2021). Women's bodies, femininity, and spacetimemattering: A Baradian analysis of the activewear phenomenon. *Sociology of Sport Journal*. https://doi.org/10.1123/ssj.2020-0171
Chen, P., Mao, L., Nassis, G. P., Harmer, P., Ainsworth, B. E., & Li, F. (2020). Coronavirus disease (COVID-19): The need to maintain regular physical activity while taking precautions. *Journal of Sport and Health Science, 9*(July), 103–104.
Clark, M., & Lupton, D. (2021). Pandemic fitness assemblages: The sociomaterialities and affective dimensions of exercising at home during the COVID-19 crisis. *Convergence: The International Journal of Research into New Media Technologies, 27*(5), 1222–1237.

Clevenger, S., Rick, O., & Bustad, J. (2020). Critiquing anthropocentric media coverage of the COVID-19 sport 'hiatus'. *International Journal of Sport Communication, 13*(3), 559–565.

Deleuze, G., & Guattari, F. (1987). *A thousand plateaus: Capitalism and schizophrenia*. University of Minnesota Press.

Drake, T., Docherty, A., Weiser, T., Yule, S., Sheikh, A., & Harrison, E. (2020). The effects of physical distancing on population mobility during the COVID-19 pandemic in the UK. *Lancet Digital Health, 2*, e385–e387. Retrieved July 15, 2020, from www.thelancet.com/pdfs/journals/landig/PIIS2589-7500(20)30134–30135.pdf

Duncan, P., McIntyre, N., & Cutler, S. (2020). Coronavirus park closures hit BAME and poor Londoners most. *The Guardian*, 10 April. Retrieved June 10, 2020, from www.theguardian.com/uk-news/2020/apr/10/coronavirus-park-closures-hit-bame-and-poor-londoners-most

Ellyatt, H. (2021). UK's Boris Johnson provokes fury over alleged 'let bodies pile high' Covid comments. *CNBC*, 27 April. https://www.cnbc.com/2021/04/27/uks-boris-johnsons-alleged-let-bodies-pile-high-covid-comments.html

Evans, A., Blackwell, J., Dolan, P., Fahlén, J., Hoekman, R., Lenneis, V., McNarry, G., Smith, M., & Wilcock, L. (2020). Sport in the face of the COVID19 pandemic: Towards an agenda for research in the sociology of sport. *European Journal for Sport and Society, 17*(2), 85–95.

Freeman, S., & Eykelbosh, A. (2020). COVID-19 and outdoor safety: Considerations for use of outdoor recreational spaces. Retrieved June 12, 2020, from https://ncceh.ca/documents/guide/covid-19-and-outdoor-safety-considerations-use-outdoor-recreational-spaces

Fullagar, S., & Pavlidis, A. (2020). Thinking through the disruptive effects and affects of the coronavirus with feminist new materialism. *Leisure Sciences*. Epub ahead of print. https://doi.org/10.1080/01490400.2020.1773996

Gallagar, K., Balt, C., Cardwell, N., & Charlebois, B. (2020). Response to COVID-19: Losing and finding one another in drama: personal geographies, digital spaces and new intimacies. *Research in Drama Education, 25*(4), 638–644.

Garmin. (2020). The effect of the global pandemic on active lifestyles. Retreived June 5, 2020, from https://www.garmin.com/en-US/blog/general/the-effect-of-the-global-pandemic-on-active-lifestyles/

Glenney, B., & O'Connor, P. (2022). Skateboarding as Discordant: A Rhythmanalysis of Disaster Leisure. *Sport, Ethics and Philosophy*, 1–13. https://doi.org/10.1080/17511321.2022.2139858

Grix, J., Brannagan, P. M., Grimes, H., & Neville, R. (2020). The impact of Covid-19 on sport. *International Journal of Sport Policy and Politics, 13*(1), 1–12.

Grossberg, L., Nelson, C., & Treichler, P. (Eds.). (1992). *Cultural studies*. Routledge.

Hokowhitu, B. (2021). Indigenous materialisms and disciplinary colonialism. *Somatechnics, 11*(2), 157–173.

Jeffrey, A., Thorpe, H., & Ahmad, N. (2022). Women yoga practitioners' experiences in pandemic: From collective exhaustion to affirmative ethics. *Sociology of Sport Journal, 39*(2), 150–159.

Johns Hopkins Coronavirus Resource Center. (2022). Mortality analysis. https://coronavirus.jhu.edu

Johnston, K. (2022). 'It's like a cult': How anti-vaccine 'mumfluencers' are fuelling the Parliament occupation. *Stuff*. Retrieved March 5, 2022, from https://www.stuff.co.nz/national/health/coronavirus/300520631/its-like-a-cult-how-antivaccine-mumfluencers-are-fuelling-the-parliament-occupation

Jonsdottir, V. (2021). Sweden's unconventional approach to Covid-19: What went wrong. *Chicago Policy Review*, 14 December. https://chicagopolicyreview.org/2021/12/14/swedens-unconventional-approach-to-covid-19-what-went-wrong/

Khan, S. (2022). Assemblage thinking in lockdown: An autoethnographic approach. *Journal of Contemporary Ethnography*, Online First.

King, S. (2021). Of companionship, curfew, and conflict: Multispecies leisure in the age of COVID. *Leisure Studies, 41*(3), 301–309.

Koch, R., & Miles, S. (2020). Inviting the stranger in: Intimacy, digital technology and new geographies of encounter. *Progress in Human Geography*. https://doi.org/10.1177/0309132520961881

Koren, M. (2020). The healthiest way to sweat out a pandemic. *The Atlantic*, 18 March. Retrieved June 2, 2020, from www.theatlantic.com/health/archive/2020/03/coronavirus-gyms-exercise-social-distancing/608278

Lefebvre, H. (2004). *Rhythmanalysis: Space, time and everyday life*. Continuum.

Lupton, D. (2022). *COVID societies: Theorising the coronavirus crisis*. Routledge.

Lupton, D., Southerton, C., Clark, M., & Watson, A. (2021). *The face mask in COVID times: A sociomaterial analysis*. Walter de Gruyter GmbH.

Lupton, D., & Willis, K. (Eds.). (2021). *The COVID-19 crisis: Social perspectives*. Routledge.

Majumdar, B., & Nahab, S. (2020). Live sport during the COVID-19 crisis: Fans as creative broadcasters. *Sport in Society, 23*(7), 1091–1099.

Margolies, D., & Strub, J. A. (2021). Music community, improvisation, and social technologies in COVID-era música huasteca. *Frontiers in Psychology*. https://www.frontiersin.org/articles/10.3389/fpsyg.2021.648010/full

Matthewman, S., & Huppatz, K. (2020). A sociology of Covid-19. *Journal of Sociology, 56*(4), 675–683.

Matthews, B., Siang Se, Z., & Day, J. (2021). Crisis and extended realities: Remote presence in the time of COVID-19. *Media International Australia, 178*(1), 198–209.

Nelson, C., Treichler, P., & Grossberg, L. (1992). Cultural studies: An introduction. In L. Grossberg, C. Nelson, & P. Treichler (Eds.), *Cultural studies* (pp. 1–22). Routledge.

Newman, J., Shields, R., & McLeod, C. (2016). The MRSA epidemic and/as fluid biopolitics. *Body & Society, 22*(4), 155–184.

Newman, J., & Thorpe, H. (2021). Sport, physical culture and new materialisms. *Somatechnics, 11*(2), 129–138.

Noah, T. (2011, January 28). Tyranny of the alphabet. *Slate.com*. https://slate.com/business/2011/01/tyranny-of-the-alphabet.html

Pavlidis, A., & Rowe, D. (2021). The sporting bubble as gilded cage: Gendered professional sport in pandemic times and beyond. *M/C Journal, 24*(1). https://doi.org/10.5204/mcj.2736

Pedersen, P. M., Ruihley, B. J., & Li, B. (Eds.). (2020). *Sport and the pandemic: Perspectives on Covid-19's impact on the sport industry*. Routledge.

Rowe, D. (2020). Subjecting pandemic sport to a sociological procedure. *Journal of Sociology, 56*(4), 704–713.

Sallis, J. F., & Pratt M. (2020). A call to action: Physical activity and COVID-19. Retrieved June 2, 2020, from www.exerciseismedicine.org/support_page.php/stories/?b=896

Scanlan, R. (2020). Doctor warns to 'steer clear' of runners. *NZ Herald*, 1 April. Retrieved May 25, 2020, from www.nzherald.co.nz/lifestyle/news/article.cfm?c_id=6&objectid=12321647

Schwenker, C. (2021). *Extreme dieting in virtual cycling: Changes to the Zwift Esports ruleset*. ZwiftInsider. Retrieved from https://zwiftinsider.com/extreme-dieting-in-virtual-cycling-4/

Sikka, T. (2021). Feminist materialism and Covid-19: The agential activation of everyday objects. *NORA-Nordic Journal of Feminist and Gender Research, 29*(1), 4–16.

Simpkins. (2017). Temporal flesh, material becomings. *Somatechnics, 7*(1), 124–141.

Smith, A. S., Smith, N., Daley, L., Wright, S., & Hodge, P. (2021). Creation, destruction and COVID-19: Heeding the call of country, bringing things into balance. *Geographical Research, 59*(2), 160–168.

Smith, J. L. (2017). I, river?: New materialism, riparian non-human agency and the scale of democratic reform. *Asia Pacific Viewpoint, 58*(1), 99–111.

Thibaut, E., Constandt, B., De Bosscher, V., Willem, A., Ricour, M., & Scheerder, J. (2021). Sports participation during a lockdown. How COVID-19 changed the sports frequency and motivation of participants in club, event, and online sports. *Leisure Studies*, 1–14.

Thoelen, J. (2020). Belgian-Dutch study: Why in times of COVID-19 you should not walk/run/bike close behind each other. Retrieved June 5, 2020, from https://medium.com/@jurgenthoelen/belgian-dutch-study-why-in-times-of-covid-19-you-can-not-walk-run-bike-close-to-each-other-a5df19c77d08

Thorpe, H., Brice, M., & Clark, C. (2021). Physical activity and bodily boundaries in times of pandemic. In D. Lupton & K. Willis (Eds.), *The COVID-19 crisis: Social perspectives* (pp. 39–52). Routledge.

Thorpe, H., Jeffrey, A., & Fullagar, S. (2023). Re-turning to fitness 'riskscapes' post lockdown: Feminist materialisms, wellbeing and affective respondings in Aotearoa New Zealand. *Gender, Place, Culture*. https://doi.org/10.1080/0966369X.2023.2195132

Thorpe, H., Jeffrey, A., Fullagar, S., & Pavlidis, A. (2022). Reconceptualizing Women's Wellbeing During Pandemic: Sport, Fitness and More-than-Human Connection. *Journal of Sport and Social Issues*. https://doi.org/10.1177/019372352211094

Thorpe, H., Jeffrey, A., Fullagar, S., and Ahmad, N. (2022). 'We Seek Those Moments of Togetherness': Digital Intimacies, *Virtual Touch and Becoming Community in Pandemic Times. Feminist Media Studies*, https://doi.10.1080/14680777.2022.2112738

Thorpe, H., Brice, J., Soltani, A., Nemani, M., O'Leary, G., & Barrett, N. (2023). *The pandemic as gender arrhythmia: Women's bodies, counter rhythms and critique of everyday life. Gender, Work and Organization*. https://doi.org/10.1111/gwao.12987

Time Lapse Global Spread of COVID-19. (2022). Yale School of Medicine. 26 April. https://medicine.yale.edu/research/covid/mapping/case-maps/global-time-lapse/

Todd, Z. (2016). An Indigenous feminist's take on the ontological turn: 'Ontology' is just another word for colonialism. *Journal of Historical Sociology, 29*(1), 4–22.

Tupekci, Z. (2020). Keep the parks open. *The Atlantic*, 7 April. Retrieved June 2, 2020, from www.theatlantic.com/health/archive/2020/04/closing-parks-ineffective-pandemic-theater/609580

Watson, A., Lupton, D., & Michael, M. (2021). Enacting intimacy and sociality at a distance in the COVID-19 crisis: The sociomaterialities of home-based communication technologies. *Media International Australia, 178*(1), 136–150.

Wheaton, B. (2022). Adventure sports, risk, and human-more than human wellbeing: Local responses to the challenges of the COVID-19 pandemic. *Sociologia del Deporte, 2*(2), 23–40.

World Health Organization. (2020). Be active during COVID-19. Retrieved June 3, 2020, from www.who.int/emergencies/diseases/novel-coronavirus-2019/question-and-answers-hub/q-a-detail/be-active-during-covid-19

World Health Organization. (2022). WHO coronavirus (COVID-19) dashboard. 25 April. https://covid19.who.int.

2

The Political Physics of an Unkicked Ball: On Diffractive No-Bodies and Pandemic Non-Matter in Footballing China

Hanhan Xue and Joshua I. Newman

In this chapter, we report on fieldwork that never happened. This is a study of no bodies, of no movement, of no (physical) culture, and ultimately of matter that wasn't and didn't. In seeking reflection upon the field of non-events brought to life by a pandemic, however, we also look at how that which never materialized and thus disappeared from public space, discourse, and consciousness *produced* significant political, cultural, and economic re-formations; that is, we explore *the matter(s) that come from the void*. More specifically, this is a study of the biopolitics that came to life as sport and physical culture, and more specifically football (soccer), was suspended in the People's Republic of China during to the COVID-19 pandemic. It is our attempt to make sense of how an enormous government-sponsored football project ceded to the virological and biological forces of a pandemic and how those forces 1) gave life to new political physics and surveillance regimes in China and 2) resuscitated Orientalist representations and tropes in the West.

H. Xue (✉) • J. I. Newman
College of Education, Florida State University, Tallahassee, FL, USA
e-mail: hxue2@fsu.edu

D. L. Andrews et al. (eds.), *Sport and Physical Culture in Global Pandemic Times*, Global Culture and Sport Series, https://doi.org/10.1007/978-3-031-14387-8_2

Prior to the onset of the pandemic, we started an extensive study aimed at examining the large-scale commercial, participatory, social, and infrastructural initiatives being undertaken by the Chinese Communist Party (CCP) and the Chinese Football Association (CFA) to grow domestic interest and business activity in football. As the central government outlined in the 50-point *Chinese Football Reform and Development Program* document (2015):

> Since Comrade Xi Jinping become General Secretary in the 18th Congress of the Chinese Communist Party, he has placed the development of football on the agenda in order to build China as a great sports nation.... Football will have a significant social impact and is adored by the masses. (Wilson, 2016).

Attending to this pronouncement, the CCP charted the guiding ideologies, fundamental principles, and reform strategies that would be used to 'transform' footballing China into a world superpower (see Yu et al., 2019).

The scale of this national football project cannot be overstated. By the start of 2017, China already had 13,381 "special football schools"—training academies that are typically attached to public primary and middle schools and brought into being with the expressed purpose of increasing the nation's footballing talent pool (according to the Chinese government, that number will be raised to 50,000 by 2025). By 2020, China was on pace to have over 30 million elementary and middle school students enrolled in organized and academy-based football training programs (Xue et al., 2020). The government also promised that the nation would maintain over 100,000 publicly-accessible football playing pitches. Football administrators vowed that by 2025 the national football infrastructure would dwarf those of established footballing nations such as Brazil, Italy, Argentina, France, Germany, and the United Kingdom.

This broad State project has been of particular interest to us given the role that sport has played in the increasingly significant and sometimes unnerving interpositions of the CCP into the lives of Chinese citizens. It has been made all-the-more exigent in sporting contexts by the extent to which capital, physical cultural practices, governance systems, science and technology, and athletic bodies have been drawn into complex association at the behest of the State. As qualitative researchers and critical scholars, we have spent the past five years tracing these associations: tracking the flows of capital and people (Yu et al., 2019), recording public football discourses and excavating quieted (censored) disquiets (Liu et al., 2021; Newman, Yan, et al., 2021a), mapping formed and forming football-related social networks (Xue et al., 2020), deconstructing state and private media representations of embodiments of the footballing nation (Newman, Xue, et al., 2021b), and engaging with the lived experiences of (emerging, in-migrating, and out-migrating) athlete-laborers. The more our multi-faceted research project evolved, the more we realized that the state of football in China was deeply (bio)political, ideological, and contingent. As we researched, the CCP and private actors continued to invest more political and financial capital into the sport and in so doing sought to incorporate domestic and distant fans, media corporations, foreign-born players, commercial partners, and political actors.

To analyze how football was both constituted by, and constitutive of, such broader geopolitical and cultural formations—specifically in spaces where footballing bodies and bodily practice were being fashioned to productively serve China's football assemblage—we planned to use the first half of 2020 to conduct observational and interview-based fieldwork at Chinese football clubs and academies. That preceding year, 2019, was perhaps the apogee of China's football project; as the State was formulating plans to bid on an upcoming Men's World Cup, world famous players such as Hulk, Oscar, and Paulinho were plying their trade in the Chinese Super League, and the nation's amateur and youth academy football population had reportedly swelled to almost 200 million players. We were planning to use the 2020 study to examine football culture and practices on the ground: interviewing coaches and CFA administrators and conducting fieldwork at the nation's residential football schools and academies.

However, as the pandemic conditions worsened in China, and the CCP took aggressive measures to limit the transmission of (bodies potentially carrying, information about) COVID-19, we were confronted by a biopolitics of corporeal life, *suspended*. In turn, we found our access to China and its football fields proscribed. Flights were cancelled, visas revoked, mobility systems disabled, and data-based human tracking proliferated. China entered what Giorgio Agamben (2005) might refer to as a geopolitically-unique 'state of exception' (even by its standards), and, to the detriment of our research project, the great football initiative was put on hold.

This chapter offers a study of what didn't happen, and of physical culture that wasn't there to be studied, during the pandemic. We undertake such task to illuminate how social institutions such as football in some ways *gave order* to pre-pandemic China (as elsewhere)—smoothing contradictions between East and West and operating as a state apparatus to form identities, ideologies, and practices. As football receded into the shadows, latent and new politics and biopolitical praxis emerged. Young academy residents were sent home and put under lockdown, stadiums were sealed off for the public, football fans were restricted from attending matches, and matches themselves were called off. For example, as the nearly 10,000 youth footballing bodies were sent home from the Guangzhou FC training academy in the early months of 2020—thus removing the sporting activities and corporeal mass that typically and increasingly came to occupy the housing units and turf-surfaces of the 100+ acre complex in South China's Guangdong Province—human bodies were replaced by dust and wind, balls sat inert and deflated, tactics left unwielded, coaching practices unperformed. It was football in a state of absence—no-thing to be studied, no-bodies to be articulated, no field to be worked.

In what remains of this chapter, we look at how football assemblages deformed, and were reformed, as the COVID-19 pandemic altered political life in the Peoples' Republic of China (and everywhere else). We turn to the notion of diffraction as an interpretive strategy to look at how discourses and discursive practices might be dialogically read "through one another" to engender creative, and unexpected outcomes (see Barad, 2007). Feminist diffraction, in the traditions of Minh-ha (1996, 1997), Haraway (1997, 1992/2004), and Barad (2007), tasks us to think about how matter, as it encounters matter, is re- and de-formed by way of its physical relationship to another matter. In contrast to reflection, the notion of diffraction supposes that a thing—such as an identity, a knowledge formation, an experience—is constituted relationally, and that researchers should stay attuned to how differences are being created in the world, and what particular effects they have on subjects and their bodies. Here we provide a dual-perspective, diffractive reading of difference as related to and through non-matter—looking at how the absence of something also forms other things, through displacement and reterritorialization (see Van der Tuin, 2019).

By looking diffractively to the void, we ask: what can we learn about sport, about physical culture, and about the political body in what appears to be a state of their absence? In this chapter, we provide a critical diffraction on what we found as players stopped running, fields emptied, grandstands were vacated, and the State game was put on hold. In this state of exception—a condition assuredly forged by State-led reterritorializations of pandemic bodies (and anti-bodies) and restricted movement/mobility, pandemic anxieties, and non-normative cultural and sporting conditions—the absence of football served as a productive form-ation through *which associations, relations, and economies of difference could be made anew*. The cultural form-ations of absence included deeply political Western media representations of China, of its people and cultural practices (including sport). The commercial side included a significant *re-formation of football reform*, whereby the CFA in conjunction with the CCP initiated a new round of modifications to further tighten oversite on player development, team ownership structures, professional wage structures, and the overall political functionalities of the game.

We do this by offering a diffractive interchange of what it was like to do fieldwork of that which wasn't, specifically by linking 1) a research actor's (Joshua) extrospective reading of pandemic-era (footballing) China as seen through the lens of English media representations, 2) a research actor's (Hanhan) lived experiences as physically immersed into 'lockdown' China during the pandemic, and 3) of the unavoidably messy, complex, and contradictory diffractions therebetween. In the place of diffractive football matter—which would allow us to chart productive differences found in the intra-actions of bodies (researching and researched), identities, politics, knowledges, and so on. Joshua's images are mediated by thousands of geographic miles and a constellation of ideological (neo-imperialist, Anglocentric, Sinophobic, US-forged) mediations on the state of things in pandemic China. Hanhan's images are forged in the material context of lockdown China, of inability to access basic services, of being in a shuttered society. In conversation, these contrasting images of emptied football fields, academies, and grandstands provide an interesting way of thinking about the relatedness of football to the State, to systems of production, labor, control, to broader cultural economies and cultural geopolitics (of what it means to sport, to be Chinese as difference), which in their existence are perhaps normalized or taken for granted, but in their absence might enable us to identify or disentangle those constitutive elements/associations/matters that in the broader ecologies of the sporting state are relationally purposed to deform, reform, reterritorialize, and redistribute power.

Ascendancy and Anxiety: The State of/and Chinese Football

Due to its size and scale, the major football development project that the CCP and CFA embarked on over the past decade became a matter of great concern for journalists, politicians, and other cultural intermediaries both inside China, across Europe, and beyond. Amongst the Chinese footballing public, the initiative was met with both optimism (e.g., improved performance of the Chinese Men's and Women's senior national teams, increased profile and profitability of the men's professional Chinese Super League) and skepticism (e.g., waisted investment in Xi Jinping's 'vanity project,' the nation's historical failures in the sport, etc.). A study by Gündoğan and Sonntag (2018) revealed that the reforms were perceived by a majority of football fans within China as primarily being driven by a 'response to a public demand to grow the game' (80 per cent), but also as an attempt to raise China's 'soft power' on the international level (59 per cent). These perceptions echo the stated goals in official reform documents, certainly in terms of growing interest in the game and promulgating influence. Relatedly, amongst the Chinese public the reform program was widely considered to be a strategy for promoting national pride and a strong sense of national identity (ibid.). Gündoğan and Sonntag (2018) argued that football fans in China had a sharpened awareness of what the reforms were intended to achieve, certainly at the levels of cultural politics and sport development.

For Anglocentric sport and political pundits outside of China, the football project was widely met with apprehensions about China's growing influence in cultural and commercial spaces previously dominated by Western business and cultural actors. The prospect of China hosting major football tournaments, of the Chinese Football Association capably wielding the footballing labor power of a 1.4 billion populace toward heightened international success, of top players from Europe, South America, or Africa choosing to play professional in China over established European leagues, or of Chinese business elites taking ownership of top European clubs all triggered a range of pronounced anxieties in the Western media. To put it bluntly, the emergence of China as a global football power was largely seen as a threat to the established order of things—both in the spheres of football and of geopolitics more generally.

At the heart of these debates were considerations about how football was being used as a political technology. Many Western commentators—most without any direct empirical engagement with football practices in China—decried the domestic features of the initiative as yet another example of 'authoritarianism' and global interconnectivity (e.g., inflow of foreign football labor, outflow of Chinese capital into the purchase of European clubs or the outflow of political influence into FIFA and other international governing bodies) as an exercise in expanding China's 'soft power.' For example, University of Michigan sports economist Stefan Szymanski (2018) argued that the Chinese football project was destined to fail due to its troubled 'authoritarian' genesis, claiming "China's soccer troubles are a case study in the limits of authoritarianism" (para. 3). As a more recent example from the *New York Times*, correspondent Andrew Keh (2021) drew upon a number of unfounded claims and polemic discourses to provide answers to his own rhetorical prompt, "do sports still need China?" Assumedly unaware that there are sports in China, the author evokes North Atlantic political tropes of China's 'totalitarian threat' and a postulated series of claims about how sport was being used by the Chinese government to cover-up human rights abuses, that the Chinese government and people more generally oppose democracy, and as such that Western sport governing bodies and commercial actors should sever ties with China to preserve their integrity and obligation to equality and free exchange of ideas and commodities.[1]

The 'soft power' discourse was perhaps the most prevailing explanation amongst Western academics and journalists as to why the CCP was seeking to expand its football industrial complex. The overarching argument went something like this: 1) China was investing in football domestically so that it could strengthen the men's and women's senior national teams, improve national team performance in major international events, and thus (like all other nations) look to use that success to galvanize nationalist sentiment within the Chinese public (Chadwick, 2020; 2) Chinese officials were incentivizing investment in foreign football clubs, brands, and in an influx of high-profile foreign players into the CSL as a way to legitimize Chinese business interests and further infiltrate those interests into the finance- and ethno-scapes of the global (sports) marketplace. The corresponding commercialization activities would thus form interdependencies that would render major clubs, leagues, and affiliated commercial partners reliant on Chinese-based capital (Xue et al., 2020); and 3) the CCP, through its investments and incentivization for private capitalists to invest in football, were seeking to place operatives in positions of influence within the sport's major governing bodies, most notably FIFA (Yu et al., 2019).

From one perspective, the underlying rhetorical function of these platitudes was to (re)center the West, neutralizing and naturalizing the idea that sport ownerships is only problematic when in the hands of non-Europeans or non-Westerners. Jacques deLisle, the Director of the Center for the Study of Contemporary China at the University of Pennsylvania, stated that:

[1] Most notably, that the CCP had detained and censored tennis player Peng Shuai after allegations of sexual coercion. Peng had posted social media that she was she was victim of an act of sexual coercion at the hands of retired Vice Premier Zhang Gaoli, with whom she on ongoing relationship for more than a decade. Peng Shuai later explained that "I have never said or written that anyone has sexually assaulted me, I have to clearly stress this point" and later stated that the post and then removal of the social media post "with regards to Weibo, it's about my personal privacy. There's been a lot of misunderstanding." The investigation of Zhang Gaoli is of this writing still ongoing, and at no point was there evidence that Peng Shuai was detained or that the CCP deleted the post.

> FIFA might be in a weaker position than the N.B.A. to put pressure on China. While the N.B.A. is dominated by wealthy American team owners, FIFA is a United Nations-like grouping of national soccer federations. Many of these soccer federations are in countries that have weak human rights records or are financially dependent on loans from China, or both. (quoted in Bradsher & Panja, 2019, para. 25)

The assumption underlying this argument is that China was anchoring football as a double pivot, to further interpose its business and political interests into both 'developing' and 'developed' national political economies, but also to forge football-specific interdependencies that could allow Chinese football's administrative aspirants to seize power of the global sport. This line of reasoning tended to assume that China's foray into global football is uniquely geopolitical—that football is genetically and banally European, that any European-based business or cultural practices naturally lie at the center of globalized interconnectivities, and that an Eastward shift in power presented a threat not only to European and North American interests but to the very core values and cultural politics of the sport itself.

Simon Chadwick, Global Professor of Sport & Director of the Centre for Eurasian Sport, Emlyon Business School, proclaimed in no uncertain terms that China was an outsider in the global/Western football order:

> There is no culture of playing football in China. Period. Someone like me—I was born and brought up in England where I had a father and grandfather who were season ticket holders. I went to a school where it was football in winter, cricket in summer. It was almost part of my DNA was football. Cricket as well. It's not part of China's DNA to play football. (Chadwick, quoted in Naik, 2021)

In seeking to naturalize Europe's place in the sport's history,[2] Chadwick evoked a common narrative: that in the world of football (as in the world of geopolitics), China is generally considered a cultural and political

[2] Specifically, by erasing the role of what many (including FIFA) believe is the original or forerunning form of the sport—the ancient Chinese sport *cuju* (a military sport that originated 2300 years ago in the Chinese city of Lin Zi and served to train the troops and check the physical condition of the soldiers, the literally meaning of which is *cu* "to kick" *ju* "a type of leather ball").

interloper, and that the game and its capital and history fundamentally belonged to Europe and its people (best captured by the English men's national team's supporters Euro 2020 anthem "football's coming home"). Chadwick was not alone in trying to position Chinese investment and expanded influence in international football as an 'incursion' into that which belonged to the West (Eckner, 2021). A 2019 CCP reformed aimed at curbing mainland and Hong Kong-based investment in European football ownership was lauded in a *Bloomberg* headline thusly: "It Looks Like China's European Soccer Invasion Is Over" (Bloomberg, 2017). These tropes of *stealing* top players (e.g., Chelsea's Oscar, the Brazilian player Hulk, former Manchester City player Carlos Tevez, etc.), *invading* the European game (by taking ownership of clubs in top leagues such as AC Milan, Espanyol, Inter Milan, West Bromwich Albion, etc.),[3] and other negative associations regarding who belongs in the global game as well as to whom the game belongs. In what could be described as a modern day *five-eyes football alliance*,[4] Western cultural intermediaries assembled a set of narratives that sought to caricaturize the People's Republic and popularize conventions that China needs to be policed, surveilled, and held to a different standard than those imposed upon business and political actors in the field of global sport and industry more generally.

Through our research, we sought to reconcile the fields of discourse and practice, to put Orientalist representations of footballing China in association with material practices of football administration, performances of sport-based spectacle nationalism, and the enacted strategies aiming to utilize the sport as a platform for telling the story of China's modernization and football's globalization. *The latter's disappearance during the pandemic, we found, gave new life to the former's import*. To

[3] Chadwick explains that this withdrawal of Chinese investment in European football came about "in conjunction with a more draconian state that is acting increasingly bullish toward entrepreneurs and its business people" (WallStreet, 2021, para. 7).

[4] The Five Eyes is an intelligence-sharing alliance consisting of the US, UK, Australia, Canada & New Zealand. As one journalist critical of pro-Western ideologies that often frame sport in China put it with respect to how these Western powers are using the 2022 Beijing Olympics to promote their interests, "The Five Eyes, constituting a majority of 'diplomatic boycott' participants, are united not just by the English language but by a common history of settler colonialism, Indigenous genocide, and violently enforced regional and global hegemony" (Xu, 2022, para. 4).

illustrate, we now turn to these competing frames of representation and action, first examining the mediated assemblage of (non-)footballing China as presented to Joshua during the COVID-19 pandemic. We follow that by exploring the material and experiential state of non-footballing China that Hanhan discovered during her time in China in 2020 and 2021.

'At What Cost'?: Framing China, and Football, in a State of Exception

The status of China has been of primary concern to Western politicians and intermediaries in recent years. Even prior to the onset of the COVID-19 pandemic—which many Western scientists and politicians have asserted originated in a market in the Chinese city of Wuhan—Western politicians and political operatives have framed China as the next great 'threat' to Western liberal democracy, a locus of human rights abuses, and the world's next great imperialist nation. A vast confederation of political actors have used their public platforms to stoke the flames of international anti-China sentimentality and governmentality (by exigently exclaiming China's 'threat' to human rights, sovereignty, and global public health). These political figures have rendered China as authoritarian state "actively pursuing crimes against humanity" (Boykoff, qtd. in Putz, 2021), uncompromisingly silencing all forms of dissent, enacting Marshal Law to hold control of the population, suppressing all forms of democratic expression, imprisoning and massacring millions of Uighurs and members of other ethnic minority groups, 'aggressively' military tensions off the eastern coast and southern border of China, and emerging as the world's 'greatest threat to the civility and peace' that define the US-led world order.

This Manichean view of China and the West, as specifically constructed in US media, has perhaps achieved its intended effects. In a recent Pew Center survey (Silver et al., 2021), the percentage of Americans who have a negative view of China increased from 36% in 2010 to 72% in 2020. Half of surveyed Americans are in favor of the US taking political or military action to curtail China's geopolitical influence. Indeed, a majority of Americans see China as "a major threat or problem" in the areas of cybersecurity, trade, human rights, climate change, and the handling of the global pandemic (Silver et al., 2021). Relatedly, and as a consequence of these negative mediations, the United States has seen a rapid increased in hate crimes against Asian, Asian American, and specifically Chinese Americans. Based on a compilation of hate crime data, published by the Center for the Study of Hate and Extremism, anti-Asian hate crime in the United States increased by 339 percent in 2021 compared to the year before (which also saw in an increase of 173% from 2019), with New York, San Francisco, Los Angeles and other cities surpassing their record numbers in 2020 (Yam, 2022). As further reflection—and indeed accelerant—of these rising tensions, US politicians have aggressively sought to impose new sanctions on China and its political affiliates, to limit pathways to US citizenship for Chinese migrants and diaspora, and to limit access into the United States for Chinese students and workers.

This was the China that Joshua came to know during the period of non-fieldwork. Keeping track of China and its politics, culture, economy, and football became an exercise in navigating a cacophony of geopolitical doublespeak, race-based essentialisms about the Chinese culture, abjectifications of the 100 million members of the Chinese Communist Party (and the Chinese population *writ large*), and war-priming narratives about China's supposed conflict-driven global ambitions. During the pandemic, Western journalists turned to the talking points fabricated for them by military-industrialists and neoconservative thinktanks. The COVID-19 pandemic has largely served to heighten these anti-China sentiments and anxieties. Of course, prior to the pandemic, China's economy was growing at a pace that was inevitably going to lead it to the top of the table of the world's largest economies (likely by 2028), and as the CCP's influence over the international political-scape expanded apace at a rate only matched by its Belt and Road initiative (Freymann, 2022), Western political forces were amassing in law and front page declarations to thwart the coming 'China threat.' The pandemic—and origin stories thereof—provided a shorthand vilification strategy resting on old Sinophobic tropes that the Chinese people were uncivilized (diet, cleanliness, etc.) and that the Chinese government was paradoxically overly repressive and too free in spreading its people, culture, and bios to the rest of the world.

To add substance to this wave of anti-China discourse, political intermediaries often simply made things up, manufactured pseudo-facts to suit political aims. For example, the American media public was inundated in 2021 with a prevailing "lab leak" theory, whereby public figures from President Joe Biden to FOX News hosts to comedians such as John Stewart speculated/postulated the unfounded and unproven 'theory' that the SARS-COV-2 virus originated in the Wuhan Institute of Virology. Even though expert analyses by both the World Health Organization (March 2021) and the US Intelligence Community (October 2021) concluded that the Chinese government did not have foreknowledge of the outbreak, and that there was no evidence that the virus was engineered in or leaked from the lab, these myths came to define how many Americans viewed China's role in the early phases of the pandemic.

In an article seeking to establish the "fact" that China was under-reporting COVID deaths and thus mishandling the pandemic, the *Economist* used machine learning techniques (based on assumptions related to how Western nations have handled the pandemic, and represents normal public health conditions and outcomes) to model "excess mortality"—presenting as fact that China had reported less than 1% of the actual Covid deaths in the country (Calhoun, 2022; The Economist, 2022a). The unnamed authors of the report speculated that, based on mortality trends in other countries, and counterfactually 'filling in gaps' in the data for China, the learned machines had predicted that the CCP was hiding millions of deaths, and that China's reported mortality rate is more than 100,000 times lower than the major Western countries. The *Economist* then doubled-down with a follow-up article seeking to illustrate how China is one of only a few nations that—by still restricting people's movement and ability to congregate during outbreaks—has 'regressed' in terms of human mobility (The Economist, 2022b). As the COVID-19 death toll in the United States neared one million people, this magazine turned its critical eye toward some restrictions China had put in place to keep its population alive. Absent any empirical evidence, this framing of China as both the source of the pandemic and—unlike the United States—incapable of tracking and handling its spread, painted for Western readers a picture of mismanagement, deception, and distrust.

These fabrications of China—supposedly rooted in scientific and data-driven truths—have been buoyed by more direct political discourses seeking to brand China/Chinese as biological threat to Western peoples, systems, and cultures. In a *Wall Street Journal* article authored by the academic Walter Russell Mead (2020) titled "China is the Real Sick Man of Asia," the author seeks to leverage the public health crisis ravaging China toward a broader critique of the CCP, of government 'secrecy,' and of the Chinese people as being complicit in the spread of the virus. In terms of the politics of embodiment, Mead also conjures a rhetorical phrasing from the Ottoman Empire era to connect the individuated and racialized Chinese human body (i.e. sick, diseased, etc.) to the body politic, and specifically renders the bodies associated with a specific nation and culture as abject, the 'real sick man' is thus rhetorically positioned at once as the body politic, the head of state (Xi Jinping), and every Chinese "man" who is ethnically or geopolitically associable to the Peoples' Republic.

Football spaces and the missing bodies therewithin became part of a larger biopolitical disappearance-assemblage: missing bodies, missing facts. As the entanglement of the global football network decoupled during the pandemic, Western commentators used the pandemic pause to 'take stock' of how football, and the global sports industry more generally, had become so reliant on the promise of Chinese consumer markets and the investment of China's venturers. For example, in a recent report on CNN, Western 'China experts' weighted in on the following interrogative: "The China market is lucrative for the sports business, *but at what cost* (italics added)?" Contributors to the piece went on to make the case that "Beijing's influence in sports is growing with its massive potential spending power and fan base. Sports organizations have to be much more delicate with China in order to not be censored or banned from the country" (Ripley, 2021).

This links to the major, almost formulaic, talking point that surfaced in the Western media with respect to China: what is the 'cost' the Western world pays to continue to sustain commercial, political, and cultural interdependencies with China? The 'at-what-cost-ism' was also often applied to the sacrifices the Chinese people are paying to remain subjects of CCP control. During the pandemic, Western intermediaries deployed the 'at-what-cost' platitudes to chasten China on everything from efforts to limit carbon emissions (Pèlegrin et al., 2021; van der Kamp, 2021) to technological development (Wakefield, 2019) to investment in foreign aid and development (Melik, 2012) to international cooperation (Pandovic, 2020), to their very efforts to limit the spread of COVID-19 and national and global deaths associated therewith (Yan & Brown, 2021).

This concerted effort to alienate China, to disarticulate the world's economies, politics, peoples, and culture from China, come at a time when Mead's and other 'sick man' yellow peril discourses are proliferating. Stories of failure, control, and the existential threat of China painted/framed/articulated populist Western understandings of the People's Republic during the pandemic.[5] Less prevalent, though not entirely absent, were stories about the positive aspects of China or the social functions that sport played during the pandemic. There was a scarcity of coverage about China's extraordinary achievements in poverty eradication, in education, in controlling the pandemic and saving lives. For example, one *TIME* article showcased the successes of newly promoted club Wuhan Zall and the role they played in restoring a semblance of normalcy and community for the people of that city following the resumption of football in 2020 (Campbell, 2020).

In both football and general political discourse, the pandemic has produced in Western media a new set of political narratives and technologies. We might describe these technologies as a sort of *speculative Orientalism*—whereby absence of information, of access to people, and to 'verifiable' 'facts' has given rise to a contextually-specific framing of state-repression. Within this framing, the Chinese political system is portrayed as inherently anti-democratic, and the Chinese people as dupes or a naturally disposed to control, complicit in their own subjugation. The void is certainly in part due to political processes and structures: most notably via an ongoing national censorship regime. It is also due to heavy government regulation and surveillance of information and bodies during the pandemic (Zero-COVID approach). However, in the absence of

[5] For example, there was considerable coverage of the State takeover of failing CSL franchises, most notably of the local government bailing out Jiangsu Suning the reigning CSL Champions, in 2021.

facts, the China Joshua came to know during the pandemic was largely one fabricated not on fact, on evidence or empirical encounter, but rather on a series of talking points wrapped in political discourse about the immanence and pervasiveness of the Chinese threat, of the danger Chinese bodies and Chinese people posed to the West.

Diffractions from Draconia: Being Chinese, Living China[6]

As we all well know, China effectively shut down in the late winter of 2020. Shopping malls were closed off, school children sent home, grocery stores made deliverable. Businesspeople and government officials shared the common burden of responding in line with strict CCP and local/provincial mandates to shutter society as the nation quarantined in the months following the Wuhan outbreak. As for football, sports officials were under pressure when it came to COVID control versus organizing and hosting sports events. In 2020, all the football games were mandated to be suspended and postponed in China. For example, as of January 30th, 2020, the Chinese Football Association (CFA) released the "Announcement on the Postponement of the 2020 Season of Domestic Football Matches" and ruled that the Chinese Super League, local amateur level games, grassroots and youth competitions and related activities would be postponed. Further, the General Administration of Sports launched the "Notice of Temporary Suspension of All Sports Events" on March 31st, 2020, cancelling all sports games and events. Yet, for Chinese sports officials, the pressure came not only from fulfilling the central government's COVID order but also from maintaining the Chinese football team's qualification in the Asian Football Conference and striving for the FIFA World Cup eligibility (given the AFC Champions League games

[6] This section is written in the first-person, by Hanhan, offering reflections of her time in China during the lockdown and pandemic. In the absence of any direct observations or co-present empirical interactions with football in China at this time, this first-hand account is intended to demonstrate what life in China—during this period of football absence and exceptional biopolitical control—was like and how the researcher whose project was put on pause was entangled in various political and social formations.

were still taking place in 2020). Under the dilemmatic pressures, the CFA officials eventually adopted a closed-loop system in which the Chinese Super League was split into two groups—one group played in a 'bubble' in Suzhou and the other in Dalian. Football was, for the moment, *closed off from an already closed society*.

When I went home in the Summer of 2020 I did so not for football research, but due to a family emergency. There was no football awaiting my homecoming, but the politics of moving bodies pervaded nonetheless. Since March 28th, 2020, the Chinese government imposed an entry ban for all foreigners, including immediate family members of Chinese citizens, and from July 20th 2020 has tightened entry restrictions for all travelers. Flights to China from abroad have been drastically reduced; Chinese citizens travelling from overseas must undergo a COVID-19 test and submit a 14-day health report prior to departure (later all passengers entering China must obtain appropriate vaccinations). In spite of the tighter travel restrictions and the global spread of COVID-19, I had to fly to China in summer 2020 as my father's health was deteriorating due to late-stage pancreatic cancer. Although there were not many options available, I was lucky/vigilant enough to find a single-trip ticket for $6,500 departing from Tallahassee (stopping in Atlanta, Amsterdam, and Seoul) to Shanghai in August 2020 (it cost over $10,000 on average to fly from the United States to China at that time). However, Joshua was not able to travel with me due to his American citizenship.

After a 48-hour trip, I finally landed in Shanghai. I took the PCR test (a combined nose and throat swab) again at the airport, after which I was transported to a hotel in Shanghai and, later, a hotel in Wuxi (my hometown) for a 14-day central quarantine. During quarantine, I was prohibited from going anywhere other than my own hotel room. Every day, I was required to do a nose and throat swab and take my body temperature. When the central quarantine was over, I was mandated by the local *ju wei hui* (residential committees–which constitute a major part of China's local government system for assisting the implementation of policies)–to undergo another seven-day home quarantine.

The quarantine I experienced was only a very small part of the "zero tolerance" policy ingrained and enacted throughout the entire country. To implement the "zero-tolerance" policy, the Chinese government imposed stringent regulations and bans on all aspects of life to curb the number of COVID-19 cases. As a result of hospital regulations, inpatients (including my father) and their families and caregivers were largely restricted in their mobility and access. My mother would not leave the hospital until my father passed away; I was not permitted entry into the hospital one week prior to my father's passing when suspicious COVID cases were reported in the local area. These restrictive measures were pervasive. I saw hundreds of red banners with anti-virus propaganda slogans spreading across roads and streets. My neighborhood, day and night, was bombarded with *ju wei hui's* loudspeaker broadcasts of the COVID-related rules and regulations to be obeyed. All mass gatherings, such as international sporting event or games, were canceled or postponed. Some important domestic games, such as the Chinese Super League, were organized using a closed-loop control system. Chinese residents were restricted from participating in mass sports and entertainment activities. In my hometown, for instance, people caught playing mahjong in public were accosted and sent to education programs by government officials.

These stringent regulations, however, did not spark complaints or public resistance in China. The Chinese people instead seemed to appreciate and commend the government's COVID "zero tolerance" policy. For instance, when I complained to my family and friends in China about the restrictions and effects they had on my dad's situation, they tried to convince me that the Chinese government is doing what's right for the people and the country, since the Chinese government prioritizes the lives of the people and takes responsibility for its people. For comparison, I often heard on TV, the news, social media, and in casual conversations with Chinese people, how little concern the U.S. government has for its citizens and how poorly the U.S. government controls the spread of COVID. This led me to wonder how the Chinese State has successfully transformed a pandemic crisis into a nation-wide political campaign that reinforces and reinvigorates the superiority of CCP ideology.

Perhaps one of the most predominant tools employed by the Chinese government to implement its COVID "zero-tolerance" policy was smartphone technology and big data analytical tracking. When I was in China, I had to make sure my individual Health Code (HC) was ready to be scanned wherever I went—train stations, shopping malls, grocery stores, and hospitals. An HC is a digital code generated for each Chinese citizen upon registering their mobile phone number and personal information with a WeChat or Alipay app (app version varies by cities and provinces via WeChat or Alipay), which allows local and central governments to gather personal data, track if the citizen travels to contaminated areas or is exposed to COVID, and measure whether and to what degree the citizen poses a risk for spreading disease. The HC system operates by categorizing citizens into three color-based groups—green, yellow, and red—which can be used to determine whether the citizen is allowed access to public spaces and transportation. Green indicates 'normal' and the user can take public transportation and go to public spaces. Yellow symbolizes a 'risk' which means the user has travelled to low- and middle-risk regions within the last 14 days and needs to take PCR tests and 'voluntarily' undergo home quarantine, while red demotes a 'danger' which requires the user to go to designated hospitals for screening test and central quarantine (Cong, 2021).

Chinese citizens, including myself, live in constant anxiety and fear that our HC might turn yellow or red and our mobility would be restricted at some point in the future. For example, two suspicious cases were found in Pudong, Shanghai in October 2020—concurrent to my visit to Shanghai to visit a medical expert for my father. My HC turned yellow, and the *ju wei hui* in Wuxi notified me to stay home and monitor my health status for a week. Meanwhile I was required to sign an affidavit confirming that I was not exposed to suspicious cases of COVID, otherwise I had to take legal responsibility for spreading the virus should that occur. This mobility restriction made me extremely frustrated because I could not visit and care for my father and, at the same time, created a sensation of fear and anxiety as it related to the government surveillance permeating every aspect of my life via technologies.

Yet the Chinese public (including the older generation many of whom do not even know how to use a smartphone and how to register for a HC) has by-and-large, and paradoxically, embraced the HC system. For most Chinese, HCs help identify and differentiate ALL potential COVID carriers (including the virally innocent) and hold the promise of ZERO cases, which offers a sense of security that they are protected by the government from the virus and from other infected people.

At this point, this smartphone technology and HC tracing system is not only a tool ostensibly used by the government to manage the transmission of infectious diseases, but more importantly it constitutes a new bio-surveillance institution that embeds a digitally empowered disciplinary regime into the motions and emotions of human bodies. Put more specifically, Chinese citizens are being reduced to two-dimensional digital codes which can be simply traced, arranged, (de)mobilized, and ruled through smartphone technology woven into an automated network spanning community government agencies (e.g., *ju we hui* and police), homes/hotels/hospitals, and technology corporations. Fears and anxieties (of the virus, mobility restriction, and infected individuals) and desires for safety and security have been reproduced and normalized through self-disciplinary practices (self-quarantine, self-monitoring, and self-subjugation) insomuch to sustain the power of the surveillance network and consolidate the state order.

As the Chinese government utilizes technological innovation to reinforce its biopolitical control and social order within the public, the COVID-19 opened fissures within the central government. The Chinese government has often been criticized by the Western media, as a collective group, for its autocracy and dictatorship in launching and implementing various 'inhumane' policies and maneuvers, including its 'zero COVID' and isolation strategies during the pandemic. However, the West is wrong in treating the Chinese government simply as a holistic entity. First, it is a complex structure comprised of a multitude of officials and administrative staffs at different administrative levels (e.g., *ju wei hui*, village/town, district, county, prefecture-level city, province, direct-administrated municipality, and special economic zone) and across different functional departments (e.g., sports, education, culture & tourism, commerce, finance, civil affairs, transport, housing and urban-rural development, etc.). In terms of the number of the government officials, China's media insiders claim that there are at least seven million government officials (cadres), as well as around 50 million employees in different levels of governments and public service sectors (Wang, 2016). Second, the tax-sharing system and the decentralization of authority reform launched since 1994 (although it was modified in 2016) had further significantly reshaped the dynamics of the economic and political power between local and central governments (Jin et al., 2005). With such structural and political complexities, internal struggles, tensions, and conflicts across various levels of the Chinese government (particularly the local government) appear unavoidable when implementing policies mandated by the central leadership (Zhu & Zhao, 2021).

The central government's "Zero COVID" order may yield such struggles and tensions as well. This can be manifested through the central leaders' ongoing efforts to tighten COVID control and maintain a closed-door policy while making local government officials fully responsible for increased COVID cases. For example, the CCP secretary of Hubei province, the CCP secretary of Wuhan, and the mayor of Wuhan (highest-ranking local government officials) were removed from their positions due to "botched outbreak response" in 2020 (Zheng, 2020). Around 70 local government officials from the cities of Guangzhou, Zhengzhou, Nanjing, Yangzhou, Zhangjiakou, and Yantai, were purged or held accountable in 2021 for the hundreds of COVID cases that arose in their jurisdictions (Shangguan, 2021). Clearly, local politicians' appointment is now closely tied to their performance on limiting COVID cases, which would inevitably put excessive pressures on government officials to prioritize COVID control over everything else (see Xi'an's and Shanghai's lockdown to halt COVID outbreak). Nevertheless, the local governments must meanwhile absorb the financial and economic pressures associated with COVID (OECD, 2020). China's local government debts, for example, reached CNY25.66 trillion (US$4.4 trillion) by December 2020 (China's Financial Ministry, 2021); whereas the hidden debts were estimated at CNY45 trillion (US$7 trillion) (Lee, 2021). The massive local financial deficiency might to some extent exacerbate the "entrenched distrust at the central government level of local governments being able to implement the party's economic policy" (Genevaz, 2019, para. 7).

These are but a few reflections of my time in China as I look back to a period of time when I was brought back home but not to 'normal conditions'—rife mass gatherings, football spectacles, and Had football been there to study, we might have been able to trace old articulations and association—to in- and outflows of capital, people, mediations (good and bad, as Joshua outlines above), discourses and disquiets about the status of Chine in the world (football) order, and so on. In football's absence, I found some features of government and culture that had been made dormant—or been hidden from public view—during China's opening up period. For example, local and provincial politicians were motivated by and rewarded in relation their ability to execute the will of the central government. But whereas in the past those governance practices tended to articulate to opening new shopping malls, growing the local GDP, building infrastructure, or even fashioning a successful football club, the pandemic gave rise to systems of regulation and control. What I found in pandemic era China was a state of exception, but one very much defined by strong levels of state control, surveillance, and biopolitical technologization. My China was still very much different than the caricatures painted for Joshua as he watched my home country from afar. These images betrayed the complexities of government, but also how those stratifications and bureaucratic structurations were working with and against the people of China during this exceptional period.

Speculative Diffractions: Footballing No-Bodies and Pandemic Non-Matter

So, what did we learn about football? Very little, as there was at first no football to be studied and no access to football spaces or footballing bodies once the games did resume. However, as metonym of globalizing China, football served as a symbolic and corporeal proximation of a nation that was closing itself to the world (for better and worse), a conduit through with the global flowed into a once closed society but was now reterritorializing in equal parts COVID precaution and geopolitical insularity. While football's disappearance was not the major turning pointing in the trajectory of the nation, its subtraction from the public sphere was consequential in reorganizing how public culture, assembled bodies, and the mediated nation would be configured for public use. In the absence of research sites and anthropological data to be rendered, what did we learn about non-footballing China? Joshua learned that the pandemic served as a catalyst to reinvigorate Western framings and misrepresentations China, its government, and its people. While China's football failures (domestic and international, on and off the pitch) served for anti-China media fodder prior to the pandemic (too much government involvement, China investment not welcome and does not belong in European football, etc.), COVID catalyzed an intensified, if formulaic, abjectification of the People's Republic, the cultures, bodies, and customs. Sport, and football—once an increasingly important vessel Western-China interconnectivity (economic, cultural, political)—was now framed a something to be disassociated from given the 'costs.' We also learned, through Hanhan's experiences, that the football-absent state of exception formed in pandemic-era China was one defined by intensified regimes of surveillance and control, and that a new biopolitical architecture had given life to the State and it power in managing the population.

References

Agamben, G. (2005). *State of exception*. University of Chicago Press.

Barad, K. (2007). *Meeting the Universe Halfway: Quantum Physics and the Entanglement of Matter and Meaning*. Duke University Press.

Bloomberg. (2017, August 18). It looks like China's European soccer invasion is over. https://www.bloomberg.com/news/articles/2017-08-18/for-european-soccer-teams-flood-of-chinese-money-seen-drying-up

Bradsher, K., & Panja, T. (2019, October 24). In China, FIFA's focus is soccer, not human rights. *The New York Times*. https://www.nytimes.com/2019/10/24/sports/soccer/fifa-china-soccer-human-rights.html

Campbell, C. (2020, December 29). 'This means a lot.' After their city was battered by coronavirus, Wuhan's soccer fans find redemption. *Time*. https://time.com/5923989/wuhan-zall-soccer-china-pandemic/

Calhoun, G. (2022, January 5). Part 2: Beijing is intentionally underreporting China's Covid death rate. *Forbes*. https://www.forbes.com/sites/georgecalhoun/2022/01/05/beijing-is-intentionally-underreporting-chinas-covid-death-rate-part-2/?sh=314c223173b8

Chadwick, S. (2020, April 8). The game must go on: global football and the geopolitics of generosity. *South China Moring Post*. https://www.scmp.com/sport/football/article/3078831/game-must-go-global-football-and-geopolitics-generosity

China's Ministry of finance (2021). Local government bond issuance and debt balance in December 2020. http://yss.mof.gov.cn/zhuantilanmu/dfzgl/sjtj/202101/t20210125_3649040.htm,2021.04.01.

Cong, W. (2021). From Pandemic control to data-driven governance: The case of China's health code. *Frontiers in Political Science, 3*, 8.

Eckner, C. (2021, April 13). China's Communist Party forcing investors to pull money out of European football. *DW*. https://www.dw.com/en/chinas-communist-party-forcing-investors-to-pull-money-out-of-european-football/a-57171818

Freymann, E. (2022). *One belt, one road: Chinese power meets the world*. Harvard University Press.

Genevaz, J. (2019). Sources of political stress in China. *War on the Rocks*. https://warontherocks.com/2019/05/sources-of-political-stress-in-china/

Gündoğan, I., & Sonntag, A. (2018). Chinese football in the era of Xi Jinping: What do supporters think? *Journal of Current Chinese Affairs, 47*(1), 103–141.

Haraway, D. (1992/2004). "The Promises of Monsters: A Regenerative Politics for Inappropriate/d Others." In *The Haraway Reader*, 63-124. : Routledge.

Haraway, D. (1997). *Modest_Witness@Second_Millenium. FemaleMan©_Meets_OncoMouse™: Feminism and Technoscience*. Routledge.

JohnWallStreet. (2021, February 22). Chinese investors flee European football after home government policy change. *Sportico*. https://www.yahoo.com/video/chinese-investors-flee-european-football-105538940.html

Jin, H., Qian, Y., & Weingast, B. R. (2005). Regional decentralization and fiscal incentives: Federalism, Chinese style. *Journal of Public Economics, 89*(9-10), 1719–1742.

Keh, A. (2021, December 1). Do sports still need China? *The New York Times*. https://www.nytimes.com/2021/11/24/sports/olympics/china-sports-peng-shuai.html

Lee, A. (2021, November 2). Is China's local government debt a concern and what role do LGFVs play in infrastructure spending? *South China Morning Post*. https://www.scmp.com/economy/china-economy/article/3154549/chinas-local-government-debt-concern-and-what-role-do-lgfvs

Liu, Z., Chen, R., & Newman, J. I. (2021). The football dream of a sleeping dragon: Media framing (s), east–west Geopolitics, and the crisis of the Chinese men's national team. *Communication & Sport, 9*(1), 55–87.

Melik, J. (2012, 27). China brings jobs to Ethiopia but at what cost? *BBC*. https://www.bbc.com/news/business-18094181

Mead, W. R. (2020, February 3). China is the real Sick Man of Asia: Its financial markets may be even more dangerous than its wildlife markets. *Wall Street Journal.* https://www.wsj.com/articles/china-is-the-real-sick-man-of-asia-11580773677

Minh-ha, T. T. (1988/1997). "Not You/Like You: Postcolonial Women and the Interlocking Questions of Identity and Difference." In *Dangerous Liaisons: Gender, Nation, and Postcolonial Perspectives*, 415-149. Edited by Anne McClintock, Aamir Mufti, and Ella Shohat. : University of Minnesota Press.

Minh-ha, T. T. (1996). An Acoustic Journey. In J. C. Welchman (Ed.), *Rethinking Borders* (pp. 1–17). University of Minnesota Press.

Naik, S. (2021, March 15). 'Football needs to be far less a state instrument in China, more a social democratic institution.' *The Indian Express.* https://indianexpress.com/article/sports/football/simon-chadwick-football-team-sports-in-china-7229102/

Newman, J. I., Yan, G., Xue, H., & Watanabe, N. M. (2021a). To Live, Play, and Die in Tianjin: Football as Biopolitical Assemblage in Contemporary China. *Sociology of Sport Journal, 1*(aop), 1–13.

Newman, J. I., Xue, H., Chen, R., Chen, Y., & Watanabe, N. M. (2021b). Football and cultural citizenship in China: A study in three embodiments. *Sport in Society, 24*(12), 2222–2245.

OECD. (2020). The territorial impact of COVID-19: Managing the crisis across levels of government. https://read.oecd-ilibrary.org/view/?ref=128_128287-5agkkojaaa&title=The-territorial-impact-of-covid-19-managing-the-crisis-across-levels-of-government

Pandovic, M. (2020, August 10). Serbia has rolled out the red carpet to China—but at what cost? *Euro News.* https://www.euronews.com/2020/10/08/serbia-has-rolled-out-the-red-carpet-to-china-but-at-what-cost

Pèlegrin, C., Shapiro, J., & Li, Y. (2021, January 16). Green transition in China: At what cost? *Green European Journal.* https://www.greeneuropeanjournal.eu/green-transition-in-china-at-what-cost/

Putz, C. (2021, August 1). Jules Boykoff on a Beijing 2022 Boycott. *The Diplomat.* https://thediplomat.com/2021/07/jules-boykoff-on-a-beijing-2022-boycott/

Ripley, W. (2021, November 24). The China market is lucrative for the sports business, but at what cost? [Video file]. *CNN.* https://www.cnn.com/videos/business/2021/11/24/china-sports-money-peng-shuai-ripley-pkg-intl-hnk-vpx.cnn/video/playlists/business-china/#:~:text=Beijing's%20influence%20in%20sports%20is,or%20banned%20from%20the%20country.

Shangguan, H. (2021, August 12). The directors of the health commissions in multiple places have been dismissed, and the official website of the Central Commission for Discipline Inspection: Serious accountability! [多地卫健委主任被免职，中纪委官网:严肃问责!]. *Shangguan News*. https://web.shobserver.com/wx/detail.do?id=395264

Silver, L., Devlin, K., & Huang, C. (2021, March 4). Most Americans support tough stance toward China on human rights, economic Issues. *Pew Research Center*. https://www.pewresearch.org/global/2021/03/04/most-americans-support-tough-stance-toward-china-on-human-rights-economic-issues/

Szymanski, S. (2018, June 18). Opinion: Why China doesn't dominate soccer. *The Washington Post*. https://www.washingtonpost.com/news/global-opinions/wp/2018/06/18/why-china-I-dominate-soccer/

The Economist. (2022a, February 27). The pandemic's true death toll: Our daily estimate of excess deaths around the world. https://www.economist.com/graphic-detail/coronavirus-excess-deaths-estimates

The Economist. (2022b, January 18). China stands alone in its attitude towards the pandemic. https://www.economist.com/graphic-detail/2022/01/18/china-stands-alone-in-its-attitude-towards-the-pandemic

van der Kamp, D. (2021, October 22). Clean air at what cost? The rise of blunt force regulation. *Chinese Politics and Economy Research Seminar Series*. https://uschinadialogue.georgetown.edu/events/clean-air-at-what-cost-the-rise-of-blunt-force-regulation

Van der Tuin, I. (2019). On research 'worthy of the present'. *SFU Educational Review, 12*(1), 8–20.

Wakefield, J. (2019, December 24). China is getting smarter—but at what cost? *BBC*. https://www.bbc.com/news/technology-50658538

Wang R. (2016, June 21). The total number of Chinese civil servants disclosed for the first time: 7.167 million [中国公务员总数首次披露:716.7万人]. *China Economic Weekly*. http://www.xinhuanet.com/politics/2016-06/21/c_129077723.htm

Wilson, C. (2016). Read Chinese football's 50-point reform plan in full—exclusive translation. https://wildeastfootball.net/2016/02/read-chinese-footballs-50-point-reform-plan-in-full-exclusive-translation/

Xue, H., Watanabe, N. M., Chen, R., Newman, J. I., & Yan, G. (2020). Football (as) Guanxi: A relational analysis of actor reciprocity, state capitalism, and the Chinese football industry. *Sport in Society, 23*(12), 2005–2030.

Xu, C. (2022, February). Beijing 2022 and China's challenge to sports imperialism. *MRonline.* https://mronline.org/2022/02/11/beijing-2022-and-chinas-challenge-to-sports-imperialism/

Yan, S., & Brown, M. (2021, January 23). Wuhan one year on: The city that appears safe from COVID—but at what cost? *The Telegraph.* https://www.telegraph.co.uk/news/0/wuhan-one-year-city-appears-safe-covid-cost/

Yam, K. (2022, February 14). Anti-Asian hate crimes increased 339 percent nationwide last year, report says. *NBC.* https://www.nbcnews.com/news/asian-america/anti-asian-hate-crimes-increased-339-percent-nationwide-last-year-repo-rcna14282

Yu, L., Newman, J., Xue, H., & Pu, H. (2019). The transition game: Toward a cultural economy of football in post-socialist China. *International Review for the Sociology of Sport, 54*(6), 711–737.

Zheng, W. (2020, February 23). Coronavirus: Beijing purges Communist Party heads in Hubei over 'botched' outbreak response in provincial capital of Wuhan. *South China Morning Post.* https://www.scmp.com/news/china/politics/article/3050372/coronavirus-beijings-purge-over-virus-takes-down-top-communist

Zhu, X., & Zhao, H. (2021). Experimentalist governance with interactive central–local relations: Making new pension policies in China. *Policy Studies Journal, 49*(1), 13–36.

3

Sporting Coronapolitics: Politics, Ideology and U.S. Nationalism in Pandemic Times

Anthony J. Weems

Proem

On January 6th, 2021, United States (U.S.) Olympic gold medalist Klete Keller was spotted among the group that stormed the U.S. Capitol building (Crouse & Mather, 2021). Wearing his Team USA jacket, Keller was joined by hundreds of other supporters of former U.S. President Donald Trump in an attempt to stop the certification of the 2020 Presidential election. Having since plead guilty to a felony charge of obstruction of Congress, the three-time Olympian stated that he "took phone photos and videos inside the Capitol, then destroyed the phone, its memory card, and *threw away the Team USA jacket* within 48 hours" (Hart, 2021, para. 5, italics added for emphasis). Keller's involvement in an insurrection attempt that resulted in several deaths at the U.S. Capitol while wearing his Team USA jacket brings with it questions about the politics of sport, athletes, nationalism, and broader political-cultural expressions

A. J. Weems (✉)
Florida International University, Miami, FL, USA
e-mail: aweems@fiu.edu

D. L. Andrews et al. (eds.), *Sport and Physical Culture in Global Pandemic Times*, Global Culture and Sport Series, https://doi.org/10.1007/978-3-031-14387-8_3

in pandemic times. As such, the purpose of this chapter is to explore the cultural politics of ethno-nationalism, how these politics relate to the sporting sphere during a global pandemic, and how uber-sport has served as a preeminent vehicle for advancing fascistic politics the U.S.

In a recent book titled *Making Sport Great Again: The Uber-Sport Assemblage, Neoliberalism, and the Trump Conjuncture* (2019), David Andrews outlines the idea of uber-sport as an analytical concept for understanding the assemblage of political, cultural, and economic function(s) of sport in contributing to "the instantiation of both US neoliberalism and Trump's authoritarian populist campaigning and presidential performativity" (p. 3). Although written before the onset of the novel coronavirus as a pandemic, the concept of uber-sport is critical to understanding the complexity of elite sport in the U.S. As Andrews's work highlights, this framing of sport has been markedly shaped by neoliberal politics while further substantiating far-right political articulations in the contemporary U.S. Yet, while the assemblage of uber-sport has played a central role in the development of contemporary neoliberal politics, it is important to also acknowledge the ways in which this project has enabled resistance to a broader system of elite-white-male dominance (see Feagin & Ducey, 2017). The space of sport itself is a highly visible and contested terrain through which the politics of domination and resistance play out. Neoliberalism necessarily creates the tensions that lead to resistance (Cannella & Lincoln, 2015), and scholarship increasingly points to how sport serves as a primary arena where this resistance materializes (see Agyemang et al., 2020; Cunningham et al., 2021).

Acknowledging this resistance within the context of uber-sport, I nonetheless focus on (white) nationalist interactions with—and mobilizations of—uber-sport as an ideological framework. Specifically, this work aims to explicate the function(s) of uber-sport in a wider political movement where mobilizing factions increasingly support the deployment of fascist political strategies during a global pandemic. This is, in essence, an extension of and contribution to the work of Andrews (2019) while situating uber-sport within the context of *coronapolitics*. According to Callison and Slobodian (2021), the term coronapolitics refers to the political climate in which loosely organized groups have mobilized around the world in efforts to oppose pandemic-related lockdowns, social distancing, guidelines, mask mandates, vaccines, and more. These groups are often characterized by a political thought structure Callison and Slobodian refer to as diagonalist:

> Born in part from transformations in technology and communication, diagonalists tend to contest conventional monikers of left and right (while generally arcing toward far-right beliefs), to express ambivalence if not cynicism toward parliamentary politics, and to blend convictions about holism and even spirituality with a dogged discourse of individual liberties. (para. 2)

In the U.S., these far-right orientations overlap significantly with, and are often co-determined by, (white) nationalistic politics.

Ethno-nationalism, U.S. Fascism, & Sport

Historical and sociological research have detailed extensively the political significance of ethno-nationalism in forming and shaping the U.S. and its institutions. From early propaganda campaigns designed to galvanize European-American colonials, to the U.S. Civil War, to the interwar period between World War I and II, to the development of neoliberalism, white nationalism has been a driving political force (see Edgar, 1977; Feagin & Ducey, 2018; Parkinson, 2016; Zeskind, 2009). Furthermore, several scholars have examined the ways white nationalist, far-right, and fascistic politics have historically interacted and co-determined one another. For example, historical writings have outlined uniquely "American" iterations of fascist thought, with much focus on the 1920s and 1930s (Ferkiss, 1957).

Steigmann-Gall (2017) referred to this interwar fascist movement as star-spangled fascism—a distinctly American formation of fascist thought and action. Whereas Steigmann-Gall (2017) suggested it is critical not to necessarily equate "fascist" with "far-right" or similar terms, we *can* sociologically disentangle nationalist engagements with far-right politics to highlight the "seedbed of fascism" (p. 119). In this sense, other scholars have noted prominent far-right nationalist movements that drew heavily upon, or outright supported, fascistic "solutions" to anti-racism, such as the politics of the National Front (Edgar, 1977). Adding to this discussion on historical developments of white nationalism in the U.S., Zeskind (2009) expertly articulated the ways nationalist politics were absorbed into mainstream political thought, forming a political climate in which the Republican Party (characterized by conservative thought) implicitly and explicitly represents the interests of white people (Feagin, 2012). As such, while we cannot and should not *equate* fascism with terms like conservative or far-right, there are historically bound relationships between these concepts in the U.S.

Still, although there is a history of fascist thought and action that have been absorbed into mainstream political thought, there is much debate as to whether the U.S. is or can be considered a fascist state, and what this means for researchers (Harris et al., 2017; Kuntz, 2021). While this debate it valid, it is not within the scope of this chapter to speculate over whether the U.S. should be considered a fascist state, particularly given the sensitivities surrounding historical genocides like that of Nazi Germany. Rather, the objective is to critically interrogate the use of ideological axioms as political mechanisms that have historically facilitated fascistic movements in the U.S. Broadly defined, ideology can be understood as a thought structure characteristic of particular individuals, groups, or cultures, often with political implications (Otto, 2019). In this sense, the uber-sport assemblage plays a key role in establishing and legitimating ideologies. Due to its naturalized material structure, uber-sport serves as a highly visible vanguard through which power can be grasped and wielded against the Other. This consolidating of power has accelerated during the novel coronavirus pandemic where white nativist groups and figures have engaged with sport as a sacred institution, organized with one another, and politically mobilized.

With the historical relationship between white nationalism and fascist politics in mind, scholars of sport have started disentangling the sport-nationalist-fascist nexus, pointing to both historical and contemporary developments. For example, Murtha et al. (2021) examined Bernarr Macfadden's engagement with Italian dictator Bennito Mussolini in the

1930s. The authors noted a turn in U.S.-based nationalism around this time partly catalyzed through Macfadden's fascist flirtation as part of a broader acceptance of, admiration for, and adoption of European fascisms within the U.S. nationalist movement:

> The kind of nationalism promoted by Macfadden was in many ways a palimpsest, one which built on prevailing trends linked to fitness, eugenics, nationalism, and American identity. Macfadden created, promoted, and sustained, an American sense of nationalism that began first and foremost with the body... [B]uilt bodies were patriotic ones. (Murtha et al., 2021, p. 1953).

Thus, as early as the 1930s, a politically significant relationship was established in the U.S. between sport, physical culture, nationalist ideology, and fascist politics.

Analyzing the intersection of sport with nationalism during the recent Trump presidency, Falcous et al. (2019) looked at engagements with white nationalist politics through the hyper-conservative media outlet, Breitbart. Noting the porous line between far-right and fascist politics, the authors argued, while "...White nationalism actually 'constitutes the movement's centre of gravity' [in far-right political thought]..., it includes new manifestations and fractures including anti-globalization, antiestablishment, and misogynist elements" (Falcous et al., 2019, pp. 591–592). As ideological axioms central to fascist political thought, these newer manifestations warrant examination. To embark on a contribution to this literature, I turn to the work of linguistic philosopher Jason Stanley and his book, *How Fascism Works: The Politics of Us and Them* (2020), to outline a framework for understanding the nature of political strategies in advancing fascism. The application of this framework to political projects in, through, and of uber-sport is a critical project for scholars looking to develop sociological understandings of the intersections between sport, ethno-nationalism, and fascism during a global pandemic.

How Fascism Works

Although *How Fascism Works* was originally published in 2018, I draw from the paperback version published in 2020 which includes an updated preface specifically addressing the advancing of fascist politics since 2018 as well as the global spread of the novel coronavirus (officially declared a pandemic by the World Health Organization on March 11, 2020). According to Stanley (2020), there are ten political strategies that coalesce form a broader ideological framework for advancing fascism: "the mythic past; propaganda; anti-intellectual; unreality; hierarchy; victimhood; law and order; sexual anxiety; appeals to the heartland; and a dismantling of public welfare and unity" (p. xxix). Overall, these ten political strategies are woven together, leading to a concerted political effort known as fascism. Sociologically examining these issues can be a difficult task for researchers for a multitude of reasons. One major reason why this can be difficult is because fascistic groups/figures depend on an inverted framing good/bad, us/them, and just/criminal to grasp power. Thus, interviews, surveys, and other popular research methods tend to be inefficient in adequately capturing the fascist assemblage. For the purpose of this research project, I drew from a bricolage-inspired form of content analysis to be able to stitch together a bigger picture on the sociopolitical function(s) of sport in fascist politics during the pandemic.

Methodology

The bricolage approach to research constitutes a multimodal form of scholarship (Lincoln, 2001). The concept of a bricolage form of research stems from the writings of Claude Levi-Strauss referring to the bricoleur as jack-of-all-trades who makes use of whatever tools are available to accomplish a particular task. Since then, qualitative scholars have drawn from Levi-Strauss's extensive discussion to conceptualize a bricolage form of research, broadly defined as "a critical, multiperspectival, multi-theoretical and multi-methodological approach to inquiry," with an emphasis on the notions of eclecticity, emergent design, flexibility, and plurality (Rogers, 2012, p. 1). Influenced by this research design, I employed a bricolage-inspired approach to content analysis.

Method

Content analysis can be defined as "a family of analytic approaches ranging from impressionistic, intuitive, interpretive analyses to systematic, strict textual analyses" (Hsieh & Shannon, 2005, p. 1277). With the current study, I drew from Hsieh and Shannon's conceptualization of *conventional* and *directed* content analysis. The research draws from the directed approach as Stanley's (2020) outlining of how fascism operates contributed significantly to the overall direction of the study. The analysis is conventional in that the data gathered is analyzed in relation to the phenomenon of fascistic politics and how the ideological structure of uber-sport was strategically activated throughout the pandemic.

Data was collected from March 11, 2020 to September 11, 2021. March 11th was chosen as the start date for data collection as this was when the WHO declared the coronavirus a global pandemic. March 11th also marked the day the NBA "shut down" or paused its 2019–2020 season after Utah Jazz player Rudy Gobert tested positive for the virus (Zillgitt, 2020). Data was then collected over the next 18 months to be able to analyze the complex relationship between the pandemic, sport, ethno-nationalism, and the politics of fascism. The chosen 18-month period served as an adequate frame of reference for collecting data as it allowed for investigation of the following issues: the scope of COVID-19 and its impact on sport and much of the world; the intersection of sport and global anti-racist movement; the continued rise and mainstreaming of far-right extremist groups; a troubled "return" of sport in the U.S.; the 2020 U.S. Presidential election; the rescheduling of the 2020 Olympic Games in Tokyo which were held in the summer of 2021; an end date of September 11, 2021, which served as a nationally significant date in the U.S. to finish collecting data; along with several other applicable points throughout the timeframe. Data logged throughout the timeframe included press articles, media interviews, empirical social science, social media posts, and governmental documents. Inclusion and exclusion decisions were made throughout the collection process to the degree that data could speak to at-hand issues to the point of saturation. Conflicting data were triangulated with other sources and reconciled in terms of reliability and relevance. Data points were then amalgamated and are presented here utilizing the work of Stanley (2020) as a framework for contextualizing and making sense of fascist political strategy.

Sport, Nationalism, & Fascist Political Stratagem

Six out of ten strategies outlined by Stanley (2020) interacted directly with the ideological structure of sporting coronapolitics during the data collection period. Specifically, this included the themes of the mythic past, anti-intellectual, unreality, hierarchy, Sodom and Gomorrah, and a stressing of subservient labor as an appropriate strategy for navigating coronapolitics in and through uber-sport. The other four themes (i.e., propaganda, law and order, victimhood, and sexual anxiety) resonated strongly throughout the broader frame of nationalistic politics during this period but did not interact with sporting coronapolitics to the same degree as the other six themes. These engagements with uber-sport included—but where not limited to—the use of sport's imagery in a propaganda video shown hours before Trump supporters stormed the U.S. Capitol (Stanley, 2021); far-right political pundits framing sport as politically lost to "woke" forces (Cancian, 2020; Castronuovo, 2021; Rolli, 2020; McVitie, 2021); the demonization and attempted controlling of athletes protesting police brutality and systemic racism (Agnew, 2021; Patrick, 2021); and roughly half of the anti-trans bills proposed or passed during the data collection period emphasizing (women's) sport (Freedom for All Americans, 2021; Save Women's Sports Act, 2021). Although these white nationalist politics are heavily related to a broader set of fascistic strategies, I focus here on the six strategies that interacted explicitly with sporting coronapolitics.

The Mythic Past

According to Stanley (2020), the strategy of *the mythic past* refers to how, historically, fascist politics draw upon narratives of a pure and mythic past that was tragically destroyed. Particularly among extreme nationalists, this glorious past is framed as having been lost to globalism, liberal cosmopolitanism, and respect for values such as equality. Contained within this strategy is an explicit effort to regain or to return to a non-existent past uniformity; a past that is characterized by a strong patriarchal bend where patriotic men fought for and protected the nation's glory.

Tied to broader, white-framed ideas on a U.S. mythic past (see Feagin, 2020) is the inherently pure and apolitical nature of sport; a mythic framing of sport (see Coakley, 2015) which has only recently been "spoiled" by athlete activism. The stoppage of elite sporting events with the onset of the novel coronavirus pandemic set a foundation for far-right political and cultural leaders to draw upon this *mythic* past of sport, as well as stress an immediate need to return to sporting normalcy—or at the very least, to allow sport's mythic nature to heal the U.S. from both the pandemic and broader social unrest. Indeed, the cultural and political quest to "Make Sport Great Again" (Andrews, 2019, p. 121)—to return to a mythic past of sport itself—was a common theme throughout the 18-month long data collection period. While the premise for this assemblage had already been substantiated through Donald Trump's populist politics and his combative approach to athlete activism in previous years (Andrews, 2019), the pandemic offered a specific and contextualized need for an authoritative resolution to and through sport.

As early as late-March and April of 2020, Donald Trump was calling for a return of sport events. In early April, it was made public that Trump had a call with several sport league owners and commissioners (e.g., Adam Silver, Gary Bettman, Roger Goodell, Rob Manfred, among others). In this call, Trump made it clear that he wanted sporting competitions to resume "as soon as we can" and that he wanted "fans back in the arenas" (as quoted in Reynolds, 2020, para. 1-2). Despite not knowing or acknowledging the irreparable damage that the pandemic would wage on the lives of millions of Americans, Trump repeatedly stressed a need to bring back sport in full force: "'We have to get back,' Trump said. 'We have to get back. Remember that. We have to get back and we have to get back soon'" (Reynolds, 2020, para. 17).

Sticking to the strategy, Trump and other political leaders continued to pressure various institutions for a full return to and of sport. Perhaps most visible was Trump's pressure to see college football return in the fall of 2020. Other figures who consistently called for a full return of college football included Representative Jim Jordan, who simply tweeted, "America needs college football," and Senator Kelly Loeffler who tweeted, "College universities and athletic conferences need to put politics aside and come together to find a way to safely play college football this season" (Boren, 2020, para. 8–9). These figureheads often played off of the political convergence of the Black Lives Matter movement and a desire by prominent athletes to *safely* return to play with little-to-no safety plans articulated by the NCAA, athletic conferences, or individual universities. However, the very politics that informed athlete solidarity in this moment were disregarded by elite politicians such as Trump who over-simplified the complex nature of what athletes were calling for at the time (Boren, 2020).

Since then, sport's "return" to its pre-pandemic, and presumably apolitical, glory has been a long and troubled journey. However, a common theme in this process was the celebration of sport, fanship, and the psycho-social sense of sporting normalcy. For example, a Texas Rangers baseball game marked a significant point in conservative coronapolitics, where the Rangers home opener in April of 2021 became one of the first full-capacity professional sporting events in roughly one year (Vera & Dotson, 2021). Despite a majority of Americans who were polled disagreeing with the decision to operate at full capacity (Star Telegram, 2021), sporting headlines captured one simple reality: sports were returning and so were fans (Vera & Dotson, 2021; Young, 2021).

Returning sport to its former glory, as a political strategy, was intertwined with broader racial (and national) politics. That is, many outlets, fans, and politicking figures engaged with sport in ways that positioned sport's return as a return to "the way things were before," racially speaking. This apolitical framing allowed far-right outlets to target and further antagonize anti-racist movement around the country. In an article for *The*

American Conservative titled 'Sport Is For Liberals?,' Rod Dreher (2020) suggested the following: "Sports used to be a unifying phenomenon in American life, but no more—not since athletes got woke" (para. 7). Dreher later argued "sports never before was politically charged," but because of woke football players, "Now it is" (para. 11). This distorted political view resembles the nature of the *mythic past* strategy outlined by Stanley (2020), whereby a glorious past of sport was manufactured and emphasized only to have been ruined by liberalism, anti-racism, and ideals such as equality or justice.

Anti-intellectual

The *anti-intellectual* prong of fascist politics focuses on attacking language and expertise, particularly as represented in and through educational institutions (Stanley, 2020). The goal of this strategy is to undermine and supplant critical public discourse with the ideological axioms of the dominant group. To illustrate this strategy, consider far-rights attacks on rich intellectual traditions in the U.S. such as critical race theory, Marxist thought, feminism, or even more recent formations like The 1619 Project.

During the pandemic, fascistic groups have relied heavily on an anti-intellectual strategy, openly attacking evidence-based policy decisions and amplifying anti-Other politics in the process. U.S. Representative Marjorie Taylor Greene's interaction with CrossFit as a nationalist project, in addition to an anti-science approach to the pandemic, has been a consistent thread weaving its way through far-right politics during the pandemic. Along with promoting a multitude of QAnon conspiracy theories about the pandemic and other nationalist talking points, Greene regularly drew upon her engagement with CrossFit workouts to ground herself within a larger set of coronapolitics. On April 1, 2021, Greene posted a video of one of her CrossFit-style workouts with a caption that read, "This is my Covid protection" and claiming, "It's time to #FireFauci" (Greene, 2021a). That same day, Greene responded to her own workout post detailing two new proposed bills, the Fire Fauci Act and the We Will Not Comply Act, aimed at evidence-based policy decisions under the guise of protecting "the freedom of the American People" (Greene,

2021b). Her consistent engagement with CrossFit to promote her own anti-intellectual political agenda was egregious enough for CrossFit to publicly respond and distance themselves from Greene (see Brooks & Jamieson, 2021).

Also of weighty significance in manufacturing an anti-intellectual response to the pandemic has been the platforming of (predominately male) athletes who have spoken out with skepticism regarding the efficacy of vaccines or those who have publicly taken a stand against vaccines. Cole Beasley, NFL wide receiver, publicly spoke on why he had not received the COVID-19 vaccine at a press conference in July of 2021. Although Beasley claimed he was not for or against vaccinations and he felt NFL players were not given adequate information about the vaccines (Jackson, 2021), his personal Twitter account sheds light on a different narrative. In June of 2021, he posted a long message explaining why he was against being vaccinated: "If your [*sic*] scared of me then steer clear, or get vaccinated. Point. Blank. Period. I may die of covid, but I'd rather die actually living" (Beasley, 2021). Despite roughly 93% of NFL players being vaccinated as of late-August (Goodbread, 2021), the Buffalo Bills formally promoted Beasley's July press conference questioning the efficacy of vaccines on Twitter, meaning the Bills paid Twitter for Beasley's message to be broadcast to a wider audience. Anti-intellectual approaches to policy and the widespread adoption of conspiracy theories throughout the pandemic have helped far-right groups destabilize evidence-based claims about the novel coronavirus, politically mobilize a carefully crafted image of the enemy, and mainstream a substantially white-framed version of unreality.

Unreality

Unreality is a fascist tactic in which the goal of political propaganda is to subvert the very foundations upon which reality is known. "When it is successful," argues Stanley (2020), "its audience is left with a destabilized sense of loss, and a well of mistrust and anger against those who it has been told are responsible for this loss" (p. 57). Of particular utility within fascist political strategy is the circulation and legitimation of conspiracy theories. The goal of these theories is not necessarily to highlight a "hidden truth" but to propagate an idea so far away from truth that it creates the need to capitulate to a fascist leader or party to reclaim reality.

Since the onset of the pandemic, far-right groups and related conspiracy theorist groups have played a significant role in creating an alternate epistemic world. This is critically important in the politics of fascism because the destabilization of reason and expertise enables groups to follow authoritative leaders while scapegoating minoritized groups, particularly in threatening moments such as a pandemic. In this context, Donald Trump often played the role of a spectacle-strongman in response to the broader destabilizations of expertise among certain conspiracy groups. For example, QAnon conspiracy theorists believe(d) Trump to be "fighting a secret war against a global cabal of Democratic elites who are Satan-worshipping, cannibalistic pedophiles" (Rogers, 2021, para. 2). Although pre-dating the onset of the novel coronavirus, coronapolitics were subsumed into QAnon thought, whereby the pandemic was framed as an evil scheme by the globalist elite, and Trump was the lone strongman willing to stand against these forces. Some even speculated that the pandemic was manufactured specifically to oust Trump from the presidency (Reuters, 2021).

Despite a lack of evidence to support these theories, they have been particularly effective in destabilizing popular consensus, especially as it relates to uber-sport. Although sport events were carefully implemented back into a regular American programming during the earlier stages of the pandemic, so too did sport seem to absorb the politics of ignoring expertise. While progressive-branded leagues such as the W/NBA opted for "bubble" seasons in 2020, more conservative-branded leagues such as the NFL and MLB chose routes that all-but-ignored the science on the spread of the virus, resulting several games being rescheduled or cancelled altogether (Selbe, 2020). The functional result of this dichotomy has been a pressing of the boundaries moving forward, and a general framing of the pandemic as something that can be waded through and overcome by sheer will. The return of uber-sport signaled progress, triumph over the coronavirus. In reality, however, leagues across the board pressed forward without well-articulated plans to curb the spread of the virus or to reconcile short- and long-term damage incurred by those who contracted the virus.

The mainstreaming of certain conspiracy theories pushed sporting coronapolitics to capitulate to white nationalist ideals. Whether it was Klete Keller's storming of the U.S. Capitol in his Team USA jacket, or Cole Beasley's public comments about the vaccines, sports are positioned at the forefront of far-right political movements and seamlessly integrated into a broader set of nationalist politics. For individual athletes, it is their *sportness* that provides necessary legitimation for the political project of creating unreality, an alter-world onto which other white-framed groups and organizations (e.g., the NFL's Buffalo Bills) can attach themselves, contributing to a webbing of fascistic thought and action.

Hierarchy

White nationalist groups have adopted a clear, hierarchical approach to resolving their own grievances in and through sport. Most notably was the gripping of power by Donald Trump and the defending thereof by groups such as the Proud Boys, Oath Keepers, boogaloo boys, QAnon followers, and (mostly) white conservatives more broadly. Throughout the pandemic, Trump was painted as a leader who was fighting widespread liberal and globalist corruption on behalf of his supporters. Primed significantly by QAnon conspiracy theories, Trump aimed much of his fight against global liberalism at the hyper-visible space of sport. It was through sport where Trump was able to continue his attacks on antiracist activists, especially at the height of the Black Lives Matter movement in 2020, and even more so throughout several sports' careful navigation of the novel coronavirus.

Despite some sport leagues such as the W/NBA being able to put together moderately successful "bubble" experiences in the fall of 2020, Trump articulated a white-framed vision of sport and athletes in this moment whereby failures to live to up to pre-pandemic numbers in viewership were blamed directly on predominantly Black athletes and liberal, accommodative leagues like the NBA (led by a Jewish-American Commissioner, Adam Silver). Amplifying a fringe argument of among far-right groups, Trump regularly referred to NBA players as "very nasty" and "very dumb" while blaming TV ratings on the Black Lives Matter movement (Robertson, 2020, para. 1). Trump characteristically took to Twitter one day, tweeting out the following message:

> People are tired of watching the highly political @NBA. Basketball ratings are WAY down, and they won't be coming back. I hope football and baseball are watching and learning because the same thing will be happening to them. Stand tall for our Country and our Flag!!! (as quoted in Guardian Sport, 2020)

Despite Trump's consistent antagonism, the W/NBA and players were able to work together to complete their 2019–2020 seasons with widespread testing for the coronavirus, social distancing, masking, and a general concern for social well-being. Contrarily, the Trump administration had repeatedly "discouraged widespread testing, promoted quack cures and urged agency officials and governors to stick their fingers in their ears and proceed with business as usual" (Robertson, 2020, para. 20).

Still, Trump's authoritative and nationalistic approach resonated with his base of supporters. This was evident, for example, at a boxing match the former president hosted on September 11th, 2021, where home viewers who paid to stream the match "also got access to a live chat in which viewers talked about QAnon, Hunter Biden, Joe Biden sucking, Pepe the frog, Trump actually winning the 2020 election, and Jeffrey Epstein not actually killing himself" (Stieb, 2021, para. 4). Weaving together the cultural fabric of white nationalism, Trump routinely drew upon uber-sport's appeal to the masses to promote a broader set of sporting coronapolitics.

Sodom and Gomorrah

Sodom and Gomorrah refers to politically manufactured tensions between more populated cities and a nation's countryside. "Whereas cities, to the fascist imagination, are the source of corrupting culture, often produced by Jews and immigrants, the countryside is pure" (Stanley, 2020, p. 144).

The rhetoric of Donald Trump drew heavily upon this dichotomy to appeal to a wider base more accepting of fascistic strategy. For example, despite several cities seeing lower crime rates than they had seen in generations and low unemployment, Trump offered the following in one of his campaign speeches:

> Our African-American communities are absolutely in the worst shape that they've ever been in before, ever, ever, ever. You take a look at the inner cities, you get no education, you get no jobs, you get shot walking down the street." (as quoted in Stanley, 2020, p. 149)

Rural life, on the other hand, is associated with a righteous ethos upon which the national mythos is constructed. Ignoring the ways in which fascistic groups cut public programs, exploit and scapegoat minoritized communities, and clamp down on democratic process such as voting, this emphasis in fascist politics becomes self-fulfilling in the sense that it affirms what some suburban communities experience in life, while simultaneously creating an enemy based on longstanding fears of the "Other." This dichotomy has been amplified during the pandemic where populated cities have struggled to contain the spread of the coronavirus. As many cities have adopted different types of restrictions to address viral spread, this has, ideologically, played into the fascist politics of demonizing cities as liberal, corrupt, and threats to Americanism.

Uber-sport provides a unique backdrop in the cultural politics of this antagonistic relationship. A recurring theme across all major sports is the dichotomy between large media market cities (e.g., Los Angeles, New York, Miami) and what are referred to as small media market cities (e.g., Milwaukee, San Antonio, Salt Lake City). This dichotomization often plays off of and into the politics of *Sodom and Gomorrah*, where large market teams are framed according to their team's star power, fan base, and organizational gravitas. On the other hand, small market teams are framed as having to outwork the large market teams, adopting more of a blue-collar branding.

In the fall of 2020, The Los Angeles Lakers won the NBA championship in the Orlando "bubble." Led by mega-star LeBron James, the Lakers have historically been known as a team with significant star power. This aligns with the general framing of Los Angeles as a city of celebrities. This is significant as QAnon believers regularly claim Hollywood as the center of child sex trafficking and that Hollywood celebrities are harvesting young children for adrenochrome, believed to be "a mystical psychedelic favored by the global elites for drug-crazed satanic rites, derived from torturing children to harvest their oxidized hormonal fear" (Hitt, 2020, para. 5). Immediately following the Lakers win, questions about a large market franchise winning the championship began to permeate the popular press, particularly framing their success as being trouble for small-market teams: "Most of [the small-market teams] are doing all they can, while teams like the New York Knicks just sit around and hope a superstar wants to play at Madison Square Garden. *That's not fair*" (Berg, 2020, para. 6, italics added for emphasis). Intrinsic to this framing is an understanding of an antagonistic relationship between bigger cities and smaller areas.

However, just one rushed season after the Lakers won the championship, the Milwaukee Bucks won the NBA championship. This was significant for multiple reasons, but especially as it relates to the racial politics of the pandemic. The Wisconsin/Minnesota region repeatedly found itself in the national news after multiple high-profile shootings of unarmed Black men by police officers happened in the area. In August of 2020, the Milwaukee Bucks team went on strike in Orlando after the shooting of Jacob Blake by refusing to play (Zagoria, 2020). However, the Bucks' triumph in 2021 appeared to wash all of that away. No longer were discussions about police brutality, as the Bucks had finally accomplished their championship mission under the leadership of the Greek superstar, Giannis Antetokounmpo. Instead, many conversations reverted to the large-market/small-market dynamic, where media outlets celebrated the win by the Bucks. A common sentiment throughout these celebrations was the notion that "The Milwaukee Bucks are Built, Not Bought" (LeVene, 2021). Calling the victory a historic win for small-market sports fans all around the world, LeVene offered the following: "The chips are stacked against the teams in the 'small' professional sports cities, yet somehow, the Bucks were able to overcome all adversity and become World Champions" (para. 23). Uber-sport normalizes a politics of high-profile liberal cities as being in contrast with everyone else—the true Americans in the heartland of the U.S. This dynamic, although not always explicit in nature, plays an integral role in the politics of fascism as it lays a foundation for uniting conservative groups against the liberal and cosmopolitan enemy of large cities, particularly with the challenges brought forth by the pandemic.

Arbeit Macht Frei

At the heart of the fascist politics of "us" and "them" is the notion that "we" are hardworking, self-sufficient, and deserving; and "they" are lazy, dependent upon the state, and undeserving. Moreover, the framing of a lazy and undeserving outgroup is grounded in the notion that "they" can be fixed of their laziness through hard labor, thus the famous slogan on the gates of the Auschwitz concentration camp, ARBEIT MACHT FRIE—work shall make you free (Stanley, 2020, p. 157). While it is not my intention to directly compare the contemporary U.S. with the atrocities committed by Nazi Germany by drawing upon this theme, the emphases on the un/deserving should not be understated as they are central to fascist political strategies.

The push to bring back sport during the pandemic, to silence athlete activism, and to wade through the pandemic at all costs has been significantly shaped by a similar predatorial approach to work and labor. Throughout the pandemic, nationalist groups crystallized an attack on supposedly lazy and undeserving athletes to mobilize a political worldview where "they" should work as voiceless workers and "we" are the deserving group—deserving of service, of leisure, of social programs, and more. This is accentuated in the world of uber-sport where elite athletes are largely painted as the privileged few, and not necessarily understood as holistic laborers with extraneous needs, interests, and desires. An existing talking point in (white) conservative politics, far-right figureheads regularly harped on elite athletes who chose to speak out such as Trump's attacks on NFL players or Laura Ingraham's attacks on LeBron James. Far-right figures regularly paint elite athletes as being spoiled, dumb, and/or undeserving: "It's always unwise to seek political advice from someone who gets paid $100 million a year to bounce a ball… Keep the political comments to yourselves… Shut up and dribble," said Ingraham about LeBron James (as quoted in Sullivan, 2018, para. 7).

In strategically crafting a hyper-visible enemy, far-right outlets regularly attacked "woke" athletes and leagues with tenacity. Take, for example, Breitbart News, a far-right nationalist outlet that saw significant expansion during the data collection process. On Instagram, Breitbart regularly deployed the phrase "Go Woke, Go Broke!" in their simplistic vilification of the Other (e.g., see Breitbart News, 2020). Often featured in their posts were images of LeBron James or other athletes kneeling during the National Anthem. Their framing was consistent in the sense that if sporting bodies work within the far-right political spectrum, they are worthy and deserving of the platform sport provides. On the other hand, progressive politics relating to race, gender, militarization, or the coronavirus are painted as undeserving and are demonized. Much of this tactic from far-right outlets relied heavily on TV viewership and ratings, pointing to a seemingly "objective" measure of (un)deservedness where the Other is being righteously judged by conservative, market-based ideals. Focusing on declining ratings for the NBA All-Star Game, Breitbart sarcastically stated the following on Instagram: "Outstanding news! Congratulations, woke BLM-NBA millionaires! You did it!" (Breitbart News, 2021). Posts such as these demonstrate the un/deserving dichotomy deployed by far-right groups, a key strategy in the overall rise in fascist political thought.

Related to the mythic past theme, it is through precarious (and, at times, forced) labor that sport's return during a pandemic was possible. From a framing perspective, far-right outlets strategically ignored the threat of the pandemic in demonizing athlete-activists. Rather than bringing into context the dangers (personally, communally, or nationally) of playing during a pandemic—or even the economic impact on many of the leagues in question—hyper-conservative figures created a narrative where subservient labor was the way for sporting figures (and, by extension, Americans as a whole) to move forward. This was the case across all levels of sport, whether athletes were or were not compensated for their labor in a physically threatening context.

Implications & Conclusion

Although the us/them dichotomy is central to fascist political strategy, it is important to observe the way in which this dichotomy has been deployed throughout the pandemic. As fascistic groups continued to organize and mobilize throughout 2020 and on into 2021, nationalistic framings of the us/them dichotomy developed a hyper-focus on uber-sport. It was through this dialectical engagement with the space of sport that a political vision of nation, race, and patriarchal power was projected by far-right outlets and figureheads. Consequently, nationalist engagements with the sporting realm throughout the pandemic have significantly contributed to a broader advancing of fascistic politics.

While the focus in this study was on sporting coronapolitics in the U.S. context, the transnational nature of far-right political movement adds significant weight to the advancement of fascistic politics. Stanley's (2020) work poignantly shows how the rise of fascist political strategies are not confined within the U.S., or any single nation for that matter. Rather, the contemporary swelling of fascist tactics is global in nature. Similarly, uber-sport largely depends on a globalized structure which interacts with a variety of locales. Fascism may take on different forms across contexts and interact with ancillary institutions in varying ways; however, sport tends to play an integral role in fascist politics, historically and contemporaneously. In the U.S. as well as other politically significant geolocations, sociological analysis should continue explicating the role of sport in society to ascertain how fascist political strategies might be engaged and, ultimately, disrupted.

References

Agnew, D. (2021, April 8). Senate democrats support conservative-backed Texas bill requiring pro-sports teams with state contracts to play national anthem. *The Texas Tribune*. Retrieved April 17, 2021, from https://www.texastribune.org/2021/04/08/star-spangled-banner-protection-act-texas/

Agyemang, K. J., Singer, J. N., & Weems, A. J. (2020). 'Agitate! Agitate! Agitate!': Sport as a site for political activism and social change. *Organization, 27*(6), 952–968.

Andrews, D. L. (2019). *Making sport great again: The uber-sport assemblage, neoliberalism, and the Trump conjuncture*. Springer.

Beasley, C. [@Bease11]. (2021, June 18). Public service announcement [Tweet]. *Twitter*. https://twitter.com/Bease11/status/1405971914607239172?ref_src=twsrc%5Etfw%7Ctwcamp%5Etweetembed%7Ctwterm%5E1405971914607239172%7Ctwgr%5E%7Ctwcon%5Es1_&ref_url=https%3A%2F%2Fwww.si.com%2Fnfl%2F2021%2F06%2F18%2Fcole-beasley-bills-blasts-nfl-covid-19-protocol-unvaccinated-players

Berg, B. (2020, October, 16). Why the Lakers' championship spells trouble for NBA's small-market teams. *The Daily Campus*. Retrieved September 10, 2021, from https://dailycampus.com/2020/10/16/why-the-lakers-championship-spells-trouble-for-nbas-small-market-teams/

Boren, C. (2020, August 10). Trump tweets 'Play College Football!' as officials consider whether to cancel the season. *The Washington Post*. Retrieved August 13, 2021, from https://www.washingtonpost.com/sports/2020/08/10/trump-play-college-football/

Breitbart News. (2020, October 1). Go woke, Go broke! [Instagram post]. *Instagram*. https://www.instagram.com/p/CF0fkcLHj3t/

Breitbart News. (2021, March 9). Outstanding news! Congratulations, woke BLM-NBA millionaires! You did it! [Instagram post]. *Instagram*. https://www.instagram.com/p/CMNFEo4n7rd/

Brooks, R., & Jamieson, A. (2021, March 11). CrossFit is finally fed up with Marjorie Taylor Greene. *BuzzFeed News*. Retrieved May 17, 2021, from https://www.buzzfeednews.com/article/ryancbrooks/marjorie-taylor-greene-qanon-crossfit

Callison, W., & Slobodian, Q. (2021, January 5). Coronapolitics from the Reichstag to the Capitol. *Boston Review*. Retrieved December 13, 2021, from https://bostonreview.net/articles/quinn-slobodian-toxic-politics-coronakspeticism/

Cancian, D. (2020, June 9). Ben Shapiro Says politics has ruined sports for him. *Newsweek*. Retrieved September 26, 2020, from https://www.newsweek.com/ben-shapiro-american-sports-politics-protests-1509555

Cannella, G. S., & Lincoln, Y. S. (2015). Critical qualitative research in global neoliberalism: Foucault, inquiry, and transformative possibilities. In N. K. Denzin & M. D. Giardina (Eds.), *Qualitative inquiry and the politics of research* (pp. 51–74). Routledge.

Castronuovo, C. (2021, August 5). Trump slams US women's soccer team: Would have gold if not 'woke'. *The Hill*. Retrieved August 6, 2021, from https://thehill.com/blogs/blog-briefing-room/news/566490-trump-us-womens-soccer-team-wouldve-won-olympic-gold-instead-of?rl=1
Coakley, J. (2015). Assessing the sociology of sport: On cultural sensibilities and the great sport myth. *International Review for the Sociology of Sport, 50*(4–5), 402–406.
Crouse, K., & Mather, V. (2021). Olympic gold medalist was part of crowd that invaded capitol. *The New York Times*. Retrieved April 13, 2021, from https://www.nytimes.com/2021/01/12/sports/olympics/klete-keller-capitol-trump.html
Cunningham, G. B., Dixon, M. A., Singer, J. N., Oshiro, K. F., Ahn, N. Y., & Weems, A. (2021). A site to resist and persist: Diversity, social justice, and the unique nature of sport. *Journal of Global Sport Management, 6*(1), 30–48.
Dreher, R. (2020, September 10). Sport is for liberals? *The American Conservative*. Retrieved September 21, 2021, from theamericanconservative.com/dreher/sports-is-for-liberals-conservative-alienation/
Edgar, D. (1977). Racism, fascism and the politics of the National Front. *Race & Class, 19*(2), 111–131.
Falcous, M., Hawzen, M. G., & Newman, J. I. (2019). Hyperpartisan sports media in Trump's America: The metapolitics of Breitbart Sports. *Communication & Sport, 7*(5), 588–610.
Feagin, J. R. (2012). *White party, white government: Race, class, and US politics*. Routledge.
Feagin, J. R. (2020). *The white racial frame: Centuries of racial framing and counter-framing*. Routledge.
Feagin, J. R., & Ducey, K. (2017). *Elite white men ruling: Who, what, when, where, and how*. Taylor & Francis.
Feagin, J. R., & Ducey, K. (2018). *Racist America: Roots, current realities, and future reparations*. Routledge.
Ferkiss, V. C. (1957). Populist influences on American fascism. *Western Political Quarterly, 10*(2), 350–373.
Freedom for All Americans. (2021). Legislative tracker: Anti-transgender legislation filed for the 2021 Legislative Session. *Freedom for All Americans*. Retrieved October 6, 2021, from https://freedomforallamericans.org/legislative-tracker/anti-transgender-legislation/
Goodbread, C. (2021, August 26). NFL says player vaccination rate at 93%; weekly testing for fully vaccinated players proposed. *NFL*. Retrieved

September 9, 2021, from https://www.nfl.com/news/nfl-says-player-vaccination-rate-at-93-weekly-testing-for-fully-vaccinated-playe
Greene, M. T. [@mtgreenee]. (2021a, April 1). This is my Covid protection [Tweet]. *Twitter*. https://twitter.com/mtgreenee/status/1377614474862006279?ref_src=twsrc%5Etfw%7Ctwcamp%5Etweetembed%7Ctwterm%5E1377703190871867397%7Ctwgr%5E%7Ctwcon%5Es2_&ref_url=https%3A%2F%2Fd-20281035307805388 89.ampproject.net%2F2109102127000%2Fframe.html
Greene, M. T. [@RepMTG]. (2021b, April 1). NEW BILL ALERT! [Tweet]. *Twitter*. https://twitter.com/RepMTG/status/1377647623339905035
Guardian Sport. (2020, September 1). Donald Trump attacks 'highly political' NBA and warns NFL over protests. *The Guardian*. Retrieved September 4, 2020, from https://www.theguardian.com/sport/2020/sep/01/donald-trump-nba-protests-nfl
Harris, J., Davidson, C., Fletcher, B., & Harris, P. (2017). Trump and American fascism. *International Critical Thought, 7*(4), 476–492.
Hart, T. (2021, September 29). Klete Keller pleads guilty to Felony charge in connection with Capitol Riot. *SwimSwam*. Retrieved September 29, 2021, from https://swimswam.com/klete-keller-pleads-guilty-to-felony-charge-in-connection-with-capitol-riot/
Hitt, T. (2020, August 14). Followers of the pro-Trump conspiracy theory QAnon believe Hollywood and democratic elites take a psychedelic drug called Adrenochrome harvested from the fear of children. *The Daily Beast*. Retrieved August 15, 2020, from https://www.thedailybeast.com/how-qanon-became-obsessed-with-adrenochrome-an-imaginary-drug-hollywood-is-harvesting-from-kids
Hsieh, H. F., & Shannon, S. E. (2005). Three approaches to qualitative content analysis. *Qualitative Health Research, 15*(9), 1277–1288.
Jackson, W. (2021, July 28). Cole Beasley says players need to have 'Proper Information' on vaccines: 'I'm Not Anti or Pro Vax'. *Sports Illustrated*. Retrieved August 1, 2021, from https://www.si.com/nfl/2021/07/28/cole-beasley-covid-19-vaccine-nfl-rules-pro-choice
Kuntz, A. M. (2021). "Piercing This wall": Truth-making in a fascist world. *Qualitative Inquiry, 27*(5), 491–501.
LeVene, M. (2021). Milwaukee bucks: Have they mastered the "Small" market blueprint? *Fansided*. Retrieved August 8, 2021, from https://dairylandexpress.com/2021/07/23/4-biggest-reasons-milwaukee-bucks-won-nba-finals/

Lincoln, Y. S. (2001). An emerging new bricoleur: Promises and possibilities—A reaction to Joe Kincheloe's "Describing the Bricoleur". *Qualitative Inquiry, 7*(6), 693–696.
McVitie, P. (2021, August 5). 'Woke means you lose'—Trump tears into USWNT's 'leftist maniacs' after failure to win Olympic gold medal. *Goal.* Retrieved August 6, 2021, from https://www.goal.com/en/news/woke-means-you-lose-trump-tears-into-uswnts-leftist-maniacs/xvac5ianuzag1f4geg7a4jpcn
Murtha, R., Heffernan, C., & Hunt, T. (2021). Building American Supermen? Bernarr MacFadden, Benito Mussolini and American fascism in the 1930s. *Sport in Society, 24*(11), 1941–1955.
Otto, K. (2019). *Applied ethics for sport managers.* Carolina Academic Press.
Parkinson, R. G. (2016). *The common cause: Creating race and nation in the American Revolution.* UNC Press Books.
Patrick, D. (2021, February, 10). @mcuban Your decision to cancel our National Anthem at @dallasmavs games is a slap in the face to every American [Tweet]. *Twitter.* https://twitter.com/DanPatrick/status/1359499692695027717
Reuters. (2021, June 29). Fact check: COVID-19 is not a hoax to eliminate Trump. *Reuters.* Retrieved July 17, 2021, from https://www.reuters.com/article/uk-factcheck-covid-hoax-eliminate-trump/fact-check-covid-19-is-not-a-hoax-to-eliminate-trump-idUSKBN27S31E
Reynolds, T. (2020, April 4). Trump talks with US pro sports leaders to discuss virus. *AP.* Retrieved April 5, 2021, from https://apnews.com/article/college-basketball-nhl-mlb-sports-general-nfl-4c63d4382453e89bd169fdbfa29fc746
Robertson, D. (2020, August 16). What the NBA could teach Trump about Coronavirus. *Politico.* Retrieved September 3, 2020, from https://www.politico.com/news/magazine/2020/08/16/nba-coronavirus-bubble-covid-politics-trump-395506
Rogers, K. (2021, March 4). Why QAnon has attracted so many White Evangelicals. *FiveThirtyEight.* Retrieved June 17, 2021, from https://fivethirtyeight.com/features/why-qanon-has-attracted-so-many-white-evangelicals/
Rogers, M. (2012). Contextualizing theories and practices of bricolage research. *The Qualitative Report, 17*, 1–17.
Rolli, B. (2020, June 9). Ben Shapiro lost his safe space because sports are political now. *Daily Dot.* Retrieved September 26, 2020, from https://www.dailydot.com/debug/ben-shapiro-sports-political-safe-space/

Save Women's Sports Act, H4153, S. C. 124th General Assembly. (2021). https://www.scstatehouse.gov/billsearch.php?billnumbers=4153&session=124&summary=B&PRINT=1

Selbe, N. (2020, October 8). Which NFL games have been rescheduled due to COVID-19? *Sports Illustrated*. Retrieved December 4, 2020, from https://www.si.com/nfl/2020/10/09/every-game-rescheduled-due-to-covid19-this-season

Stanley, J. (2020). *How fascism works: The politics of us and them*. Random House Trade Paperbacks.

Stanley, J. (2021, February 4). The movie at the Ellipse: A study in fascist propaganda. *Just Security*. Retrieved February 5, 2021, from https://www.justsecurity.org/74504/movie-at-the-ellipse-a-study-in-fascist-propaganda/

Star Telegram. (2021, April 28). New poll asks fans about Texas Rangers allowing full capacity. *Start Telegram*. Retrieved September 22, 2021, from https://account.star-telegram.com/paywall/subscriber-only?resume=251004724&intcid=ab_archive

Steigmann-Gall, R. (2017). Star-spangled fascism: American interwar political extremism in comparative perspective. *Social History, 42*(1), 94–119.

Stieb, M. (2021, September 11). Trump Guest-hosting a boxing match on 9/11 was a vision from an alternate reality. *Intelligencer*. Retrieved September 11, 2021 from https://nymag.com/intelligencer/2021/09/trumps-9-11-boxing-match-was-a-vision-from-another-reality.html

Sullivan, E. (2018, February 19). Laura Ingraham told LeBron James to shut up and dribble; he went to the hoop. *NPR*. Retrieved July 15, 2021, from https://www.npr.org/sections/thetwo-way/2018/02/19/587097707/laura-ingraham-told-lebron-james-to-shutup-and-dribble-he-went-to-the-hoop

Vera, A., & Dotson, K. (2021, April 5). Texas Rangers sell over 38,000 tickets to home opener, marking one of the first full-capacity sporting events in a year. *CNN*. Retrieved June 7, 2021, from https://www.cnn.com/2021/04/05/us/texas-rangers-home-opener-stadium-full-capacity-spt-trnd/index.html

Young, M. (2021, March 10). Texas Rangers to allow full capacity on opening day. *Houston Chronicle*. Retrieved March 11, 2021 from https://www.chron.com/sports/astros/article/Texas-Rangers-full-capacity-stadium-COVID-masks-16015464.php

Zagoria, A. (2020, August 26). Milwaukee Bucks players make history by boycotting NBA playoff game after Jacob Blake shooting; multiple games postponed. *Zags*. Retrieved October 2, 2020, from https://www.zagsblog.

com/2020/08/26/milwaukee-bucks-players-make-history-by-boycotting-nba-playoff-game-after-jacob-blake-shooting/

Zeskind, L. (2009). *Blood and politics: The history of the white nationalist movement from the margins to the mainstream*. Farrar, Straus and Giroux.

Zillgitt, J. (2020). NBA shuts down after Rudy Gobert tests positive for coronavirus. *USA Today*. Retrieved May 11, 2021, from https://www.usatoday.com/story/sports/nba/2020/03/11/coronavirus-nba-shuts-down-after-rudy-gobert-tests-positive/5028026002/

4

Lockdown Cartographies: Active Bodies, Public Spaces and Pandemic Atmospheres in Italy

Nicola De Martini Ugolotti, Antonio Donato, and Leonardo Tonelli

During the first wave of the Covid-19 pandemic in Italy, conceptualisations of sport and physical activity as contested (bio)political domains acquired new layers of meaning and intensity. As the country became the pandemic epicentre in Europe and put in place restrictive lockdown measures, *already-existing* concerns and processes related to the government of practices and bodies deemed illegitimate in public spaces swiftly extended

N. De Martini Ugolotti (✉)
Bournemouth University, Poole, UK

Associazione Frantz Fanon, Turin, Italy
e-mail: ndemartiniugolotti@bournemouth.ac.uk

A. Donato
University of Bologna, Bologna, Italy

Associazione Leib, Bologna, Italy

L. Tonelli
Associazione Leib, Bologna, Italy

D. L. Andrews et al. (eds.), *Sport and Physical Culture in Global Pandemic Times*, Global Culture and Sport Series, https://doi.org/10.1007/978-3-031-14387-8_4

to the entire population. This chapter takes cue from the intensified and *spectacular* processes of surveillance of (active) bodies in public spaces during the first lockdown to interrogate how the body/space/health/security nexus has been experienced, understood and (re)assembled within and beyond this timeframe in Italy. Our discussion contends that the first responses to the pandemic in Italy intensified and exposed the shortcomings of existing, individualised health imperatives and priorities. Consequently, we address how public debates informed by neoliberal understandings of (un)healthy, autonomous, and self-responsible subjects made *invisible* other bodies-spaces-health-security entanglements: those of workers *having to* operate in Covid-unsafe conditions, those for whom "home" was dangerous or non-existent, and those of prisoners and (forced) migrants *stuck* in overcrowded penitentiaries, detention and reception centres. Articulating the different physical, spatial and health domains that the public and political focus foregrounded or made inaccessible, we reflect on how the pandemic event contributed to exacerbate existing boundaries of deservingness and worth in Italy. Finally, we consider how addressing the pandemic as a bio-social event constitutes a necessary starting point to approach the entanglement of (active) bodies, spaces and health in ways that can register the "intrusion of Gaia" (Stengers, 2015 [2009]) as a political subjectivity in the late-capitalist world-order.

Introduction

Towards the end of March 2020, at the height of the devastating first wave of the Sars-Cov2 epidemic in Italy, a *meme* appeared on one of the authors' social media timeline. The meme had been posted by a friend, a young man born in Morocco who have been living in Italy for most of his life, and stated:

> *People are suspicious of you at the markets, the police control you every day.*
> *Calm down, it's just two weeks that you are an Arab.*

The spatial and temporal context to which the meme hinted was the draconian lockdown put in place in Italy in early March 2020 until mid-May 2020. The lockdown measures saw the implementation of curfews and the prohibition of any non-essential activities and movement of people between and within cities and towns. These measures were enforced by a pervasive military and police presence which heightened and materialised a widespread *feeling* of an invisible, yet ever-present enemy that made *any body* a suspect in the public health catastrophe that was unfolding. In this scenario, existing conceptualisations of sport and physical activity as contested (bio)political domains in urban spaces arguably acquired new and unexpected layers and implications; particularly so, as between March and May 2020 the figure of the recreational runner/jogger became associated with widespread narratives of disruptive, illegitimate, *polluting* bodies contributing to the diffusion of the virus. Yet, as the Italian government applied pervasive processes of surveillance to scrutinise and question individuals' presence and practices in public spaces across the national territory, the meme above reminded something important and widely disavowed. What was now being applied to the entire Italian population constituted the extension and intensification of *already existing* concerns and processes related to the control of practices and bodies deemed dangerous, suspicious and/or illegitimate in public spaces in Italy (see Palmas, 2009; De Martini Ugolotti & Moyer, 2016; De Martini Ugolotti, 2022; Tulumello & Bertoni, 2019).

Taking cue from this *apparently* casual, yet emblematic observation ("*calm down, it's just two weeks that you are an Arab*"), this chapter interrogates the extensive and spectacular processes of surveillance of (active) bodies in public spaces during the first lockdown. From this starting point, we advance some considerations on how the body/space/health/(in)security nexus has been understood, narrated, and re-assembled within and beyond this timeframe in Italy. In doing this, we outline a cartography of some of the *lines and folds* that characterised the events and processes that took place between late February and end of May 2020. We engage with a cartographic approach as "a theoretically based and politically informed reading of the present" (Braidotti, 2013, p. 164) that accounts for our location in terms of both space (political, and ecological dimensions), and time (historical and genealogical dimensions).

Our aim in focusing on the Italian context during the first wave of the pandemic is to tease out the multiple processes, contingencies and agencies that continue to shape the "history of the present" (Garland, 2014). In this sense, and following Roth (1981, p. 43) we contend that "writing a history *of* the present means to write history *in* the present; consciously writing in a field of power relations and political struggles" (emphasis added) as they link to, manifest in, and emerge with physical cultural spaces and practices.

In advancing this perspective, we address the body, and more specifically, the reciprocally constitutive domains of body, space and place, as key sites of articulation where different political scales, domains and registers overlapped and (e)merged during the pandemic, often exacerbating existing inequalities and social fault-lines, but also opening possibilities of critical interrogation and praxis. This ontological, epistemological, and political positioning compels us to articulate the multifaceted and entangled relationalities and political registers that underpinned *and shaped* the unfolding of the pandemic event in Italy: from (neoliberal) State policies and infrastructures to individualising discourses on (un)healthy bodies, from pervasive concerns surrounding urban decorum/decay, to more-than-human agencies and planetary transitions.

Following these premises and after an overview of the first wave of the pandemic in Italy, this chapter broadly explores two main lines of discussion. We start by examining how public debates informed by neoliberal understandings of (un)healthy, autonomous, and self-responsible subjects made *(in)visible* specific bodies-spaces-health entanglements and contributed to exacerbate existing hierarchies of deservingness and worth in Italy. We then expand this focus by advancing a discussion of *pandemic atmospheres* to address the multiple sites, scales, registers, and agencies through which the events that have marked the first lockdown unfolded and are still unfolding. We conclude by considering how such approach can contribute to register the "intrusion of Gaia" (Stengers, 2015 [2009]) as a political subjectivity in the late-capitalist world-order. In doing this, we draw on Isabelle Stengers' engagement with conceptualisations of the Earth as a dynamic system whose life-sustaining, biotic/abiotic couplings can elude, displace, and subvert human knowledge and agency and are "capable of assemblages that are very different from the ones on which we depend" (Stengers, 2011 [2002], p. 163; see also Clarke, 2017).

The First Sars-Cov2 Wave in Italy

The Sars-Cov2 virus was first detected in Italy when its diffusion was still widely perceived as a distant issue, whose origin and spreading was mostly related to the "backward" cultural and health practices of the "Orient" and could be managed by tighter controls on incoming travellers from China. A week after the first case of Covid-19 emerged in the small town of Codogno on the 28th February 2020 the governor of the Veneto region, Luca Zaia, argued that Italians' health, hygiene, and food standards had successfully contained the spread of the virus. This had not been the case in China, Mr. Zaia added, because "everybody knows that people eat live rats there" (RAI News, 2020). On the 8th March 2020, among soaring cases, hospitalisations and deaths, the Italian government put the whole Italian territory and population in a lockdown to control the spread of the virus. The nation-wide lockdown closed schools and universities, prohibited all commercial activities except for supermarkets and pharmacies and restricted the movement of people for non-essential purposes. On the night between the 18th and the 19th March, the Italian Army was deployed to Bergamo, the city worst hit by the pandemic, as the local authorities could no longer process the number of bodies in the city's mortuaries. Army trucks transported coffins to crematoriums in several other towns, as the dedicated city's structures were unable to cope with the number of deceased arriving from local hospitals, care and private homes. On the 20th March, with the health services under immense strain nation-wide and close to collapsing in the Lombardy region (Nacoti et al., 2020), lockdown regulations were further tightened. New measures included closing parks and playgrounds and banning open-air sports and running, except individually and in "close proximity"[1] of one's residence. The Army was from then deployed to assist the police forces in strictly enforcing the lockdown on the national territory. This was at the time the largest lockdown in Europe as well as the most aggressive response taken in any region beyond China. Despite these measures,

[1] The Decree Law did not define what constituted "close proximity", leaving local authorities the powers to decide on that. This brought to restrictive interpretations of the Decree delimiting the proximity to one's residence to a distance between 100 and 300 meters.

between mid-March and mid-April 2020 Italy became the world epicentre of the pandemic, with Covid-related deaths higher than anywhere else in the world (Indolfi and Spaccarotella, 2020). In 2021 National Institute for Statistics (ISTAT) recorded 2020 as the year with the highest number of deaths (including non-Covid related) since 1945, when Italy was fighting World War Two on its soil (ISTAT, 2021).

The unfolding of these events was marked by a succession of images that became worldwide symbols of a nation at the verge of collapse and of the individual and community efforts made in the "fight against the virus". These included health workers' faces bruised by wearing protective equipment for long hours or sleeping exhausted on their desks; people coming together on their balconies to sing, play music and clap to show support to health workers and each other; the widespread presence of the Italian Army in the streets enforcing the "stay at home" mandate for the population.

As it would soon happen also in other countries, these images, affective registers, and the public messages exhorting everyone to "play their part" to support those on the *frontlines* in the fight against the virus, shaped cultural and public narratives and feelings of a nation at war against an invisible enemy (De Martini Ugolotti, 2020). While fitting to an extent the catastrophic scenarios and consequences of the epidemic, these widespread narratives had nevertheless several significant implications. As we discuss in the sections below, while continuously claiming that "we are all on the same boat", these processes made *visible* the moral boundaries between (un)healthy and (ir)responsible bodies in the nation-at-war. At the same time, they also defined and made *invisible* the processes and infrastructures that facilitated the virus' diffusion, and the lives deemed to be "worth less" amid the pandemic. Relatedly, as the meme with which we started this discussion hinted to, the processes, narratives and interventions just outlined did not constitute the inevitable and *unprecedented* responses to a catastrophic health crisis. Rather, we can understand what happened between (and beyond) March and May 2020 in Italy as the extension and intensification of prevailing and overlapping political processes, cultural narratives and "affective regimes" (Gilbert, 2008) that marked Italian public life and polity in the last three decades. In this sense, the controversial figure of the runner/jogger in urban spaces constituted a significant site from where to unpack how these overlapping registers surrounding health, (in)security, nationhood and responsibility re-assembled in and through bodies and spaces during the first lockdown.

Pandemic Genealogies

Seen from the perspective of scholarly works that underlined the affinities between contemporary physical cultures and neoliberal political, economic, and cultural sensibilities, the pervasive concerns surrounding active bodies in public spaces, (in)security and responsibility during the first lockdown in Italy should not come as a *complete* surprise. The national obsession with individual behaviours and practices in urban spaces during a public health catastrophe could be arguably seen as the other-side-of-the-coin of long consolidated neoliberal narratives that regularly framed systemic health issues and inequalities as individual responsibilities (Andrews & Silk, 2018; Donato et al., 2019; Fullagar et al., 2019). Concurrently, these narratives converged during the first lockdown with other neoliberal rationales regarding the management of urban and national (in)security that have increasingly blurred the distinction between military interventions, risk prevention, surveillance, and public order to preserve economic flows and growth (Graham, 2010; Tulumello & Bertoni, 2019). In this sense, in the context of the first Italian lockdown, existing cultural articulations around health, responsibility, physical activity and (in)security simultaneously converged and changed in scope and intensity in two significant and related ways. The first regarded the spectacular extension of individual health responsibilities from one's body to the national body politic. As individual bodies became increasingly aligned with the national collective body, the concept of *responsibility* strengthened its double grip in relation to the *capacity to control* one's behaviours and as the *culpability* associated to the violation of a (moral) prohibition (Moretti, 2020). The second related to how the individualised, therapeutic perspectives that widely prescribed the health benefits of an active lifestyle were turned around by definitions of physical activity in public spaces as dangerous, irresponsible, and immoral. In fact, extending well beyond the domain of moral judgements, widely shared public narratives between March and May 2020 ascribed a direct correlation between a run, or a walk, and the spread of the virus on the national territory. Within this timeframe, a discursive constellation of politicians' declarations, "instructional" videos, advertising, and local/national by-laws composed a widely shared focus on what and whose bodies were supposedly to surveil and blame for the catastrophic spreading of the virus. Now widely identified as the enemy-within-the-nation-at-war, joggers and "non-essential" walkers would be pro-actively chased by police and media drones in live-TV pursuits, and when attacked in public spaces, politicians would implicitly justify their aggressions based on what they did (not) wear (e.g., a facemask).

At the same time, what remained constantly concealed by a pervasive focus on physical practices such as jogging or walking was the fact that throughout the first lockdown the main drivers of contagion in Italy remained hospitals and workplaces (Nava, 2020; Da Mosto et al., 2021; Nacoti et al., 2020). In this sense, the tragic paradox of health services acting as drivers of contagion while trying to cure the ill could be arguably linked to three decades of neoliberal welfare "reforms" which cut 100.000 hospital beds, one-third of general practitioners, and suppressed 759 hospital wards from the late 1990s (Indolfi and Spaccarotella, 2020). The most significant of these "new public management" reforms took place in Lombardy, the region that would be worst hit by the pandemic; under the aegis of a "more efficient" health provision, these included the erasure of general health practitioners and prevention services in the community and the *privatisation and centralisation of health services* in hospitals focused on state-of-the-art, patient-centred therapeutic activities (Nava, 2020). While not directly citing these processes, the doctors of the Giovanni XXIII hospital in Bergamo clearly outlined their implications in an open letter on the 21st March 2020 as they detailed the role of centralised care in hospitals in the spread of the Covid-19, called for community-based health services and warned that "the more medicalized and centralized the society, the more widespread the virus." (Nacoti et al., 2020, p. 3).

Relatedly, while the *un-detailed* definition of "essential activity" in the Decree Laws implemented between March and May 2020 enabled police forces and local authorities to capillary scrutinise activities like jogging or walking, it also provided significant leeway for businesses to qualify as "essential" and require employees to go to work in warehouses and factories (Nava, 2020). In this sense, the framing of national "stay at home" orders as a moral gesture of solidarity for the frontline heroes and heroines fighting against the virus disavowed the precarious conditions of workers who *had to* go to work in often Covid-unsafe environments. Simultaneously, these responsibilising narratives also concealed how often workers *felt compelled to go to work* because without any substantial welfare support, any closure of economic production raised the spectre of crisis, unemployment, and social disaster (Nava, 2020). The neoliberal imperatives and affective regimes which placed concerns over economic productivity and competitiveness *ahead of anything else*, even in the epicentre of a catastrophic health crisis were captured by Nava (2020) who argued that "[during the first lockdown] in Lombardy it was impossible to stop the production, in Lombardy it was only possible to die" (Nava, 2020, p. 184).

Yet, political, and public debates informed by neoliberal understandings of (un)healthy, autonomous, and self-responsible subjects did not only conceal how economic imperatives, political reforms, and the *infrastructures of circulation that they shaped* drove the spreading of the virus. They also intensified the distinction between what Judith Butler (2004) defined *grievable and ungrievable lives* in the context of the pandemic. When between 8th and 12th March 2020 detainees in Italian penitentiaries revolted against containment measures and the health risk posed by systemic overcrowding, the response was the military-enforced isolation of the rioters: 14 people, 12 inmates and 2 prison guards would die by the end of the revolt. Amid countless episodes of covid-outbreaks in informal camps and buildings occupied by (forced) migrants (many working in essential sectors like agriculture and food delivery), in April 2020 asylum seekers in Rome set fire to the reception centre in which they were confined. They did so to protest the lack of health responses to a covid-outbreak among the 130 people in the overcrowded building. Until then, the main public response to the outbreak had been the heightening of the perimeter walls of the building to avoid escapes (Mellino, 2020). Overall, the lockdown implementation resulted in the widespread, yet publicly disregarded exacerbation of health issues and social exclusion (including sheer hunger) for hundreds of thousands of asylum seekers, undocumented migrants and people experiencing homelessness[2] as the operations of community organisations supporting them were forced to stop without any relevant alternatives in their place (Da Mosto et al., 2021). While the Italian government took "unprecedented" economic measures to assuage the socio-economic impacts of the epidemic on "Italian families" and the nation seemed to re-discover a sense of shared solidarity and purpose, conditions of destitution, hunger and endangerment continued to be considered more tolerable for some than for others.

Cartographies of Differential Vulnerability and Pandemic Atmospheres

Recent commentaries on the pandemic responses enacted in Italy and elsewhere meaningfully highlighted how the bio-political processes of "nationalization of the biological" (Foucault, 1990 [1978], p. 244) (not exclusively) evoked by lockdown measures imply a politics of *differential vulnerability* (Lorenzini, 2021); a politics that structurally relies on the establishment of hierarchies in the value of lives that produces, and multiplies vulnerability to death and illness *as a means of governing people* (Lorenzini, 2021, p. 44). Roberto Esposito (2011, 2013) has argued that the consolidation of these (already existing) hierarchies of the value of life accompanied the contemporary expansion of an *immunity paradigm* which seamlessly applied bio-medical models of prevention, isolation, and immunisation to a wide range of political issues (from terrorism to migration flows, from digital security to epidemics). Operating "at the intersection of law and biology, medical and legal procedure" (Esposito and Hanafi, 2013, p. 85) an immunity paradigm understands both individual and collective bodies (e.g., nations) as sites whose boundaries/borders must be protected from the invasion of (in)visible foreign entities. Yet,

[2] At the start of the pandemic, there were about 600,000 undocumented migrants in Italy, soon to become about 800,000 because of legal restrictions introduced with the 2018 Salvini Security Decree-Law. The number of people experiencing homelessness in 2020 have been estimated between 49,000 and 52,000 (Barbieri, 2020).

Newman et al. (2016) underlined the paradox of biopolitical/immunitary understandings of (active) bodies as at once bounded and fluid, as entities whose boundaries need to be secured from "any external element that threatens" (Esposito and Hanafi, 2013, p. 85) and as "leaky" sites of transmission of such threats. This paradox arguably emerged in the first lockdown in Italy, during which pervasive surveillance and security measures have been justified to protect the nation's collective body from individuals' "leaky bodies" (Newman et al., 2016). However, the increasingly pervasive application of "immunitary" rationales during the first lockdown did not only reinforce and redrew the boundaries between the inside and the outside of the nation. Nor it simply legitimised the increased *surveillance of anyone* as a potential "living pathological vessel" (Newman et al., 2016, p. 155) *for the sake of everyone*. Rather, it exacerbated and legitimated the differential definition of *what and who is worth preserving* within the collective body of the nation.

Following these considerations and what discussed in the previous section, we could see a politics of differential vulnerability being applied during the first lockdown in Italy through (at least) two simultaneous and intersecting processes. The first saw the enactment of pandemic responses that aimed to protect the nation from the virus, but in ways that arguably defended the nation by prioritising "its markets, not its people" (Butler, 2020; see also Nava, 2020). The second related to the intensification of an already existing public and political consensus regarding whose lives are worth less amid recurring "crises" (De Martini Ugolotti & Caudwell, 2022). This was made evident by the fact that the framing of the "household" as a space of protection in the government's "stay at home" restrictions completely ignored the circumstances of those for whom "home" was overcrowded, dangerous or non-existent.

The analyses mentioned so far have insightfully articulated the links between bio-, and necropolitical forms of pandemic management and the affective politics that centred on responsibilising subjects to "do their part" in the war against the virus; this, all the while concealing other processes and infrastructures of circulation that enabled and accelerated its spread. These discussions have been fundamental to pose critical questions on the pandemic responses and their implications. Yet, they also implicitly privileged the relationships between the *corporeal subjectivities* (Newman et al.,

2016) of citizens, denizens, patients, workers, (recreational) runners and the state as the only agents shaping the nexus of health, space and (in) security in pandemic times. In doing so, these perspectives reproduced a distinction between nature and culture, the human and non-human, and between agents and non-agents that the pandemic event arguably complicated (see Latour, 2021). To address how bodies in urban spaces became so central in the affective politics of the pandemic we explore and engage with the idea of (pandemic) *atmospheres*. More specifically, through the notion of atmosphere we attend to and articulate two issues that we consider fundamental to address the entanglement of bodies, health, (in)security and (urban) spaces during the first pandemic wave in Italy: moral and aesthetic concerns surrounding urban decorum (and indecorous bodies and spaces) and Gaia's intrusion in late-capitalist social and spatial order.

Atmospheres of Decorum/Decay and (Infectious) Urban Bodies

In the frame of the "preventive turn" that marked global trends in the securitisation of urban spaces, the Italian context was specifically characterised in the last three decades by the emergence and consolidation of the notion of "decorum" (and its discursive opposite "decay") as a keyword and a tool for urban governance (Pitch, 2013).

Scholars (Tulumello & Bertoni, 2019; Barchetta, 2021) have highlighted that while wider politics of urban securitisation focused on preventing urban practices and behaviours as potential sources of threat (e.g., crime, terrorism, disorder, violence, etc.), the politics of decorum operate and intervene specifically on *urban bodies*. In this sense, although focusing on the same urban groups (the urban poor and the homeless, undocumented migrants, Roma minorities, racialised youth, street vendors, drug addicts, etc.) the politics of security and decorum differ as the latter focus and intervene directly on specific bodies *as causes* of urban decay. This, because of such bodies' supposed lack of adherence to never clearly defined, but always assumed as "common-sense" moral and aesthetic criteria (Tulumello & Bertoni, 2019). Importantly, these "common-sense" moral and aesthetic criteria tend to inevitably embody the classed, racialised and gendered characteristics of economically independent, "healthy", and (conspicuously) consuming urban subjects (De Martini Ugolotti & Silk, 2018). In other words, within the frame of the politics of decorum, the bodies of specific "indecorous" urban dwellers are assumed to inherently carry with themselves *impressions of disorder* and *feelings of insecurity* that contribute to produce landscapes and sensations of urban decay (Tulumello & Bertoni, 2019). Expanding on Sarah Ahmed's (2004) work, Barchetta (2021) addressed through the notion of atmosphere the intensities of evoked or visceral feelings of decay that *stick* on bodies and urban spaces/surfaces, and the ideas, narratives and practices (e.g. media depictions, urban by-laws and interventions, Decree Laws etc.) that simultaneously address and produce them.

In this sense, with Brighenti (2016) an atmosphere can be thought as the air that is breathed, at the same time a subjective perception and an ecological element that is constantly *shared with* and *defined by* human and non-human forces. For this reason, while it may at first seem encompassing and enveloping, an atmosphere always also has an interstitial character to it; like, air, an atmosphere's capacity to connect and stick-on things, spaces and bodies is intimately linked to its constant *infiltration* through barriers such as doors, walls, and other infrastructures. According to Brighenti (2016), the notion of atmosphere can thus contribute to understand cities as *spaces of respiration*, and to understand respiration as the *rhythmic component of every atmosphere*. Notably enough, as a floating signifier, the concept of decorum can be arguably understood as a perception that is at the same time subjective and ecological; one that has enveloped and infiltrated the political narratives, urban policies and everyday practices and rhythms of Italian cities (Pitch, 2013). The idea of decorum is indefinable, only perceivable through its opposite, decay (Tulumello & Bertoni, 2019). As a result, the city can never be understood, experienced, or *felt* as "decorous", as decorum emerges only from the absence of decay. The idea and politics of urban decorum thus implies a process of ever-expanding surveillance, containment, deterrence on specific "indecorous" urban bodies, and infiltration in apparently mundane domains of urban life (e.g., the regulation of dress-codes and informal social gatherings in Italian cities, see O'Sullivan, 2017). Further, in line with the wider preventive turn analysed in the literature, atmospheres of decorum imply a pervasive and compelling dimension of responsibility that is at the same time individual ("avoid contributing to, or being the victim of urban decay") and collective; the latter implying the mobilisation of the "community" to enact social surveillance and draw the boundaries between decorous and indecorous bodies/spaces. In this sense, through the notion of atmosphere we can grasp and articulate the intersection of visceral, discursive, material, and political registers through which rhetoric, feelings and practices of decorum/decay could be impressed on specific bodies and urban spaces.

Following these considerations, the pervasive and specific focus on (active) bodies in urban spaces during the first lockdown can be understood as the re-assembling of intensities, narratives and practices of prevailing urban politics and atmospheres with the socio-political and ecological shifts impressed by the Sars-Cov2 epidemic. During the first lockdown, perceptions of health and security thus converged and aligned with existing affective, moral, and aesthetic judgements that associated specific bodies with the infection of urban spaces, cities, and the nation at large (Barchetta, 2021). The focus of public concerns moved from "aesthetically unpleasing" and "morally indecorous" bodies to the irresponsible and selfish bodies of runners and walkers. The latter "non-essential" presence in urban spaces was pervasively perceived as undermining the *moral conduct* and *aesthetics* of the nation-at-home (and at war), and *as such* a threat to the collective body of the nation. In other words, while interpellating health-related rationales, the visceral, discursive, and practical perception of bodies in urban spaces during the first pandemic wave implied the intensification of urban atmospheres in which contagion was already understood, lived, and felt[3] as much a *moral and aesthetic process* as a physical and molecular one (see also Moretti, 2020).

It is here that the notion of atmosphere can contribute and expand insights focused on the bio-, and necro-political rationales that underpinned the pandemic responses. These analyses have importantly focused on bodies as political, sensual, and biological sites through which it is

[3] Moretti (2020) has provided insightful analogies between the systematic search and harassment of individuals as supposed plague-spreaders during the first lockdown with the cosmologies of witchcraft.

possible to illuminate the irreconcilable tensions and hierarchies in the value of life that underpin contemporary understandings of health, responsibility and (in)security. However, the notion of atmosphere as a field of forces in which different bio-social bodies actively participate in assembling specific intensities, meanings, and processes expands a specific focus on bodies and corporeal subjectivities (Newman et al., 2016) by addressing and repositioning them as part of wider ecological registers and relationalities. An atmospheric reading of the first lockdown in Italy can thus illuminate and keep together the entrenched forms of differential vulnerabilities intensified by the pandemic responses *and* the non-human forces that exercised their agency independently of human priorities and intentions. Agreeing with Barchetta (2021), we contend that illuminating these socio-ecological connections is fundamental to understand the pandemic event as the combination of historical phenomena and the agencies of unexpected political subjectivities. In this sense, the notion of atmosphere as a sensorial register of bio-social life invites us to extend our focus to other relationalities, forces and agencies that contributed to shape the spatial, temporal, and physical cultural sites explored in this work.

From Bio-politics to Cosmopolitics? Pandemic Atmospheres and the Intrusion of Gaia

Bacteria and viruses can also call the shots. (Lundi-Matin, 16th May, 2020)

Following Denowski and Viveiros de Castro (2017, p. 15) we could argue that if the Euro-American *Weltanshaung* posed that the social structure of modernity stands on its ground floor, the economy, the pandemic event has reminded that such vision has forgotten the foundations: the Earth (System). In this sense, some scholars have argued that the term Anthropocene, notwithstanding the important critiques directed to its use to define the current geological era,[4] carries the significance of a meaningful

[4] As posed through the notions of Capitalocene (Moore, 2016) and Plantationocene (Haraway, 2015). Assessing the content of these critiques is beyond the remit of this chapter, but we contend that all these terms in different ways enable us to (re)think ecological relations at the scale of the planetary.

reminder. According to these perspectives, the meaningfulness of this formulation stems from the explicit acknowledgement that the transformation of our species from a mere biological agent "into a geological force" (Chakrabarty, 2009) tangibly questions the dichotomies between environment and society, ecology and economy, nature and culture that have started to be problematised from the second half of the twentieth century. It could be argued that the implosion of these dichotomies has been made even more evident by the diffusion of a virus that has not attacked or made ill the (late)capitalist social order, but has *hacked* it, literally using highly networked global infrastructures (e.g., transportation, health, economy) *as an exoskeleton* to fulfil its main biological function: reproduce itself. Relatedly, acknowledging that the acceleration of time and the related compression of space are not anymore exclusively an *existential prerogative* of Western modernity but are *bio-social features* of a pandemic phenomenon, makes increasingly *real* the brusque, abrupt, and relentless "intrusion of Gaia" (Stengers, 2015) into the horizon of human history.

With the figure of Gaia, Isabelle Stengers drew on Lovelock and Margulis' notion of an Earth System arising from biotic/abiotic couplings and co-productions that sustain the biosphere (Clarke, 2017). From this starting point, Isabelle Stengers suggested 'the new figure of Gaia indicates that it is becoming urgent to create a contrast between the earth valorized as a set of resources and the earth considered as a set of interdependent processes, *capable of assemblages that are very different from the ones on which we depend*' (2011 [2002], p. 163, emphasis added). In other words, according to Stengers (2015), the figure of Gaia encapsulates the paradox of a present and inconvenient truth; that one way or another the time is over for "us" (read, the Western/modern *anthropos*) to consider ourselves the true actors of our history, freely discussing if the Earth is available for our use or should be protected. In this sense, as the Euro-American incarnation of humanity transformed itself in a "geological force", the notion of Gaia's intrusion has given the Earth System the menacing form of a *historical subject and a political agent* (Latour, 2013; Denowski & Viveiros de Castro, 2017). In fact, as Stengers (2015 [2009]) argued, the brutality of the intrusion of Gaia corresponds to the brutality of what has provoked her, that of a "development" (or progress, modernity, etc.) that is blind to its consequences, or which, more precisely, only takes its consequences into account from the point of view of the new sources of profit they can bring about. If the pandemic event can be arguably seen as the latest manifestation of Gaia's intrusion in the horizon of Western modernity, we contend that the notion of atmosphere can constitute a useful analytical lens to address the planetary transformations that we are witnessing. The concept can help us to situate our perspectives between different scales by articulating the spatial, temporal, and visceral manifestations of entangled ecological, socio-political, and biological change (see Barchetta, 2021). In other words, the notion of atmosphere contributes to address how the inconvenient truth of Gaia's intrusion, as manifested through the pandemic event, tangibly materialises *in and as* the air we can(not) breathe, the spaces we can(not) inhabit, the temporalities that we can(not) control, and the intensities we can(not) feel.

To come back at the focus of this chapter, the notion of atmosphere as an *ecological feeling* (Barchetta, 2021) that displaces any separation between the visceral, the social and the ecological, can be useful to start (re)thinking the reciprocal constitution of bodies and spaces during the first wave of the pandemic in Italy. From such a perspective, observing how bodies, spaces, health, and (in)security have been re-assembled during the pandemic implies recognising, keeping together, and making visible the political dynamics, affective regimes, and bio-social processes that operate at different but entangled speeds and scales and converge in and through the same physical cultural sites (e.g., the city, its public spaces and infrastructures, running/walking, un/healthy bodies, intimate, yet ecological feelings). Such a perspective can allow for a political reading of pandemic processes of surveillance, containment and control that underlines the "radical ecological interdependency" (Escobar, 2019) between scales, registers, temporalities and knowledges generally assumed and interpreted as separated.

Put it differently, acknowledging the intrusion of Gaia in understanding how the body/space/health/security nexus has been (re)assembled during the first lockdown in Italy can produce different folds to the binary understandings and narratives that emerged in this timeframe (active bodies in public spaces as pathological vessels of contagion *or* as means of individualised health and resilience). In this sense, this perspective highlighted how runners/walkers' bodies and urban landscapes impressed and carried ecological feelings of fear and contagion that could not *exclusively* be ascribed to the widespread imposition and acceptance of bio-political discourses and interventions of "protective negation of life" (Esposito, 2011). Acknowledging the intrusion of Gaia expanded these perspectives by registering how the "cold panic" (Stengers, 2015) of these ecological feelings *also* re-assembled and intensified existing concerns over *morally and aesthetically* polluting bodies and spaces, and the forgotten and inconvenient truth that "viruses can also call the shots". We contend that this perspective can expand fundamental socio-cultural approaches that understand sport and physical culture as sites of relation to the body that are imbued in power relations[5] by addressing *the physical* as a domain that (literally) put in place and enable the creation of atmospheric and (political) ecological relationalities in, with, and through the body.

In this sense, an atmospheric reading of the political, cultural, and ecological changes brought to the fore by pandemic event can meaningfully contribute to important work addressing the more-than-human constitution of physical cultures (see Newman et al., 2020). It can do so by articulating the important lines of enquiry raised by this body of scholarship with the inconvenient truth that Gaia's intrusion is not yet another "crisis" to be overcome but is a transcendence that is here to stay (Stengers, 2015 [2009]). Acknowledging the intrusion of Gaia as a formidable, yet forgotten force that is shaping the future of life on earth poses what we contend is a fundamental question: what kind of physical cultures (can) emerge from the ruins left by anthropic devastations and Gaia's agencies?

Is There a World to Come? For a Physical Cultural (Cosmo)Politics of the Ruins

> *The white people, they do not dream as far as we do. They sleep a lot but only dream of themselves.* (Kopenava & Albert, 2013, p. 3)

---

[5] We refer here to Bourdieu's evocative definition of sport as a "relation to the body" (1978, p. 833) and to Silk and Andrews' formulation of physical culture (2011, p. 6).

Starting from the pervasive concerns that recreational physical activities in public spaces attracted in the spatial and temporal context of the first lockdown in Italy, this chapter articulated apparently disconnected body/space/health/security entanglements that the public and political focus foregrounded or made inaccessible during the first pandemic wave in Italy. In doing so, we drew on and contributed to work on sport, leisure and physical culture that has underlined the relevance of understanding bodies and spaces as co-constituted and intra-acting with wider ecologies and socio-economic infrastructures operating at different speeds and scales (Newman et al., 2020). Firstly, our discussion reminded how the pervasive and *spectacular* processes of surveillance of (active) bodies in public spaces during the first lockdown in Italy implied the extension *to everybody* of existing processes of surveillance and control of bodies deemed dangerous, suspicious and/or illegitimate in public spaces (e.g. racialised minorities, people on the move and seeking asylum, the urban poor, political activists, etc.); all the while, an already existing public and political consensus regarding whose lives are worth less amid recurring "crises" implied the legitimation of processes of abandonment, destitution and endangerment of those for whom the association between "home" and "safety" was impossible (e.g. prisoners in penitentiaries and detention centres, people experiencing homelessness and domestic violence, etc.).

Yet, an atmospheric reading of the first lockdown enabled us to keep together the entrenched forms of differential vulnerability intensified by bio- and necro-political (in)actions, moral and aesthetics concerns over indecorous bodies, and the non-human forces that are imposing themselves so clearly to our attention "that they can no longer treated as elements of an inert Earth" (Ghosh, 2020, p. 197). Through this perspective, we addressed the significance of registering and articulating the different scales, speeds and intensities through which socio-ecological transformations entangle with regimes of bordering, expulsion and extraction, embodied feelings attune to planetary transitions, and the temporalities of lockdown lives merge with those of molecular reproduction.

After all, as Barchetta (2021) contended, when facing the disasters generated by centuries of accumulation by dispossession, human and non-human exploitation, and environmental devastation, what is the Anthropocene if not an *atmospheric diffusion* of toxicity, pollution and differential vulnerabilities to illness and death at a planetary scale?

The space-time tangles (Barad, 2007) that such a perspective underlines complicate many of the public and political narratives that continue to shape the pandemic phenomenon as they represent it in Italy and pretty much elsewhere: the linearity of a pre vs. post pandemic time, of crisis vs. normality or as sport and physical culture as means of contagion vs. "healthy habits". As the sounds of clapping, balcony chants and the hopes of a more equitable "post-pandemic great reset" fade away and give space to exacerbating social divisions and unrest, political narratives keep on ensuring that the Sars-Cov2 intrusion constituted a temporary interruption of "the ways things have been"; including the ways in which sport, leisure and physical cultures have been practiced, consumed, and managed.

Disavowing the extended spatial-temporal tangles of the pandemic, the focus of political and public (including sporting) narratives fail to consider how the pandemic event constituted the manifestation of an unfolding process rather than an(other) "unprecedented" crisis: to borrow from Davi Kopenawa, the Western/modern and white-centred *anthropos* keeps dreaming only of itself.

However, the introduction of a new invisible character able to reverse the order and hierarchy of agencies (Latour, 2013) forces us to re-locate discussions surrounding the "depths and possibilities of physicality" (Newman et al., 2020, p. 7) in the context of planetary ecological transitions. We contend that it does so by placing physical cultural domains and analyses *amid the ruins* caused by ongoing regimes of extraction and private accumulation, the intensification of entrenched forms of differential vulnerabilities, *and* the intrusion of Gaia.

In this sense, with Navaro-Yashin (2009) we intend the ruins not just as the debris of socio-ecological devastation, and not as the negative counterpart ('the other') to the subjective realm or the social order, but as what is intrinsically constitutive of it. The abject, the ruin is not (only) that which is packed away in the garbage bin (or the waste management centre), the toilet, or the graveyard to maintain personal or social integrity. As Evers addressed discussing "polluted leisure" (2019), *ruination*, though not only related to pollution, is right here, in one's vicinity, environment and domestic space, in one's midst.

However, the point of placing physical cultural domains and analyses amid the ruins is not (only) about illuminating the fault-lines and consequences of ideas of progress, growth and (self)development that constitute physical cultural domains and industries. It is not, to use an oft-cited Antonio Gramsci's quote, taking stock that "the old is dying, and the new cannot be born" (Gramsci, 1971, p. 271).

Rather, to address what physical cultures (can) emerge amid the ruins we consider necessary to engage with ways of being "human" that have been subjugated and violated by modern conceptions of humanity, that have endured amid the ruins *of ending worlds*, but have nevertheless continued to live other relations with time-space-matter implied by other possible and existing forms of being-with-the-world. It is about the necessity to bear witness and support a plurality of "actually existing" ways in which the domain of *the physical* is embedded amid wider socio-ecological relations, as well as ontological and cosmological pluralities (see Fox & McDermott, 2019; McGuire-Adams, 2020).

The notion of atmosphere and the acknowledgement of Gaia's intrusion have afforded us to attune to the bio-social composition of the bodies/spaces/health/(in)security nexus during the first lockdown in Italy in ways that we see advancing some productive questions and insights to scholars and practitioners in sport, leisure, and physical culture.

Yet, while framed as "contributions" these ideas are far from new from perspectives grounded in non-Western ontologies, and in fact could contribute to *silence them* (see Todd[6], 2016). In this sense, placing physical cultural domains and analyses *amid the ruins* means explicitly acknowledging that "we" (Western, Euro-American and white scholars) are *only now* starting to come to terms with the instances that multiple silenced, devalued yet undocile *bodies of knowledge* have been addressing before and after the emergence of modernity. As these knowledges and worldviews are currently informing and inspiring multiple socio-ecological struggles around the world (Kopenava & Albert, 2013; Escobar, 2019; Estes, 2019), our question, and ultimately commitment is how we can connect these instances and support those who are already doing it, in the highly commodified, yet contested and "lively" domains of sport, leisure and physical culture.

---

[6] Todd's reflections on *Sila* as climate, life force and atmosphere points to our own lack of knowledge about non-Western ontologies in the specific case of our discussion.

References

Ahmed, S. (2004). *The cultural politics of emotion*. Routledge.

Andrews, D., & Silk, M. (2018). Sport and neoliberalism: An affective-ideological articulation. *Journal of Popular Culture, 51*(2), 511–533. https://doi.org/10.1111/jpcu.12660

Barbieri, A. (2020). CoViD-19 in Italia: la popolazione senza fissa dimora ha bisogno di protezione. Report, Medici per i Diritti Umani (MEDU). Retrieved from: https://mediciperidirittiumani.org/medu/wpcontent/uploads/2020/05/33301_Editoriale-Barbieri_ITA_Web.pdf Last Accessed 14th November 2022.

Barad, K. (2007). *Meeting the universe halfway: Quantum physics and the entanglement of matter and meaning*. Duke University Press.

Barchetta, L. (2021). *La Rivolta del Verde. Nature e Rovine a Torino*. Agenzia X.

Bourdieu, P. (1978). Sport and Social Class. *Social Science Information, 17*(6), 819–840.

Braidotti, R. (2013). *The Post-Human*. Cambridge: Polity Press.

Brighenti, A. M. (2016). The public and the common: Some approximations of their contemporary articulation. *Critical Inquiry, 42*(2), 306–328. https://doi.org/10.1086/684355

Butler, J. (2004). *Precarious life: The powers of mourning and violence*. Verso Books.

Butler, J. (2020, March 30). Capitalism has its limits. https://www.versobooks.com/blogs/4603-capitalism-has-its-limits

Chakrabarty, D. (2009). The climate of history: Four theses. *Critical Inquiry, 35*(2), 197–222. https://doi.org/10.1086/596640

Clarke, B. (2017). Rethinking Gaia: Stengers, Latour, Margulis. *Theory, Culture & Society, 34*(4), 3–26. https://doi.org/10.1177/0263276416686844

Da Mosto, D., Bodini, C., Mammana, L., Gherardi, G., Quargnolo, M., & Fantini, M. P. (2021). Health equity during COVID-19: A qualitative study on the consequences of the syndemic on refugees' and asylum seekers' health in reception centres in Bologna (Italy). *Journal of Migration and Health*. https://doi.org/10.1016/j.jmh.2021.100057

De Martini Ugolotti, N. (2020, April 8). "We are in this together": Covid-19, the politics of emotions and the borders of humanity. https://discoversociety.org/2020/04/08/we-are-in-this-together-covid-19-the-politics-of-emotions-and-the-borders-of-humanity/.

De Martini Ugolotti, N. (2022). Contested bodies in a regenerating city: post-migrant men's contingent citizenship, parkour and diaspora spaces, Leisure Studies, https://doi.org/10.1080/02614367.2022.2085775

De Martini Ugolotti, N., & Caudwell, J. (2022). Leisure and forced migration: Lives lived in asylum systems. In N. De Martini Ugolotti & J. Caudwell (Eds.), *Leisure and forced migration: Lives lived in asylum systems* (pp. 1–18). Routledge.

De Martini Ugolotti, N., & Moyer, E. (2016). 'If I climb a wall of ten meters': Capoeira, parkour and the politics of public space among (post)migrant youth in Turin, Italy. *Patterns of Prejudice, 50*(2), 188–206. https://doi.org/10.1080/0031322X.2016.1164435

De Martini Ugolotti, N., & Silk, M. (2018). Parkour, counter-conducts and the government of difference in post-industrial Turin. *City, 22*(5–6), 763–781. https://doi.org/10.1080/13604813.2018.1549849

Denowsky, D., & Viveiros de Castro, E. (2017). *The ends of the word.* Polity Press.

Donato, A., Tonelli, L., & Galak, E. (2019). *Le Pieghe del Corpo.* Mimesis.

Escobar, A. (2019). *Designs for the pluriverse: Radical interdependence, autonomy and the making of worlds.* Duke University Press.

Esposito, R. (2011). *Immunitas: The protection and negation of life.* Polity.

Esposito, R., & Hanafi, Z. (2013). Community, immunity, biopolitics. *Angelaki, 18*(3), 83–90.

Estes, N. (2019). *Our history is the future: Standing Rock versus the Dakota Access Pipeline, and the long tradition of Indigenous resistance.* Verso.

Evers, W. C. (2019). Polluted leisure. *Leisure Sciences, 41*(5), 423–440. https://doi.org/10.1080/01490400.2019.1627963

Foucault, M. (1990 [1978]). *The will to knowledge: The history of sexuality, volume one.* Penguin.

Fox, K., & McDermott, L. (2019). The Kumulipo, Native Hawaiians, and well-being: How the past speaks to the present and lays the foundation for the future. *Leisure Studies, 39*(1), 96–110. https://doi.org/10.1080/02614367.2019.1633680

Fullagar, S., O'Brien, W., & Pavlidis, A. (2019). *Feminism and a vital politics of depression and recovery.* Springer.

Garland, D. (2014). What is a "history of the present"? On Foucault's genealogies and their critical preconditions. *Punishment & Society, 16*(4), 365–384. https://doi.org/10.1177/1462474514541711

Gilbert, J. (2008). *Anticapitalism and culture: Radical theory and popular politics.* Routledge.

Ghosh, A. (2020). *The Nutmeg Curse: Parables for a Planet in Crisis.* Chicago: University of Chicago Press.

Graham, S. (2010). *Cities under siege: The new urban militarism.* Routledge.

Gramsci, A. (1971). *Selections from the prison notebooks of Antonio Gramsci* (Q. Hoare & G. Nowell-Smith, Ed. and trans.) (p. 276). Lawrence & Wishart.

Haraway, D. (2015). Staying with the Trouble: Making Kin in the Chthulucene. Chicago: Duke University Press.

Kopenava, D., & Albert, B. (2013). *The falling sky. Words of a Yanomami shaman* (N. Elliott & A. Dundy, Trans). Harvard University Press.

Indolfi & Spaccarotella. (2020). The Outbreak of COVID-19 in Italy Fighting the Pandemic, *JACC Case Reports, 2*(9), 1414–1418. https://doi.org/10.1016/j.jaccas.2020.03.012

ISTAT. (2021). Una terza guerra mondiale? Retrieved from: https://www.istat.it/it/files//2020/04/Report_Una-terzaguerra-mondiale.pdf, Last accessed 14th November 2022.

Latour, B. (2013, March 2). *Facing Gaia: Six lectures on the political theology of nature*. Gifford lectures on Naural Religion, version 10-3-13. http://www.bruno-latour.fr/sites/default/files/downloads/GIFFORD-SIX-LECTURES_1.pdf

Latour, B. (2021). Is this a dress rehearsal? *Critical Inquiry, 47*(2), 25–27. https://doi.org/10.1086/711428

Lorenzini, D. (2021). Biopolitics in the time of coronavirus. *Critical Inquiry, 47*(2), 40–45. https://doi.org/10.1086/711432

McGuire-Adams, T. (2020). *Indigenous feminist Gikendaasowin (knowledge) decolonization through physical activity*. Palgrave Macmillan.

Mellino, M. (2020, March 28). Restate a casa, ma per sempre. Decreti d'emergenza e razzismo di stato. https://www.dinamopress.it/news/restate-casa-sempre-decreti-demergenza-razzismo/

Moore, J. W. (2016). Anthropocene or Capitalocene? Nature, history, and the crisis of capitalism. Oakland: PM Press.

Moretti, C. (2020, March 20). Storie Virali. Responsabilità e Consapevolezza. https://www.treccani.it/magazine/atlante/cultura/Storie_Virali_Responsabilita_e_colpevolezza.html

Nacoti, M., Ciocca, A., Giupponi, A., Brambillasca, P., Lussana, F., Pisano, M., Goisis, G., Bonacina, D., Fazzi, M., Naspro, R., Longhi, L., Cereda, M., & Montaguti, C. (2020). At the epicenter of the Covid-19 pandemic and humanitarian crises in Italy: Changing perspectives on preparation and mitigation. *New England Journal of Medicine*. https://doi.org/10.1056/CAT.20.0080

Nava, F. (2020). *Il Focolaio. Da Bergamo al contagio nazionale*. Laterza.

Navaro-Yashin, Y. (2009). Affective spaces, melancholic objects: Ruination and the production of anthropological knowledge. *Journal of the Royal Anthropological Institute, 15*(1), 1–18. https://doi.org/10.1111/j.1467-9655.2008.01527.x

Newman, J., Shields, R., & McLeod, C. M. (2016). The MSRA epidemic and/as fluid biopolitics. *Body & Society, 22*(4), 155–184.

Newman, J., Thorpe, H., & Andrews, D. (2020). *Sport, physical culture and the moving body: Materialisms, technologies, ecologies*. Rutgers University Press.

O'Sullivan, F. (2017, July 31). Why Italy is banning everything. Bloomberg CityLab. https://www.bloomberg.com/news/articles/2017-07-31/italy-cracks-down-on-tourist-behavior-incentral-cities

Palmas, Q. L. (2009). Dentro le Gang: Giovani, Migranti e Nuovi Spazi Pubblici [Inside the Gangs: Youth, Migrants and New Public Spaces]. Verona: Ombre Corte.

Pitch, T. (2013). *Contro il decoro. L'uso politico della pubblica decenza*. Laterza.

Rai News. (2020). Zaia: "Cinesi mangiano topi vivi", ambasciata protesta, lui si scusa. Retrieved from: https://www.rainews.it/archivio-rainews/articoli/zaia-cinesi-mangiano-topi-vivi-ambasciata-protesta-lui-si-scusa-6630af83-073d-49b3-8e60-0f47339f672d.html

Roth, M. (1981). Foucault's "History of the Present". *History and Theory, 20*(1), 32–46.

Silk, M., & Andrews, D. (2011). Toward a physical cultural studies. Sociology of Sport Journal, 28 (1), pp. 4–35.

Stengers, I. (2011 [2002]). *Thinking with Whitehead: A free and wild creation of concepts* (M. Chase, Trans.). Harvard University Press.

Stengers, I. (2015 [2009]). *In catastrophic times: Resisting the coming barbarism* (A. Goffey, Trans.). Open Humanities Press.

Todd, Z. (2016). An Indigeneous feminist's take on the ontological turn: "Ontology" is just another word for colonialism. *Journal of Historical Sociology, 29*(1), 4–22. https://doi.org/10.1111/johs.12124

Tulumello, S., & Bertoni, F. (2019). Nessun decoro sui nostri corpi: sicurezza, produzione di margini e movimenti indecoros*. *Tracce Urbane, 5*. https://doi.org/10.13133/2532-6562_3.5.14561

5

Women Sport and Fitness Professionals in Pandemic Times: Feminist Ethics, Digital Connection and Becoming Community

Holly Thorpe, Allison Jeffrey, and Nida Ahmad

The COVID-19 pandemic has disproportionately affected women, emotionally, socially, physically and economically (Masselot & Hayes, 2020; Paskin, 2020). It has been well-document that women around the world have carried much of the unpaid, invisible labor required to care for their families and broader communities (Banu Özkazanç-Pan & Pullen, 2020; Power, 2020), often while simultaneously managing paid employment (many on reduced hours and/or salaries) (O'Reilly, 2020). Research has shown that women lost more than 64 million jobs globally in 2020 alone, resulting in an estimated $800 billion loss of income (Oxfam, 2021). In these conditions, women's physical and mental health has been heavily impacted, with high rates of depression and anxiety, and increased experiences of gender-based violence (Thibaut & van Wijngaarden-Cremers, 2020). Despite such challenging conditions, "new forms of gender and inter-gender solidarity are emerging, making the COVID-19 pandemic an important time for gender-related research" (Alcadipani, 2020, p. 734)

H. Thorpe (✉) • A. Jeffrey • N. Ahmad
School of Health, University of Waikato, Hamilton, New Zealand
e-mail: hthorpe@waikato.ac.nz

D. L. Andrews et al. (eds.), *Sport and Physical Culture in Global Pandemic Times*, Global Culture and Sport Series, https://doi.org/10.1007/978-3-031-14387-8_5

and potential political mobilization. Feminist researchers are both calling for, and identifying examples of, a cultural shift towards relational ethics of care in pandemic times (Branicki, 2020; De Coster, 2020; Jeffrey et al., 2021; Manzo & Minello, 2020). In this chapter, we draw upon our previously published research (Thorpe, Jeffrey, Fullagar & Pavlidis, 2022; Thorpe, Jeffrey, Fullagar & Ahmad, 2022; Thorpe, Jeffrey & Fullagar, 2023) to discuss the gendered dimensions of the pandemic, the influence on women working in the sport and fitness sector as an industry that was greatly impacted by COVID-19, and describe how some women responded with creative solutions to some of the challenges they faced both personally and professionally.

The international sport and fitness industry is one of many significantly impacted by the pandemic. For example, a loss of 300,000 jobs in the sport and fitness sector was predicted in the United Kingdom (Wilson, 2020). Similarly, in the United States, 17% of gyms and fitness centers closed permanently, and 44% of the fitness industry workforce lost their jobs (Rodriguez, 2021). Of particular note, the effect of the pandemic on the sport and fitness industry has been highly gendered. Emerging research evidences the devastating effects of COVID-19 on professional women's sport (Bowes et al., 2020; Clarkson et al., 2020). With most sports organizations and events prioritizing the continuation of men's sport, many sportswomen faced a difficult conundrum: continue training with heavily reduced human and financial resourcing without a clear future of professional sport returning in the near future, or retire. Similarly, many women working in the fitness sector (i.e., instructors, personal trainers, studio owners) lost their jobs, left the industry, or 'pivoted' to offer their services via digital technologies.

While research is revealing the impacts of the pandemic on women athletes, very little scholarship has considered how other women working in the sport and fitness industry responded to the rapidly changing financial, social and emotional environment of sport in the pandemic. In this chapter we draw upon interviews and object-oriented methods with 17 women working in the Aotearoa New Zealand sport and fitness sector (i.e., athletes, coaches, fitness instructors, studio owners) about their experiences during the various stages of strict social restrictions throughout 2020. Engaging with feminist new materialisms, we explore the women sport and fitness professionals' initial affective respondings to the pandemic, their use of digital technologies to support their communities during lockdown(s), and how the re-turn to social life post-lockdown(s) prompted new feminist ethics in their ways of working. In so doing, this chapter brings together findings from our larger collaborative project to highlight the gendered impacts of the pandemic, focusing particularly on how women in the sport and fitness sector responded with creativity and care to support their colleagues, teammates and communities during times of great uncertainty and upheaval.

Context: The Gendered Pandemic in Aotearoa New Zealand

While the pandemic is far from over, at the time of writing, Aotearoa New Zealand had led a highly successful campaign against COVID-19, 'flattening the curve', avoiding overcrowded hospitals and mass deaths, and pursuing the ambitious goal of virus elimination for almost 18 months (Baker, Wilson, & Anglemyer, 2020; Henrickson, 2020). Commencing in March 2020, the New Zealand government response included a full national "lockdown" for at least four weeks, daily updates, and messaging that encouraged solidarity, all influencing how the population responded to the threat of a global pandemic (Jamieson, 2020). Regular use of the traditional Māori saying "he waka eke noa" (we are all in this together) (Watene, 2020), and nationalistic (and sporting) discourse, such as the "team of five million" (Morton, 2020), encouraged citizens to (temporarily) reflect on their roles and responsibilities amidst the shared experience of pandemic. At the time of our research (late 2020), Prime Minister Jacinda Ardern was receiving international praise for her leadership as an approach that addressed the crisis through the use of compassion, empathy, and communication (Friedman, 2020).

From the outside, it may have seemed that the nation of Aotearoa was riding the waves of COVID-19 with relative grace. From the inside, however, the country, like so many others, was experiencing the ongoing stressors that accompany any lengthy lockdown: an uncertain economic future and vast inequities experienced differently by various social groups, particularly Māori and Pacific communities. Mirroring international trends, the pandemic exposed longstanding inequities and injustices (i.e., poverty, a housing crisis, health disparities) in Aotearoa society. As various scholars and commentators have highlighted, the negative effects of COVID-19 in Aotearoa were being felt disproportionately by women, and especially women in marginalized groups (Masselot & Hayes, 2020). Congruent with global trends (Paskin, 2020; Power, 2020), women in Aotearoa faced greater economic, social, and health concerns when compared with men. During the COVID restrictions of 2020, 90 percent of pandemic-related redundancies were positions held by women, and the following year, many more women were working in 'precarious jobs' (Stats NZ, 2020; Kendall, 2020). While the 2021 Wellbeing Budget launched by the Ardern government included an objective to "support into employment those most affected by COVID-19, including women", the strong prioritization on industries related to physical infrastructure (i.e., construction, roading) and lack of any specific initiatives for women workers, were critiqued as lacking a gender responsive approach (Curtin et al., 2021).

In May 2020, Sport New Zealand created a $25M (NZ) Relief Package, which was followed by a further governmental investment of $264.6M (NZ) to support sport and active recreation organisations to "respond to the disruption caused by the COVID-19 pandemic and associated lock down measures" (Ihi Aotearoa, 2021). Similar to the overall governmental recovery framework, however, the Sport New Zealand 'Recovery Package' also lacked any gender-specific response. It failed to acknowledge the gendered impacts of the pandemic on women's sporting and physical activity participation, or the challenges for women working in the sector. As this chapter reveals, future sport, work and social policy and recovery strategies would do well to acknowledge the intersectional gendered complexities of the COVID-19 pandemic, and to learn from the lived experiences and creative solutions developed by women for their communities.

Re-Turning with the Literature: COVID-19, New Materialisms and Sport

The COVID-19 pandemic has prompted a growing number of scholars to turn to new materialisms to help with making meaning of, and finding ways of responding to, the affective, environmental, technological, and biological entanglements present in this unique moment in time (Braidotti, 2020; Lunstrum et al., 2021; Lupton et al., 2021; Lupton & Willis, 2021; Sikka, 2021). Of particular relevance here are feminist engagements with new materialisms to examine the gendered affects of COVID-19, and feminist reimaginings of the posthuman condition within the pandemic (Bozalek et al., 2020; Braidotti, 2020; Fullagar & Pavlidis, 2020; Jeffrey et al., 2021).

Writing early in the pandemic, Fullagar and Pavlidis (2020) drew upon feminist new materialisms to explore the affective, embodied and gendered experiences generated by the COVID-19 disruption, powerfully arguing that "the disruptive biocultural force of the coronavirus highlights the value of more-than-human perspectives for examining the gendered effects and affects on our everyday lives and leisure practices" (p. 152). In so doing, they also acknowledge the limitations of humanist notions of 'agency' for understanding "what the coronavirus 'does' as a gendered phenomenon" (p. 152). In Braidotti's (2020) discussion of the "posthuman condition" (p. 1) and the pandemic, she described the limitations of approaches that focus solely on human agency and encouraged the inclusion of non-human forces (including viral formations) to be considered as agentic. In this chapter, we take inspiration from feminist materialist scholars, and build upon our previous work, to explore how women working in the sport and fitness sector navigated their affective and embodied experiences, and re-turned to training and working (mostly digitally) with their sporting and fitness communities during the pandemic. As well as revealing the emergence of new feminist respondings and ethics of care in the sport and fitness sector, our analysis also reveals the need for more gender-responsive policies and recovery investments.

While broadly framed under feminist new materialisms, the specific theoretical inspiration for this chapter comes from our recent intra-actions with Barad's agential realism, and our various collaborative engagements with the resulting concept of "becoming community" (Cassar, 2020, p. 12), as well as their writing on 'closeness' (Barad, 2014) (also see Thorpe, Jeffrey, Fullagar, & Pavlidis, 2022; Thorpe, Jeffrey, Fullagar, & Ahmad, 2022). Drawing upon the work of Barad and Braidotti, Cassar

(2020) proposes a posthuman perspective of “becoming community”, as “a stabilizing and destabilizing process” (Barad, 2007, p. 210) that is “dynamic and enmeshed with material-discursive practices of transitioning from one state to another” (Barad, 2007, p. 142). According to Cassar (2020, p. 12), the process of “becoming community” develops “simultaneously with past, present and future reconfigurings of the world. It happens between the ‘no longer’ and the ‘not yet’ and is fueled by a force that ‘traces the possible patterns of becoming’ (Braidotti, 2012, p. 32)”. As women navigate the complexities of social life during pandemic (i.e., social isolation, mental health, precarious work), and as discussed by Braidotti (2020), coming together to understand an existence that is intricately interconnected will allow for new creative and thoughtful responses to the challenges that are faced in more-than-human sporting and fitness communities.

Nikolić and Skinner (2019) also take up new materialist and posthumanist onto-epistemologies and ethico-politics to explore how community might be rethought in a more-than-human world. In doing so, they move us from human-oriented understandings of community towards commoning and assemblage, exploring what they refer to as “community of material-discursive commoning”: “In a more-than-human world… there is no distance between a subject and multispecies in/organic commoning-community; there are only patterns of care and their un/making” (p. 11). Although they were not writing specifically about community during the pandemic, we see much value in Cassar (2020) and Nikolić and Skinner’s (2019) posthuman and new materialist understandings of community as entangled, made through non-human relations and “patterns of care”, and always in a process of becoming. In particular, we were interested in exploring the ways in which women sport and fitness professionals became entangled with their athletes, colleagues, clients, and communities—through more-than-human connection, and shared embodied movement—during the pandemic.

Towards Feminist Relational Methods in Pandemic

Following an online call for participants and purposive sampling among our existing networks in the Aotearoa sport and fitness sector, we conducted semi-structured digital interviews with 17 women who were living in Aotearoa during the pandemic and working in the sport or fitness industry. Interviews commenced in August and finished in November 2020. With intention, our participants were not a homogenous group; they ranged in age (34–50), body shapes and sizes, ethnicities and cultural backgrounds (i.e., Pākehā/NZ European, Māori, Samoan, Muslim, Asian), and varied living situations (i.e., living alone, with young children, flat-mates, and in multi-generational homes with elderly parents and/or extended family). All of the participants were working in the sport and fitness industry before and during the pandemic; some operated and ran fitness studios (i.e., CrossFit, Yoga) or their own training programs (i.e., running, functional fitness, boxing), whereas others were trainers at gyms, coaches for other athletes or participants. A few were elite athletes in a range of sports (i.e., rugby, football, surfing, running, cycling).

Most interviews were approximately one hour in duration, with all interviews conducted online (the majority via Zoom) and professionally transcribed. The interviews were semi-structured, and we discussed a range of topics, including how COVID-19 had affected their sporting and physical activity participation; where/who they participated with, and reasons for their participation during this difficult time; engagement with digital technologies for their sport, fitness and social connectivity; and how their participation enabled or constrained their sense of connection to people, places and/or the environment. Recognizing the unique socio-materialities being lived and felt during COVID-19 (Clark & Lupton, 2021; Sikka, 2021; Watson, Lupton, & Michael, 2021), we also invited women to bring images and/or objects to the interview in the hope that this might evoke affective moments and different dimensions of experience that may elude more normalised human interview methods. Inspired by recent feminist posthuman and new materialist research (Brice & Thorpe, 2021; Fullagar et al., 2021; Hickey-Moody, 2020), this optional object-oriented method provided an opportunity to explore some of the non-human relations being lived and felt by the women during the pandemic. Participants brought along a range of personally meaningful objects and images (i.e., teacup, ornaments, weights, photos) that evoked affective responses related to their lived experiences and memories of pandemic (see Jeffrey et al., 2022; Thorpe, Jeffrey, Fullagar & Pavlidis, 2022). The method of object interviews was further developed in a subsequent project relating to women's wellbeing and physical activity during the pandemic (see Thorpe, Brice, Soltani, Nemani & O'Leary, 2022). Elsewhere we also discuss the relational ethics required of us doing feminist research during pandemic times (Jeffrey & Thorpe, In Press).

Women Sport and Fitness Professionals Respondings in Pandemic Times

Bringing the interview material into lively dialogue with feminist new materialist theory, the remainder of this chapter is organized into three parts. In the first, we describe the women sport and fitness professionals' affective respondings during the initial stages of the Aotearoa New Zealand lockdown(s) of 2020. We then discuss their engagements with digital technologies, particularly how many women 'pivoted' to offer free classes and sessions as an act of care and response-ability to their communities. In so doing, the women came to new understandings of touch, connection and community. Finally, we illustrate how the women's more-than-human entangled and affective relations during the pandemic encouraged them to rethink their collective responsibility, with some seeking new strategies to better support others in the face of uncertain futures. Each section draws upon some of our previous writing on this topic, bringing the insights together here to offer an overview of our key findings across the broader project (see Jeffrey, Thorpe & Ahmad, 2021; Thorpe, Jeffrey, Fullagar & Pavlidis, 2022; Thorpe, Jeffrey, Fullagar & Ahmad, 2022).

Initial Affective Respondings: From Individualized Fear to Collective Care

In 2020, Aotearoa experienced two 'waves' of COVID-19, with an initial "go hard and go early" national lockdown strategy that included an isolation period (Levels Four and Three) of just over 7 weeks from late March to mid-May (Jamieson, 2020). During this time, citizens were legally required to stay within their household 'bubble', with only essential travel allowed (i.e., food, medical supplies or essential work). Many of the women in our study described the intensity of their affective respondings that they identified as feelings of fear and anxiety. The following comment from Stella is reflective of the deeply affective feelings of many of the women in our study, particularly fears for vulnerable family members, as the country transitioned into lockdown:

> I worry about my husband because he has three life threatening conditions [...] so he is my first concern [...] and I've got mum here and she is in her 70s so one of those at-risk demographics as well. (Stella, PT business owner)

During the initial stages of COVID-19 in Aotearoa, immune systems (and those of loved ones), housing and job insecurity, poverty, government policies, access to medical supplies and care, scientific modeling, daily briefings on infection rates, and more, influenced women's experiences of fear.

By the time of the interviews (late 2020), Aotearoa had remained one of the most successful countries in terms of protecting its citizens from COVID-19 infections and deaths, due mostly to strict border controls and lockdowns (Henrickson, 2020; Jamieson, 2020). This meant that although mobility continued to be highly restricted, infections were largely contained and thus fear transitioned to worry about future careers, as well as care for others. Many of the women expressed new and ongoing concerns about uncertain futures and economic instability. For example, the competitive athletes in our sample wondered about the impacts on international sport, and particularly for New Zealand athletes unable to travel due to border restrictions:

> The biggest thing for us, as surfers, is like we surf every single day. So for that to all of a sudden be taken away from us, yeah, I guess we were sad and angry and all the emotions came through. I guess at the moment it is so unknown [...] the fear is if it doesn't happen next year, then I will obviously have to start thinking about retirement and thinking about a new career. (Gina, professional surfer)

> I guess a fear would be that it kind of stays around and we can't do anything from our side of things and we are just kind of stuck in this bubble almost away from the rest of the world. I mean we are pretty safe here so we are lucky, but I guess if everything is cancelled you kind of get unmotivated because there is nothing to work towards. So I guess that would be the biggest fear, that international sport doesn't resume. (Ruby, football athlete)

In this way, the concerns expressed by the athletes in our sample mirror those in recent research on the impact of COVID-19 on professional women's sport (Bowes et al., 2020; Clarkson et al., 2020). Interestingly, however, some of our participants were more worried about the impact of the pandemic on the health and wellbeing of their teammates, colleagues and clients:

> I was feeling quite relieved [when lockdown was announced], but also obviously fearful. Like, what would it mean, ultimately? Like, in our sport, people normally run long distances, and so there's a lot of people battling with mental health issues. And so that was really concerning for me.... (Joan, ultra-runner and coach)

> ... once it became obvious that it [the pandemic] was going to impact New Zealand, I was fearful. But I think as time went on, I became less fearful for myself and my own business, but more worried about... my clients, about how they were all going to cope with lockdown ... I was mostly concerned for other people. Those that had kids, and had a 9-5 job to do, and all that kind of stuff. (Jolene, PT studio owner)

Whereas the athletes in our sample were most concerned about their future careers, as seen in the quotes above from Ruby and Gina, many of those working in the sport and fitness industry (i.e., coaches, instructors) expressed an ethics of care for the physical and mental health of their movement communities (see Jeffrey et al., 2021). Many of the fitness professionals we spoke to had been exploring a range of strategies as respondings to the unique problems their communities were facing during the pandemic (i.e., loneliness, increased stress, financial and mental health concerns). As we illustrate in the remaining sections, for all of the women in our study, connection, community and care revealed themselves as important during pandemic and came to be known and felt in and through the moving body, which was often digitally mediated.

Digital Technologies and Communities of Care

Digital technologies played (and continue to play) a critical role in connecting humans—families, friends, students and teachers, classmates, colleagues, health professionals—during the pandemic (Matthews et al., 2021; Watson, Lupton, & Michael, 2021). Each of our participants spoke of the important role of digital technologies for maintaining their connection with others. For many, digital platforms (i.e., Zoom, WhatsApp, Messenger) allowed them to reach out, support and share experiences with their friends, colleagues and teammates. For example, Michael, a yoga teacher, found that she prioritized "physical activity, kindness to others, connecting with friends and family" during the lockdown, adding that such relations of care were mostly facilitated "through Zoom and WhatsApp." Similarly, Sarah, a fitness studio owner, describes using email and other digital technologies to share messages of support and care with her staff and clients:

> …how to keep your immunity up, good winter soup things, so yeah, just flick them messages, keeping in touch and whatever is happening with their family, keep in touch with that, you know, just keep in the loop. If someone is not feeling well, I let them know I am here and I can chat with you, and I am around for a call.

The women's experiences of technology in the pandemic troubled passive/active, present/absent, digital/physical binaries that are persistent in sport and physical cultures, and instead revealed how women's active embodiment materialised through digital technologies (seeing and being seen moving on screens together-apart) (see Thorpe, Jeffrey, Fullagar & Ahmad, 2022).

For the women in our study, their relations with family, friends, colleagues and clients (re)produced through screens and technologies enabled new sensorial experiences of connection and care. For example, for the athletes in our group, Zoom workouts and social gatherings were important in supporting one another through challenging workouts while isolated from the physical team environment:

> Our sport scientists would run a group session and a lot of the girls found that really good. Because even though you are not physically there with each other, you *can still push each other through the screen*. And just knowing that there are people doing the same thing as you that are trying to work hard through this time was nice. (Ruby, football athlete)

> Yeah, so for the team they did a few zoom sessions regularly and they did some with our wellbeing coach. The team had a few online sessions to keep in touch with what is happening and how they are dealing with it. And they had daily zoom meetings for work to see how things are going on. We had Friday virtual drinks and staff quiz and stuff like that … We tried a few things… just to stay connected. (Mackenzie, national sport team manager)

For each of our participants, digital technologies offered opportunities to maintain connections with their families, friends, teammates and colleagues during a time of disruption and uncertainty. It is worth noting that this was also occuring during a time when mental health and wellbeing were increasingly becoming part of a broader conversation in Aotearoa about kindness and care, as led by Prime Minister Ardern (see Craig, 2021; Jeffrey et al., 2021).

Prior to the pandemic, few of these women were offering online fitness or coaching classes. The focus of their everyday practices were in-person training and shared movement. The lockdown, however, prompted them to quickly transition to providing services through various digital platforms. Of the 17 women in our study, 13 offered online classes (mostly free-of-charge) during the initial Aotearoa lockdown. In so doing, the women described experiencing a range of technological challenges, with an initial period of rapid self-teaching and upskilling to set up the online classes, and to continue their communication with fellow athletes, clients and wider communities. Claire-Lee remembered, "within days I had my stuff going online and all of a sudden I'm becoming this Zoom master." Others, particularly those with young children in the home, discussed the challenges of managing these new online environments alongside their caring responsibilities. For example,

> Yeah it [training clients online] really gave me that sense of purpose and obviously at the same time I was trying to juggle being a mother and trying to juggle being a school teacher and then housework and being a wife and all of the other things … that was hard [because these] two different environments that you would normally be in (the gym and home), and then they go like this [demonstrates fingers weaving together] that don't necessarily go well together, yeah it was hard. (Naomi, PT business owner)

As well as navigating family responsibilities and routines, some also went to great lengths to create spaces in their home that they felt were suitable (i.e., welcoming but professional, and not too personal) for offering online classes. Elsewhere we explore the digital intimacies of offering live online fitness classes during the pandemic (Thorpe, Jeffrey, Fullagar, & Ahmad, 2022).

Importantly, an ethic of care informed the women's initial efforts and ongoing digital encounters with clients, friends and community members. That is, they offered (mostly free) online sport and fitness sessions as an act of care—to support the physical and mental health and wellbeing—of their communities:

> [I offered free online boxing classes because] we need to keep people active, one for their mental health because this was something affecting everybody, but it was more about keeping that kind of consistency and habit going so and having that one thing that they could still do that *makes it a little bit normal.* (Teresa, boxing coach and facility manager)

> I think for me the Zoom stuff was more of a mental health thing […] because it felt like I was able to keep in touch with my clients. Like I said, I am quite invested in my clients and who they are and their journey and

> their lives outside the gym […] so for me it was a really great way of keeping in touch and keeping that line of communication going and not feeling quite so much that feeling of isolation. (Naomi, PT)

Some of the women went to great lengths to support the wellbeing of their community by not only offering free online physical activity sessions (i.e., yoga, pilates, boxing, running, CrossFit), but also creating space within their classes for caring conversations:

> Expressing things publicly [in online classes] felt like it was a way to give other people permission to do the same. Rather than have to just "soldier on" and "button up" and "everything is going to be okay". Just being okay with acknowledging that this is unchartered territory and it is a bit scary. (Michael, yoga teacher)

> We did a daily squad WOD (Workout of the Day) online and set a time each morning, but it was more fun, social [thing] rather than a work hard out. … At the start, we had 10 or 15 minutes where we all chatted and said hello to people and their pets. I think that was one of the things that really helped us get it through as well. You know, you have your connections. (Joan, ultra-runner & coach)

A number of our participants acknowledged how these online workout spaces, and related get-togethers with human and nonhuman co-participants (i.e., pets, household objects), created a new everyday digital infrastructure for movement-based routines that contributed to different flows and "formations of community" (Cassar, 2020, p. 12). These digital-physical flows emphasized intimacies and vulnerabilities as moments of connection and differentiation as "shared understandings" of their more-than-human condition (Cassar, 2020, p. 12).

For many of the women in our study, these human and nonhuman digital intimacies and the sharing of personal challenges and vulnerabilities through moving together, prompted new understandings of community as "dynamic, unfinished and in a process of 'becoming'" (Cassar, 2020, p. 12):

> It has been beautiful to see the care in our [yoga] community [...] And just the strength of so many of those relationships in our community, students and our teachers, how it all weaves together. (Aurora, yoga studio owner)

> This year we have seen a lot of inhumane things unfortunately, but people have really looked out for each other. I feel like communities have come together a lot more, which is really nice to see and I saw this in some [fitness] studio spaces. (Hannah, yoga teacher)

Some of the women explicitly acknowledged their virtual encounters with others—particularly through familiar faces and comforting voices—as enabling processes of becoming communities of care:

> There was something about the voice of familiarity and the voice of the home studio and people seeing the same people that they knew and I really think that was soothing and a number of people said "this has been a big life saving thing to have these practices". (Winifred, yoga studio owner)

> People did comment on those videos. Things like, "it's really nice to hear your voice" and "thank you for being there". (Michael, yoga teacher/senior sport coordinator)

These comments evoke particular infrastructures and practices of care (de La Bellacasa, 2017) that were produced through technologies with digital-physical flows materialised as felt and imagined communities of bodies moving together-apart finding connection through human (i.e., voice, muscles, skin) and nonhuman (i.e., pixels, fitness objects, books, pets, furniture) encounters.

In this section we have explored how screens and technologies co-constituted women's shifting relations with family, friends, colleagues and clients, producing new sensorial experiences of connection and care. Through these various instances, we observed women enacting an ethos of care with kindness and compassion for their virtual communities. These practices of care were practiced through offering free online classes and ensuring there was time to chat and share personal experiences and vulnerabilities before/after such classes. Through this care orientation, the women were exploring different modes of responding to their communities in terms of their professional capacity and response-ability for the affective contours of pandemic life.

As Barad (2014) writes, touching (reaching out for encounter) is a "matter of response. Each of 'us' is constituted in response-ability. Each of 'us' is constituted as responsible to the other, as being in touch with the other" (p. 161). Each of these intra-actions (i.e., offering free online classes; making time to chat; inviting others into their home spaces) was a small gesture—a fine detail—in these women's everyday lives during the pandemic. As singularities, these moments were enacted as an affective dimension of their work as fitness professionals that made visible care for others' wellbeing during an emotionally challenging time. For the women in our study, sharing (digital) movement practices was the enactment of care that produced a different—more than fitness—dynamic of community formation. Importantly, this ethos of care was entangled in COVID-19 as gendered phenomena (Fullagar & Pavlidis, 2020). As seen in many other aspects of pandemic society (i.e., the home, essential workers, nursing), the responsibility to enact the emotional, physical and digital labor and (often invisible unpaid or lowly paid) care for others were affective respondings felt and practiced predominantly by women in the sport and fitness sector.

Re-Turning: Post-Lockdown Respondings

As Aotearoa transitioned out of a strict lockdown, many of the women spoke of an affective overload and feelings of becoming socially 'overwhelmed' as they returned to social life. Some of the women were experiencing individual and 'collective exhaustion' (see Jeffrey et al., 2021) from the stress and fatigue of the prolonged lockdown, with many of our participants managing child and family caring responsibilities alongside their new online work arrangements and community care relations. Some found the haptic encounters of everyday life too stimulating, particularly after a prolonged period of social isolation. For example, a boxing coach described her anxieties of 'hugging' upon returning to her work environment and the need to reestablish her own bodily boundaries:

> I liked that COVID gave me the barrier that I needed so people no longer, you know, hugged and tried to hug and kiss you. You know? And especially when they haven't seen you for seven weeks and everyone just wanted to come and hug and kiss and I had lovely male older members they'll be like, can I just give you a hug? I am like no. I was using COVID as an excuse but really it was just like, no. I wanted that space. (Teresa, boxing coach)

As a recently converted Muslim, Teresa's experience of lockdown and isolation, and the ongoing threat of COVID-19, meant that she worked to maintain some sense of space from others (asserting boundaries of touch) when and as she needed, while navigating her Māori culture and the community she was still coaching. Renegotiating this 'space' from others was needed by many in our study. In the following comments from Claire-Lee, a yoga studio owner, we hear of the high levels of personal and collective exhaustion being experienced upon reentering social life:

> By the time it got to about 3 or 4 o'clock in the afternoon I started to get overwhelmed by the everything-ness. Just the traffic, the driving, the face-to-face interaction. I mean I love people but just that whole realisation like, "whoa! Life is full on!"

> Those evening class numbers were definitely impacted. People were conditioned to "home is safe" and we were in winter. So when people got to the end of the day it was like, go home and re-hibernate.

Some described the emotional upheavals during this 'return' to the 'routines' of social life as prompting new social anxieties and feelings of uncertainty, or what participants referred to as 'social awkwardness' (Aurora) during a 'very sensitive' and 'wobbly' time (Winifred). Some of the women worked to reimagine the classes and spaces that they offered their participants with the intention of better supporting both themselves and others in the renegotiation of boundaries that had materialised in the lockdown bubble:

> I feel in many ways this COVID thing, on a more esoteric level, has really highlighted how impermanent everything is and that all we really have is

> the present moment […] So, [I have been] looking at our studio and thinking about what practices, what styles, what teachers can we bring in that can really emphasize that and support that for the community. (Aurora, yoga studio owner)

As Aurora illustrates, and as other women described, experiences of living during pandemic prompted many individuals to face the limitations of mortality, a concept that is often not considered or discussed with such regularity or at such a large scale. Recognizing and responding to "how quiet people felt when they first started coming back", Aurora designed a class where "they weren't expected to be social", they could just "be quiet" and "reconnect with their bodies". For those women providing physical activity opportunities for others, many considered these complexities and adjusted their programming, where possible, to attend to the range of physical and emotional issues emerging in their communities.

With the lowering of social-restrictions and the return to in-person sport and fitness training, some of the women also discussed the implementation of new rules and regulations to navigate risk in their sporting and fitness environments (see Thorpe, Jeffrey & Fullagar, 2023), including new objects of risk management:

> It was a matter of changing up our classes and what we offer and how they were offered… making sure that there's that one meter difference between everybody. When they're doing their workouts together, everybody has to wear gloves. So it's not just the normal cotton gloves, but they have to wear these cotton gloves with plastic where the palm is *so there is no transferring of sweat*. (Teresa, boxing coach)

> [When we train] we wear GPS units. So we usually wear a bib that we have that in and usually they would wash all of that for us, but we had to take all of that home and wash it ourselves and only use our own bib and *we weren't allowed to touch any of the gear or anything, like we weren't allowed to pick up cones*. So there were a few different rules. (Ruby, football player)

Exploring the agential activation of 'everyday objects' during COVID-19, Sikka (2021) examines the face mask and toilet roll as agentic, "nodal technologies within the assemblages of objects (human and non), relations, institutions, and structures" (p. 12) (also Lupton et al., 2021). For many of the women in our study, the socio-material intra-actions with objects of health (i.e., sanitizer) and fitness (i.e., bibs, cones, gloves) prompted new affective relations, sensory experiences, embodied routines and strange new intimacies with sporting human and non-human matter post-lockdown. Such objects, while seemingly mundane, 'do' something in that they prompt new haptic encounters of touch and contact in and through moving bodies.

Importantly, various objects (i.e., hand sanitizer, masks, gloves) also reemerged as significant in the women's relations of care for their communities following the lockdown/s. For example, a number of the women spoke about hand sanitizer and masks as small but important gestures of care for their clients:

> I spent like 200 dollars on this bulk thing of hand sanitizer. I was in that kind of panic mode. And I think many of us were just thinking about all of these new things that we have to be doing and these new precautions and *looking after my community* and making sure that *they felt safe* and looked after in this time of chaos. (Claire-Lee, yoga studio owner)

> I definitely sent out a lot of emails… just to try and reassure people… if they wanted me to wear gloves I would wear gloves. If they wanted me to wear a mask, I'd wear a mask. We could train outside. Just trying to make people feel as comfortable as I could make them feel under the circumstances. (Naomi, PT)

For the sport and fitness professionals in our study, the affective intensities of connection (with humans, objects, technologies) were reinvigorated when they reentered social life post-lockdown/s, and began moving again with their friends, teammates, clients and colleagues. Importantly, however, these relations were not the same as before the pandemic, but rather entangled in human, nonhuman, environmental and affective forces of becoming together, differently, across time and space. This movement of bodies re-turning together-apart can be understood as a diffractive motion that "allows pasts to fold back into presents in unexpected ways, bodies are pushed to become other than who they have been, and corporeal forms are changed physically and emotionally" (Hickey-Moody, Palmer, & Sayers, 2016, p. 217).

Most of our participants recognized the many possibilities for connection (pixels, voices, faces, personal objects and spaces) offered through digital technologies during the lockdown/s. However, through the re-turning of social life, many came to realize how much they value connecting with others through the immediacy of their own and others' physically moving (non-pixelated) bodies. They spoke about the joys of the affective and corporeal relations associated with 'being' in the physical presence of others post-lockdown:

> When you are in a room and people are moving together there is that *shared energy*. I mean you could do the same movements online all you like, but it is not the same. (Hannah, yoga teacher)

> It was such a relief being able to *see* other people's faces up close again [...] I really missed it. I think there's something different about seeing pixels on a screen to *seeing someone's face up close*. As soon as we were allowed, I did a group run with some of my girlfriends....we went out to the local trail in the forest and watched the sunrise... it was really nice to *see* people again. (Joan, ultra-runner & coach)

Participating in shared physical activity experiences again, some of the women acknowledged new noticings and affective respondings to both the natural environment (i.e., the forest, sunsets) and the built spaces of physical movement (i.e., yoga studio, boxing gym). For example, Winifred recalled the joys of moving with others again in her yoga studio:

> Lots of people said that they are happy to be back in the shala [yoga studio], you know, just that sanctified space. Between those walls and with that light and with one another, physically *with* one another [...] one of the most profound things was lying down in savasana [relaxation pose] next to a person a meter and a half away, either side and in front and behind you, en masse, in a room, just lying down together.

For the women in our study, they came to new ways of knowing closeness (i.e., "seeing someone's face up close"; the "shared energy" of moving together in the same room; "watching the sunrise and hang[ing] out") through their human and more-than-human encounters during and after lockdown periods, which they articulated through a visceral sense of loss and connection, proximity and distance. While digital entanglements offered an important infrastructure of care for moving bodies, the desire to return to co-present activities is also a longing for the "aliveness of the universe" (Barad, 2017, p. 403) that materialises through intra-actions of the sensory body with particular places and other bodies (both human and non), each with distinctive atmospheres, histories and ecologies. Embodied movement requires thinking through these entangled relations (rather than in terms of individuated selves) in order that we might accord greater value to the ethos, infrastructures and practices of care that sustain sporting intimacies.

In contrast to dominant discourse, many of the women in our study had little desire to return to a 'new normal' based on updated versions of neoliberal, patriarchal, and colonialist pre-COVID models of governance. They each saw this moment as an opportunity to live differently, in big and small ways (i.e., career changes, moving from the city to rural communities, finding greater contentment in their flawed and vulnerable selves, growing gardens, everyday practices to live more sustainably, relationships with neighbors). Instead, they experimented with different modes of relating and living with non/human others and objects to reconceptualize their work in the sport and fitness sector as an orientation—a direction, an ethos, response-ability—bound up with uncertain futures (also see Jeffrey et al., 2021). Some of the women in our study were moved by the affective capacities and their entangled human and non-human relations in and through COVID-19 towards new practices as sport and fitness professionals. For example, many described how sharing free online classes during the lockdown prompted them to reflect on their values, and ultimately adjust their business models to better support those with diverse socio-economic needs:

> Offering free classes online felt really good. So when it came time to promote memberships, we decided to try something a little different. We offered three pricings for the one membership and just said "choose what is right for you." ... Most people opted for the most expensive options, and some messaged to say they actually paid more because of our offer. Others

> messaged to say thank you because they were hardly making rent and were grateful for the cheaper option. … it just seemed to bring out the good in people. (Aurora, yoga studio owner)

> A couple of things I had going on [included] offering a price range for people. Like, you want to do zoom but you don't have much income at the moment, just offer a donation if you can, that sort of thing. And just giving people the option to have a refund if they need it. (Michael, yoga contractor & regional sport coordinator for seniors)

Importantly, for the women in our study, such renewed business models were prompted by an ethos of care—respondings and response-ability—that considered the new and vastly different worlds that they were now forced to operate within. The women's lives were greatly altered by the restrictions that accompanied the pandemic, and their respondings through communal solutions involved more-than-human aspects of everyday lives. The women's creative gestures revealed opportunities for movement cultures in their processes of "becoming community" together-apart both during and following long periods of social isolation and physical distancing.

Conclusion

In this chapter we drew upon interviews with 17 women working in the sport and fitness sector in Aotearoa New Zealand, to explore the gendered impacts of COVID-19 on women's embodied experiences and affective respondings, as well as the creative strategies they are developing to renew a sense of connection and community amidst disruption and uncertainty. Engaging both theoretically and methodologically with feminist materialisms, we considered the various ways women sport and fitness professionals in Aotearoa were moved by the pandemic. A key finding in this research was how many of the women turned to digital technologies, offering free online classes as a feminist act of care for their communities (see Thorpe, Jeffrey, Fullagar & Ahmad, 2022).

Building upon our recent research in which we take inspiration from feminist materialist understandings of closeness *and* community, we considered how women sport and fitness professionals' affective, practical and political respondings (i.e., trying to minimize risk in their classes and studios, offering free online classes, providing emotional support to their colleagues and clients) prompted new ways of knowing, intimacies and connections through their relations with other humans and digital technologies. For many of the women in our study who turned to offering their classes through digital technologies, experiencing moving bodies in, through and beyond virtual particles prompted "yearning[s], as desire, as reaching toward, as affecting and being affective", thus igniting new ways of knowing what moving bodies can be and do, and how communities of movement might become together, differently (Bozalek et al., 2020, p. 850). For some, these digitally-mediated 'condensations' of socially-distanced closeness prompted the becoming of community through shared movement experiences, with hope, longing and desire for connection evoking ethics of care and creative communal solutions.

As Braidotti (2020) writes, the conditions of the pandemic can prompt us all to consider "how and how fast can we transform the way we live" (p. 4). The examples of the women sport and fitness professionals in our study highlight the capacity for movement communities to change within a matter of days, with some re-turning to feminist ethics and exploring new practices to support others through crisis. For some, these new ethical modes of responding to the world around them prompted new feminist models of working in the sport and fitness sector. In so doing, our research also illustrates the highly gendered impact of COVID-19 on women's sporting and fitness lives and livelihoods. Arguably, COVID-19 recovery investment strategies aimed at supporting athletes, staff and sports organizations during and beyond the pandemic should be gender-responsive in that they acknowledge the embodied, affective and gendered impacts of the pandemic on women working in the sport and fitness industry. Such policy initiatives would also do well to create space for the reflections and respondings of women. Without doing so, sports organizations risk overlooking invaluable more-than-human learnings and creative strategies devised by women to support their communities during the pandemic. Furthermore, without gender-responsive policies, support structures and investment strategies, there is also a very grave risk of losing many highly talented, passionate and experienced women from the sport and fitness sector.

References

Alcadipani, R. (2020). Pandemic and macho organizations: Wake-up call or business as usual? *Gender, Work and Organization, 27*(5), 734–746.

Baker, M., Wilson, N., & Anglemyer, A. (2020). Successful eliminatoin of COVID-19 transmission in New Zealand. *The New England Journal of Medicine, 383*(8), e56.

Barad, K. (2007). *Meeting the universe halfway: Quantum physics and the entanglement of matter and meaning*. Duke University Press.

Barad, K. (2014). Diffracting diffraction: Cutting together-apart. *Parallax, 20*(3), 168–187.

Barad, K. (2017). Troubling time/s and ecologies of nothingness: Re-turning, re-membering, and facing the incalculable. *New Formations, 92*(92), 56–86.

Bowes, A., Lomax, L., & Piasecki, J. (2020). The impact of the COVID-19 lockdown on elite sportswomen. *Managing Sport and Leisure*, AOP, 1–17.

Bozalek, V., Newfield, D., Romano, N., Carette, L., Naidu, K., Mitchell, V., & Noble, A. (2020). Touching matters: Affective entanglements in coronatime. *Qualitative Inquiry, 27*(7), 844–852.

Braidotti, R. (2012). The notion of the univocity of Being or single matter positions difference as a verb or process of becoming at the heart of the matter: Interview with Rosi Braidotti. In Dolphijn, R., & Van der Tuin, I., *New Materialism: Interviews & Cartographies* (pp. 19–37). Ann Arbor. MI: Open Humanities Press.

Braidotti, R. (2020). "We" are in this together, but we are not one and the same. *Journal of Bioethical Inquiry, 17*(4), 465–469.

Branicki, L. (2020). COVID-19, ethics of care and feminist crisis management. *Gender, Work and Organization, 27*(5), 872–883.

Brice, J., & Thorpe, H. (2021). New materialisms, material methods, and the research process: A creative experiment in cutting together-apart. *Leisure Sciences*. https://doi.org/10.1080/01490400.2021.1981504

Cassar, J. (2020). Becoming community: A posthuman perspective. *Societas. Expert*, (2), 12–13.

Clark, M., & Lupton, D. (2021). Pandemic fitness assemblages: The sociomaterialities and affective dimensions of exercising at home during the COVID-19 crisis. *Convergence*. https://doi.org/10.1177/13548565211042460

Clarkson, B., Culvin, A., Pope, S., & Parry, K. (2020). Covid-19: Reflections on threat and uncertainty for the future of elite women's football in England. *Managing Sport and Leisure*, AOP, 1–12. https://doi.org/10.1080/23750472.2020.1766377

Craig, G. (2021). Kindness and control: The political leadership of Jacinda Ardern in the Aotearoa New Zealand COVID-19 media conferences. *Journalism and Media, 2*(2), 288–304. https://doi.org/10.3390/journalmedia2020017

Curtin, J., Bickerton, S. H., Morrissey, S., & Herath, U. (2021). NZ Budget 2021: Women left behind despite the focus on well-being. *The Conversation.* https://theconversation.com/nz-budget-2021-women-left-behind-despite-the-focus-on-well-being-161187

De Coster, M. (2020). Towards a relational ethics in pandemic times and beyond: Limited accountability, collective performativity and new subjectivity. *Gender, Work and Organization, 27*(5), 747–753.

de La Bellacasa, M. P. (2017). *Matters of care: Speculative ethics in more than human worlds.* University of Minnesota Press.

Friedman, U. (2020). *New Zealand's Prime Minister May Be the Most Effective Leader on the Planet.* The Atlantic, April 19. Accessed 29 April 2020: https://www.theatlantic.com/politics/archive/2020/04/jacinda-ardern-new-zealandleadership-coronavirus/610237/?fbclid=IwAR2yQdgbbcHn8fm2MVRaUbBtHF3a-8HmkSR-h5Kb3hOrTAg57hN4N_k2hw

Fullagar, S., & Pavlidis, A. (2020). Thinking through the disruptive effects and affects of the Coronavirus with feminist new materialism. *Leisure Sciences, 43*(1–2), 152–159.

Fullagar, S., Pavlidis, A., Hickey-Moody, A., & Coffey, J. (2021). Embodied movement as method: Attuning to affect as feminist experimentation. *Somatechnics, 11*(2), 174–190.

Henrickson, M. (2020). Kiwis and COVID-19: The Aotearoa New Zealand response to the global pandemic. *The International Journal of Community and Social Development, 2*(2), 121–133.

Hickey-Moody, A. C. (2020). New materialism, ethnography, and socially engaged practice: Space-time folds and the agency of matter. *Qualitative Inquiry, 26*(7), 724–732.

Hickey-Moody, A., Palmer, H., & Sayers, E. (2016). Diffractive Pedagogies: dancing across new materialist imaginaries. *Gender and Education, 28*(2), 213–229.

Ihi Aotearoa. (2021). Sport New Zealand COVID-19 recovery funds. https://sportnz.org.nz/funding/covid-19-recovery-funds

Jamieson, T. (2020). "Go hard, go early": Preliminary lessons from New Zealand's response to COVID-19. *American Review of Public Administration, 50*(6–7), 598–605.

Jeffrey, A., Thorpe, H., & Ahmad, N. (2021). Women yoga practitioners' experiences in the pandemic: From collective exhaustion to affirmative ethics. *Sociology of Sport Journal, 39*, 150–159.

Jeffrey, A., & Thorpe, H. (In Press). Relational ethics of care in pandemic research: Vulnerabilities, intimacies and becoming together-apart. *Qualitative Inquiry*. https://doi.org/10.1177/10778004231163497

Kendall, L. (2020). *Uneven results: The economic impacts of COVID-19 on women*. ANZ. Retrieved from https://news.anz.com/new-zealand/posts/2021/03/covid-impact-on-women

Lunstrum, E., Ahuja, N., Braun, B., Collard, R., Lopez, P., & Wong, R. (2021). More-than-human and deeply human perspectives on COVID-19. *Antipode, 53*(5), 1503–1525.

Lupton, D., Southerton, C., Clark, M., & Watson, A. (2021). *The face mask in COVID times: A sociomaterial analysis*. Walter de Gruyter GmbH.

Lupton, D., & Willis, K. (Eds.). (2021). *The COVID-19 crisis: Social perspectives*. Routledge.

Manzo, L., & Minello, A. (2020). Mothers, childcare duties, and remote working under COVID-19 lockdown in Italy: Cultivating communities of care. *Dialogues in Human Geography, 10*(2), 120–123.

Masselot, A., & Hayes, M. (2020). Exposing gender inequalities: Impacts of COVID-19 on Aotearoa | New Zealand employment. *New Zealand Journal of Employment Relations, 45*(2), 1–14.

Matthews, B., Siang Se, Z., & Day, J. (2021). Crisis and extended realities: Remote presence in the time of COVID-19. *Media International Australia, 178*(1), 198–209.

Morton, J. (2020). *What exactly united the 'team of 5 million' to quash COVID-19?* New Zealand Herald. Retrieved from https://www.nzherald.co.nz/nz/what-exactly-united-the-team-of-5-million-to-quash-covid-19/E4XA77T6NDXOJM6C3AHPC22IOE/

Nikolić, M., & Skinner, S. (2019). Community. *Philosophy Today, 63*(4), 887–901.

O'Reilly, A. (2020). 'Trying to function in the unfunctionable': Mothers and COVID-19. *Journal of the Motherhood Initiative for Research and Community Involvement, 11*(1). https://jarm.journals.yorku.ca/index.php/jarm/article/view/40588

Oxfam. (2021). COVID-19 cost women globally over $800 billion in lost income in one year. https://www.oxfam.org/en/press-releases/covid-19-cost-women-globally-over-800-billion-lost-income-one-year

Özkazanç-Pan, B., & Pullen, A. (2020). Gendered labour and work, even in pandemic times. *Gender, Work and Organization, 27*(5), 675–676.

Paskin, J. (2020, March 11). Women are bearing the brunt of coronavirus disruption. *Bloomberg Businessweek*. https://www.bloomberg.com/news/articles/2020-03-11

Power, K. (2020). The COVID-19 pandemic has increased the care burden of women and families. *Sustainability: Science, Practice and Policy, 16*(1), 67–73.
Rodriguez, M. (2021). Fitness industry still feels COVID's negative impact. *The Global Health and Fitness Association*. https://www.ihrsa.org/improve-your-club/fitness-industry-still-feels-covids-negative-impact/
Sikka, T. (2021). Feminist materialism and Covid-19: The agential activation of everyday objects. *NORA-Nordic Journal of Feminist and Gender Research, 29*(1), 4–16.
Stats NZ. (2020). *Covid-19's impact on women and work*. Stats NZ. Retrieved from https://www.stats.govt.nz/news/covid-19s-impact-on-women-and-work
Thibaut, F., & van Wijngaarden-Cremers, P. (2020). Women's mental health in the time of COVID-19 pandemic. *Frontiers in Global Women's Health*. https://doi.org/10.3389/fgwh.2020.588372
Thorpe, H., Brice, J., Soltani, A., Nemani, M., & O'Leary, G. (2022). Methods for more-than-human wellbeing: A collaborative journey with object interviews. *Qualitative Research*. https://doi.org/10.1177/14687941221129374
Thorpe, H., Jeffrey, A., Fullagar, S., & Ahmad, N. (2022). "We seek those moments of togetherness": Digital intimacies, virtual touch and becoming community in pandemic times. *Feminist Media Studies*. https://doi.org/10.1080/14680777.2022.2112738
Thorpe, H., Jeffrey, A., Fullagar, S., & Pavlidis, A. (2022). Reconceptualizing women's wellbeing during the pandemic: Sport, fitness and more-than-human connection. *Journal of Sport and Social Issues*. https://doi.org/10.1177/01937235221109438
Thorpe, H., Jeffrey, A., & Fullagar, S. (2023). Re-turning to fitness 'riskscapes' post lockdown: Feminist materialisms, wellbeing and affective respondings in Aotearoa New Zealand. *Gender, Place, Culture*. https://doi.org/10.1080/0966369X.2023.2195132
Watene, K. (2020, April 24). Caring for community to beat coronavirus echoes Indigenous ideas of a good life. *The Conversation*. https://theconversation.com/caring-for-community-to-beatcoronavirus-echoes-indigenous-ideas-of-a-good-life-136175
Watson, A., Lupton, D., & Michael, M. (2021). Enacting intimacy and sociality at a distance in the COVID-19. crisis: The sociomaterialisties of home-based communication technologies. Media International Australia, 178(1). https://doi.org/10.1177/1329878X2096156
Wilson, J. (2020). Job losses in sport could reach 300,000 due to COVID-19. *The Telegraph*. https://www.telegraph.co.uk/sport/2020/09/25/job-losses-sport-could-reach-300000-due-coronavirus-10000/

6

Meeting the Physical Online: Thinking with Agential Realism About Digitally Entangled Becoming in the Time of Corona

Kathrine Liedtke Thorndahl,
Lasse Nørgaard Frandsen, and Sine Agergaard

Prelude

> This 'beginning', like all beginnings, is always already threaded through with anticipation of where it is going but will never simply reach and of a past that has yet to come. It is not merely that the future and the past are not 'there' and never sit still, but that the present is not simply here-now. (Barad, 2010, p. 244)

All beginnings are cuts, and just like a beginning that is always already threaded through with anticipation of where it is going, such cuts are always already threaded through with questions: Where do we begin? What does it even mean to begin? What is it that has begun? Is it even possible to begin? In the specific case of the COVID-19 pandemic, the questions that come to the fore may be: When did the pandemic begin?

K. L. Thorndahl (✉) • L. N. Frandsen • S. Agergaard
Aalborg University, Aalborg, Denmark
e-mail: klt@hst.aau.dk

D. L. Andrews et al. (eds.), *Sport and Physical Culture in Global Pandemic Times*, Global Culture and Sport Series, https://doi.org/10.1007/978-3-031-14387-8_6

Where did it begin? How? Why? Since answering these broad questions is far beyond the scope of what we aim to do in this chapter, we ask another even more specific question, namely: What does COVID-19 do? We do so in an effort to show how the COVID-19 pandemic affected the everyday lives and physical activity of adolescents in Denmark.

Meeting the Physical Online

October 21, 2021

"How awkward is this?" Thomas, a 14-year-old boy, thinks to himself as Gray, a tall, skinny, middle-aged man, sits down next to him at the desk by the window in Thomas's room. Gray sends Thomas a warm smile, having just drawn back the heavy curtains to allow the autumn sunlight to enter the second-floor room.

"Okay, now that we can actually see each other, are we good to go?" Gray asks. Thomas nods and mirrors the friendly facial expression even though the feeling of awkwardness persists. The two of them sit in front of a large computer screen on which two pairs of curious eyes, one green, the other brown, have appeared from out of nowhere. Thomas knows that the eyes belong to Gray's two co-researchers, whose names Thomas has forgotten, and so he secretly decides to dub them Mr. Green and Mrs. Brown, and yet he cannot shed the feeling of extreme awkwardness. Thomas shifts uneasily in his seat. His comfy gaming chair suddenly feels like a bed of nails underneath him. The intently staring eyes on the screen make him nervous. Like skilled dancers, the four eyes move in perfect synchronicity as if guided by a well-rehearsed choreography, following him, tracing his every move, taking note of even the slightest change in posture, gesture, or tone of voice. At least so Thomas imagines. The intruding cascades of natural light gushing unapologetically through the window as if revenging the days of darkness when the unwelcoming curtains prevented its rays from illuminating the room only serve to aggravate the pervasive strangeness of the situation. Indeed, combined with the invasive presence of Mr. Green's and Mrs. Brown's probing gazes dancing across the screen in front of him, the hostile brightness of sunlight makes everything seem strange and unfamiliar.

Life in the Time of Corona

This chapter is written in the aftermath of the first two waves of the COVID-19 pandemic in Denmark and at the beginning of a third. In that sense, this text is itself threaded through with the lived experiences of a myriad of intra-actively constituted embodied and embedded agencies that weave in and out of each other, past events, in addition to anticipation of the future. It is also written in the process of making sense of the ways in which the past two years, marked by lockdowns and regulations, have shaped and still are shaping our lives, including those aspects of our lives that are related to our embodied becoming.

When the COVID-19 pandemic broke out in Denmark in March of 2020, regular schooling, including the compulsory physical education classes, was suspended and replaced with online alternatives, first for two months (March 16, 2020–May 18, 2020) and later for three months (December 21, 2020–March 15, 2021) with an additional period of online classes for the oldest students (11–16-year-olds). During the period when COVID-19 was defined as a critical threat to society, some schools tried to keep students physically active by offering physical education classes online. However, in a survey conducted during the second lockdown in January and February of 2021, one-third of the 6–16-year-olds said they had not received any physical education or other physical activities in the winter of 2021 (Pawlowski & Schmidt, 2021). Furthermore, 80.3% of the 6–16-years-old said they had not participated in organized sports activities in the same period (Pawlowski & Schmidt, 2021). Thus, it appears as if physical activity was left for children and adolescents to pursue mainly on their own or together with peers and/or family members. The period when no organized sports and physical education activities were available neither in nor out of school was further prolonged because physical education classes were among the last to be reintroduced when students returned to school due to the risk such activities inevitably involve of spreading the virus. Therefore, for a great many adolescents in Denmark, who were used to being physically active every day during school hours, and who often participated in sports and recreational physical activities after school, COVID-19 thus came to matter a great deal.

Beginning Anew: Tardy Introductory Remarks

Although several months have passed since the reopening of Danish society, and although our everyday lives in Denmark are by now only slightly influenced by the consequences of the pandemic, COVID-19 still seems to linger, not only in our thoughts as memories and misgivings but also in our bodies, where the late complications of having been infected with Coronavirus are not the only way the pandemic has materialized as embodied sensations. Thus, while some struggle to rebuild normal lung capacity, others have experienced bodily changes in the shape of lost physical fitness and/or athletic abilities, weight gain, skin problems, long and permanently tangled hair, etc. Despite the widespread prevalence of such problems, the pandemic has not affected everyone in the same way. Indeed, because we are all embodied and embedded (Braidotti, 2013), we experience the effects of the pandemic differently, in general, and with regards to physical activity, depending on how specific circumstances influence our lives and lived experiences according to the specific conditions that constitute them.

The purpose of this chapter is to show how COVID-19 and the drastic changes of life as we knew it materialized and became embodied in the life of an adolescent boy. Considering the changes described above in particular, we ask: What does COVID-19 do to adolescents' bodies and their processes of becoming? Using Barad's agential realist theory in conjunction with the narrative account of one Danish adolescent boy, we aim to illustrate how the pandemic and the preventive measures put in place to stop the virus from spreading affected and continue to affect processes of becoming. In the context of the present study, the relational understandings of the nature of reality inspire a shifting of perspectives from one concerned with what the COVID-19 pandemic *was* and *meant* to a performative perspective that encourages us to take an interest in what COVID-19 *did* and *still does*.

Thus, our chapter will not just turn attention to how matter matters in matters of loss of athletic ability due to weight gain and decreased physical fitness. Instead, we argue and show how the pandemic can be said to function as a critical disruption, highlighting that the loss of physical fitness and athletic ability has also contributed to cultivating a new and heightened awareness of the entangled nature of nonhuman technologies and humans to the extent that this entanglement now appears highly conspicuous. This newfound awareness, in turn, brings about new possibilities for realizing/experiencing how the entangled nature of everything works.

Our hope is that thinking with agential realism will allow us to create and inspire a heightened awareness of how adolescents' bodies are entangled with all kinds of nonhuman technologies, from chairs and tables to laptop computers and cell phones. Importantly, we argue that these entangled relations did not emerge *as a consequence of* the pandemic. Instead, they were always already there. This leads us to the next section in which we explain our understanding of Barad's agential realism and how this perspective facilitates a different way of thinking and writing in studying the material-discursive reconfigurations that enact the world.

Becoming and Thinking with Agential Realism

> It matters what matters we use to think other matters with; it matters what stories we tell to tell other stories with; it matters what knots knot knots, what thoughts think thoughts, what descriptions describe descriptions, what ties tie ties. It matters what stories make worlds, what worlds make stories. (Haraway, 2016, p. 12)

Barad's agential realist perspective is a performative, non-dualist, relational ontology (Kaiser & Thiele, 2014; Murris & Bozalek, 2019) in which no hierarchies exist between the human and non-human, culture and nature, being and knowing, matter and meaning, etc. In fact, nothing exists as separate entities at all. Instead, everything exists in a continual state of intra-active relational becoming. According to Barad, the basic unit of reality is not separate, individual entities because there *are* no ontologically separate entities. Instead, what exists are *phenomena* that, according to Barad (2007), are "the ontological inseparability of agentially intra-acting components" (p. 33).

Human physical activity only emerges as a phenomenon in and by itself thanks to the intra-actions that ensue from the relations that produce what *appears* as separately existing entities in the shape of subjects and objects. Indeed, it is due only to the so-called agential cuts that cut things together and apart that we become capable of drawing boundaries around the entities within phenomena. Therefore, material objects such as cups and cupboards as well as computers and other digital technologies along with human bodies matter and should not be ignored, disregarded, or excluded from our research efforts. Instead, we might think of research as a so-called *assemblage*. According to Fox and Alldred (2015),

> The research-assemblage (Fox & Alldred, 2013; Coleman & Ringrose, 2013, p. 17; Masny, 2013, p. 340) comprises the bodies, things and abstractions that get caught up in social inquiry, including the events that are studied, the tools, models and precepts of research, and the researchers. (p. 400)

Starting from such a non-dualist and relational ontology results in a radically different way of thinking not only about sports and physical and digital activity but also about subjectivity more generally. A relational ontology requires us to understand subjectivity, not as something bound to individuals but rather, as Braidotti (2019) has pointed out, as a transversal and co-operative trans-species effort that takes place "in-between nature/technology; male/female; black/white; local/global; present/past—in assemblages that flow across and displace the binaries" (p. 33).

The implications for research of beginning from a point of departure inspired by Barad's agential realism are far-reaching. Hence, the agential realist point of departure spills over into our methodological framework, not least because agential realism dissolves the distinction between being and knowing and thus between ontology and epistemology, which in turn entails that "knowledge practice is a practice of worlding; the world and "us" with it, are continuously performed; that is, continuously coming into being" (Juelskjær et al., 2021, p. 14). According to Barad (2007), it follows that there can be no distinction between theory, methods, researcher, and the object of research. All of them are implicated in complex processes of inquiry. Thus, as researchers, we are "always entangled" (Wiszmeg & Mellander, 2016, p. 10) with the phenomena we study.

Taking our point of departure in an agential realist position may contribute to the production of a different encounter with the empirical material when we include as part of our research efforts not only an examination of our own positioning but also an examination of our intra-active becoming as researchers with the empirical material. It follows that an agential realist position entails that theory and data constitute researchers just as much as researchers constitute theory and data. Once this idea has been accepted, it only takes a small leap to realize that this signals a profound transformation of the (imagined) divisions that separate theory, writing, thinking, data, participants, and researcher selves (Jackson & Mazzei, 2012).

Readingwriting a-Part-Together

By making just a few very minor adjustments, Barad's description of how matter comes to matter can easily be adapted to produce a telling description of how (the act of) writing comes to matter. Thus, like matter, we might say that writing is itself diffracted, dispersed, threaded through with materializing and sedimented effects of iterative reconfigurings of reading and writing, thinking and doing. Writing, like matter, is a sedimented intra-acting, an open field. Sedimenting does not entail closure (adapted from Barad, 2014, p. 168). On the contrary, the evocative style of writing employed asks, demands even, that readers allow themselves to become involved with what they read and that they contribute to the meaning-making process by engaging deeply with the insights, feelings, and emotions described in and through the textual accounts. We employ this style of writing as an act of therapeutic sense-making that we hope will serve to cleanse our minds of the sticky residue of habitual patterns of thinking and normativity that hamper the ability to imagine different differences differently. In the case of the adolescent boy in this study, thinking with agential realism allows us to map intra-acting material and discursive agencies and look at the differences such entanglements made for him during the COVID-19 pandemic.

Escape Room with a Digital View

Also October 21, 2021

So there they are. Two researchers behind each of their laptops, sitting at home in their studies, waiting to warp into the lobby to join the other two, Gray and Thomas, a 14-year-old boy, whom the three researchers have invited to be interviewed about his experiences during the COVID-19 pandemic. The three researchers have carefully planned how the setup around the interview is to be arranged. But because none of them are familiar with the technology to be used, they struggle to connect on Zoom, and when they finally succeed, they can't figure out how to record the interview nor how to turn the camera on. After several feeble failed attempts on the part of the researchers, Thomas solves both problems for them. The camera in Thomas's room is set up so that the two researchers joining the interview online view Gray and Thomas from an odd sideways position which gives them a clear view of the impressive computer setup on the desk in front of Thomas and Gray. Flashy flashing gaming gear. The Logitech G502 lightspeed hero wireless gaming mouse that can dance across the smooth surface of the Odin gaming zero gravity 2XL Alex Otos V3 limited edition mousepad. No unnecessary friction. Next to the mouse is a red and black G915 TKL wireless mechanical gaming keyboard with keys that actively pop back to the starting position after being pressed down to direct a movement when directing characters in the games he plays. There is also a professional-looking microphone, held by an arm as if for a musician in a recording studio. But Thomas is not a musician. Rather, he is a schoolboy deprived of his usual possibilities for being physically active as both his school and the sports club where he used to practice at least three times a week have been closed as part of a nationwide lockdown to prevent the spread of the Coronavirus. Although Gray is skinny, he blocks the other researchers' view of Thomas behind Gray.

"What day is it today?" Thomas asks in a hoarse, barely audible voice when the technology finally complies. The double absurdity of the question is not lost on the researchers. They smile. Mrs. Brown is reminded of her own comic confusion about what day it was during the lockdowns. The absurdity of the situation has Mr. Green thinking of a famous scene from an absurd play by Beckett in which the characters find themselves clueless about what day of the week it is. What used to be funny because of how odd the idea of losing track of what day it is seemed to most people now no longer seems neither far-fetched nor absurd, since many of us can now relate to the experience.

Having briefed Thomas about the purpose of the interview, Gray opens the conversation by asking Thomas to describe in as much detail as possible what an average day would look like for him during the lockdowns. Thomas clears his throat and answers,

"Yes. I got up as late as possible to have a little extra sleep. I then went downstairs to get breakfast. I would usually bring the food to my room so I could eat it during the first online class of the day. We had fewer classes during the lockdowns, so I would often be finished by the early afternoon." Thomas pauses, which allows Gray to follow up with another question.

"How were the online classes? Were you able to focus?"

"The classes would usually start with the teacher introducing the assignments we needed to complete. Then we would either be on our own or work in small groups. After that, we would all meet up again before we were allowed to log off."

"So were you able to focus on the teaching?" says Gray and adds, "Or did you do other things during classes?" Thomas smiles crookedly.

"I participated in the classes, but sometimes during math classes, for example, my friends and I would finish the assignments really quickly to give us time to play OverWatch," Thomas continues.

"Sometimes I play after school as well."

"How many hours on average would you say you spend playing OverWatch?" Mr. Green asks.

"No more than two hours a day," Thomas quickly replies. There is a short intermezzo of silence before Thomas continues, correcting his previous statement. "Yeah, okay, I sometimes play maybe three or four hours after school. I like to sit here. It's fun. I play with my friends, and I like that I don't have to worry about what's happening outside. It's like an escape, and we are always online in Discord.

"In what?" Mr. Green asks.

"Discord," Thomas repeats and adds to educate the clueless adults, "It's a program like Zoom or Teams or something like that. Only it's for gaming."

"All right, so you can see each other when you play?" Mrs. Brown asks.

"We can hear each other." Discord appears to be the place where Thomas and his group of friends make their game strategy and help each other.

"So what character are you in the game? Can you describe it in a way so that even those of us who are unfamiliar with OverWatch can understand it?" Thomas proceeds to describe the game, the different characters, and the different roles he has played, first as a so-called "damage dealer" and eventually as a kind of medic which he calls a "healer." Talking about the game makes Thomas excited. His vivid description of the minute details of the game is so animated that it almost seems as if he is more alive inside the computer game in his role as a healer than in the world outside it.

Now, instead of meeting his friends in the locker room of the sports club, Thomas is now meeting them in the digital lobbies of OverWatch. Lobby after lobby. Game after game. Day in and day out. His body posture has no other option than to be formed by the chair it is becoming with. But today, before he can join another lobby with his friends to play a game, he has to tell the researchers about his life during Corona.

"How do you remember the first lockdown?" Mrs. Brown asks. Thomas hesitates, which gives the researchers time to think about their own experiences.

"What I am about to say here tonight will have huge consequences for all Danes." That was the message from Prime Minister Mette Frederiksen on the evening of March 11, 2020. Sitting in front of the TV in disbelief reminded Mrs. Brown of how she experienced the events of 9/11 almost twenty years earlier. Both of these landmark events seemed utterly surreal, each in its own way marking the beginning of a new era—of a new reality and world order.

"Corona is here, and it's spreading," the Prime Minister concluded. Thomas interrupts Mrs. Brown's thoughts.

"I remember that I returned from practice. My whole family was sitting in front of the TV. They looked very serious. When my dad told me about the lockdown, I just couldn't believe it."

"Do you remember what you felt when you first heard about the lockdown?" Mrs. Brown asks.

"It all felt… I mean, it was unbelievable." Thomas looks past Gray into the camera to the right of him, "To be honest, I remember feeling relieved because we were not going to school. I thought it would be like an extra vacation." Thomas laughs as if to say, "Boy, was I wrong about that!"

"But when I found out that it was not just the schools that would be closed but shops and sports facilities as well, I was kind of sad because I thought I might get bored."

"So did you? Get bored, that is," Gray asks.

"No, not really. I like to play OverWatch, and I talk to my friends all the time when we play."

During the summer, the restrictions were finally beginning to be lifted. Belonging to the oldest group of students, however, Thomas only attended school once a week, and it took a while before school was back to normal.

"So how was it to return to school," Mr. Green asks.

"Well, it was a bit weird. I realized that many things had changed. It was strange seeing each other again, and some of my classmates had really grown."

"But hadn't you grown as well?" Gray asks. Thomas looks down.

"Well, maybe, but I used to be first when we raced up the flights of stairs to the classroom. Now I can't even keep up with Brian, one of my classmates. Brian of all people! He practically used to move at the speed of a snail!"

"How did that happen?" Mrs. Brown asks.

"Well, obviously, I am not as fast as I used to be because I've been sitting down the whole time during the lockdown, and now I am a bit heavier than I was before. I mean, I'm out of shape." Thomas's comment about being out of shape leads the conversation towards what it means to be out of shape. Thomas describes how he has lost the ability to perform particular skills that he used to be able to do easily.

"How was it to start practicing your breakdance again?" Mr. Green asks.

"Well, it's really nice to be back at the gym and to feel the atmosphere again, but other than that, it's been tough! It's been really hard, actually." Thomas lets out a sigh.

"Why has it been so hard, you think?"

"Well, for one, I used to be able to do all my moves like it was nothing, but now I really struggle with a lot of them, and I can't even land the standing tuck properly! I used to be able to do that so easily." Mr. Green is just about to ask Thomas for more details, but before he can do so, Thomas continues without prompting.

"Also, the coaches have decided to put me in the second-best team this season. I used to be on the best team."

"Is that what bothers you most? Being cut from the team?"

"No… not really, it's okay, I mean. The worst part is actually the muscle aches. It's pretty much there all the time now that I've started practicing three times a week again, and even after months, my body is so unbelievably sore from the training because I'm not used to it anymore."

Becoming Together-Apart

But what about us? The researchers, that is. The increased use and presence of digital devices and technologies were certainly also evident in our own practices, for better or worse. During the process of writing the present text(s), the three of us became what Haraway (2016) describes as "companion(s) throughout tentacular thinking" (p. 5) as we thought and read and wrote together. But COVID-19 also caused us to do different work differently, to use our tentacles differently than we would have under other circumstances. In particular, as our means of communication were exiled to online platforms, the subtle feeling of always being slightly out of step with one another prevalent during collaborative writing projects suddenly came to feel not so subtle anymore. It was as if the mediating function of the variety of digital devices such as Google Docs, Outlook, Messenger, Word, Chrome, Safari, Teams, Zoom, Wikipedia, Gmail, eBooks, online dictionaries, online library, Stanford Encyclopedia of Philosophy that we employed and which enabled us to work at all also introduced a new layer of noise in the communication between us. What is more, these things also enact agency—they are not only affected by humans; rather, humans are also affected by them.

Although we never imagined our collaborative work to be neat and ordered, following a strict plan, nor did we anticipate how the migration to a fully digital form of collaboration would affect our work. Different matters mattered differently at different points in the process for each of us, which complicated the process of writing in unforeseen ways. While these complications sometimes rendered the process tedious, they also opened up new and generative vistas as our different opinions and perspectives met.

Discussion: Beginning Over and Over Again

This chapter has allowed three modes of heightened awareness of how knowing and being are mutually implicated to fold into one another. First, the way it is *experienced and described* by Thomas, the adolescent boy, testifies to the existence of what we might call an *embodied* mode of awareness of how knowing and being are mutually implicated. Second, the process of *researching* Thomas's embodied awareness has produced what we might refer to as an *articulated* mode of awareness of how knowing and being are mutually implicated. Third, *reading* about the embodied and articulated modes of awareness may (we hope) provide readers with what might be characterized as a *vicarious* mode of awareness of how knowing and being are mutually implicated. In that sense, our approach of thinking with agential realism resonates with Barad's (2007) description of diffraction when she posits that diffractive methodologies can be used to "highlight, exhibit, and make evident the entangled structure of the changing and contingent ontology of the world, including the ontology of knowing" (p. 73).

In fact, the idea of this newfound experience and (perhaps) realization of entanglement resonates with Barad's argument about the nature of and relation between knowing and being. Barad (2007) writes that

> knowing is a matter of part of the world making itself intelligible to another part. Practices of knowing and being are not isolable; they are mutually implicated. We don't obtain knowledge by standing outside the world; we know because we are of the world. We are part of the world in its differential becoming. (p. 185)

Because ontology and epistemology are understood as mutually co-constituted in the ethicoontoepistemological framework proposed by Barad (2003), it follows that knowledge-building processes cannot be considered isolated activities directed towards producing accurate representations or illustrations of reality. What is more, subscribing to this theoretical perspective entails a rejection of traditional representationalist ideas about the existence of and relationship between words and things according to which the notion of truth is directly dependent on the possibility for connecting what is seen as individual entities by establishing correct correspondence between them. Barad's decidedly nonrepresentationalist alternative eschews the idea that realism must imply that what is real are independently existing entities with inherent attributes (Barad, 2007). Instead, Barad advocates in favor of conceptualizing reality as monist and intra-active, constituted by phenomena, that is, by entangled material agencies such as the material entangled practices of knowing and becoming. Thus it is that knowledge(s) of the world are "produced by and contribute to engendering material-semiotic processes of change" (Nardini, 2014, p. 21).

The significant changes that ensued due to the outbreak of the COVID-19 pandemic have not been limited to the personal sphere. Rather, in the wake of the COVID-19 pandemic, a number of institutional changes followed. These changes significantly affected everybody whose everyday lives used to be structured by the daily routines in and of such institutions. The most significant change in this regard might have been the reorganization of all schooling to online alternatives, which radically transformed the everyday lives of children and adolescents in Denmark and elsewhere. In addition, many children and adolescents were also affected by the decision to discontinue all recreational activities, which led to further disruption of their habitual practices. The interview with the adolescent boy, Thomas, clearly illustrates how the radical structural changes seriously affected Thomas's everyday life and how the changes manifested in his body and social relations with his peers.

Based on the interview with Thomas, who used to be physically active, doing sports almost every day of the week, it is clear that the COVID-19 pandemic as a whole and online teaching and the limited possibilities for being physically active in particular have had a significant impact. While the pandemic has significantly reinforced the importance of digital devices and technologies in adolescents' daily lives, Thomas's vivid descriptions also provide insight into how the COVID-19 pandemic has materialized on several other levels of his lived experience, including but not limited to the physical, the psychological, the social, the educational, and the material. In that sense, the COVID-19 pandemic has made evident how the digital, material, discursive, physical, and social spheres are intra-actively entangled.

Furthermore, the interview with Thomas also illustrates how the inertia of COVID-19 materialized in Thomas's life in the shape of substantial bodily changes that suddenly made themselves felt and known as limited physical fitness and abilities. Interestingly, in the online universe of OverWatch, these changes were not noticeable. Here everything remained the same, and in that sense, it not only allowed Thomas to escape from the chores and activities dictated by his parents, it also allowed him to escape the physical limitations of his own body even if it did not necessarily occur to him until after the end of lockdown. At that time, he realized that the sedentary lifestyle that caused him to almost wholly neglect his body in favor of becoming a character in the online universe of OverWatch turned out to actually have very real consequences for him once it was time to return to his normal activities.

The COVID-19 pandemic has exposed numerous social issues that have been quietly converging for decades. In the world of adults, it has brought to light wealth disparities in which the ability to work from home via technology is available only to the wealthy; the poor are forced to continue working in unsafe conditions, potentially exposing them to the virus. Similarly, in the world of children and adolescents, certain kinds of technological equipment may easily become prerequisites for participation in online communities, thereby excluding those without the means to purchase the necessary equipment. Thus, there is a new risk of exclusions because of our embodied and embedded existence. While such exclusions might well have happened prior to the pandemic, the lockdowns have exacerbated both the number and severity of consequences of not being able to participate in online communities.

While adolescents' everyday lives may quickly be reestablished, the pandemic is still present. Indeed, it is as if the pandemic has left a sticky residue behind that makes it hard to rid oneself of the sensual, emotional, and physical consequences of COVID-19. In that sense, COVID-19 is not just in the past. Rather, it still lingers in the present. Unlike the late complications of COVID-19 that are recognized in the medical system, however, the lived experiences of the pandemic have not been given much attention.

We are well aware that COVID-19 is undoubtedly not the only factor affecting our everyday lives. Nevertheless, focusing on the pandemic and the changes that ensued in Thomas's life may bring about fresh understandings of how the digital and the physical matter for the technologically entangled bodies of adolescents and how they become matters of concern.

As a further consequence of the agential realist position, it follows that there is an increasing need for ways of understanding the world, capable of accounting for its intra-active nature and differential becoming. Thus, it is increasingly apparent how human activity, materiality, and digital spaces are entangled in ways that allow human-material situatedness to present itself while leaving traces in our virtual as well as face-to-face interactions. Such new and different ways of thinking and doing require new kinds of inquiry for researching the emerging phenomena that ensue from new practices. Alaimo and Hekman (2008) write that

> We need ways of understanding the agency, significance and ongoing transformative power of the world—ways that account for myriad "intra-actions" (in Karen Barad's terms) between phenomena that are material, discursive, human, more-than-human, corporeal, and technological. (p. 5)

If there was ever any doubt about the agency of Nature, that is, if we had somehow managed to convince ourselves that Nature is merely the "invisible background conditions against which the 'foreground' achievements of reason or culture (provided typically by the white, western, male expert or entrepreneur) take place" (Plumwood, 1993, p. 4), the outbreak of COVID-19 certainly feels like a rude awakening, reminding us that Nature is neither passive nor non-agentic.

Postlude

It would go against our philosophical point of departure to claim that this journey has reached its final destination as if this postlude signals our arrival on a metaphorical beach of white sand where meaning and message can go hand and hand. Such a final destination does not exist except perhaps in the wild dreams of representationalism. Indeed, we do not want to spur on such canards by pretending that it does (Jackson & Mazzei, 2008). Instead, we want the journey to continue. Put differently—it must continue, only differently, in the intra-action with readers when the text, of which we can only take partial ownership, becomes text, and readers become readers. Indeed, according to Barthes (2001), "the true locus of writing is reading," because as he argues,

> As soon as a fact is *narrated* no longer with a view to acting directly on reality but intransitively, that is to say, finally outside of any function other than that of the very practice of the symbol itself, this disconnection occurs, the voice loses its origin, the author enters into his own death, writing begins. (p. 1466)

At the same time, not least because we became readers of our own texts multiple times through the journey of the present inquiry, we were repeatedly reminded that all narratives inevitably tell one story while leaving others untold. Try not to forget.

References

Alaimo, S., & Hekman, S. (2008). Introduction: Emerging models of materiality in feminist theory. In S. Alaimo & S. Hekman (Eds.), *Material feminisms* (pp. 1–19). Indiana University Press.

Barad, K. (2003). Posthumanist performativity: Toward an understanding of how matter comes to matter. *Signs, 28*(3), 801–831.

Barad, K. (2007). *Meeting the universe halfway: Quantum physics and the entanglement of matter and meaning*. Duke University Press.

Barad, K. (2010). Quantum entanglements and hauntological relations of inheritance: Dis/continuities, spacetime enfoldings, and justice-to-come. *Derrida Today, 3*(2), 240–268.

Barad, K. (2014). Diffracting diffraction: Cutting together-apart. *Parallax, 20*(3), 168–187.

Barthes, R. (2001). The death of the author. In V. Leitch et al. (Eds.), *The Norton anthology of theory and criticism* (pp. 1466–1470). Norton.

Braidotti, R. (2013). *The posthuman*. Polity Press.

Braidotti, R. (2019). A theoretical framework for the critical posthumanities. *Theory, Culture & Society, 36*(6), 31–61.

Fox, N., & Alldred, P. (2015). New materialist social inquiry: Designs, methods and the research-assemblage. *International Journal of Social Research Methodology, 18*(4), 399–414.

Haraway, D. (2016). *Staying with the trouble: Making kin in the Chthulucene*. Duke University Press.

Jackson, A., & Mazzei, L. (2008). Experience and "I" in autoethnography: A deconstruction. *International Review of Qualitative Research, 1*(3), 299–318.

Jackson, A., & Mazzei, L. (2012). *Thinking with theory in qualitative research: Viewing data across multiple perspectives*. Routledge.

Juelskjær, M., Plauborg, H., & Adrian, S. (2021). *Dialogues on agential realism: Engaging in worldings through research practice*. Routledge.

Kaiser, B., & Thiele, K. (2014). Diffraction: Onto-epistemology, quantum physics and the critical humanities. *Parallax, 20*(3), 165–167.

Murris, K., & Bozalek, V. (2019). Diffraction and response-able reading of texts: The relational ontologies of Barad and Deleuze. *International Journal of Qualitative Studies in Education, 32*(7), 872–886.

Nardini, K. (2014). Becoming otherwise: Embodied thinking and the "transformative matter" of (new) feminist materialist theorizing. *Artnodes, 14*, 18–24.

Pawlowski, C. S., & Schmidt, T. (2021). Børn og unges bevægelse i krise: En spørgeskema-undersøgelse om 6-16-åriges fysiske aktivitet under COVID-19 nedlukning. *Forum for Idræt, 36*(2) https://tidsskrift.dk/forumforidraet/article/view/128112

Plumwood, V. (1993). *Feminism and the mastery of Nature*. Routledge.

Wiszmeg, A., & Mellander, E. (2016). Interfering with others: Re-configuring ethnography as a diffractive practice. *Kulturstudier, 1*, 93–115.

7

Dreaming of "Level Free": Lockdown and the Cultural Politics of Surfing during the COVID-19 Pandemic in South Africa

Glen Thompson

End the lockdown! Let us surf! So, yeah, I'm front of line to take back our freedom.
—Surfer, May 18, 2020 (comment in Davis, 2020b)

Introduction: Surfing with COVID-19

Surfing was shut down due to a beach ban during the first wave of the COVID-19 pandemic in South Africa. Beaches were empty, the surf shops were shut, organised surfing cancelled amateur and professional surf contests, and the surf media was starved of content. "The Coronavirus is a massive wave that has momentarily overwhelmed us," observed Mami Wata (personal communications, 2020, March 20). The South African surf brand was correct about the scale of the COVID-19 crisis yet overly

G. Thompson (✉)
Cape Town, South Africa

D. L. Andrews et al. (eds.), *Sport and Physical Culture in Global Pandemic Times*, Global Culture and Sport Series, https://doi.org/10.1007/978-3-031-14387-8_7

optimistic about being "momentarily overwhelmed". The pandemic has persisted globally, South Africa has remained in lockdown for 21 continuous months, and waves went (seemingly) unridden during the local beach ban.

This chapter explores COVID times from the perspective of surfers as a specific group of beach-users for the period March to August 2020 during the first wave of the pandemic in South Africa. It focuses on the cultural, social and material determinants for the May 5, 2020 beach protest against the ban on ocean-based activities and how surfers imagined or lived a "level free" during the pandemic. The social attitudes of recreational surfers and the surfing cultural industry (the surf media and national surfing body) provides a lens into how the lockdown shaped the experience of those participating in surfing among the largely white, middle-class groups living at the coast. To surface surfer consciousness, I consider how the cultural politics of surfing informed the making of a politics of refusal centered on the beach.

The work of writing this pandemic present is tentative. I find it particularly unsettling as an historian who surfs and my reflections on this period remain partial. My own COVID-19 illness infects my narrative and my voice can be found in the archived collection I make reference to here. Methodologically, I sourced digital source material and archived these texts on the Zotero and Evernote digital platforms. These sources were supplemented by print surfing magazines published during the period as well as ethnographic research (telephonic and in-person conversations with surfers as well as observations of beaches via webcam live feeds). I took a cultural studies approach to media analysis to contextualise these primary sources. While I am cognizant of pandemic histories in South Africa (e.g., Phillips, 2012), this chapter is not historiographic in its intent but part of a wider socio-cultural study on the beach in COVID-times attentive to subaltern and decolonizing trends within surfing in post-apartheid South Africa.

South African Politics and Society during Lockdown

Like many other countries globally, South Africa imposed a shutdown of society and the economy in response to the COVID-19 crisis. Following the disease outbreaks in Asia and then Europe, South Africa saw its first cases of the SARS-CoV-2 virus in early February 2020. For the period under review to August 18, 2020, COVID-19 infections increased to 592,144 cases, with 12,264 recorded deaths (Department of Health, 2020). At the time of writing, South Africa has experienced three waves of the pandemic and entered a fourth wave in December 2021.

After the World Health Organisation declared COVID-19 a pandemic on March 11, 2020, the South African President Cyril Ramaphosa, leader of the governing African National Congress (ANC), announced on March 15, 2020 that the country was placed under a national state of disaster to "flatten the curve" of coronavirus transmissions. This was made law through section 27(2) of the Disaster Management Act, Act 52 of 2002. A raft of lockdown regulations followed in the course of 2020, including a risk-adjusted approach of five lockdown levels from most severe (Level 5: shutdown of the economy and society) to most relaxed (Level 1: limited social controls). Beach closures were part of the severe lockdown measures implemented. They were first imposed by local city councils, with Durban initiating beach restrictions on March 18, 2020 and Cape Town following on March 24, 2020. With the national lockdown imposed on March 26, 2020, the beach ban was enforced along the country's coastline as part of a stay-at-home order.

Collective public support for the restrictions was evident in the initial two months of the lockdown but public frustration with anti-contagion measures became louder as the return to "normality" was deferred with subsequent lockdown extensions (Harris, 2021, pp. 580 & 587–589). Yet, the socio-economic and political climate in South Africa was already tense by the start of the COVID-19 crisis—the nation was in an economic recession, exacerbated by two decades of state capture, and protests were a part of the political climate (Simpson, 2021, pp. 411–469). In this context, Long (2021) has argued that South Africans lived within a political psychology of alienation that has shaped social misrecognition (pp. 11 & 27–37). In COVID times, this social misrecognition was intensified. For the middle classes, this dis-ease was broadened when taken for granted social and economic privileges were seen to be challenged by the bio-power of the South African state. Two months into lockdown, the historical racial and class divide was exacerbated; the largely white suburban middle class "want[ed] the opening of the economy and an end to authoritarian restrictions on their personal liberties" while predominately poor black people sought "jobs, grants and additional welfare state interventions to support their precarious lives" in the townships (Robbins, 2020). As Meth and Charlton (2020) have explained for middle class social reality during the pandemic, "the invisibility of poverty and everyday experiences of lockdown are reinforced by lockdown measures, structural inequalities, online in/exclusions, and cultures of home-space privacy, in a context of relative privilege" (p. 121). And emerging from the viral substrate of locked down suburbia were "kneejerk" and "alarmist perspectives" on "authoritarian creep" by a neo-colonial and bureaucratic government from among white conservatives and libertarians who felt politically disempowered under a majority rule black government, as well as some progressives (Robbins, 2020). This bifurcated view of South African society, which Friedman (2021, pp. 13–24) has posited as "one virus, two countries", provides a materialist explanation for the social realities and political landscape in COVID times and frames elite anti-lockdown protest at the beach.[1]

Surf Frothing: Towards a Politics of Refusal

Two themes stand out in the study of sport and physical cultures in COVID times. Firstly, the social, affective and cultural impacts of the negation of movement have become a category of analysis (Thorpe et al., 2021). Secondly, it was "the total shutdown of sport" that brought

[1] There are similarities between the anti-lockdown attitudes of white, middle-class South Africans and the anti-lockdown protests in the North, pointing to the transnational circulation of conservative and libertarian political ideologies.

COVID-19 home for many people (Hain & Odendaal, 2021, p. 405). Both themes bring to the fore the importance of sport, exercise and well-being in contemporary society. The curtailment of the movement of people outdoors meant that exercising was limited to the physical confines of one's home during the initial months of hard lockdown. For surfers in South Africa, the beach ban closed off access to the ocean and the embodied practice of riding waves.[2] As such, sporting pleasure—defined by Rinehart (2015) "to mean something that gives positive meaning to an individual or collective life" (p. 18)—was deferred indefinitely and social identities tied to the surfing lifestyle were shown to be unstable.

Surfing identity has a history in modern surfing that is able to subsume both the genealogies of non-conformist bohemianism from late 1960s youth counterculture (Booth, 2001, pp. 112–118) and more recent mainstream surf culture's commodification of a countercultural ethics (Stranger, 2011, p. 81). Within these processes, as Estes (2020) has stated, "[t]he subcultures spawned by surfing tended toward antiestablishment libertarianism" (pp. 850–851). These historically and culturally constructed identities and dispositions washed up on South African shores to shape local surfing culture (Thompson, 2017). Yet, it is this counterculture image of *the surfer* that has become transhistorical within both surfing and public imaginations. This image is located in a discourse of freedom and care-free living and as a result, "[s]urf culture and counterculture are linked in affinity and in cultural connections … The surfer signifies the same thing … the memory of something particular—pleasure" (Lawler, 2011, pp. 107–108). Yet, surfing pleasure is embodied in identity. As Stranger (2011) has stated, "[s]urfers are people with a particular orientation, a particular set of priorities; their lifestyles are constructed around maximizing access to the surf, and a defining theme for surfers themselves is the level of commitment to this prioritization" (p. 52). Following Wheaton (2013), there are further lifestyle sport elements structuring the surfer identity: the pursuit of stoke (an embodied aquatic pleasure stimulated by thrill, risk or danger) in the experience of riding waves; surfing as an individualistic activity; surf spots become cultural spaces in nature and provide refuge from the urban edge; an

[2] I use the term surfing inclusively for all ocean-based wave-riding boardsports.

aversion for the regulation and institutionalisation of sport; and a transnationally orientated and "predominately, middle-class, white and Western" social identity "associated with 'youth'" despite "wider-based age ranges and ... less gender-differentiation than institutionalised sports" (pp. 29–30)—although surfing remains largely white and male-dominated in post-apartheid South Africa.

Fiske adds another cultural dimension when considering the construction of surfing identities at the beach. The invitation to transgression in the everyday is part of the embodied experience of moving from the coastal urban edge to the beach and then into the waves. Semiotically, this is a transition from culture to nature, where nature denotes freedom from social controls and cultural norms. This transgression embodied pleasure, "it creates a privatized domain beyond the scope of a power whose essence lies in its omnipotence, its omnipresence. Showing that life is liveable outside [power] denies it" (Fiske, 1989, p. 64). Refusal emerges here as an individualistic politics of withdrawal with affective agency analogous to libertarian impulses emphasising personal autonomy. Using Baudrillard (1981) in neo-Marxist mode, surfing pleasure can then be seen as "the *contents of thought* that come into play in real situations. In sum, ideology appears as a sort of cultural surf frothing on the beachhead of the economy" (p. 144, emphasis in the original).

Taken together, these cultural, social and ideological configurations provide the basis for a politics of refusal at the beach. But this mode of refusal does not necessarily have the radical intent of the Marcusian Great Refusal—to question cultural domination and "protest against unnecessary repression" (Marcuse, 1969, p. 125). Rather, refusal is a more nebulous and individuated response in COVID times: it forms fleeting coalitions around social issues; may float across ideological leanings; and directs social action towards non-adherence with lockdown rules. These are discursive responses to material conditions. With the economy shutdown and society locked down by governments, a politics of refusal emerged from alienation; "[a]ll over the world this massive interruption of normality stirred, in various degrees, incomprehension, indignation, resistance, noncompliance, and protest" (Tooze, 2021, p. 27). Yet, as Markula (2019) has recognized for physical cultures, "identity-based group resistance can turn out to be a reactionist investment" (p. 91), therein promoting entitlement and privilege. The mythologies configuring a politics of refusal are a perceived right to leisure and an individuated pursuit of happiness found in physical cultures made possible by consumptive leisure and sporting practices within the contemporary neoliberal era. It is a cultural politics informed by the transnational and online mediated narratives of individuals pushing against the social control of lockdown—in the practice of everyday life, in circulating social media petitions, or protesting as an interest group. Theorizing a politics of refusal opens up a means to approach the anti-lockdown beach protest in South Africa.

Framing the Beach Protest

The May 5, 2020 beach protest in South African has received only a few mentions in academic scholarship. In sport and leisure studies, both Young (2020), in discussing the impacts of lockdown on the leisure pursuits, and Martin-Gonzalez et al. (2021), in exploring the socio-economic impacts of the COVID-19 crisis on surf tourism in Cape Town, described the protests as led by surfing community interests. In Africanist political studies, Melber (2020) saw the surfer protests as an elitist "frustration" for a return to outdoor recreation couched as "a violation of their civil liberties" (p. 476). Where surfer-driven beach protests usually do get attention in scholarly literature it is in relation to environmental issues such as marine pollution (see Wheaton, 2007) or the conservation of waves as a natural resource under threat from coastal development (see Lazarow, 2007). The beach has also been cited as a politicized space within critical surfing studies (e.g., Evers (2008) on the 2005 Cronulla race riots in Sydney, Australia).

The South African surfer responses to lockdown, however, were not anomalous within the transnational surfing community. In many countries, especially in the initial months of the COVID-19 pandemic, beach closures and a ban on ocean-based activities were imposed as part of lockdown restrictions, including in: Africa (Cape Verde, Morocco); Asia (China); Europe (France, Italy, Portugal, Spain); Central America (Costa Rica, Panama); the Middle East (Israel); Oceania, (Aotearoa New

Zealand, Australia); North America (the coastal states of the U.S.A.); and South America (Brazil, Peru) (e.g. Surfline, 2020). As Wheaton et al. (2021) have observed, "[t]he unusual circumstances of the lockdown showed how surfers had previously taken-for-granted their mobility and access to the coast" (p. 913). In many of these regions, surfers surreptitiously ignored lockdown rules and went surfing despite the legal risk of arrest or fines. In Aotearoa New Zealand and the U.S.A. states of Florida and California, recreational surfers used online petitions to call on their local government to open the beaches, primarily for three reasons: on the basis that surfing was seen as "essential exercise" for physical and mental well-being in contexts where walking, jogging or cycling were permitted; that "surfers practice social distancing always" as surfing was seen as an individualistic sport; and to allow "responsible surfing" due to the low risk of a surfer, as an experienced ocean-user, needing rescuing by emergency services due to serious injury (Marlo, n.d.; Pike, 2020b). Several predominately white and affluent coastal communities in southern California, U.S.A., as part of the wave of national anti-lockdown protests in April and May 2020, gathered at local beachfronts to demonstrate against state restrictions and assert their freedom to individual liberty—including surfers voicing opposition to beach bans (see Hernandez, 2020). However, what distinguished the South African surfer response from that in other surfing nations was how the spectre of the past and present social realities politicized the beach in COVID times.

There are some historical and contemporary examples that provide for the possibility of the beach as a site of political protest in South Africa. In November 1966, white surfers protested against the summer surfing ban at Surfers Corner, Muizenberg Beach (Masterson, 2019). The surfing prohibition by local authorities aimed to protect sea-bathers from injury from the heavy longboards to safeguard beach tourism. While the outcome of how the surfer protest influenced the authorities was uncertain, in early 1967 government sentiment changed in the face of a tourism downturn at Muizenberg and the surfing prohibition was lifted. In the struggle against apartheid's racially segregated laws, the beach had another meaning; that of white domination. Peaceful political protests by anti-apartheid campaigners at white designated beaches in various coastal cities from the mid-1980s to late 1989 included bathe-ins, wade-ins, mass gatherings, and picnics (Rogerson, 2017, pp. 105–106). However, the racial oppression of black people has cast a long shadow and beach apartheid remains a painful memory for many people. In the democratic era after 1994, the legacy of beach apartheid has remained and the beach retains citations of racism and the maintenance of white privilege despite racial desegregation. In Cape Town in mid-December 2018, the Clifton Beach protest by apartheid struggle veterans and African popularists over the securitisation of white beach residents' interests and the removal of black people from the beach, is the most recent example of the politicization of the beach before the pandemic (Trotter, 2019, pp. 5–11).

In COVID times it is important to see the beach protest as one among many other protests by people attempting to engage the South African government over civic issues. Of note, however, was that the May 5, 2020 beach protest did not explicitly feature in the Institute of Security Studies review of protests during lockdown for the period of March, 27 to July, 31 2020 (Lancaster & Mulaudzi, 2020). Of the total 511 protests reported—with 51 protests, two per day on average, in the month of May—most were peaceful but, in some cases, disproportionate police force was used to break up non-violent protests.[3] The main reasons for lockdown protests were: policing lockdown and crime, labour issues (including the supply of personal protective equipment), electricity supply, and municipal service delivery. In the sporting world, while South African sportspersons took the knee before a game in some major sports, South African surfers did not show solidarity publicly with the Black Lives Matters (BLM) anti-racism movement.[4]

Seen historically, the novelty of the South African beach ban was such that this was the first time since the demise of beach apartheid that national restrictions on access to the beach were proclaimed by the South Africa state. For surfers born in a democratic South Africa this was their first experience of a ban on surfing. Nevertheless, under lockdown, the idea of the beach as a place of freedom and well-being remained and was informed by cultural, economic, political, and sporting processes in the

[3] There were on average 2.26 protests per day reported for the seven-year period from 2013.

[4] While *Zigzag* called for solidarity with the BLM global paddle out protests in June 2020, no local protest occurred due to the beach ban. Surfer-led BLM protests took place in Aotearoa New Zealand, Australia, Costa Rica, France, Indonesia, Senegal, U.K. and U.S.A.

neoliberal era: sport had been declared as a constitutional right in South Africa (Department of Sport and Recreation, 2012); global trends in the consumption of leisure and sport had created a demand for outdoor lifestyles, including surfing (Wheaton, 2013); the therapeutic turn in associating exercise and fitness with physical and mental well-being, especially by immersing in blue spaces such as the ocean (Jellard & Bell, 2021); and the concomitant benefits of "surf therapy", as expounded within surf development non-profit organisations (Benninger et al., 2020), circulated within global surf culture. With these meanings associated with the beach and the consumption of waves, the beach ban therefore became a sign of lockdown social control and an impetus for its refusal.

The curtailing of individual freedoms in the pursuit of pleasure by means of government lockdown measures was undertaken within a public health crisis. The government's intent in implementing the beach ban as part of lockdown regulations was that "[c]ontrol measures must be put in place in relation to public spaces, facilities and offices to ensure social distancing" so as to contain the spread of contagion among people (see section 6.5.1 in Republic of South Africa, 2020). The South African government "took the virus seriously" and its lockdown directives erred on the side of caution in a context where the scientific understanding about the SARS-CoV-2 virus was evolving during the initial stages of the pandemic (Friedman, 2021, p. 26). The rationale for lockdown was to reduce the risk of contagion and to enable national public health facilities to prepare for increased hospitalizations due to COVID-19.

The official lockdown discourse of the state was proclaimed at local and national levels and provided the rationalization for the national beach closures and a ban on water-based activities in the ocean. On March 23, 2020 the City of Cape Town (2020), stated that "we will be closing beaches … to limit public contact and to assist our residents with respecting the National Government's call to practice social distancing … Until further notice, beaches along Cape Town's coastline will be closed for all activities be it on the beach itself or in the water." The City of Cape Town (2020) then observed in reference to television and online media news broadcasts:

> We have seen around the world how members of the public have flocked to beaches during this critical time and we want to ensure that residents and visitors are not placing themselves at increased risk by congregating in large numbers at beaches.

Nationally, lockdown policy was directed by the National Coronavirus Command Council and, as the chair of that council, President Cyril Ramaphosa communicated the South African government's stance on the lockdown to the country. His pronouncements included references to positive lessons drawn from the lockdown in the Wuhan, China and, on the day before the May 5 beach protests, that "[t]he regulations we have put in place are founded on that commitment to life and dignity, and which justify—in these extreme circumstances—temporary restrictions on other rights, like freedom of movement and association" (Ramaphosa, 2020).

The beach ban also had public beach and water safety implications, especially at the local level where these functions were government-managed. In the period under review lifesavers were not on duty, the shark nets on the East Coast were not by deployed the KwaZulu-Natal Sharks Board, and the Shark Spotter programme in Cape Town paused its services until late June, 2020. The upholding of near-shore ocean safety also fell to the South African Maritime Safety Authority (SAMSA). In late April 2020, SAMSA denied Canoeing South Africa's request to allow its members to paddle in the ocean under Level 4 restrictions, justifying its decision with reference to lockdown rules allowing limited land-based exercise and that ocean-based activities were dangerous for participants and may require emergency search and rescue services (Pike, 2020c).

The Making of the Beach Protest

This official discourse framed how surfers responded to the beach ban. Several factors need to be taken into account in the period from late March to early May to explain the reasons for the May 5, 2020 beach protest. The following causes worked together, in varying degrees of influence, to produce the anti-lockdown beach protest, namely: surfers went surfing regardless of the beach ban; surfer petitions to open beaches circulated on social media; surfer expectations of a return to surfing were raised when government eased lockdown restrictions; and a social media call to protest the beach ban. The circulation of knowledge of these events among the local surfing community was undertaken by means of social media or online surf media sites.

The first signs of surfer push-back against the beach ban were individual acts of surfer defiance by going surfing. These acts, however, came at a price. Under hard lockdown, the police enforced lockdown regulations. Two surfers in their early twenties were arrested and each fined R5000 (US$278) for surfing in Jeffreys Bay (Wilson, 2020) and a middle-aged surfer was arrested in Cape Town (King, 2021).

The second factor was the publication of surfer petitions on social media. On March 27, 2020 a petition on Facebook titled "Please Let Kouga Residents Surf" called for the Kouga municipality to allow surfing in Jeffreys Bay and the Cape St Francis area in the Eastern Cape. The petition gained only 48 signatures (Pike, 2020a). On April 10, another petition titled "Surfing is an essential activity" was posted to social media and gathered 3425 signatures within four days. Composed by a surfer from Mossel Bay in the Western Cape, the petition was addressed to the premier of the Western Cape provincial government and the South African President. It define surfing in lockdown language as an "essential activity". The surfer noted that the petition was his attempt "to extend my right to practice my own way to handle this lockdown," that he was "not alone feeling isolated from going surfing," and that surfing had health benefits (quoted in Pike, 2020b). However, the petition was not unique. In an example of transnational slippage and the flattening of online spaces for social activism, a surfer petition to the governor of Florida, USA was adopted as a blueprint for South Africa (despite the factual errors in importing American considerations into the local context). While this petition found sympathy with many South African surfers, it did not influence government and other surfer groupings opposed this expression of surfie libertarianism. The Democratic Alliance's Premier of the Western Cape government stated, "While we understand that people miss their regular activities, we all need to make some personal sacrifices during the lockdown period to ensure that we are able to stop the spread and save many lives" (quoted in Grobler, 2020).[5] Surfing South Africa (SSA, 2020a), the national surfing body, distanced itself from the petition and stated, "the top-down regulations should be complied with and surfers are accordingly encouraged to comply". Surfers with a social conscience publicly criticised the petition in the online surf media, "I think it is in bad taste and incredibly tone-deaf to demand the right to surf when the country is literally fighting for people's lives and to prevent nationwide starvation" (quoted in Pike, 2020b). Surf journalist Pike (2020b) commented, "Sometimes self-identity becomes so ingrained, it starts to resemble entitlement."

A third factor was the changing social attitudes of surfers in response to government announcements to ease lockdown levels. In the two weeks leading up to the move from Level 5 to Level 4 lockdown on May 1, 2020 the hope of lifting the beach ban was raised among the surfing community. Ahead of this date, the government announced some relaxation of the stay-at-home order (South African Government News Agency, 2020). Outdoor exercise was permitted but limited to walking, jogging or cycling within a 5-kilometre (3.1 miles) radius of one's home between the hours of 6 a.m. to 9 a.m. The beach ban remained in place and adherence to the new regulations would be policed. Surfer responses were two-fold in the middle-class suburb of Kommetjie in Cape Town: poetic and pragmatic in their lockdown refusal. Surfer and political cartoonist Chip Snaddon (2020) lampooned the government's new exercise regime in a digitally edited image published to social media of a female longboard surfer saying to a black, male police officer, "Just going for a walk, officer ..." while riding a wave on a longboard. At dusk on April 30, 2020, the last day of Level 5 lockdown, surfers paddled out at the Outer Kom surf spot. May 1, 2020 dawned with the new morning exercise rules in place and "about 30 surfers" surfing at the nearby Long Beach (Wavescape, 2020). *Zigzag* surfing magazine explained why the surfers paddled out:

[5] Nationally, the Democratic Alliance (DA) is the official opposition to the ruling ANC. Of the nine provinces in South Africa, the Western Cape is governed by the DA while all the other provinces are governed by the ANC.

> But as the days have meandered on, more and more who are directly affected by the economic stranglehold of the lockdown have changed or fortified their views against such an authoritarian governance. After five weeks of suppressing the personal freedoms we all took for granted—things like surfing, the controversial moral, ethical and the religious question of the week had to be answered. To surf or not to surf? Today we decided. (Van Gysen, 2020)

The surf session, however, was short-lived. A large delegation of police arrived shortly before the 9 a.m. curfew. Surfers quickly exited the sea; some were given a warning by police to stay out of the waves but no arrests were made.

Surfers across the country reacted strongly to the Kommetjie paddle out, reflecting both refusalist and conformist stances. Those for going surfing stated: it was seen a matter of personal conscience; the lockdown rules were pointless and imposed by an authoritarian state; that exercise provided physical and mental well-being; and that surfing promoted social distancing in the surf—as one surfer noted, in a context where the science on the transmission of the virus in the ocean environment was debated in surfing circles, "[s]urfing by its very nature involves social distancing and viruses can't swim" (comments in Van Gysen, 2020). Those adhering to the beach ban noted: compliant actions supported the social collective; show respect for the law, family and community by making personal sacrifices to curb the coronavirus; going surfing was entitled and irresponsible and puts an unnecessary burden on law enforcement; and to support humanitarian work in underprivileged communities instead of "paddling out to pleasure themselves" (comments in Van Gysen, 2020).

The fourth factor was the May 4, 2020 #Backinthewater campaign that was disseminated via Facebook and WhatsApp and received national news media attention. A call for a "national peaceful protest" at South African beaches, reportedly originating from Durban, was extended to "individualised sport ocean users" to demonstrate at beaches along the South African coastline the next morning (quoted in Davis, 2020a). There was a willingness to conduct the protest within the bounds of lockdown rules: it was to be held between 8 a.m. to 8.30 a.m. during the exercise period and was to comply with public health protocols by wearing a face-mask and adhering to social distancing. *Zigzag* was not in favour of this appeal to protest and indicated that they had received a notice "that the protest is illegal under Alert Level 4 because it constitutes a 'gathering'" (Davis, 2020a). Furthermore, the planned protest was seen as a pointless exercise that would not sway the government to further relax lockdown rules. Rather, by referencing the humanitarian work of local surf icons in supporting feeding schemes, *Zigzag* encouraged readers to "do something positive with all that pent up ~~rage~~ energy" (Davis, 2020a, strikethrough in the original) or follow official channels to make representations to government to re-open the beach. There were several online responses from surfers to the *Zigzag* article with viewpoints for and against the protest. Two issues defined the rationale for refusing to adhere to the lockdown rules, echoing surfer sentiment from elsewhere in the world: experienced surfers had the ability to self-manage water safety and therefore there was no need for emergency rescue services, and as surfing promoted social distancing outdoors it was an activity with a low-risk of transmitting COVID-19.

On Tuesday morning May 5, 2020 the beach protest took place and received wide coverage in the national news and on social media. There were three focal points for the peaceful beach protest across the nation, each attracting a small number of surfers and other ocean sport enthusiasts. In the Western Cape, "about 30" protesters gathered on the beach promenade in the southern Cape Town suburb of Muizenberg (Jordan, 2020) while on the city's western seaboard "about 70" protesters lined up the on the pavement above Blouberg Beach (Cape Times, 2020). In KwaZulu-Natal, in the coastal town of Ballito north of Durban, some twelve protesting surfers took to the streets with their surfboards (Fourie, 2020; numbers estimated from photograph). These locations had symbolic significance for surfing. Muizenberg and Ballito are cultural centers for South African surfing—Surfers' Corner at Muizenberg Beach has a Sixties surfing heritage and provides evidence of a local "rainbow nation" surf culture; Ballito, since 2009, has been home to the annual Ballito Pro surf contest which is part of the world surfing tour. Blouberg Beach has a local surf culture with strong kite-boarding tourism links since the 1990s. Beside the evident whiteness of the protestors at these beaches, they were inclusive of sex and age groupings—although more representative of adult surfers. Despite the heavy policing at Muizenberg Beach, only two protesters were arrested for allegedly contravening the lockdown laws (Siyo, 2020). The national surfing body publicly distanced itself from the beach protest (Siyo, 2020).

Surfboards were used as placards to display protest slogans, three of which summed up protester voices: at Muizenberg Beach, the question of when the beaches will be reopened (slogan: #WHEN) and that the activity of surfing itself promotes social distancing (slogan: "Surfing √, Social Distancing √"); and at Blouberg Beach, the perceived irrationality of the lockdown laws preventing ocean sport (slogan: "Are your Rules to Punish or Protect"—stated without a question mark) (CapeTalk, 2020a).

While social media and online comments from the South African public were generally divided into for or against camps, many situated the protesters as white, privileged surfers disconnected from the social realities of the COVID-19 crisis. National media coverage also highlighted this social difference. The progressive political cartoonist Zapiro included a panel in his "Corona Contradictions" editorial cartoon with an illustration of the surfer with the #WHEN slogan and the criticism that "privileged protests look ridiculous" (2020, p. 78). The "surfer's protest" also received political scrutiny and was referred to by Brett Herron of the Good Party in a provincial government debate as an example of anti-lockdown attitudes undermining adherence to public health protocols (Hansard, 2020, p. 106). Common to these representations of surfer entitlement was the association with the idea of the pursuit of individual freedom. Surfing thus became a trope within wider South African society for an anti-lockdown libertarianism with conservative tendencies that disregarded the collective good in COVID times.

Surfing in the Interregnum

After the beach protest, from early May to mid-August 2020, two paths toward the return to the waves were evident among the surfing community; appeals to authorities by compliant groups to allow the resumption of surfing, or non-adherence to lockdown rules by going surfing. Surfing

South Africa (SSA), the national surfing association, and the surf media appealed, along with other ocean-related sporting bodies, to the government's National Coronavirus Command Council, the national Department of Sport, Arts and Culture and the South African Sports Council Olympic Committee (SASCOC) to permit ocean sports. In making its May 2020 appeal SSA stated it represented "over 20,000 competitive and recreational surfers (all disciplines) in South Africa" (SSA, 2020b, p. 1).[6] SSA made further advances in June to the sports minister to open up the beaches to surfing, alongside calls by other ocean-based sports. Yet, these minor, technical sports did not have much political influence at SASCOC compared to the mainstream sports of rugby, cricket, soccer, athletics and swimming, with their mass appeal and large number of participants. It was only in early August 2020 that the sports ministry announced the resumption of non-contact sport events with COVID protocols in place during level 3 lockdown, a move that re-opened organised ocean sport, including competitive surfing—but not recreational surfing.

The second path was that the small but nationally visible beach protest gave momentum to surfer disaffection with lockdown rules, which was fueled by ambiguous lockdown messaging from government. Prompted by the protest some surfers illicitly took to the waves (e.g., Moir, 2020). At the end of May and the beginning of June, as the government eased regulations to Level 3, surfer expectations were again raised that the beaches were to be re-opened. In the Western Cape, the provincial premier had made public calls to the national government to re-open the beach under Level 3 (Hansard, 2020, p. 106). Adding further confusion to matters, the Deputy Minister of Cooperative Governance and Traditional Affairs (COGTA) stated on a Cape Town radio station that while there was a ban on "social surfing", competitive surfers with permits could surf (CapeTalk, 2020b). In addition, the Level 3 regulations, while allowing physical exercise at any time in the day, omitted to mention that the beach ban remained in force. Another motivation for wider public questioning of the rationality of lockdown was a legal challenge to

[6] However, it was estimated that there were some 60,000 surfers in the country in 2007 (Pike, 2007, p. 37).

the state from civil society. In the case of De Beer and Others v Minister of COGTA, the court ruled on June 2, 2020 that aspects of Level 3 and 4 lockdown measures were unconstitutional and invalid, among other, the limitations on exercise (North Gauteng High Court, 2020, clauses 7.8–7.9).

When the lockdown eased to Level 3 on June 1, 2020 surfers used this regulatory uncertainty to go surfing. The editor of the surfing magazine *Boardtalk* (2021, p. 106) termed it "WATERSHED DAY". Pike (2020d) reported, after 67 consecutive days of hard lockdown it was now "Level Free!" but "while hundreds, if not thousands, of South African surfers went surfing in the bright blue yesterday, [the beach ban] remained wrapped in a grey area, a ham-fisted land of schizophrenic interpretation and mind-numbingly incongruous application of Level 3 laws." Officially, the beaches were closed yet general police inaction—reported as due to a lack of clarity of the new lockdown rules—enabled many "renegade surfers" to enter the waves (Mazin, 2020). Two surfers, however, were arrested on the day at Muizenberg.

It was this June 1, 2020 event, more so than the May 5, 2020 beach protest, that ushered in a return to surfing despite the beach closures. In many surfing centers from early June 2020, and especially in those places where law enforcement did not patrol the beach ban, surfers openly rode waves. By mid-June, the beach-going public followed surfers to the beach in Cape Town—although the beach ban was still enforced at uMdloti Beach in KwaZulu-Natal in early August. On August 18, 2020 the government eased lockdown measures to Level 2 and the beaches were officially re-opened.

Conclusion: Masking Surfing

Edelman (2020) has argued that while sport can tell us about culture and society, it "can also mask historical realities" and therefore "we need the wisdom to know when sport is a mirror and when it is a mask" (p. 2). In narrating the beach protest and the surreptitious return to surfing, this chapter has shown how these refusalist surfer responses mirrored anti-lockdown attitudes among the coastal white, middle-class groupings during COVID times. The events leading up to the May 5, 2020 beach protest, and specifically surfer frustrations due to the extension of hard lockdown measures, explain how the contents of surfer thoughts and dissenting social acts nurtured a politics of refusal in a desire to reclaim their personal freedom to exercise in the ocean. This refusal sought to affirm the surfer identity and a commitment to the surfing lifestyle.

The beach protest did not proceed from material deprivation but rather from the psychosocial alienation of lockdown. While only about 112 protesters in total demonstrated at three South African beaches on May 5, 2020, their ideologically conservative and libertarian slogans gained attention nationally in the news and social media and *the surfer* came to signify white, privileged entitlement and anti-lockdown discontent at the loss of civil liberties during the South African COVID-19 crisis. Surfing, used here in a reactionary register to politicise the beach, cited oceanic freedom to bring attention to disaffected undercurrents in society. Yet, deployed in this way, the online representations of surfers going surfing opened the possibility for lockdown non-adherence and an impetus for many more surfers to begin to return to the waves openly, without fear of reprisal, before the state officially re-opened the beaches.

Other meanings of surfing, however, were closed off by refusalist tendencies. The beach protest masked how surfer identity could be mobilized for progressive purposes, such as advancing the collective good and social justice or supporting feeding schemes and surf development organizations in marginalized communities. Rather, during the first wave of the COVID-19 pandemic in South Africa, the beach was fixated on by many surfers as a pleasuredome somehow outside of history and seemingly immune from the virus.

Postscript: a national beach ban was imposed during the second wave of the pandemic in the summer of 2020/2021. In late January 2021 beach protests again took place, yet, they involved different social dynamics, broader participation, and anti-lockdown demands were expanded beyond narrower surfer interests to include COVID denialism. Further lockdown restrictions during the third and fourth waves of the pandemic in 2021 did not include beach closures.

Acknowledgements I am grateful to David Andrews, Holly Thorpe, David Johnson and Karen Graaff for their comments on this chapter.

References

Baudrillard, J. (1981). *For a critique of the political economy of the sign* (C. Levin, Trans.). Telos. (Original work published in 1972).

Benninger, E., Curtis, C., Sarkisian, G., Rogers, C., Bender, K., & Comer, M. (2020). Surf therapy: A scoping review of the qualitative and quantitative research evidence. *Global Journal of Community Psychology Practice, 11*(2), 1–26. http://www.gjcpp.org

Boardtalk. (2021). Klapped by Covid: The hidden stories. *Boardtalk Surfing Magazine, 21*(July), 104–106.

Booth, D. (2001). *Australian beach cultures: The history of sun, sand and surf*. Routledge.

Cape Times. (2020, May 5). Arrested Muizenberg protester makes getaway on bike, woman doing yoga 'verbally abused'. *IOL*. https://www.iol.co.za/cape-times/news/watch-arrested-muizenberg-protester-makes-getaway-on-bike-woman-doing-yoga-verbally-abused-47557486

CapeTalk. (2020a, May 5). Surfers arrested at Muizenberg beach for #BackInTheWater protest. *CapeTalk*. http://www.capetalk.co.za/articles/382696/videos-surfers-arrested-at-muizenberg-beach-for-backinthewater-protest

CapeTalk. (2020b, May 29). Non-contact sports allowed but because the beaches are still regulated, Bapela says surfers must have permits to access the beach. *CapeTalk*. https://www.capetalk.co.za/articles/385210/exercise-still-only-5km-radius-from-home-says-cogta-dep-minister

City of Cape Town. (2020, March 23). City closes beaches to advance social distancing. *City of Cape Town*. https://resource.capetown.gov.za/document-centre/Documents/Speeches%20and%20statements/23_March_2020_Beaches_Closed.pdf

Davis, A. (2020a, May 4). Kicking against the lockdown. *Zigzag*. https://www.zigzag.co.za/news/kicking-against-the-lockdown

Davis, A. (2020b, May 12). Surfing under lockdown. *Zigzag*. https://www.zigzag.co.za/featured/surfing-under-lockdown

Department of Health. (2020, August 18). Update on COVID-19. *SAcoronavirus*. https://sacoronavirus.co.za/2020/08/18/update-on-covid-19-18th-august-2020/

Department of Sport and Recreation. (2012). The white paper on sport and recreation for the Republic of South Africa. *Department of Sport and Recreation*. https://web.archive.org/web/20170509172018/http://www.srsa.gov.za/MediaLib/Home/DocumentLibrary/23%20WHITE%20PAPER%20FINAL%20August%202012.pdf

Edelman, R. (2020). Sport is the new film. *The International Journal of the History of Sport, 37*(1–2), 1–4. https://doi.org/10.1080/09523367.2020.1782161

Estes, S. (2020). Surfing the Sun Belt South: An oral history. *Journal of Southern History, 86*(4), 849–876. https://muse.jhu.edu/article/772291

Evers, C. (2008). The Cronulla race riots: Safety maps on an Australian beach. *South Atlantic Quarterly, 107*(2), 411–429. https://doi.org/10.1215/00382876-2007-074

Fiske, J. (1989). *Reading the popular*. Routledge.

Fourie, P. (2020, May 6). Surfers march through Ballito for surfing rights. *North Coast Courier*. https://northcoastcourier.co.za/152627/surfers-march-through-ballito-for-surfing-rights

Friedman, S. (2021). *One virus, two countries: What COVID-19 tells us about South Africa*. Wits University Press.

Grobler, R. (2020, April 15). Lockdown: Western Cape surfer claims surfing is "essential activity", in cut-and-paste of US petition. *News24*. https://www.news24.com/news24/southafrica/news/lockdown-western-cape-surfer-claims-surfing-is-essential-activity-in-cut-and-paste-of-us-petition-20200415

Hain, P., & Odendaal, A. (2021). *Pitch battles: Sport, racism and resistance*. Rowman & Littlefield.

Hansard. (2020, May 14). Proceedings of the Western Cape Provincial Parliament. *Western Cape Provincial Parliament*. https://www.wcpp.gov.za/sites/default/files/hansarddocs/Hansard%2014.05.2020%20revised%20%20edited.pdf

Harris, J. (2021). Confronting legacies and charting a new course? The politics of coronavirus response in South Africa. In S. Greer, E. King, E. Massard da Fonseca, & A. Peralta-Santos (Eds.), *Coronavirus politics: The comparative politics and policy of COVID-19* (pp. 580–599). University of Michigan Press. https://doi.org/10.3998/mpub.11927713

Hernandez, J. (2020, June 4). BLM protests, COVID-19 beach protests, and what they say about American inequality. *The Inertia*. https://www.theinertia.com/news/blm-protests-covid-19-beach-protests-and-what-they-say-about-american-inequality/

Jellard, S., & Bell, S. (2021). A fragmented sense of home: Reconfiguring therapeutic coastal encounters in Covid-19 times. *Emotion, Space and Society, 40*(100818), 1–8. https://doi.org/10.1016/j.emospa.2021.100818

Jordan, B. (2020, May 5). Cops not so stoked as beached surfers launch waves of protest. *Times Live*. https://www.timeslive.co.za/news/south-africa/2020-05-05-cops-not-so-stoked-as-beached-surfers-launch-waves-of-protest/

King, P. (2021, July). My stealth surfing story. *Boardtalk Surfing Magazine*, 21(July), 107.

Lancaster, L., & Mulaudzi, G. (2020, August 6). Rising protests are a warning sign for South Africa's government. *Institute of Security Studies*. https://issafrica.org/iss-today/rising-protests-are-a-warning-sign-for-south-africas-government

Lawler, K. (2011). *The American surfer: Radical culture and capitalism*. Routledge.

Lazarow, N. (2007). The value of coastal recreational resources: A case study approach to examine the value of recreational surfing to specific locales. *Journal of Coastal Research*, 12–20. https://www.jstor.org/stable/26481547

Long, W. (2021). *Nation on the couch: Inside South Africa's mind*. Melinda Ferguson Books.

Marcuse, H. (1969). *Eros and civilization*. Sphere Books. Originally published in 1955.

Markula, P. (2019). *Deleuze and the physically active body*. Routledge.

Marlo, W. (n.d.). Allow responsible surfing in New Zealand [petition]. *Change.org*. https://www.change.org/p/new-zealand-public-and-government-stop-discriminating-against-surfers

Martin-Gonzalez, R., Swart, K., & Luque-Gil, A. (2021). The covid-19 crisis and the "new" normality of surf tourism in Cape Town, South Africa. *African Journal of Hospitality, Tourism and Leisure, 10*(1), 194–213. https://doi.org/10.46222/ajhtl.19770720-95

Masterson, M. (2019, June 19). 1960s surfing prohibition: The Muizenberg banning saga. *John Whitmore Book*. https://johnwhitmorebook.wordpress.com/2019/06/19/surfing-prohibition-the-muizenberg-banning-saga

Mazin, N. D. (2020, June 8). Poynton Shute's perfect storm, episode 7 of Poynton Shute's Coronavirus Novel. *Wavescape*. https://www.wavescape.

co.za/surf-news/breaking-news/coronovirus-novel/coronavirus-novel-episode-6-2.html
Melber, H. (2020). Covid-19 and southern Africa. *The Round Table, 109*(4), 476–477. https://doi.org/10.1080/00358533.2020.1790776
Meth, P., & Charlton, S. (2020). Seeing in the suburbs. *Transformation: Critical Perspectives on Southern Africa, 104*, 113–124. https://doi.org/10.1353/trn.2020.0037
Moir, C. (2020). Lost at sea. *Zigzag, 44*(4), 35–36.
North Gauteng High Court, Pretoria. (2020). De Beer and Others v Minister of Cooperative Governance and Traditional Affairs (case no. 21542/2020) ZAGPPHC 184. *Southern African Legal Information Institute.* http://www.saflii.org/za/cases/ZAGPPHC/2020/184.html
Phillips, H. (2012). *Plague, pox and pandemics: A Jacana pocket history of epidemics in South Africa.* Jacana Press.
Pike, S. (2007). *Surfing in South Africa.* Double Storey.
Pike, S. (2020a, March 30). I fought the law … an' the law won. *Wavescape.* https://www.wavescape.co.za/surf-news/breaking-news/i-fought-the-law-.-an-the-law-won.html
Pike, S. (2020b, April 14). Despite times. *Wavescape.* https://www.wavescape.co.za/surf-news/breaking-news/desperate-times.html
Pike, S. (2020c, April 28). Ocean ban looks set to stay. *Wavescape.* https://www.wavescape.co.za/surf-news/breaking-news/ocean-ban-looks-set-to-stay.html
Pike, S. (2020d, June 2). Level Free! *Wavescape.co.za.* https://www.wavescape.co.za/surf-news/breaking-news/level-free.html
Ramaphosa, C. (2020, May 4). From the desk of the president. *The Presidency: Republic of South Africa.* https://www.thepresidency.gov.za/from-the-desk-of-the-president/desk-president%2C-monday%2C-4-may-2020
Republic of South Africa. (2020, March 25). Disaster Management Act (57/2002): Directions made in terms of Section 27(2) by the Minister of Cooperative Governance and Traditional Affairs. *Government Gazette*, Vol. 657, No. 43147. https://www.gov.za/sites/default/files/gcis_document/202003/4314725-3cogta.pdf
Rinehart, R. (2015). Pleasures small and large. In R. Pringle, R. Rinehart, & J. Caudwell (Eds.), *Sport and the social significance of pleasure* (pp. 12–28). Routledge.
Robbins, S. (2020, May 4). Is the lockdown authoritarian creep or "proportionate response"? *Daily Maverick.* https://www.dailymaverick.co.za/article/2020-05-04-is-the-lockdown-authoritarian-creep-or-proportionate-response

Rogerson, J. (2017). "Kicking sand in the face of apartheid": Segregated beaches in South Africa. In K. Rogatka & D. Szymańska (Eds.), *Bulletin of geography.* Socio-economic Series, 35. Nicolaus Copernicus University (pp. 93–109). https://doi.org/10.1515/bog-2017-0007

Simpson, T. (2021). *History of South Africa: From 1902 to the present.* Penguin Books.

Siyo, A. (2020, May 6). Two surfers to appear in court after demonstration at Muizenberg beach. *IOL.* https://www.iol.co.za/capetimes/news/two-surfers-to-appear-in-court-after-demonstration-at-muizenberg-beach-47590692

Snaddon, C. (2020, April 29). Just going for a walk, officer .... [Image attached]. *Facebook.* https://www.facebook.com/andrew.snaddon/posts/10158408127668993

South African Government News Agency. (2020, April 29). SA's level 4: The new normal. *South African Government News Agency.* https://www.sanews.gov.za/south-africa/sas-level-4-new-normal

Stranger, M. (2011). *Surfing life: Surface, substructure and the commodification of the sublime.* Ashgate.

Surfing South Africa (SSA). (2020a, April 28). Surfing and the current national state of disaster. *Surfing South Africa.* https://www.surfingsouthafrica.co.za/surfing-and-the-current-national-state-of-disaster

Surfing South Africa (SSA). (2020b, May 11). Appeal for consideration of surfing and other ocean sports to be permitted as exercise under lockdown. *Surfing South Africa.* https://www.surfingsouthafrica.co.za/wp-content/uploads/2019/12/SURFING-SOUTH-AFRICA-LOCKDOWN-APPEAL-MAY-11th-2020.pdf

Surfline. (2020, April 10). A global update on beach closures due to coronavirus. *Surfline.* https://www.surfline.com/surf-news/global-update-beach-closures-due-coronavirus/82461

Thompson, G. (2017). Pushing under the whitewash: Revisiting the making of South Africa's surfing sixties. In D. Z. Hough-Snee & A. S. Eastman (Eds.), *The critical surf studies reader* (pp. 155–176). Duke University Press.

Thorpe, H., Brice, J., & Clark, M. (2021). Physical activity and bodily boundaries in times of pandemic. In D. Lupton & K. Willis (Eds.), *The COVID-19 crisis: Social perspectives* (pp. 39–52). Routledge.

Tooze, A. (2021). *Shutdown: How COVID shook the world's economy.* Viking.

Trotter, H. (2019). *Cape Town: A place between.* Catalyst Press.

Van Gysen, A. (2020, May 1). To surf or not to surf. *Zigzag.* https://www.zigzag.co.za/featured/to-surf-or-not-to-surf-3/

Wavescape [@wavescapesa]. (2020, May 1). Oops. Saffa surfers have cracked. Busted en mass. Long Beach, South Africa this morning. Believed to be about 30 people [Image & video attached]. *Instagram*. https://www.instagram.com/p/B_o4OcNpcGh/

Wheaton, B. (2007). Identity, politics, and the beach: Environmental activism in Surfers Against Sewage. *Leisure Studies, 26*(3), 279–302. https://doi.org/10.1080/02614360601053533

Wheaton, B. (2013). *The cultural politics of lifestyle sports*. Routledge.

Wheaton, B., Waiti, J. T. A., Olive, R., & Kearns, J. (2021). Coastal communities, leisure and wellbeing: Advancing a trans-disciplinary agenda for understanding ocean-human relationships in Aotearoa New Zealand. *International Journal of Environmental Research and Public Health, 18*(2), 1–20. https://doi.org/10.3390/ijerph18020450

Wilson, G. (2020, March 30). J-Bay surfers slapped with R5,000 fines for breaking lockdown. *Dispatch Live*. https://www.dispatchlive.co.za/news/2020-03-30-watch-j-bay-surfers-slapped-with-r5000-fines-for-breaking-lockdown/

Young, M. (2020). Leisure pursuits in South Africa as observed during the COVID-19 pandemic. *World Leisure Journal, 62*(4), 331–335. https://doi.org/10.1080/16078055.2020.1825252

Zapiro. (2020). *Do the Macorona: Cartoons from the Daily Maverick*. Jacana.

8

Proximity to Precarity: Confronting the COVID-19 Pandemic as Graduate Apprentices in Physical Cultural Studies

Eric A. Stone, Anna Posbergh, and Brandon Wallace

Part I: Introduction

The COVID-19 pandemic has provoked considerable disruption to the world, demonstrating the fragility of the institutions, systems, and norms that underpin our everyday lives (Asonye, 2020; Blum, 2021; Braidotti, 2020; Grant, 2021). While there has emerged a widespread awareness of global and systemic issues such as climate change, structural racism, and oppressive regimes, so too have we mourned losses of life, routine, and work-life balance. Inevitably, the COVID-19 pandemic effects will be felt for years, if not decades, to come, thereby necessitating new ways of thinking and living. In this vein, feminist theorist Rosi Braidotti (2020) contends that this moment should not be about "grand theorizing, but for collective mourning, affective resistance, and regeneration. We need to mourn the dead…[b]ut over and above all else, we also need to develop different ways of caring, a more transversal, relational ethics" (p. 2). That

E. A. Stone (✉) • A. Posbergh • B. Wallace
University of Maryland, College Park, MD, USA
e-mail: estone14@umd.edu

D. L. Andrews et al. (eds.), *Sport and Physical Culture in Global Pandemic Times*, Global Culture and Sport Series, https://doi.org/10.1007/978-3-031-14387-8_8

is to say, it is vital for all to come together and generate ways of thinking that respond compassionately and justly to the significantly altered conditions of our lives, relations, and institutions.

Indeed, academia is one such place where scholars have urged a reimagination to incorporate a "culture of care," further advocating for an academic praxis that embraces forms of productivity and success that enhance wellbeing and compassion (Barad, 2014; Braidotti, 2020; Corbera et al., 2020). Many have written about the pressures placed upon academics (especially those in early career stages) to produce work that fits within the scope of acceptable scholarship and research dictated by the neoliberal university[1] (Shore, 2010; Silk et al., 2010). Within this growing academic industrial complex, graduate students have especially felt the effects of the COVID-19 pandemic on their vulnerable states of existence. As they already find themselves positions that encompass complex intra-actions formed from their roles as mentors, teachers, students, and burgeoning scholars, the COVID-19 pandemic has induced further stress on their precarious financial, professional, and personal situations (Elfman, 2021; Stewart et al., 2021). Currently, graduate students face the following challenges: a shrinking job market (Carey, 2020; Zahneis, 2021); growing political hostility towards academics, academia, and higher education more broadly (Baker, 2021; Hett, 2021); antipathy by university administration towards graduate student unionization and collective bargaining as unrecognized employees of the institution (including at our own university, see Lumpkin, 2021); unlivable stipends and declining funding opportunities (DiBella & Hoyle, 2021); and growing student debt (Hess, 2021). Such precarious conditions, we argue, were magnified as universities cut budgets in the wake of decreased enrollment following the emergence of COVID-19 as the 2020–2021 academic year commenced (Hubler, 2020). Consequently, during the course of the pandemic, graduate students were compelled to re-define their work schedules, workspaces, and trajectories to navigate the "new

[1] We adhere to King-White's (2018) definition of the neoliberal university as "an educational environment and administrative structure that more closely represents a private enterprise…the primary result of this transformation is that students have come to be regarded as customers, academic researchers are thought of as entrepreneurs competing for external grant funding, and the university itself more closely resembles a business model than an institute of higher learning" (p. 7).

normal" while also wondering what futures would arise when the pandemic "ended" (if, indeed, it will?) (Asonye, 2020; Elfman, 2021; Stewart et al., 2021).

Despite the unique crossroads that graduate students find themselves in, there remains limited scholarship on graduate students' lived experiences and even less reflection by graduate students. In this chapter, we "re-turn" to our individual physical cultural experiences before and during the onset of the COVID-19 pandemic to explore the possibilities of moving forward in post-pandemic futures (Barad, 2014). As graduate students at various stages of completing our doctoral programs, we reflect on and share our lived realities during the 18 months (and counting) of isolation during the pandemic while concurrently grappling with the complexities of graduate student-ness during this moment. While reflecting on and writing this chapter separately and together, we discovered shared commonalities across our experiences, yet were also inspired by the ways in which they differed. For Anna, the enforced severance of (physical) interactions with training partners and academic "teammates" presented challenges for maintaining community while simultaneously offering innovative forms of sociality. For Eric, the importance of necessary physical-distancing exposed the complex relationship between embodied pedagogy and the (in)active body, and fundamentally altered how we aid and assess undergraduate students' shared yet personal understandings of their corporealities in relation to physical culture and society. For Brandon, being largely restricted from engaging with the outdoors has provoked critical reflections on the spatial physicalities of the *indoors*, igniting new perspectives on empathy and pedagogy. In what follows, we examine and explore our diffractive experiences during the COVID-19 pandemic.

We present our stories as narratives, or "vignettes" wherein we adopt an auto-ethnographic approach (see Norman et al., 2019; Thorpe et al., 2011) to reflect on moments of our lived experiences. Our vignettes differ in focus and style to faithfully illustrate our interpretations and emotions during this turbulent period, ranging from stream-of-consciousness to more theoretically-grounded. We further incorporate specific elements related to the focus of this Anthology that we found most pertinent to our experiences: *people* (Anna), *pedagogy* (Eric), and *place* (Brandon).

However, in our conversations together, we also discovered shared elements within and between our experiences—*precarity and proximity*—which we also incorporate into our vignettes. These reflections are more than navel-gazing, however, for in embracing our perspectives as precarious graduate apprentices, laborers, and students, we aim to highlight under-discussed issues relevant to the aforementioned elements of precarity at the heart of academia's pasts, presents, and futures, and especially as we begin to rethink what the world will be as we move further from the height of the pandemic. Furthermore, we argue, the COVID-19 pandemic forces us to address these issues while pursuing more critical, caring, and humane changes to systems and institutions with which we interact.

Throughout our experiences, we engage with Barad's (2014) idea of "diffraction" to map the similarities and differences of our COVID-shaped pasts, presents, and futures, and "re-turn" to specific moments and memories. While wrestling with our own pandemic experiences, we have found the concept of diffraction a helpful one, even as we have realized that though the calls for accepting and embracing a new normal have continued to sound:

> there is no moving beyond, no leaving the 'old' behind. There is no absolute boundary between here-now and there-then. There is nothing that is new, there is nothing that is not new. Matter itself is diffracted, dispersed, threaded through with materializing and sedimented effects of iterate reconfiguring of spacetimemattering, traces of what might yet (have) happen(ed). (Barad, 2014, p. 168)

These experiences we have shared will continue to alter how we understand our position as graduate students, as scholars, and as people invested in helping to enact a better world. By sharing these vignettes, we offer (along with the other scholars in this excellent book) a way of considering how the effects of the COVID-19 pandemic have been felt, and how these effects offer new opportunities for scholars at any stage of their career. The chapter concludes in a brief discussion of how we can respond to this uncertain moment by moving beyond written platitudes and enacting the world we wish to see.

Part II: Vignettes

Anna:

March 15, 2019: Rise and shine.

I throw my running shoes in my bag and begin the walk across campus to the track. It's 7:00am on the dot and I'm rushing out the door. It's a busy day today, full of teaching, meetings, and colleagues. I hope to see and chat with my friends during my morning run (or maybe even hop in for a repetition!), but still make my meetings. It's a day full of people, and it gives me energy.

As I arrive at the track, I look around and see emptiness. I love the temporary silence. It feels like the silence before the starting gun, followed by a rush and exhilaration. I lace up my running shoes and begin my warm-up. Soon, the silence is broken when my friends (training partners) arrive at the track. Their workout is much longer and more intense than mine today, but there is comfort and joy in being around other track-and-field aficionados. As we all push through our respective workouts, we cheer loudly during the hard repetitions and high-five after every set. They are my teammates and I am theirs, even though we only see each other at the track. We share an unspoken bond that is renewed every time we endure a workout together. At the end, we cool-down and part ways, until tomorrow.

I enter the School of Public Health, heading straight to my desk in the graduate student office. I smile, wave, and cheerfully say hi to the all that I pass on my way to the office. When I arrive at my desk, my cubicle buddy (as we call ourselves) is already there, preparing for a day of assays, blood draws, and other scientific techniques that I hope he will explain to me later. We fist-bump—our usual greeting—before I grab my "work clothes" to go and get ready for the day.

I return to my desk and prep my lecture, specifically adding questions for students to answer together in small groups. After teaching, I chat with a former student on my way to my office hours and she tells me about her recent acceptance to the physical therapy school of her dreams. I smile widely and congratulate her, quietly ecstatic that she shared this personal news with me.

During my office hours, I pack my backpack to prepare for the walk to the Writing Center to review a grant proposal, followed by a check-in with my advisor, and then a co-author meeting at a coffee shop. I will take my final meeting of the day at home on Skype with a collaborator overseas: the time difference can be difficult, which is why we don't "meet" very often, but I enjoy these rare virtual opportunities. At the end of the day, I sit on the couch with my partner and we reflect on our joys and our frustrations. What we learned and what we look forward to.

I feel fulfilled as I move through my day; my day filled with people who are my teammates, professional and personal. And I am theirs.

* * *

March 15, 2020: Rise and shine.

I throw my running shoes in my bag and begin the walk across campus to the track. It's 7:00am on the dot and I'm moseying out the door. It's a strange day today, full of navigating this new virtual world as a teacher, learner, and graduate student. I make a mental note to check in on my friends and family. It's a day full of solitude, and it gives me confusion.

As I arrive at the track, I look around and see emptiness. I loathe the never-ending silence. It feels like the silence of a ghost town: empty, devoid, longing. I lace up my running shoes and begin my warm-up. The silence continues through my warm-up and run, only broken up by the sound of my breaths and footsteps. As I push through my workout, I end each repetition with my hands on my knees, out-of-breath, and count out loud after every set so I don't lose track. I have no teammates and I feel my isolation, even though I am told that this is a "temporary" shut-down. At the end, I cool-down and leave the track, until tomorrow.

I return home to prepare for the day. My partner is in the kitchen, eating breakfast. I half-smile and blandly tell him about my solo morning workout before going upstairs to prepare for my day. I change into my "comfy clothes" to get ready for the day.

I sit at my desk and prep my lecture, specifically making sure my room is quiet for when I record my lecture. I record and re-record and re-record my voice over my PowerPoint slides, unsatisfied with each take. A stutter, a mispronounced word, an embarrassingly long "ummm." Finally, I begrudgingly upload a version to Canvas, along with lecture-specific questions on a discussion board for my students to consider and respond to. After recording, I open Zoom to host my office hours and stare at the empty meeting room.

During my office hours, I send some emails before settling in to research, read, and write for the remainder of the day. I will take my only meeting at the kitchen table: sitting at my desk can be monotonous, which is why I try to change locations inside the house, but I miss the walking-across-campus-for-meetings opportunities. At the end of the day, I sit on the couch with my partner and we reflect on our fears and our hopes. What we learned and what we look forward to.

I feel uncertain as I move through my day; my day filled with a virtual world without my teammates. And I feel alone.

* * *

March 15, 2021: Rise and shine.

I throw my running shoes in my bag and begin the walk across campus to the track. It's 7:00am on the dot and I'm rushing out the door. It's a busy day today, full of online teaching, Zoom meetings, and colleagues forgetting to unmute their microphones. I hope to see my new pandemic-made friends on my way—the groundskeeper, the construction worker, the turf technician—while still making my meetings. It's a day full of people, and it gives me cautious optimism.

As I arrive at the track, I look around and see emptiness. I listen to the familiar silence. It feels like the silence during a sunrise: peaceful and full of hope. I lace up my running shoes and begin my warm-up. I hear the background noises to the silence: the chirping of the morning birds, the construction vehicles, the cars on the nearby highway. I take a selfie of myself at the track and send it to my training partners along with the message "Track Tuesday digs": a reference to our pre-pandemic training sessions. The silence is broken by my text message alert as I receive replies: a picture of a teammate at a different track; a message from another that reads "I'll be out there later today!". As I push through my workout, I pretend to race alongside them, in anticipation and preparation for our post-pandemic return. They are my teammates and I am theirs, even though we "see" each other virtually. We share an unspoken bond that not even our COVID-19 isolations could break. At the end, I cool-down and leave the track, until tomorrow.

I return home to prepare for the day. My partner is in the kitchen, eating breakfast. I smile and happily show him the messages from my training partners before going upstairs to prepare for my day. I change into my "comfy clothes" to get ready for the day.

I sit at my desk and prep my lecture, channeling my energy and enthusiasm into my lecture. After recording, I open Zoom to host my office hours and see a student in the waiting room. We chat about his current classes and he tells me that he misses talking with people in-person, but has learned how to build connections in our new virtual world. I smile widely and congratulate him for his persistence and creativity, quietly grateful that I am not alone in feeling this way.

During my office hours, I send some emails before settling in to research, read, and write for the next couple hours. I read through some documents to prepare for my virtual meetings today: one with my advisor, another with a coauthor, and a third with the Writing Center. I will take all three meetings at my desk: I still miss the walking-across-campus-for-meetings opportunities, but I don't notice the monotony of my days as much when I am able to share part of them with my colleagues. At the end of the day, I sit on the couch with my partner and we reflect on our joys and our hopes. What we learned and what we look forward to.

I feel contentment as I move through my day; my (virtual) day filled with people who are my teammates, professional and personal. And, once again, I am theirs.

Eric:

I. Before…

I'm always uneasy walking into a classroom; a heady mix of anxiety and excitement as I prepare for the upcoming lecture. I feel protected knowing I've worked hard preparing to instruct my students; yet I also fear their blank stares, their (sometimes) judgmental glances.

Full disclosure. I love teaching. I love the look students get when they figure out a tough concept, or when they discover they've learned something new about themselves. These are the moments that keep me motivated during my progress towards my doctorate. In the weeks before shutdown, I felt at home in the classroom; that vulnerable feeling of standing in front of 200 students, completely exposed, had dissipated, and I was enjoying feeling calm perseverance replacing the rush of adrenaline.

Our last week of in-person class focused on the idea of cyborgs, the mixture of skin and technology usually depicted in science-fiction, but in actuality represents our lived-experiences as beings ensorcelled by tools enabling our lives (Hoberman, 1992). The students sat incredulously as I asked them to raise their hands if they wore glasses, or contacts, or were using pens to take notes. "You are cyborgs," I said, "We all are." I shared the story of my knee injury, and the complex surgery that repaired it, a fusion of flesh and scientific technology that allows me to walk. I was nervous about sharing my story, my body, but I could see the difference in their expressions.

When next we met, through my own embodied performance I explained our topic: gender performance and masculinity. The students showed looks of interest and leaned forward as we discussed my long hair, my speech and gait. Through my performance, they came to understand that Butler (2014) had a point about gender and its social construction. As class ended, I stood at the front of the room answering curious questions about the lecture and gearing them up for our upcoming discussion on class and habitus. None of us realized that when they left at the end of class, we would not meet again.

II. COVID sends us home

Over the next several weeks, as we learned more about COVID-19, its deadly outcomes, and the dangers of gathering in person, nearly every aspect of our lives changed, including teaching. Uncertainty about returning to the classroom was replaced with the realities of online teaching and learning, along with the daunting task of engaging with my students in ways I had never imagined. Where before I was anxious about teaching in person, I now longed for the familiarity of the classroom and the anonymity of my non-academic life.

I felt exposed in front of the camera, constantly aware of my appearance and movements. Gone were the confidence and composure I had, now replaced by hyper-awareness of my voice and the concern for my partner's privacy in our tiny apartment. I also felt trapped by the unspoken expectation to exude competency and flexibility, while also serving as a source of normalcy in a moment of abnormality. Did I look happy? Could people see my messy office? Should I dress more formally? The tyrannical nature of the camera and its constant state of on-ness seemed to serve as an omnipresent reminder of my role as purveyor of positivity, yet perversely, also as a window into the students' lives (King, 2006). Understandably, students eliminated their interactions with the camera and its audience by leaving it off. I had no such luxury and learning to teach in this new environment began to take its toll, as tired faces were replaced by happy pictures, or more frequently, black boxes.

I was left sitting behind my desk, delivering lectures with as much enthusiasm as I could muster. Moving in my cluttered office in front of my camera was impossible. Rather than feeling open to sharing aspects of myself to enhance class, I was afraid that students were learning too much about who I was and how I lived. This window into my life was typically one way, and I couldn't blame students for their reluctance to share.

The distance between us, whether five miles or five thousand, was palpable, yet in those last weeks of the semester we found rare moments of joy. My dog jumping into my lap during class was the first time I had seen my students smile in weeks. It was an important moment reminding me of when my jokes would land (more likely not) and working through complex ideas felt more like it had before. Other events elicited laughter, such as the disembodied belch from the kitchen, or the music I played at the start of each class. I grew less concerned about what they were learning, and more concerned about how they were managing.

In rediscovering this "classroom community," we had made the best of untenable circumstances, yet uncertainty remained. For me, it was a loss of the connections between concept and reality that eluded many of my students. I was afraid that in easing our standards, the students missed out on the "a-ha!" moments I had promised. As the pandemic evolved with vaccines released, these concerns continued shifting.

III. Back into the classroom:

Rumors began in the spring semester that we would return to in-person instruction that fall. Details were limited and little communication was forthcoming as we waited for information about vaccines, research restrictions, and the lifting of pandemic protocols. As graduate students, we knew our status as educators meant that we would receive our vaccines, but our questionable status as university employees left us uncertain about when we would receive our appointments and largely unable to argue for concessions or considerations due to existing labor laws (Douglas-Gabriel, 2019; Douglas-Gabriel, 2021). Even vaccinated, I was concerned about potentially spreading COVID-19 in the classroom, or during my long commute on public transportation. How would I teach with a mask on? Would students be able to hear me as I moved around the room? Are there classrooms big enough for us all to sit together safely? Others were open to the return, longing for a "normal school year" without Zoom, or masks, or staying at home. While I couldn't begrudge them their views, I couldn't help but think what it meant for all the changes we had made, the ground we had gained in compassion for each other, and learning new ways to facilitate students' learning.

These anxieties reflect the sacrifices we make as we move about in a post-COVID (?) world. As Braidotti (2020) contends, this moment is one in which we can reimagine and reinvent our relations with the world around us, recognizing that our "shared exhaustion" illuminates possibilities for deeper reflection on who we are, what we do, and how we do it. We have an opportunity to recognize the university as a place for safely failing and asking questions about how we learn about and interact with the world through our bodies. We can reflect on the nature of grades and assignments, reminding students that we are enlivened by their struggle to understand the world even as we fumble through our own. We can recognize that care, compassion, and intention should be at the heart of our pedagogical interactions, and revel in watching our students find their way.

I've received more emails about how much fun classes have been in the last year than in my previous three, and it reminds me that my commitment to teaching is not about how I look at the front of the classroom. Rather, it is about how my students come to know the world differently than how they did before. My pedagogy is less about making tests easier to grade and concepts easier to digest and more about seeing students realizing that gender is a social construction, or that preferences are shaped by our socialization. Instead, my pedagogy is about helping my students to be more open and understanding of the world around them. What does it say about our sacrifices for our neighbors, family, and friends if we simply return to a "normal" that wasn't working for us all?

We cannot lose sight of this, craving a return to "normal" and ignoring the strides we made in crafting a more caring and flexible course experience. Less rigid deadlines, more convenient office hours, and less pressure to attend in-person lectures contributed to students worrying less about their grades and focusing more on engaging challenging ideas. A classroom does not need to be face-to-face with inflexible content. Instead, our embodied pedagogy and praxis demands that we commit ourselves to our craft and to lessening our students' burdens so that they can continue to redefine what normal should be in their post-covid futures.

Brandon:

When the spirit of public safety prompted my community to detach the rims from the backboards at my favorite basketball court, my encounter with the COVID-19 pandemic jolted from the abstract to the personal and the physical. I was always willing to adhere to public ordinances to avoid non-essential outdoor pursuits, especially as my built environment morphed to largely prevent those pursuits altogether. Ever since, however, the underlying theme of my pandemic experience has been my daily existential confrontation with the indoors, and how it has reformulated my relationship to pedagogy.

Scholars have used color as an effective metaphor for conveying the visual and affective dimensions of space. In doing so, they have highlighted the co-constitutive relationships and interactions between the corporeal, psychological, and ecological that underlie physical culture. For instance, parks and other outdoor spaces have commonly been designated "green" spaces, representing not only the visual greenness of the grass, plants, and trees found in the environment, but the concomitant feelings of health, peace, and refreshment—values often linked to the color green (van Braam, 2021)—that accompany immersion into nature (Roberts et al., 2021; Twohig-Bennett & Jones, 2018). Beaches, lakes/oceans, and other spaces that contain water have commonly been designated "blue" spaces, referencing both the blueness of water and the color blue's associated characteristics of strength, tranquility, and harmony that are often evoked by proximity to water (Booth, 2020; Olive & Wheaton, 2021). While useful, the space-color metaphor—and arguably spatial analyses in general—has almost exclusively been applied to outdoor spaces, or at least the spaces encountered once one steps outside of the home. I argue that the isolation sparked by the COVID-19 pandemic necessitates the identification of a similar space-color metaphor: the "grey" space of the *indoors*.

Greyness has pervaded my pandemic experience. It has also, I contend, been the predominant milieu within which physical cultural educators have been forced to engage students in critical conversations about sport, health, embodiment, and social structures. The indoors exude "grey" for reasons beyond the fact that it is the literal color of the walls that have surrounded me as I adapted my work, leisure, and social life to the confines of my private indoors. As noted by cognitive psychologist Hailey van Braam (2020), while the color grey is linked to largely positive characteristics of modesty, reliability, and calmness, I surmise that more have found resonance with its negative characteristics: boredom, monotony, isolation. These feelings—that higher education evokes in many even in "normal" circumstances—have been exacerbated by quarantine and relegation to the indoors. As such, there is need for critical engagement with the indoors as an affected and affecting space that provokes crucial considerations on embodiment, physical activity, and mental/social/emotional wellbeing.

The grey space of the indoors has ramifications for pedagogy, and also prompts questions about the power dynamics of sociocultural education for undergraduates regarding sport and physical culture. On a personal level, what does it mean to embody a grey space, and how is physicality altered, limited, reimagined, and/or rearticulated in the grey space of the indoors? On a professional level, how is critical physical cultural pedagogy advanced or restricted when administered/received within the grey indoors? On a broader political level, what inequalities that impact learning are exacerbated, alleviated, and/or disrupted in grey spaces?

My inability to play basketball pales in comparison to the issues that COVID caused for many. Yet, in aggregate, these personalized idiosyncrasies demonstrate the effects of indoor relegation on physical and mental health. Basketball—in the form 5-on-5 live action, shooting hoops individually, or anything in between—was my preferred mode of physical activity. However, to think of basketball only in terms of its physical health benefits would overlook its purpose as an exuberant venture of escapism that was fundamental for easing the stresses and anxieties that accumulate over the duration of my week of graduate life. One can—and should—be sympathetic to efforts to reduce the risk of contagion through large gatherings while also recognizing how these changes have beget widespread disruptions in physical, mental, social, and emotional health practices. This ironically occurred at a time when people most needed physical activities to manage their mental health and wellbeing.

As intimated earlier, the relegation to grey spaces also impacted pedagogy. The Zoom-ification of the academy ruptured the delicate balance of dialogue and corporeal communication that educators use to guide the learning and reflection process. The transfer of these discussions to the digital screen limited the ways that mannerisms and physical movement facilitate the communication of knowledge, as well as how the nuances of body language and emotional intelligence can promote the peer empathy and solidarity that is integral for critical pedagogy.

Linked to and demonstrated within these micro-level changes are broader, systemic evolutions. Like all space—green, blue, or any other color—the grey indoors is a contested space, often structured by sociopolitical context and thus emanates the power differentials the manifest in educational outcomes. Students demonstrated an immediate awareness of this, taking steps to manipulate their indoor spaces displayed via Zoom classes. I have seen students strategically placing pictures or words in the background space to express ideas about their politics or identity, flaunting the opulence of their rooms or special indoor spaces to convey their socioeconomic status deploying virtual backgrounds or shutting off the lights completely to conceal the background of their room (and these exclude cases where students refuse to ever turn their Zoom camera on). Whereas Goffman (1959) argued that social actors constantly engage in "impression management" of the self as they negotiate power and status in public spaces, the pandemic has seen the necessity of impression management creep into the private space of the home. The Zoom background has thus become a visual marker of class; a modality of displaying (for the privileged) or obfuscating (for the underprivileged/precarious) one's grey space of the indoors.

The pandemic has also revealed how socioeconomic inequalities shape students' academic (in)dependence. My critical pedagogical method requests vulnerability from my students, asking them to reflect on things such as their upbringing, their exposure to power and cultural influences, and how their experiences in life and sport shape their current self. Where the in-person classroom implies a space of focused discussion—wherein one could largely share their experiences and observations without worry that family or friends are listening in—administering class via Zoom to students living in their family homes has meant that critical discussion has lacked complete freedom from outside familial influences. The quality and substance of critical discussion has often depended upon the privacy students can access. It soon became clear to me that indoor academic privacy is linked to socioeconomic status. From my particular anecdotes, many privileged students had their own rooms or own spaces within which they could listen, focus, and participate in class discussion unencumbered. Disadvantaged students (disproportionately from minority ethnic backgrounds) seemed more likely to share spaces with their parents or siblings, have obligations to help out around the house during class time, or have background noise that hindered their ability to listen and learn. These manifested in instances where students felt it necessary to whisper when reflecting on childhood experiences so that their family did not overhear, type out their contributions instead of vocalizing them, or stop abruptly mid-sentence if they sensed a parent or sibling nearby in the house (let alone the instances where these factors combined to discourage participation altogether).

I share these experiences with indoor pandemic pedagogy because it is clear that private indoor spaces will remain, in some capacity, a factor in higher education going forward. As physical cultural scholars work to re-incorporate sport and embodied physicality into the learning process, we must recognize the spatial barriers to equitable pedagogy produced by the indoors and work to overcome them with empathy and creativity. Rather than falling into the trap of hopelessness or viewing the ramifications of the pandemic as insurmountable, scholars can identify the aspects of the pandemic that in themselves have been pedagogical to promote the importance of education and advocate for a more humanizing politics. As noted by Giroux (2021), the pandemic perhaps more than any phenomenon in recent life has highlighted the inhumanity and structural contradictions of neoliberal capitalism. As such, pedagogy of the indoors can be used to expose physicality and community—ironically, through over a year of its general widespread absence—as key mediators of human existence and cognition. Simultaneously, reflections of learning in the pandemic can be fruitful for what Freire (2017) termed "problem-posing" education, which highlights the dehumanizing aspects of one's reality, leading to conscientious intervention in pursuit of liberation and humanization. The end of the pandemic will obviously not equate to the end of precarity. However, the monotony, isolation, and inequalities present in the grey indoors can be translated into praxis, as educators can harness the disruptions to our "normal" to encourage a reimagining and reshaping of what the "normal" many of us yearn for should entail.

Part III: Conclusion, or Together, Apart, and Together Again

Taken together, our narratives reflect our distinct yet shared experiences during COVID-19. While highlighting our unique actions and reactions to the onset of pandemic times, our (forced) separation in these moments has revealed the ways in which we are together-yet-apart, in addition to revealing the fragility of previously taken-for-granted institutions and structures. Through being apart, we have become aware of the ways that we can be, and remain, (inter)connected through our yearning for closeness: physically, intellectually, emotionally, pedagogically. At the same time, the pandemic has continued to reinforce (and, in some cases, magnify) structural barriers, exploitations, and norms that continue to disproportionately impact graduate students. This prompts our central question: how do we move forward in ways that challenge the (new) status quo, resisting the very precarity we have decried?

This is surely a daunting goal, especially for graduate students who spend a limited amount of time at an institution before moving on with their careers. However, to borrow from Cheryl Cooky's (2017) call for public sociology of sport, we must actively "ensure knowledge is publicly translatable with the potential for change" (p. 9). In the case of graduate students and the 'ivory tower,' this means there is an imperative for us to act and find ways to come together that reimagine pre-pandemic norms and structures while confronting the same old problems. Though solutions are elusive, this process of writing, reflecting, collaborating, and learning has taught us that, to move forward, we must be vulnerable; we must value collaborations over competitions; we must find solidarity with other graduate students and laborers, especially those who are currently fighting for fair wages and collective action. We must look beyond ourselves and recognize that "We-who-are-not-one-and-the-same-but-are-in-this-convergence-together," before, during, and after(?) pandemic times (Braidotti, 2020, p. 5). We also encourage other early career researchers as well as established academics to recognize the precarity of this moment, not only for us, but for themselves as well, and commit more effort to collective action that supports the very apprentices they have trained.

Processing and reflecting on the impact of the COVID-19 pandemic separately and then together has enabled us to think about our "responsibility," as Barad (2014) puts it, for we have sought to explore and

> respond to, to be responsible, to take responsibility for that which we inherit (from the past and the future)... to put oneself at risk, to risk oneself (which is never one or self), to open oneself up to indeterminacy in moving towards what is to-come. (p. 183)

For each of us, our experiences invited deep and sometimes previously-realized feelings of isolation, frustration, and uncertainty as we sought to make sense of what has been called the "new normal." At the same time, we are more than these vignettes and they do not convey the fullness of our experiences over the last 18 months (Asonye, 2020). Yet "normal" for us as graduate students has always been entwined in the precarity of student-apprenticeship: a rite of passage or vehicle to (eventually or for some, ideally) join the ranks of academia. Despite this precarity we face, we have sought "to take responsibility for that which we inherit (from the past and the future)…to put [ourselves] at risk" and move forward into a future where we as scholars, as teachers, indeed as humans are able to facilitate the emergence of a more caring, compassionate, and equitable world (Barad, 2014, p. 183).

This ability to respond also leads to the question of 'so what?' What about the graduate student experience during the COVID-19 pandemic can help us to rethink how we understand graduate students in relation to the people in their lives, the pedagogy they develop, and the places they move in and through? We would argue that embracing the pandemic as an opportunity to revisit and reexamine the graduate student "role" in the academy helps to demonstrate a potential path forward for altering the current state of graduate student development. How can we develop healthier relationships that do not force us to overwork ourselves or our students? How can we advocate for a more equitable society beginning in our own institutions? How do we care for ourselves and others in a time where our once private places are now open to the world? In this opportunity, we can look to the hopefulness of the future, and embrace our duty to engender care, compassion, and intention in the act of being in this particular spacetimemattering, as well as others (Barad, 2014).

Across these vignettes, we have also sought to identify the nature of our embodied diffractions, examining the very effects of difference in our experiences of the pandemic. We do this despite the precarity of graduate student life, and seek to, as Blum (2021) puts it, flourish rather than languish. Yet flourishing looks differently for different people, and indeed for us as graduate students, our definitions of flourishing differ amongst ourselves. But what matters, we argue, is that we continue to collaborate with our colleagues and friends, both professionally and in our private lives, to work for collective justice, rather than competition for limited opportunities. We continue to develop our pedagogies (both embodied and digital) in the service of generating more care-oriented student interactions. And we continue to recognize that the spaces in which we live, work, and play are anything but "normal"; that we are able, in any space gray or otherwise, to reshape what equity looks like in "normal" times as we move towards uncertain futures.

References

Asonye, C. (2020, June 5). There's nothing new about the 'new normal' – and here's why. *World Economic Forum*. https://www.weforum.org/agenda/2020/06/theres-nothing-new-about-this-new-normal-heres-why/

Baker, R.K. (2021, October 22). There is no academic freedom without academic tenure. Professors need job protection. *USA Today Opinion*. https://www.usatoday.com/story/opinion/2021/10/22/tenure-universities-professors-academic-freedom/6120514001/?gnt-cfr=1

Barad, K. (2014). Diffracting diffraction: Cutting together-apart. *Parallax, 20*(3), 168–187.

Blum, D. (2021, May 6). The Other Side of Languishing is Flourishing. Here's How to Get There. *New York Times*. https://www.nytimes.com/2021/05/04/well/mind/flourishing-languishing.html

Booth, D. (2020). Entangling corporeal matter and geomatter: Making and remaking the beach. In J. I. Newman, H. Thorpe, & D. L. Andrews (Eds.), *Sport, physical culture, and the moving body: Materialisms, technologies, ecologies* (pp. 246–266). Rutgers University Press.

Braidotti, R. (2020). "We" are in this together, but we are not one and the same. *Journal of Bioethical Inquiry, 17*(4), 465–469.

Butler, J. (2014). *Bodies that matter: On the discursive limits of "sex"*. Routledge.

Carey, K. (2020, March 6). The Bleak Job Landscape of Adjunctopia for Ph.D.s *New York Times*. https://www.nytimes.com/2020/03/05/upshot/academic-job-crisis-phd.html

Cooky, C. (2017). "We cannot stand idly by": A necessary call for a public sociology of sport. *Sociology of Sport Journal, 34*(1), 1–11.

Corbera, E., Anguelovski, I., Honey-Rosés, J., & Ruiz-Mallén, I. (2020). Academia in the time of COVID-19: Towards an ethics of care. *Planning Theory & Practice, 21*(2), 191–199.

Dibella, S., & Hoyle, A. (2021, November 16). UMD just raised the minimum graduate stipend. It's not even close to enough. *The Diamondback*. https://dbknews.com/2021/11/16/graduate-students-stipend-compensation-salary-administration/

Douglas-Gabriel, D. (2019, September 20). NLRB reverses course on graduate students' right to organize as employees. *Washington Post*. https://www.washingtonpost.com/education/2019/09/20/nlrb-reverses-course-graduate-students-right-organize-employees/

Douglas-Gabriel, D. (2021, March 21). Labor board withdraws rule to quash graduate students' right to organize as employees. *Washington Post*. https://www.washingtonpost.com/education/2021/03/12/nlrb-graduate-student-workers-unions/

Elfman, L. (2021, March 18). A new normal: Graduate schools making adjustments to meet COVID-19 related challenges. *Diverse Issues in Higher Education, 37*(26), 14–17.

Freire, P. (2017). *Pedagogy of the oppressed*. Penguin Random House.

Giroux, H. A. (2021). *Race, politics, and pandemic pedagogy: Education in a time of crisis*. Bloomsbury Publishing Place.

Goffman, E. (1959). *The presentation of self in everyday life*. Bantam Doubleday Dell Publishing Group.

Grant, A. (2021, July 29). There's a Name for the Blah You're Feeling: It's Called Languishing. *New York Times*. https://www.nytimes.com/2021/04/19/well/mind/covid-mental-health-languishing.html

Hess, A. J. (2021, July 16). Only 25% of those with student loans went to graduate school- but they owe around 50% of all student debt. *CNBC*. https://www.cnbc.com/2021/07/16/graduate-students-owe-around-50percent-of-all-student-debt.html

Hett, B. C. (2021, November 5). Op-Ed: When politicians claim professors like me are the enemy, what are they really attacking? *Los Angeles Times*. https://www.latimes.com/opinion/story/2021-11-05/jd-vance-professors-are-the-enemy-politics

Hoberman, J. M. (1992). *Mortal engines: The science of performance and the dehumanization of sport*. Free Press.

Hubler, S. (2020, November 2). Colleges Slash Budgets in the Pandemic, With 'Nothing Off-Limits'. *New York Times*. https://www.nytimes.com/2020/10/26/us/colleges-coronavirus-budget-cuts.html

King, S. (2006). *Pink ribbons, inc.: Breast cancer and the politics of philanthropy*. University of Minnesota Press.

King-White, R. (Ed.). (2018). *Sport and the neoliberal university: Profit, politics, and pedagogy*. Ser. The American Campus. Rutgers University Press.

Lumpkin, L. (2021, March 5). Workers and universities at odds as labor movements unfold on Maryland campuses. *Washington Post*. https://www.washingtonpost.com/local/education/university-maryland-system-labor-movements/2021/03/05/8181cca2-7ddc-11eb-a976-c028a4215c78_story.html

Norman, M., Esmonde, K., & Szto, C. (2019). Public sociology of sport and digital media: A self-reflexive analysis of public engagement in the "hockey blogosphere". *Sociology of Sport Journal, 36*(2), 135–143.

Olive, R., & Wheaton, B. (2021). Understanding blue spaces: Sport, bodies, wellbeing, and the sea. *Journal of Sport and Social Issues, 45*(1), 3–19.

Roberts, J. D., Ada, M. S. D., & Jette, S. L. (2021). NatureRx@UMD: A review for pursuing green space as a health and wellness resource for the body, mind and soul. *American Journal of Health Promotion, 35*(1), 149–152.

Shore, C. (2010). Beyond the multiversity: Neoliberalism and the rise of the schizophrenic university. *Social Anthropology, 18*(1), 15–29.

Silk, M. L., Bush, A., & Andrews, D. L. (2010). Contingent intellectual amateurism, or, the problem with evidence-based research. *Journal of Sport and Social Issues, 34*(1), 105–128.

Stewart, D. W., Davoren, A. K., Neumeister, J. R., Knepler, E., Grigorian, K., & Greene, A. (2021). *Graduate Schools respond to COVID-19: Promising pathways to innovation and sustainability in STEM education.* NORC at the University of Chicago. https://www.norc.org/PDFs/Graduate%20Studies%20COVID/NORC_COVIDWhitePaper_2021_FINAL.PDF

Thorpe, H., Barbour, K., & Bruce, T. (2011). "Wandering and wondering": Theory and representation in feminist physical cultural studies. *Sociology of Sport Journal, 28*(1), 106–134.

Twohig-Bennett, C., & Jones, A. (2018). The health benefits of the great outdoors: A systematic review and meta-analysis of greenspace exposure and health outcomes. *Environmental Research, 166*, 628–637.

van Braam, H. (2020). Gray color psychology and meaning. *Color Psychology.* https://www.colorpsychology.org/gray/

van Braam, H. (2021). Green color psychology and meaning. *Color Psychology.* https://www.colorpsychology.org/green/

Zahneis, M. (2021, February 15). The shrinking of the scholarly ranks – The pandemic may do lasting damage to the pipeline of academic researchers. *The Chronicle of Higher Education.* https://www.chronicle.com/article/the-shrinking-of-the-scholarly-ranks

9

Black Bodies and Green Spaces: Remembering the Eminence of Nature During a Pandemic

Jennifer D. Roberts, Shadi Omidvar Tehrani, and Gregory N. Bratman

9.1 Introduction

From the enslaved African on a southern American plantation, who used nature as a place of deliverance, healing and route to freedom, to the Central Park bird watcher, whose green space presence was perceived as a threat to White physical safety in the midst of a pandemic, systemic racism has shaped the experience, connection, and relationship to the natural world among African Americans. Over the past two years, the

---

J. D. Roberts
University of Maryland, College Park, MD, USA
e-mail: jenrob@umd.edu

S. Omidvar Tehrani
Vanderbilt University, Nashville, TN, USA
e-mail: Shadi.Omidvar.Tehrani@Vanderbilt.edu

G. N. Bratman
University of Washington, Seattle, WA, USA
e-mail: bratman@uw.edu

D. L. Andrews et al. (eds.), *Sport and Physical Culture in Global Pandemic Times*, Global Culture and Sport Series, https://doi.org/10.1007/978-3-031-14387-8_9

COVID-19 pandemic revealed not only the true value of nature and open public spaces, but it reified the presence and persistence of racism in and throughout American institutions. The racism of 'wilderness', an early construct of Whiteness to reinforce White supremacist ideology and the oppressive servility of Black, Indigenous and People of Color (BIPOC) in natural environments, whether that be parks, trails, pools or beaches, has and still poses a threat to the physical and mental health benefits than can be deservingly received from nature among BIPOC. Many have even argued that racism fueled the COVID-19 pandemic and left many BIPOC communities exceptionally vulnerable to experiencing disparities in COVID-19 morbidity and mortality. Headlines such as "Segregated parks linked to higher COVID-19 deaths for Black and Latino Americans" (USA News) or "What outdoor space tells us about inequality" (BBC) articulated a significant nature gap with respect to green space distribution and the unjust experiences that many BIPOC have in the outdoors. Low-income and BIPOC, distinctly African American and Hispanic communities, are nearly three times more likely to reside in "nature deprived" areas, or those with no access to parks, paths and green space, in comparison to White communities. Through an examination of built, social and natural environments, this chapter will delve into historical and contemporary inequities stemming from structural racism that are experienced by African or Black Americans and other marginalized communities. Specifically, disparities related to these environments as well as COVID-19 health outcomes will be discussed. Finally, the toxic interrelationship between race-/class-based privilege and place or space and its impact on natural space access, particularly throughout the pandemic will be critically assessed.

9.2 Unnaturally Enslaved

The slave starts for Canada, the North Star is his guide. When the clouds intervene, and thus obscure the flickering light of this 'beautiful star', nature has a substitute. A smooth soft substance called moss, which grows on the bark of the trees is thicker on the north side of the tree, and thus serves as a guide northward, till the heavenly guide again appears. **Reverend W.M. Mitchell**

The Atlantic slave trade, beginning in the late 1400s, pilfered bodies, established colonial rule, fractured societal structures, and dismantled the earthly connection with Black bodies throughout West Africa. Between 1525 and 1866, the years that span the history of slave trade to the New World, 12.5 million bodies were shipped from Africa. However, only 10.7 million survived the Middle Passage, an 80-day voyage from West Africa to North America where human beings were savagely packed together on or below ship decks without space, proper ventilation, or water (Gates Jr., 2013a, 2013b; NPS, 2020). Among the men, women and children who survived the journey, approximately 388,000 were delivered to territory forming into the United States and forced into the chattel slave system. As Europeans continued to penetrate the rainforests, savannas, forests and arid grounds of West Africa over the course of the transatlantic slave trade, the inhabitants, who were hunter-gatherers, farmers, as well as sheep, goat and cattle herders, were forced to develop a new pact with America, a land that represented betrayal, brutality, exploitation, and subjugation.

9.2.1 Sun, Stars and Moss

Although the African slave trade was outlawed by the U.S. Congress in 1808, internal trading flourished by tripling the enslaved population over the next five decades. With land possession, wealth in southern American society was measured by the extend of slave ownership. Throughout the antebellum, the labor of enslaved Africans was capitalized for the production of several commodities (e.g., tobacco, cotton) and nearly every aspect of their chattel experience put them into direct contact with the natural environment. Any and all nature learnings gained from this new land as well as the wisdom carried over from Africa gave the enslaved a knowledge that was both detailed and practical. As plantation owners gained more prosperity through the accruement of acreage, they increasingly became more removed from the land and the natural world. Consequently, this removed relationship reduced their ability to control and decreased their chances of finding fugitives throughout the uncultivated landscapes.

In the nineteenth century, race, class, and gender governed perceptions of nature. White planters viewed nature as a product to be dominated and used for profit while enslaved Africans perceived nature as "good use" and recognized that everything on earth, from the plants to the animals, had a "soul and place in the world" (Blum, 2002). Christianity, a foundational doctrine availed to slavery's defense, was also used to buttress the notion of White supremacy and the elevation of White men over the natural world. This sentiment ultimately justified the exploitation of natural resources, especially the land (Claborn, 2017; Blum, 2002). The enslaved community or rather the burgeoning African American population harmonized their existence with nature and developed a conservative use of environmental resources that were a hybrid of African traditions and practices produced by the conditions of bondage. Many of these included using the sun, stars, or even moss on trees, for direction and landmarking. Furthermore, these earthly resources were also used as a wellspring of power among enslaved women as they were able to acquire natural resource knowledge to support and protect their families (Blum, 2002). As an example, natural elements, including roots, tree bark, and plant leaves, were used by many enslaved women to bring color and life to their shabby clothes, particularly for Sunday best church wear (Fabien, 2014).

9.2.2 Nature Retreat and Revolt

As the land of this new world fought cultivation and taming, enslavers and the enslaved used nature to reinforce their own class interests. Controlling nature was necessary for the political power, social standing and economic success of the planters and equally so, they also invested heavily to build, maintain, and control their land and enslaved community (Turner, 2012). By creating a 'geography of containment', the slaveholding elites were able to control the movements and activities of enslaved people by space and time (Camp, 2002). All enslaved individuals throughout every plantation were prohibited by law and common practice from leaving their enslaver's property without passes. Slave patrols, organized groups of armed men who were compensated in pay, rewards, or exemptions, attempted to ensure obedience by apprehending and punishing runaways and monitoring the restrictive pass requirements for the enslaved traveling off plantations (Hadden, 2001; Reichel, 1988). Even though this geography of containment limited the land knowledge of many enslaved people, particularly those that worked in the planter's residence or rather the "Big House" and not in the field, enslaved laborers persistently engaged in truancy and absenteeism.

Conversely, many enslaved people created a 'rival geography' both on and off the plantation that included quarters, outbuildings, woods, swamps and neighboring farms (Camp, 2002). Unlike the enslaver's mapping of the plantation, which was defined and anchored by structures, the rival geography was not a fixed spatial formation. Rival geography was characterized by truant movement, a behavior that facilitated independent activity and denial of labor (Camp, 2002). Nature provided a haven to escape the realities of bondage for many enslaved men and women. Through their knowledge of nearby woods, fields, and waterways, many enslaved people would seek these areas as hiding places for a temporary retreat from White control and the horror of slavery (Blum, 2002). In addition to the truants, who ran away for short periods, the 'escapees' sought permanent freedom up North. Finally, the 'maroons', another group of enslaved fugitives, intended to permanently leave the plantations, but not the American South (Turner, 2012). Ranging from ten to more than one hundred members, maroon societies often engaged in highly organized militant forms of resistance, lived together deep in the woods or swamps for many years and even generations and became thriving counter-culture regions for fugitives.

9.3 Dirt on Our Hands

Southern trees bear strange fruit, blood on the leaves and blood at the root, black bodies swinging in the Southern breeze, strange fruit hanging from the poplar trees. **Abel Meeropol**

One of the most turbulent times in American history was the reconstruction era from 1865 to 1877. During this period, following the Civil

War, national efforts were directed on reunifying the South with the Union. It required seeking reconciliation between White and African Americans, especially in the South, where slavery had established the racial hierarchy for centuries. As part of reconstruction, amendments to the U.S. Constitution were enacted, including the Thirteenth Amendment, which abolished slavery, and the Fourteenth and Fifteenth Amendments, which guaranteed citizenship and the constitutional right to vote for African Americans, respectively. These amendments intended to guarantee freedom, citizenship, and voting, but with ambiguous language they lacked clarity for implementation. As such, reconstruction did not usher in the improvements or equality that many African Americans expected (Chandra, 2011). With all the promises bestowed upon African Americans, reconstruction served only to provoke White supremacy violence and facilitate the establishment of future discriminatory regulations (Cross, 2011).

9.3.1 Neoslavery and Strange Fruit

After the emancipation of African Americans, sharecropping became one of the most effective farming choices due to the fact that enslavers no longer had free labor to cultivate their land and millions of the formally enslaved needed employment. From the 1870s to the 1950s, sharecropping, an agricultural system instituted in southern American states, continued to perpetuate inequalities between White and African Americans. Leveraging the reality that formerly enslaved people possessed no residence, job, land, livestock or farm equipment, the White landowners sold these necessities and supplies on credit to the sharecroppers. With sharecropping contracts, African American farmers were mandated to turn over a portion of the crop yield in order to compensate for these supplies and against any other debts the landowners would uncover. While this agricultural system had placed the newly freed African Americans in perpetual servitude and thwarted their ability to thrive economically, sharecropping sustained the unique connection of the land and nature with African Americans (Chandra, 2011). In the mid 1930s, Zora Neale Hurston, a pre-eminent author of twentieth century African

American literature, published literary works that spoke of a deep respect and pride for nature's seasonal forces. During this period many African Americans regarded the creation of earth as a space of freedom, humanity, and spirituality despite it often being the gist of indignity (Fabien, 2014). In Hurston's *Their Eyes Were Watching God*, two characters referenced nature as a vessel that holds the essence of omnipotence and omniscience; "It's de strongest thing dat God ever made, now. Fact is it's de onliest thing God ever made. He made nature and nature made everything else" (Hurston, 1937).

The "Jim Crow" era refers to a period of history when oppressive and discriminatory laws and customs were used to restrict African American rights, promote racial segregation, and maintain a social hierarchy characterized by White supremacy. Numerous acts of violence were committed during this time by White nationalists, including the Ku Klux Klan, a terrorist group that used violence against African Americans and sympathizers, in the name of preserving the values of White civilization. African Americans were frequently denied a trial for alleged Jim Crow law violations and instead killed by lynching. Lynchings, the violent public execution of an individual, were generally carried out by lawless White mobs with the sanctioning of police officers. Held particularly in the South, lynchings often involved torture, mutilation, decapitation, desecration and ended with men and women hanging ablaze from trees. While these public spectacles were often attended by the White community as festivities in triumph of White supremacy, the terror of these events in parks, on farms, near rivers, or in any outdoor space loomed among African Americans (Mock, 2016). Although many lynchings have not been document, it has been determined that between 1877 and 1950, there were over 4,084 lynchings of African Americans in 12 southern states and most of these events occurred in some of the most majestic areas of nature (EJI, 2017; Dunning, 2021). Unfortunately, the darkness of this legacy still lingers today.

9.3.2 The Warmth of Other Suns

Richard Wright, a prolific American writer, published a memoir titled, *Black Boy: A Record of Childhood and Youth*. Wright compared his childhood on a plantation near Natchez, Mississippi and other areas of the South, including Memphis, Tennessee and Elaine, Arkansas, to his migration to Chicago, Illinois as an adult in 1927 (Duffus, 1999). As a final insertion in the restructuring of *Black Boy*, Wright was able to poignantly and poetically speak of his journey in this migration (Wilkerson, 2010).

> *I was leaving the South to fling myself in the unknown…I was taking a part of the South to transplant in alien soil, to see if it could grow differently, if it could drink of new and cool rains, bend in strange winds, respond to the warmth of other suns and, perhaps, to bloom.* **Richard Wright**

As result of poor economic conditions, racial discrimination, and Jim Crow terror, African Americans fled the rural South to urban centers in the northeastern, midwestern and western parts of the United States. This massive exodus, known as the Great Migration, occurred over six decades and began as a quiet pilgrimage approximately in the early twentieth century. Initially unnoticed with only few families leaving the South, the numbers migrating would swell to approximately six million. When the First Great Migration (1915–1940) began, 90% of African Americans were living in southern states, but by the time the Second Great Migration (1940–1970) ended 47% of African Americans were living in northern and western cities, resulting in a significant redistribution of the African American population. Both the First and Second Great Migrations had a profound and significant effect on race relations, politics, and the transformation of urban America throughout the country (Boustan, 2010). As Wilkerson writes in her Smithsonian Magazine (2016) article, "A rural people had become urban, and a Southern people had spread themselves all over the nation."

Segregation represented a significant deviation from the former social order of the antebellum South and the psychology of racial relations after the emancipation of enslaved people. During slavery, White Americans used physical proximity to strengthen and retain control over their assets (e.g., enslaved African Americans), but with the collapse of slavery the order was reversed (Woodward & McFeely, 2002). The segregation of the formerly enslaved became a function of keeping African Americans "in place"—a continuous and contemptuous reminder of their alleged inferiority (Birkett, 2020).

While segregation was not legalized in the North as it was in the South, racism and prejudice were nonetheless widespread. Through practices and policies steeped in racism, housing opportunities were significantly diminished for African Americans. Housing was segregated through the use of racial covenants and governmentally sanctioned actions, such as "redlining." The "redlining" maps of the United States federal government were one of the most well-defined and provable examples of racial discrimination in housing throughout American history. With the goal of increasing homeownership and reducing foreclosures, the federal government enacted the 1934 National Housing Act, which also established the Federal Housing Administration (FHA). By decreasing interest rates, the FHA insured private mortgages in order to make real estate more accessible and affordable for most White Americans. Specifically, the FHA entrusted the Home Owners Loan Corporation with developing "Residential Security Maps" for 239 American cities (Coates, 2014; Lipsitz, 2011). These maps rated neighborhood mortgage risk levels throughout cities whereby "low risk" areas were given an "A" rating and depicted in green on a map, while those deemed "highest risk" were redlined and rated "D". In essence, neighborhoods that inhabited African Americans, immigrants, or poor White Americans were redlined and homes in these areas failed to gain significant equity in comparison to the higher ranked neighborhoods. This practice significantly impacted the African American institutional division of capital and the disinvestment of redlined homes and neighborhoods affected the socio-spatial pattern of services (e.g., healthcare), amenities (e.g., parks), opportunities (e.g., schools), as well as other social determinants of health within the United States. Social determinants of health, or rather the constellation of environmental and socioeconomic conditions (e.g., housing; food; schools; parks) affecting where individuals are born, live, learn, work, and play, can cascade along a pathway to improve or worsen health and wellbeing over the life course.

9.3.3 Separate But Unequal from Nature

Just as the First Great Migration was beginning to swell, the United States National Park Service (NPS), a bureau in the Department of the Interior subject to preserving national parks and monuments, was signed into law on August 25, 1916 by President Woodrow Wilson. Most of the national parks, such as Yellowstone National Park, were initially located in the western part of the country and until the 1930s the racism displayed was in the form of ejecting Indigenous People from the parks. However, during this decade and under the direction of federal legislation, several new parks were created in the South where segregation was legalized. With low-cost entry and a boost in automobile ownership, the number of campers and park visits increased substantially for Americans. While the law, also known as the "Organic Act", stated that the purpose of the NPS was to "conserve the scenery and the natural and historic objects and the wildlife therein and to provide for the enjoyment", the reconciliation of this purpose with legalized segregation as well as southern laws and customs was challenged (NPS, 2018). For example, NPS Director Arno B. Cammerer embraced plans for racially separate facilities at the Shenandoah National Park in Virginia despite pushback from African American citizens and leaders in the National Association for the Advancement of Colored People. In so many words, Cammerer admitted to NPS Associate Director, Arthur E. Demaray, that segregation, although inequitable, in the parks was the best option (Young, 2009).

> *There will be some criticism by colored people against segregation. But I think we would be subject to more criticism by the colored people as well as the white people if we put them in with the white people.* **Arno B. Cammerer**

Both the NPS Organic Act and the subsequent Wilderness Act of 1964 used language in a comparable fashion that described the preservation of resource integrity. It was Congressional intent in both acts to "conserve" and "secure" the wilderness for the enjoyment and benefits of present and future generations. The Wilderness Act, which also created the National Wilderness Preservation System to protect over 100 million acres of wilderness throughout the country, is considered one of America's greatest conservation achievements, yet, the act "presumed a universality of ideals" without an acknowledgement of the structural and systemic inequities born out of racism (Finney, 2014). As a segregated and White supremacist American society, Black bodies were forbidden from "the benefits of an enduring resource of wilderness" (US.Congress, 1964). Many others have also argued that the Wilderness Act "materially and symbolically" erased the presence of African Americans in ecosystems, outdoor spaces, and "wilderness", a concept created by and for White men which bifurcates humans from nature and narrowly defines mankind (Davis, 2019; Smith, 2005). To illustrate, John Muir, the "Father of Our National Parks" and founder of the environmental organization Sierra Club, perpetuated a whitewashed wilderness doctrine steeped in anti-Black racism with declarations such as "one energetic White man, working with a will, would easily pick as much cotton as half a dozen Sambos and Sallies"; "but idle Negroes were prowling about everywhere, and I was afraid"; and "seen anywhere but in the South, the glossy pair would have been taken for twin devils, but here it was only a Negro and his wife at their supper", in *A Thousand-Mile Walk to the Gulf*, his travel memoir across the southeastern United States (Muir & Badè, 1916). Anti-Black and anti-Indigenous racism and elitism were embedded within wilderness ideology and subsequently framed the development of the Wilderness Act, policy which permitted "opportunities for solitude or a primitive and unconfined type of recreation" in areas "where man himself [was] a visitor who does not remain" (SierraWild.gov, n.d.). With such language, this policy ignored working class men, women, and BIPOC since they were always defined as primitive from the lens of Whiteness. Furthermore, this legislation externalized the unequal and inequitable development of Black and White spaces by reserving federally protected lands, which were brutally seized from Indigenous Peoples, to now be designated as wilderness according to the institutions, coalitions, social relations and rules of the American White middle class and elite constituencies (Davis, 2019).

The quest to preserve American wilderness, a classified White space, began in response to the social transformations of emancipated African Americans and the influx of immigrants toward the end of the nineteenth century (Davis, 2019). In order to secure and uphold White racial identity, purity and supremacy, the creation of impenetrable racialized spaces for recreation or living was essential. Notwithstanding the disruption of White equilibrium by the country's social transformations, efforts to maintain the status quo were put in place through policy and investment and were rigorously maintained by local, state and federal governments. For instance, in areas of the country that were redlined and hence occupied predominately by BIPOC, distinctly African Americans, investments in ecosystems, namely parks, green spaces, and trees were diverted away from these neighborhoods. An analysis of 37 metropolitan areas throughout the United Stated revealed that formerly redlined areas have nearly 50% less tree canopy compared to areas formerly graded A which were predominately occupied by American born White residents (Locke et al., 2021). Consistent with this analysis, other research has shown that redlined neighborhoods have far fewer parks and green space in comparison to other neighborhoods (Nardone et al., 2021). Furthermore, many of these formerly redlined areas, which were also subject to the blowback dynamics of White Flight and suburbanization also lack blue spaces in the form a municipal swimming pools and surface water (Napieralski et al., 2022; Plumer and Popovich, 2020). Other policies, such as urban renewal, to preserve or restore White equilibrium have also adversely impacted the access and connection of nature with BIPOC throughout the country. Until its destruction by 1950s and 1960s urban renewal efforts, Watts Branch Stream Valley Park was a natural environment in the Washington DC metropolitan area visited by many African Americans (NRPA, 2011). Through similar urban renewal programs, the Mahlon Stacy Park in Trenton, New Jersey as well as the Humboldt Parkway in Buffalo, New York (Fig. 9.1) were demolished (Antebi, n.d.; PFLWN, 2017). As a result of these and other nature inequities, many previously redlined neighborhoods or those impacted by racist planning policies, have been found to be unhealthy due to excess heat, air pollution and other environmental hazards (Cusick, 2020). Despite mounting evidence, the adverse impacts of nature gaps and inequitable access for BIPOC were underrecognized and overlooked, that is, until a pandemic made green spaces and other natural environments popular to visit (Cirruzzo, 2021; Spotswood et al., 2021).

HUMBOLDT PARKWAY, BUFFALO, NY – C.1912

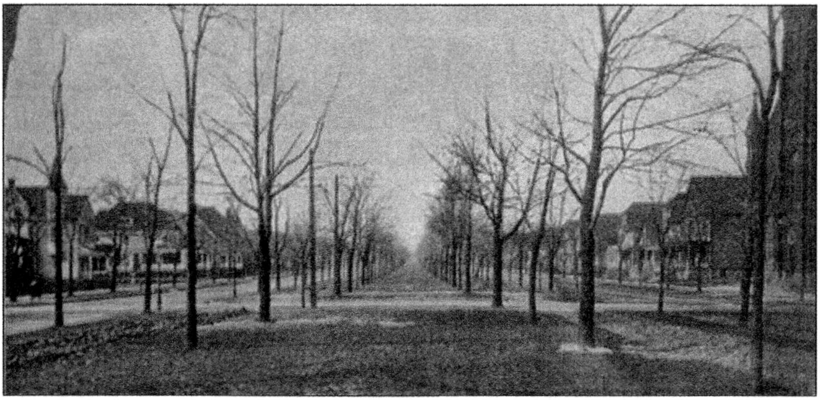

KENSINGTON EXPRESSWAY, BUFFALO, NY – PRESENT DAY

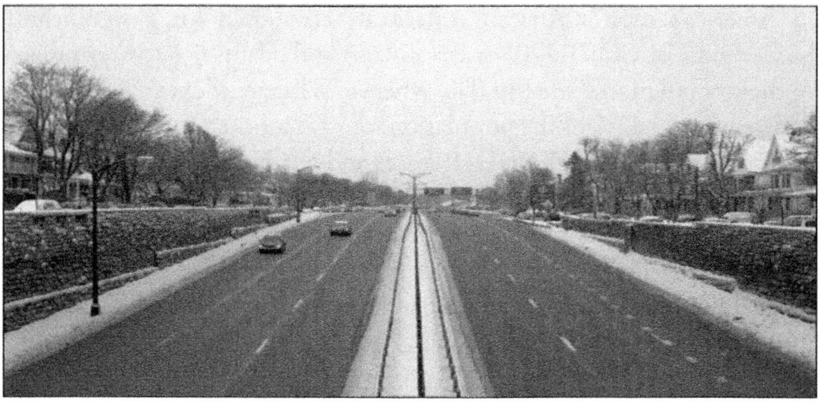

Fig. 9.1 Buffalo, New York Urban Renewal. (Source: Puma, Mike. Developing: Bringing Black an Olmsted Parkway, Buffalo Spree, April 1, 2015)

9.4 Pandemic and Park Inequities

Parks are good for health, and during the pandemic they have been particularly important places for people to get physical activity and stay connected to one another, with lower risk of COVID transmission compared to indoors. Residents of the most racially privileged neighborhoods were able to take the greatest advantage of those benefits. **Jonathan Jay**

Historically, epidemics have disproportionately harmed marginalized members of societies, and there is no exception for the COVID-19 pandemic (Dee et al., 2011; Quinn et al., 2011). The notion that race, ethnicity, and culture significantly impact health disparities is not novel. Within the United States, COVID-19 morbidity and mortality rates disproportionately affect many BIPOC, resulting in a death rate that is at least double that of White Americans. Even though disparities in infection and death rates had declined by early 2022 throughout the country, African Americans still accounted for a slightly higher share of deaths (13.5%) as well as a lower share of vaccination (9.9%) compared to their population share (12.5%) (Fig. 9.2) (Artiga et al., 2021; CDC, 2021a, 2021b). Furthermore, Hispanic Americans also experienced an elevated infection rate (24.0%) in comparison to their population share (17.0%). In some regions the disparity and is still more pronounced. For example, in America's capitol African Americans accounted for a significantly higher share of COVID-19 cases (58.0%) and deaths (71.0%) compared to their population share (45.0%) whereas White residents, who make up approximately 37% of the population, only accounted for 19% and 13% of Washington, DC's COVID-19 cases and deaths, respectively (Fig. 9.3) (KFF, 2021).

These racially and ethnically based disparities in COVID-19 morbidity and mortality reflect systemically racist policies and practices that drive and influence social determinants of health within the United States

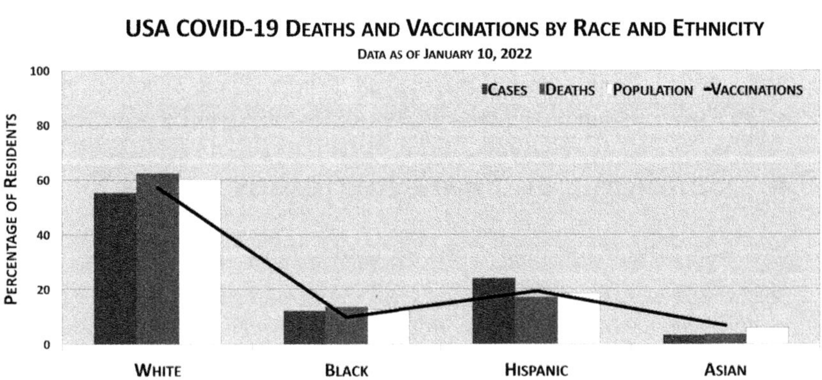

Fig. 9.2 USA COVID-19 Rates by Race and Ethnicity

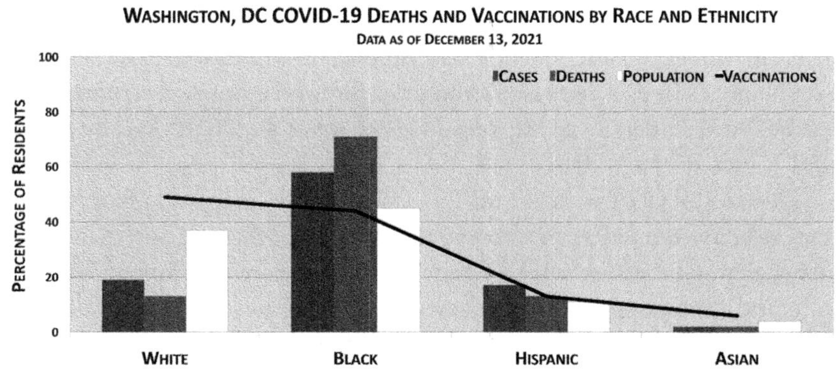

Fig. 9.3 Washington, DC COVID-19 Rates by Race and Ethnicity

(Dickinson et al., 2021). It has been shown that the cumulative, aggregate and synergistic impact of deleterious social determinants increases COVID-19 health risk. One such social determinant, the access to nature and green space, left many BIPOC communities exceptionally vulnerable throughout the COVID-19 pandemic. As mentioned previously, low-income and BIPOC, distinctly African American and Hispanic communities, are nearly three times more likely to reside in "nature deprived" areas, or those with no access to parks, paths and green space, in comparison to White communities, which ultimately limits their ability to receive the physical and mental therapeutic benefits of nature (Borunda, 2020; Rowland-Shea et al., 2020; Slater et al., 2020).

9.4.1 Health of Nature

Evidence from multiple disciplines has demonstrated the health benefits of nature experiences for a variety of populations and under many different circumstances (Bratman et al., 2021; Frumkin et al., 2017; Meidenbauer et al., 2020). Methodologies from psychology, exposure science, and environmental epidemiology have informed the analytic approaches and framing of results in support of these associations (Bratman et al., 2019). Studies have employed a variety of designs, from controlled experiments to observational and cross-sectional studies

(Bratman et al., 2012). Through this research, documented outcomes from nature exposure include assessments of increased psychological wellbeing, as well as decreased stress and risk for the onset of certain mental health disorders (e.g., depression) (Bezold et al., 2018; Egorov et al., 2017; Hartig et al., 2014).

Due to the fact that most of human evolution has taken place within natural environments, psycho-evolutionary hypotheses posit that there are direct associations between time spent in nature and human wellbeing, and that a deprivation of these experiences may be maladaptive for our mental and physical health (Berman et al., 2012; Kaplan & Kaplan, 1989; Ulrich et al., 1991). This framing relies to some degree on the notion that humans share an "innate connection to nature", a concept supported by the biophilia hypothesis, and one that has heavily informed two dominant theories in the field (Kellert & Wilson, 1995). The first of these theories, attention restoration theory (ART) posits that the demands of urban environments deplete our directed attention resources due to the need to overcome distractions, and natural environments provide an opportunity for a replenishment of this capacity when an alternative, less taxing facet of attention is engaged (Kaplan, 1995; Kaplan & Berman, 2010). Second, stress reduction theory (SRT) posits that nature contact benefits well-being through the restorative activation of the parasympathetic nervous system (the "rest and digest" system), and a corresponding reduction of sympathetic nervous activation (the "fight or flight" system) (Ulrich et al., 1991). Through this pathway, nature contact may help reduce the effects of an acute stressor, and potentially buffer against the toxic effects of chronic stress and its wear and tear on the mind and body. Other posited causal pathways include the ways in which enhanced immune function, physical activity, and social cohesion from nature contact may explain many observed benefits (Hartig et al., 2014; Jennings & Bamkole, 2019; Kuo, 2015). These explanations are not mutually exclusive, nor are they exhaustive when it comes to potential mechanisms.

Many approaches to measure nature exposure exist in the literature (Holland et al., 2021). Some studies involve the use of satellite imagery and maps that capture the proximity of residences to green space, or a calculation of total greenness around a point as a "cumulative opportunity" metric (Ekkel & de Vries, 2017). These studies often use cross-sectional analyses that link survey responses with objective measures of vegetation, mostly from satellite data, many of which estimate how much total vegetation is within a certain distance of one's residence (Balseviciene et al., 2014). Some of these approaches are limited insofar as cross-sectional data cannot rule out reverse causation, or by the confounding factor that more privileged, wealthier, and healthier individuals may move to more natural areas as they have the capability to do so. To some degree, experimental approaches address these concerns, but these designs have limitations regarding generalizability as they are often conducted within laboratory settings and with limited sample sizes (Bratman et al., 2021). With all of these approaches, it is important to specify what is meant by nature "exposure" or "contact" in each instance, including the socio-cultural context of the experiences, and the specificities of the nature with which individuals interact. This includes visual, olfactory or auditory stimuli characteristics and the details of the human-nature interaction patterns (Lev et al., n.d.; Buxton et al., 2021; Kahn et al., 2018). For example, ART and SRT tend to focus on the visual pathway, whereas research in shinrin-yoku (known as forest bathing in the United States) posits an olfactory pathway for observed benefits (Ikei et al., 2016; Lee et al., 2011; Park et al., 2010). Research has shown that the auditory pathway likely plays a role as well (e.g., loud urban noise vs. softer bird song) (Annerstedt van den Bosch et al., 2016; Ratcliffe et al., 2013). Taken together, these areas of research are beginning to demonstrate how different kinds of nature experiences impact different people differently.

Access to nearby residential green space is highly skewed, with less access often associated with social and financial disadvantage (Nesbitt et al., 2019). Even in cases when the access itself is not unequal, often the quality of the accessible green space is inversely associated with socioeconomic factors (Mears et al., 2019). In a United Kingdom study researchers found that green space availability within a reasonable proximity to one's home decreased rapidly with declining household income (Pearce et al., 2010). Moreover, the Trust for Public Land released a report, partly in response to the COVID-19 pandemic, documenting the ways in which park access, size and quality differ vastly by a community's racial, ethnic, and socioeconomic characteristics within the United States (Chapman et al., 2021). With such a statement as "this past year has proved that parks are not just a nicety—they are a necessity", the report documented substantial discrepancies in access to the amount of green space acreage and the degree of crowding in parks that were within 10-minute walks of residences within BIPOC versus majority White neighborhoods (McKoy, 2021).

9.4.2 Proximity of Nature

The nature deprivation experienced by BIPOC is the result of racism and discrimination in the United States. The policies and practices intended to design and plan neighborhoods throughout the country have had far-reaching effects on residential settlement patterns and subsequent green space access and quality (Rowland-Shea et al., 2020). Decades of redlining, discriminatory mortgage lending practices, and racist urban planning that used streets and highways as barriers to divide communities have preserved residential segregation and designed an interlocking system of housing and neighborhood disinvestment in which BIPOC reside (Dickinson et al., 2021; Hendricks & Van Zandt, 2021). As a result, other neighborhood amenities, including parks, parkways and green space in general were also disinvested. These practices on human health and ecological aspects of biodiversity have been substantial (Schell et al., 2020). These actions have left behind neighborhoods with decreased tree canopy coverage, more impervious surfaces, fewer parks, and increased levels of air pollution for low-income and BIPOC communities across the country (Jennings et al., 2021) (Locke et al., 2021; Nardone et al., 2021).

On the morning of May 25, 2020, during the continuing assent of COVID-19 cases and deaths, a woman named Amy Cooper was walking her dog unleashed in the Ramble of New York City's Central Park. The Ramble, an area where leashing is required, is a major center for birdwatching. Christian Cooper (no relationship to Amy Cooper) was birdwatching and noticed that Amy's dog was unleashed and running free. Christian asked Amy to leash her dog and she allegedly refused. By Christian's account he stated "look, if you're going to do what you want, I'm going to do what I want, but you're not going to like it" and beckoned her dog with a treat. At that point, Amy yelled "don't you touch my dog" and that is when Christian started to video record the incident with his cell phone (Sheehy, 2020). Amy began approaching Christian and asked him to stop recording while she also pointed her finger in his face. Considering that this incident was occurring at the height of the COVID-19 pandemic, he said to her "Please don't come close to me" (Aguilera, 2020). On the footage, Amy was caught saying "I'm calling the cops…I'm gonna tell them there's an African American man threatening my life". Subsequently, the video was posted on social media by Christian and his sister. With over 40 million views, the toxic interrelationship between race based privilege, or specifically White privilege, and nature access was exposed (Stewart, 2020).

The Centers for Disease Control and Prevention and other public health officials encouraged people to visit "parks that are close to your home", as a way to be safe against COVID-19 transmission (CDC, 2021c; Ingraham, 2020). While this pandemic revealed the true value of nature and open public spaces, it unfortunately reified the toxic presence and persistence of racism in America. As exemplified in the Christian Copper incident, for many African Americans, nature and park access is more than just proximity because often these spaces are racialized and stained with a historically complex and collective trauma experienced over time and across generations (Lee & Scott, 2016). Furthermore, it has been contested that the human relationship with nature is affected "by the justice or injustice of their social surroundings" (Smith, 2007; Turner, 2012). Many scholars, including W.E.B. DuBois, Frederick Douglass, and Booker T. Washington, have argued that slavery and the continued oppression of racism, negatively distorted the relationship and interaction with nature for African Americans" (Turner, 2012). Until the history of land acquisition and cultivation, the toxic interrelationship between oppressed modalities of identity, and the expression of wilderness as a privilege for White and elite constituencies within the United States is fully recognized and atoned, the access, connection and benefits or nature for many will continued to be defined by the past and present atrocities of this country.

References

Aguilera, J. (2020). *White woman who called police on a black man at central park apologizes, says 'I'm Not a Racist' – May 26, 2020.* TIme. Retrieved December 3, from https://time.com/5842442/amy-cooper-dog-central-park/

Annerstedt van den Bosch, M., Mudu, P., Uscila, V., Barrdahl, M., Kulinkina, A., Staatsen, B., Swart, W., Kruize, H., Zurlyte, I., & Egorov, A. I. (2016). Development of an urban green space indicator and the public health rationale. *The Scandinavian Journal of Public Health, 44*(2), 159–167. https://doi.org/10.1177/1403494815615444

Antebi, J. (n.d.). *Bridging the divide: Citizen participation versus urban renewal, and the struggle for community in Trenton, New Jersey*. Princeton University. Department of History. Retrieved November 24, from https://proces.princeton.edu/sites/cbli/files/media/jantebidobinprizeapplication.pdf

Artiga, S., Hill, L., & Haldar, S. (2021). *COVID-19 cases and deaths by race/ethnicity: Current data and changes over time – October 8, 2021*. Kaiser Family Foundation. Retrieved November 28, from https://www.kff.org/racial-equity-and-health-policy/issue-brief/covid-19-cases-and-deaths-by-race-ethnicity-current-data-and-changes-over-time/

Balseviciene, B., Sinkariova, L., Grazuleviciene, R., Andrusaityte, S., Uzdanaviciute, I., Dedele, A., & Nieuwenhuijsen, M. J. (2014). Impact of residential greenness on preschool children's emotional and behavioral problems. *The International Journal of Environmental Research and Public Health, 11*(7), 6757–6770. https://doi.org/10.3390/ijerph110706757

Berman, M. G., Kross, E., Krpan, K. M., Askren, M. K., Burson, A., Deldin, P. J., Kaplan, S., Sherdell, L., Gotlib, I. H., & Jonides, J. (2012). Interacting with nature improves cognition and affect for individuals with depression. *The Journal of Affective Disorders, 140*(3), 300–305. https://doi.org/10.1016/j.jad.2012.03.012

Bezold, C. P., Banay, R. F., Coull, B. A., Hart, J. E., James, P., Kubzansky, L. D., Missmer, S. A., & Laden, F. (2018). The relationship between surrounding greenness in childhood and adolescence and depressive symptoms in adolescence and early adulthood. *The Annals of Epidemiology, 28*(4), 213–219. https://doi.org/10.1016/j.annepidem.2018.01.009

Birkett, C. (2020). *America's revolutionary great migration*. Retrieved September 21, from https://journals.univie.ac.at/index.php/oezg/article/download/4044/3766

Blair, E. (2012). *The strange story of the man behind 'Strange Fruit'*. NPR. Retrieved July 20, from https://www.npr.org/2012/09/05/158933012/the-strange-story-of-the-man-behind-strange-fruit

Blum, E. D. (2002). Power, danger, and control: Slave women's perceptions of wilderness in the nineteenth century. *Women's Studies, 31*(2), 247–265.

Borunda, A. (2020). *How 'nature deprived' neighborhoods impact the health of people of color*. National Geographic. Retrieved November 28, from https://www.nationalgeographic.com/science/article/how-nature-deprived-neighborhoods-impact-health-people-of-color

Boustan, L. P. (2010). Was postwar suburbanization "White Flight"? Evidence from the black migration. *The Quarterly Journal of Economics, 125*(1), 417–443.

Bratman, G. N., Anderson, C. B., Berman, M. G., Cochran, B., de Vries, S., Flanders, J., Folke, C., Frumkin, H., Gross, J. J., Hartig, T., Kahn, P. H., Jr., Kuo, M., Lawler, J. J., Levin, P. S., Lindahl, T., Meyer-Lindenberg, A., Mitchell, R., Ouyang, Z., Roe, J., Scarlett, L., Smith, J. R., van den Bosch, M., Wheeler, B. W., White, M. P., Zheng, H., & Daily, G. C. (2019). Nature and mental health: An ecosystem service perspective. *Science Advances, 5*(7), eaax0903. https://doi.org/10.1126/sciadv.aax0903

Bratman, G. N., Hamilton, J. P., & Daily, G. C. (2012). The impacts of nature experience on human cognitive function and mental health. *The Annals of the New York Academy of Sciences, 1249*, 118–136. https://doi.org/10.1111/j.1749-6632.2011.06400.x

Bratman, G. N., Olvera-Alvarez, H. A., & Gross, J. J. (2021). The affective benefits of nature exposure. *Social and Personality Psychology Compass, 15*(8).

Buxton, R. T., Pearson, A. L., Allou, C., Fristrup, K., & Wittemyer, G. (2021). A synthesis of health benefits of natural sounds and their distribution in national parks. *Proceedings of the National Academy of Sciences of the United States of America, 118*(14).

Camp, S. M. H. (2002). 'I Could Not Stay There': enslaved women, truancy and the geography of everyday forms of resistance in the antebellum Plantation South. *Slavery and Abolition, 23*(3), 1–21.

CDC. (2021a). *Demographic characteristics of people receiving COVID-19 vaccinations in the United States*. Centers for Disease Control and Prevention. U.S. Department of Health and Human Services. Retrieved November 28, from https://covid.cdc.gov/covid-data-tracker/#vaccination-demographic

CDC. (2021b). *Demographic trends of COVID-19 cases and deaths in the US reported to CDC*. Centers for Disease Control and Prevention. U.S. Department of Health and Human Services. Retrieved November 28, from https://covid.cdc.gov/covid-data-tracker/#demographics

CDC. (2021c). *Participate in outdoor and indoor activities*. Centers for Disease Control and Prevention. Retrieved December 3, from https://www.cdc.gov/coronavirus/2019-ncov/daily-life-coping/outdoor-activities.html

Chandra, M. V. (2011). *The black/white wealth gap: The transgenerational effects of post-reconstruction sharecropping and racial systems on African Americans today*. University of British Columbia. Retrieved September 12, from https://open.library.ubc.ca/soa/cIRcle/collections/ubctheses/24/items/1.0072197

Chapman, R., Foderaro, L., Hwang, L., Lee, B., Muqueeth, S., Sargent, J., & Shane, B. (2021). *Parks and an equitable recovery: A Trust for Public Land special report – May 27, 2021*. Trust for Public Land. Retrieved November 28, from https://www.tpl.org/parks-and-an-equitable-recovery-parkscore-report

Cirruzzo, C. (2021). *Green spaces tied to smaller black-white gap in coronavirus rates*. U.S. News. Retrieved November 24, from https://www.usnews.com/news/health-news/articles/2021-05-04/green-spaces-tied-to-smaller-racial-gap-in-coronavirus-infections

Claborn, J. (2017). *Civil Rights and the Environment in African-American Literature, 1895–1941*. United Kingdom: Bloomsbury Publishing.

Coates, T. (2014). *The case for reparations. The Atlantic*. Retrieved September 21, from https://www.theatlantic.com/magazine/archive/2014/06/the-case-for-reparations/361631/

Cross, A. B. (2011). *Violence and social unrest: Implications of the reconstruction amendments for African Americans in the post civil war south, 1863–1877. History at digital commons, history master's thesis, 150*. History at Digital Commons, History Master's Thesis. Retrieved September 12, from https://www.semanticscholar.org/paper/Violence-and-Social-Unrest%3A-Implications-of-the-for-Cross/71556930941855eda9a98a999938b0f242a16c38

Cusick, D. (2020). *Past racist "Redlining" practices increased climate burden on minority neighborhoods – January 21, 2020*. Scientific American. Retrieved September 29, from https://www.scientificamerican.com/article/past-racist-redlining-practices-increased-climate-burden-on-minority-neighborhoods/

Davis, J. (2019). Black faces, black spaces: Rethinking African American underrepresentation in wildland spaces and outdoor recreation. *Environment and Planning E: Nature and Space, 2*(1), 89–109.

Dee, D. L., Bensyl, D. M., Gindler, J., Truman, B. I., Allen, B. G., D'Mello, T., Perez, A., Kamimoto, L., Biggerstaff, M., Blanton, L., Fowlkes, A., Glover, M. J., Swerdlow, D. L., & Finelli, L. (2011). Racial and ethnic disparities in hospitalizations and deaths associated with 2009 pandemic Influenza A

(H1N1) virus infections in the United States. *The Annals of Epidemiology, 21*(8), 623–630. https://doi.org/10.1016/j.annepidem.2011.03.002

Dickinson, K. L., Roberts, J. D., Banacos, N., Neuberger, L., Koebele, E., Blanch-Hartigan, D., & Shanahan, E. A. (2021). Structural racism and the COVID-19 experience in the United States. *Health Security, 19*(S1), S14–S26. https://doi.org/10.1089/hs.2021.0031

Duffus, M. (1999). *The Mississippi writers page: Richard Wright.* University of Mississippi. Retrieved September 19, from http://mwp.olemiss.edu//dir/wright_richard/

Dunning, S. K. (2021). *Black to nature: Pastoral return and African American culture.* University Press of Mississippi.

Egorov, A. I., Griffin, S. M., Converse, R. R., Styles, J. N., Sams, E. A., Wilson, A., Jackson, L. E., & Wade, T. J. (2017). Vegetated land cover near residence is associated with reduced allostatic load and improved biomarkers of neuroendocrine, metabolic and immune functions. *Environmental Research, 158,* 508–521. https://doi.org/10.1016/j.envres.2017.07.009

EJI. (2017). Lynching in America. At: https://eji.org/wp-content/uploads/2005/11/lynching-in-america-3d-ed-110121.pdf

Ekkel, E. D., & de Vries, S. (2017). Nearby green space and human health: Evaluating accessibility metrics. *Landscape and Urban Planning, 157,* 214–220.

Fabien, V. (2014). *African American environmental ethics: Black intellectual perspectives 1850–1965. Doctoral dissertation.* ScholarWorks@UMass Amherst. Retrieved September 14, from https://scholarworks.umass.edu/cgi/viewcontent.cgi?article=1210&context=dissertations_2

Finney, C. (2014). *Black Faces, white spaces.* The University of North Carolina Press.

Frumkin, H., Bratman, G. N., Breslow, S. J., Cochran, B., Kahn, P. H., Jr., Lawler, J. J., Levin, P. S., Tandon, P. S., Varanasi, U., Wolf, K. L., & Wood, S. A. (2017). Nature contact and human health: A research agenda. *Environmental Health Perspectives, 125*(7), 075001. https://doi.org/10.1289/EHP1663

Gates Jr., H. L. (2013a). *100 amazing facts about the Negro – How many slaves landed in the U.S.?* The African Americans – Many Rivers to Cross. Public Broadcasting Service. Retrieved August 11, from https://www.pbs.org/wnet/african-americans-many-rivers-to-cross/history/how-many-slaves-landed-in-the-us/

Gates Jr., H. L. (2013b). *How many slaves landed in the U.S.?* The African Americans: Many Rivers to Cross. PBS. Retrieved September 1, from https://www.pbs.org/wnet/african-americans-many-rivers-to-cross/history/how-many-slaves-landed-in-the-us/

Hadden, S. E. (2001). *Slave patrols: Law and violence in Virginia and the Carolinas. Harvard Historical Studies*. Harvard University Press.

Hartig, T., Mitchell, R., de Vries, S., & Frumkin, H. (2014). Nature and health. *The Annual Review of Public Health, 35*, 207–228. https://doi.org/10.1146/annurev-publhealth-032013-182443

Hendricks, M. D., & Van Zandt, S. (2021). Unequal protection revisited: Planning for environmental justice, hazard vulnerability, and critical infrastructure in communities of color. *Environmental Justice, 14*(2), 87–97.

Holland, I., DeVille, N. V., Browning, M. H., Buehler, R. M., Hart, J. E., Hipp, J. A., Mitchell, R., Rakow, D. A., Schiff, J. E., & White, M. P. (2021). Measuring nature contact: A narrative review. *The International Journal of Environmental Research and Public Health, 18*(8).

Hurston, Z. N. (1937). *Their eyes were watching god*. J. B. Lippincott & Co.

Ikei, H., Song, C., & Miyazaki, Y. (2016). Effects of olfactory stimulation by α-pinene on autonomic nervous activity. *Journal of Wood Science, 62*(6).

Ingraham, C. (2020). *Pandemic underscores how public parks shape public health – July 31, 2020*. Washington Post. Retrieved December 3, from https://www.washingtonpost.com/business/2020/07/31/public-parks-health-coronavirus/

Jennings, V., & Bamkole, O. (2019). The relationship between social cohesion and urban green space: An avenue for health promotion. *The International Journal of Environmental Research and Public Health, 16*(3), 452.

Jennings, V., Reid, C. E., & Fuller, C. H. (2021). Green infrastructure can limit but not solve air pollution injustice. *Nature Communications, 12*(1), 1–2.

Kahn, P. H. J., Weiss, T., & Harrington, K. (2018). Modeling child–nature interaction in a nature preschool: A proof of concept. *Frontiers in Psychology, 9*.

Kaplan, R., & Kaplan, S. (1989). *The experience of nature: A psychological perspective*. Cambridge University Press.

Kaplan, S. (1995). The restorative benefits of nature: Toward an integrative framework. *Journal of Environmental Psychology, 15*(3), 169–182.

Kaplan, S., & Berman, M. G. (2010). Directed attention as a common resource for executive functioning and self-regulation. *Perspectives on Psychological Science, 5*(1), 43–57.

Kellert, S. R., & Wilson, E. O. (1995). *The biophilia hypothesis*. Island Press.

KFF. (2021). *State COVID-19 data and policy actions – November 16, 2021*. Kaiser Family Foundation. Retrieved November 28, from https://www.kff.org/coronavirus-covid-19/issue-brief/state-covid-19-data-and-policy-actions/#raceethnicity

Kuo, M. (2015). How might contact with nature promote human health? Promising mechanisms and a possible central pathway. *Frontiers in Psychology, 6*(August), 1–8.

Lee, J., Park, B. J., Tsunetsugu, Y., Ohira, T., Kagawa, T., & Miyazaki, Y. (2011). Effect of forest bathing on physiological and psychological responses in young Japanese male subjects. *Public Health, 125*(2), 93–100. https://doi.org/10.1016/j.puhe.2010.09.005

Lee, L. J., & Scott, D. (2016). Bourdieu and African Americans' park visitation: The case of Cedar Hill State Park in Texas. *Leisure Sciences, 38*(5), 424–440.

Lev, E., Kahn, P. H., Jr., Chen, H., & Esperum, G. Relatively wild Urban Parks can promote human resilience and flourishing: A case study of Discovery Park, Seattle, Washington. *Frontiers in Sustainable Cities, 2*, 2.

Lipsitz, G. (2011). *How racism takes place*. Temple University Press.

Locke, D. H., Hall, B., Grove, J. M., Pickett, S. T. A., Ogden, L. A., Aoki, C., Boone, C. G., & O'Neil-Dunne, J. P. M. (2021). Residential housing segregation and urban tree canopy in 37 US Cities. *NPJ Urban Sustainability, 1*(15).

McKoy, J. (2021). *During COVID, park use was higher in majority-white neighborhoods*. Boston University. Retrieved July 20, from https://www.bu.edu/sph/news/articles/2021/during-covid-park-use-was-higher-in-majority-white-neighborhoods/

Mears, M., Brindley, P., Maheswaran, R., & Jorgensen, A. (2019). Understanding the socioeconomic equity of publicly accessible greenspace distribution: The example of Sheffield, UK. *Geoforum, 103*, 126–137.

Meidenbauer, K. L., Stenfors, C. U. D., Bratman, G. N., Gross, J. J., Schertz, K. E., Choe, K. W., & Berman, M. G. (2020). The affective benefits of nature exposure: What's nature got to do with it? *The Journal of Environmental Psychology, 72*, 101498. https://doi.org/10.10616/j.jenvp.2020.101498

Mitchell, W. M. (1860). *The under-ground railroad from slavery to freesom*. William Tweedie.

Mock, B. (2016). *For African Americans, park access is about more than just proximity*. Bloomberg CityLab. Retrieved September 17, from https://www.bloomberg.com/news/articles/2016-06-02/a-legacy-of-racism-in-america-s-parks

Muir, J., & Badè, W. F. (1916). *A thousand-mile walk to the gulf*. Houghton, Mifflin Company. http://vault.sierraclub.org/john_muir_exhibit/writings/a_thousand_mile_walk_to_the_gulf/

Napieralski, J., Sulich, C., Taylor, A., & Draus, P. (2022). Mapping the link between outdoor water footprint and social vulnerability in Metro Phoenix, AZ (USA). *Landscape and Urban Planning, 226*, https://doi.org/10.1016/j.landurbplan.2022.104498

Nardone, A., Rudolph, K. E., Morello-Frosch, R., & Casey, J. A. (2021). Redlines and greenspace: The relationship between historical redlining and 2010 greenspace across the United States. *Environmental Health Perspectives, 129*(1), 17006. https://doi.org/10.1289/EHP7495

Nesbitt, L., Meitner, M. J., Girling, C., Sheppard, S. R., & Lu, Y. (2019). Who has access to urban vegetation? A spatial analysis of distributional green equity in 10 US cities. *Landscape and Urban Planning, 181*, 51–79.

New York Times. (2020). How Decades of Racist Housing Policy Left Neighborhoods Sweltering. At: https://www.nytimes.com/interactive/2020/08/24/climate/racism-redlining-cities-global-warming.html

NPS. (2018). *Quick history of the national park service*. National Park Service. Retrieved September 29, from https://www.nps.gov/articles/quick-nps-history.htm

NPS. (2020). *The middle passage*. National Park Service. U.S. Department of Interior. Retrieved August 11, from https://www.nps.gov/articles/the-middle-passage.htm

NRPA. (2011). *Rejuvenating neighborhoods and communities through parks – A guide to success*. National Recreation and Park Association. Retrieved November 24, from https://www.nrpa.org/uploadedFiles/nrpa.org/Publications_and_Research/Research/Papers/Rejuvenating-Neighborhoods-White-Paper.pdf

Park, B. J., Tsunetsugu, Y., Kasetani, T., Kagawa, T., & Miyazaki, Y. (2010). The physiological effects of Shinrin-yoku (taking in the forest atmosphere or forest bathing): Evidence from field experiments in 24 forests across Japan. *Environmental Health and Preventive Medicine, 15*(1), 18–26. https://doi.org/10.1007/s12199-009-0086-9

Pearce, J. R., Richardson, E. A., Mitchell, R. J., & Shortt, N. K. (2010). Environmental justice and health: The implications of the socio-spatial distribution of multiple environmental deprivation for health inequalities in the United Kingdom. *Transactions of the Institute of British Geographers, 35*(4), 522–539.

PFLWN. (2017). *Humboldt Parkway makes list of 'Five places America should have saved*. Partners for a Livable Western New York. Retrieved December 2, from https://livablewny.org/2017/09/18/humboldt-parkway-list-5-places-america-saved/

Quinn, S. C., Kumar, S., Freimuth, V. S., Musa, D., Casteneda-Angarita, N., & Kidwell, K. (2011). Racial disparities in exposure, susceptibility, and access to health care in the US H1N1 influenza pandemic. *The American*

Journal of Public Health, 101(2), 285–293. https://doi.org/10.2105/AJPH.2009.188029

Ratcliffe, E., Gatersleben, B., & Sowden, P. T. (2013). Bird sounds and their contributions to perceived attention restoration and stress recovery. *Journal of Environmental Psychology, 36*, 221–228.

Reichel, P. L. (1988). Southern slave patrols as a transitional police type. *American Journal of Police, 7*(2), 51–77.

Rowland-Shea, J., Doshi, S., Edberg, S., & Fanger, R. (2020). *The nature gap: Confronting racial and economic disparities in the destruction and protection of nature in America.* Center for American Progress. Retrieved July 5, from https://www.americanprogress.org/issues/green/reports/2020/07/21/487787/the-nature-gap/

Schell, C. J., Dyson, K., Fuentes, T. L., Des Roches, S., Harris, N. C., Miller, D. S., Woelfle-Erskine, C. A., & Lambert, M. R. (2020, Sep 18). The ecological and evolutionary consequences of systemic racism in urban environments. *Science, 369*(6510) https://doi.org/10.1126/science.aay4497

Sheehy, K. (2020). *Christian Cooper recounts incident with Amy Cooper before Central Park video – May 26, 2020.* NY Post. Retrieved December 3, from https://nypost.com/2020/05/26/christian-cooper-recounts-amy-cooper-incident-before-video-footage/

SierraWild.gov. (n.d.). *The Wilderness Act.* Sierra Wild. Retrieved November 24, from https://www.sierrawild.gov/resources/wilderness-act/

Slater, S. J., Christiana, R. W., & Gustat, J. (2020). Recommendations for keeping parks and green space accessible for mental and physical health during COVID-19 and other pandemics. *Preventing Chronic Disease, 17*, E59. https://doi.org/10.5888/pcd17.200204

Smith, K. K. (2005). What is Africa to me? Wilderness in black thought, 1860–1930. *Environmental Ethics, 27*(3), 279–297.

Smith, K. K. (2007). *African American environmental thought foundations.* University Press of Kansas.

Spotswood, E. N., Benjamin, M., Stoneburner, L., Wheeler, M. M., Beller, E. E., Balk, D., McPhearson, T., Kuo, M. C., & McDonald, R. I. (2021). Nature inequity and higher COVID-19 case rates in less-green neighbourhoods in the United States. Nat Sustain. *Nature Sustainability.* https://doi.org/10.1038/s41893-021-00781-9

Stewart, N. (2020). *The White Dog Walker and #LivingWhileBlack in New York City – May 30, 2020.* NY Times. Retrieved December 3, from https://www.nytimes.com/2020/05/30/nyregion/central-park-video.html

Turner, M. W. (2012). *Hiding, hunting, and habitat: An environmental re-analysis of the slave narratives*. Boise State University Theses and Dissertations. Retrieved September 8, from https://scholarworks.boisestate.edu/cgi/viewcontent.cgi?article=1304&context=td

Ulrich, R., Simons, R., Losito, B., Fiorito, E., Miles, M., & Zelson, M. (1991). Stress recovery during exposure to natural and urban environments. *Journal of Environmental Psychology, 11*(3), 201–230.

US.Congress. (1964). *Wilderness Act (16 U.S.C. 1131 (note)*. Retrieved November 23, from https://www.fsa.usda.gov/Assets/USDA-FSA-Public/usdafiles/Environ-Cultural/wilderness_act.pdf

Wilkerson, I. (2010). *The warmth of other suns: The epic story of America's great migration*. Vintage Books.

Wilkerson, I. (2016). The Long-Lasting Legacy of the Great Migration. Smithsonian Magazine. Available at: https://www.smithsonianmag.com/history/long-lasting-legacy-great-migration-180960118/

Woodward, C. V., & McFeely, W. S. (2002). *The strange career of Jim Crow*. Oxford University Press.

Young, T. (2009). "A Contradiction in Democratice Government": W.J. Trent Jr. and the struggle to desegregate National Park campgrounds. *Environmental History, 14*(4), 651–682.

10

Experimenting with Research Creation During a Pandemic: Making Time Capsules with Girls in Sport

Adele Pavlidis, Simone Fullagar, Erin Nichols, Deborah Lupton, Kirsty Forsdike, and Holly Thorpe

Introduction

We are living through a pandemic. Many millions have already lost their lives or their livelihoods as the novel coronavirus SARS-CoV-2 spreads and mutates. Its effects are multiple, as factors such as race, ethnicity, gender, disability, geography, age, and health status intersect. Community

A. Pavlidis (✉) • S. Fullagar • E. Nichols
Griffith University, Southport, QLD, Australia
e-mail: a.pavlidis@griffith.edu.au

D. Lupton
University of New South Wales, Sydney, NSW, Australia

K. Forsdike
LaTrobe University, Melbourne, VIC, Australia

H. Thorpe
School of Health, University of Waikato, Hamilton, New Zealand

D. L. Andrews et al. (eds.), *Sport and Physical Culture in Global Pandemic Times*, Global Culture and Sport Series, https://doi.org/10.1007/978-3-031-14387-8_10

sport activities shifted from fields and clubhouses, to homes, parks, screens and the imagination during COVID-19 lockdowns. While sporting activities for some people are beginning to return to normal, for many others, lack of access or resources continue. There is a need to understand the ripple effects of this major disruption on sporting participation across regions and social groups.

As feminist scholars interested in embodiment, materiality and affect as well as in experimenting with novel approaches to social research, we have come together to explore and reveal the COVID-sport-assemblages that fell-apart/were held together/transformed over the course of the first year and a half of the pandemic in Australia. This was a period (between March 2020 and October 2021) which was characterised by a lengthy national lockdown from March 2020 followed by subsequent lockdowns of varying lengths in different cities, regions or states across the continent: implemented to contain local COVID-19 outbreaks. In particular, in our project on girls' participation in community sport during COVID-19, we were interested in thinking about how the transition to a different future has been experienced, and what in these moments will be important to carry over into future generations. In doing so, we conceived of the time capsule as an arts-based process of research-creation (Springgay & Truman, 2019) that sought to involve girls in 'making with' to produce different ways of knowing, doing and diffracting this moment in time. This project builds upon and extends international research that has used creative methods (i.e., taking photos, making cellphilms) to explore the 'distinctive experiences of girls' during the pandemic (Thompson et al., 2020).

A time capsule is traditionally a material object that contains a collection of things that are assembled with the purpose of signifying or representing a specific time and place. The idea is that once assembled, the time capsule will be put aside and opened at some point in the future, as a way of educating future generations about the time in which the capsule was made. Drawing on feminist materialisms, including DeluzoGuattarian work on affect and Baradian notions of intra-action and spacetimemattering, we saw the potential in the time capsule as a way of thinking-feeling in uncertain times. The time capsule method is future oriented, but can also support the embodied exploration of difficult to articulate affective experiences and sense-making amidst the disruption. When approached through feminist questions about embodied matters, the time capsule works with and against linear notions of time and binaries (us and them, now and then) to think about how the present might be part of the future, entangled with memories, objects and practices. In this sense, the time capsule can be mobilised as a research-creation method that provides a generative process for thinking about the future, past and present together, and for eliciting lively conversations about people's memories of past experiences or their understandings of current experiences. It also allows for multiple spaces (sporting, home, digital) to be thought together, and for the complex effects and affects of COVID-19 experiences to be materialised.

In what follows, we describe the process of implementing the time capsule method: first piloting it with our research group, and then using it with two groups of Australian girls (aged 14 to 17) who play club sport. The girls who participated in our time capsule workshops were committed to sport, but their reasons for playing were not simply to win, but for the experience of playing, of belonging and moving their bodies. The girls—one group from football (soccer) and one group from field hockey—played competitively, but as juniors their sporting lives were shaped around school, friends and parents. These were not elite nor professional athletes. As active and engaged footballers and hockey players, their sporting practice was a key site of the disruption to their everyday lives wrought by COVID restrictions.

In experimenting with the time capsule method for this project, we were interested in methodologies and processes that work to surface the affective relations that enabled or impeded girls' participation in movement practices, such as sport (Fullagar et al., 2021). Our hope is that work like this can then inform design orientated processes to improve gender equity in the return to community sport. As noted above, COVID-19 and lockdowns have disrupted and transformed sport participation and delivery at all levels and the re-turn to sport has largely focussed on managing risk (Fullagar, 2020). Through the production of a time capsule, the teenage athletes who took part in our study become part of a collaborative (re)making of the boundaries (what is in) and exclusions (what is out) of the COVID-19 pandemic. In doing so, they were returning to the past that was already being enfolded into their present experience which in turn, oriented them towards imagining their individual and collective futures beyond COVID-19. This chapter writes *with* the experiences of thinking-feeling and the affective intensities generated by the research creation process that involved researchers and participants in producing this text.

Pandemic Sport and Gender

Sport is going through a period of instability and transition, with its future unknown. Trends away from organised sport towards more individualised sports and physical activities have emerged in recent times (Harris et al., 2017), with girls' sport participation and retention an ever-present issue (Eime & Harvey, 2018). Gendered issues pertaining to inclusion, diversity, and safety that cut across topics such as wage inequality, transgender athletes and transphobia, and interpersonal violence continue to be at the forefront of research and policy in sport (Forsdike & Fullagar, 2021).

The introduction and ongoing presence of COVID-19 in our lives has exacerbated existing gender inequalities, with women experiencing even greater economic, health, unpaid care work, and gender-based violence disparities than they did prior to the pandemic (Boxhall & Morgan, 2021; United Nations, 2020). In some parts of the world women in sport were experiencing new and significant gains prior to COVID-19 such as greater recognition, accessibility, and wage parity campaigns, however professional women's sport was still considered more 'fragile' (Bowes et al., 2021). COVID-19 has highlighted the continued underlying inequalities between the genders in relation to sport, with women's sport remaining dependent upon and 'subordinate' to prioritised men's sport (Bowes et al., 2021, p. 457).

Despite an initial cessation, professional sport has been able to continue albeit without, or at least reduced, spectators. The commercial enterprise that is professional sport overcame the threat of a pandemic with extensive strategies that included biosecurity measures for sports teams in the form of sport bubbles, although incidentally mostly only for male teams (Pavlidis & Rowe, 2021). Meanwhile, community sport was shut down and opened up multiple times, disrupting the lives of all those participating. COVID-19 has therefore dramatically altered people's physical engagement with sport (Mutz & Gerke, 2021), with the lockdowns preventing access to sport facilities and social networks as experienced in organised team sport. However, emotional engagement with sport has also changed as a result of fear of leaving the house, and ultimately fear of catching the virus (Thorpe et al., 2021), as well as a decrease in motivation to participate in sport because of additional pressures during lockdown (Staley, Seal, et al., 2021a). For example, in Victoria, Australia, there was a significant downturn in physical activity during lockdown, particularly for young women aged 18-24 years (Victorian Health Promotion Foundation, 2020).

Staley, Seal, et al. (2021a) identified a paradox relating to the return to sport in Australia. Respondents to a concept mapping exercise indicated their concerns around 'staying safe whilst staying together'. Despite Sport Australia's (2020) COVID-19 Return to Sport Toolkit and the Australian Institute of Sport (2020) Framework for Rebooting of Sport (Hughes et al., 2020) offering resources to support clubs in meeting their public health requirements, Staley, Seal, et al. (2021a) found that participants' perceptions of what it means to be safe in returning were far more 'broad and complex', including fear of becoming ill from COVID-19 and injured as a result of returning to physical activity after a period away. Community sports clubs have also raised more broad and complex challenges than the toolkits and frameworks address, particularly with regards to impacts on social interactions and meeting communities' social needs when adhering to the Australian Institute of Sport's principle of '*get in, train, get out*' (Australian Institute of Sport, 2020, p.3; Staley, Randle, et al., 2021b). Physical distancing, as a strategy to prevent the spread of the virus, has had a negative impact on the athletic identity and psychological well-being of young athletes involved in team sport, although this has also been ameliorated by 'social (un)distancing' through ongoing online connection with team-mates (Graupensperger et al., 2020).

The increasing trend in individualised physical activity participation as opposed to organised sport is likely to be sustained post COVID-19 for young people (Teare & Taks, 2021). Even if they re-engage with sport and their community club, the affective relationships with their bodies, others at the club, as well as the physical infrastructure and equipment they necessarily interact with, may be forever changed (Fullagar, 2020; Fullagar & Pavlidis, 2021). As Elliott et al. (2021) argue, the consequences of COVID-19 for youth in sport can be encapsulated across '*recognition* of emotional struggle, the *reconnection* of family units and social networks, the complex issues surrounding the *re-engagement* of sport participants and volunteers, and the careful *re-imagining* of the purpose and meaning of youth sport' (p.12). Drummond et al. (2020) have gone so far as to predict a generation of Australian youth 'lost' from sport because of COVID-19. However, the future of sport post COVID-19, including its existing inequalities and affective assemblages, is essentially unknown (Fitzgerald et al., 2020). Furthermore, while research has explored the impact of the pandemic on women's sport, very little has considered the impact on girls sporting experiences.

Girls, Covid-19 and Creative Research Methods

Since the emergence of COVID-19, there has been a surge of research in youth, childhood and women's studies. However, very little research has explored the impacts of the pandemic on the everyday lives, and future hopes, of girls and young women. Of the literature focused on girls and young women's wellbeing, researchers have revealed gendered differences, with the pandemic affecting girls' mental health more than boys (Mendolia et al., 2021). Some have explored the heightened risks for girls from lower socioeconomic communities and young women experiencing the transition to adulthood while confined to the 'home'-- often an unstable and unsafe environment—without peer support and where food insecurity and gender-based violence are inescapable (Bellerose, et. al., 2020). Others are examining how teen girls' are navigating new and existing relationships (i.e., friendships, online dating) in digital environments, also with a series of safety concerns (Goldstein & Flicker, 2020).

An important feminist contribution to girl studies in pandemic times is the work of Thompson and colleagues, who explored a range of arts-based methods to contribute towards the 'positioning of girls and young women as knowers and agents of change in depicting, acting on, and reframing their circumstances during a COVID-19 lockdown' (p. 60). Building upon a growing body of research exploring creative 'girl methods' (Mitchell & Reid-Walsh, 2009), Thompson and colleagues had girls living in Quebec (Canada) taking photos and producing cell-phone based films (cellphilms) about their lived and embodied experiences of pandemic. These authors note that:

> In producing and co-analyzing visual texts together, girls and young women engaged with the worlds around them to assert their concerns and questions about the politics of the pandemic. Girls have a lot to say and feel that they should be heard, that they can contribute, and that they can make a difference.(p. 61).

Reflecting on the process of creative research with girls as intervention during the pandemic, the authors explain:

> Discussing their ideas together with other participants and the researchers helped girls and young women to address the challenges they described in relation to solitude and the heaviness, as it were, of self-isolation. Participating in the research interrupted the mundane that had set in during quarantine. Many of them first-time filmmakers, the girls liked learning how to make a cellphilm (Thompson et al., 2020, p. 59).

The pleasure and creativity in the arts-based method was appreciated by the girls in Thompson and colleagues' study. Similarly, in this chapter we describe our turn towards creative research methods with girls about their past-present-future sporting and social lives beyond pandemic times. In particular, we explore feminist new materialist reconceptualisations of the time capsule.

Reconceptualising the Time Capsule

Time capsules as collections of objects are not commonly used for social research purposes. Instead, they operate as community repositories or archives to preserve materials that are representative of a specific time and place, used in one form or another for thousands of years. The act of assembling a time capsule forces those involved to consider what elements of their cultural era are most representative or significant of the times (Jarvis, 2015). Those who assemble the time capsules usually configure a projected audience for the materials contained within, such as a future archivist or historian. Occasionally time capsules may also be constructed as warnings for future generations. One example is the AIDS Foundation Time Capsule constructed in 1990 in San Francisco, containing messages for people living 50 years into the future (Oravec, 2013).

If adopted for social research purposes, time capsules can be considered as contributing to the body of creative material methods that has been developing in scholarly literature. As Woodward explains in her book *Material Methods* (Woodward, 2019), such approaches incorporate a focus on how things elicit memories, sensations and feelings: in short, why they contain and generate significance for people. Material methods depart from a human-centred approach that focuses only on language or relationships with other people by directing attention at the everyday (or sometime extraordinary) things, spaces and place in and through which people move through their lives.

Some researchers using material methods have begun to engage with new materialism theories to consider the more-than-human dimensions of people's engagements with objects. For scholars adopting a feminist materialism approach, the affective forces, relational connections and agential capacities that are generated with and through human/nonhuman assemblages are of central interest. Objects are considered to come together with humans to create vibrancies and vitalities (Bennett, 2009). For example, exploring feminist new materialist approaches to material methods in the context of sport and physical culture, Brice and Thorpe (2021) engage an array of creative methods with objects (clothing) to explore women's more-than-human fitness practices.

Artefacts such as time capsules can be considered as 'research-creations': materials generated through research assemblages of researchers, research participants and things that can be powerful in opening capacities for understanding, thought or action. Rather than focusing on 'gathering data', scholars engaged in research-creations are interested in the vitalities and relations generated with and through these assemblages (Renold & Ringrose, 2017; Springgay & Truman, 2019).

In relation to lived experiences of the COVID-19 crisis, social researchers have been experimenting with material/arts-based methods to understand the situated contexts of the pandemic. In one example of the use of the time capsule approach, the Social Science Research Council (UK), requested prominent social researchers to select a visual artefact that would help future researchers understand the COVID crisis. These artefacts, along with interviews with the researchers about why they had chosen them, were displayed on a dedicated website (Social Science Research Council, 2021). Images included a photograph of a person taking part in a Zoom meeting, a checkout operator in a supermarket, police officers confronting a black man with his child, rolls of toilet paper, and parents waiting in a queue with their children to be allowed admitted into a school. These images, and the researchers' reflections on what they represented, bring into sharp focus how the mundane became extraordinary and consequential during the COVID crisis.

In another COVID-related example, a research team sought to configure a 'viral time capsule' as a photo-elicitation study. The resultant archive was comprised of images and texts recorded using smartphones, messaging apps and voice recording apps submitted across the globe by mental health professionals working with children about what it was like to conduct their work during the pandemic in different parts of the world. The researchers wanted to know how the health professionals coped with the challenges posed by the crisis and how clinical practice could respond in the future (Herrington et al., 2021)

A time capsule allows us to imagine a future time and the objects, ideas, places and practices that might be important to share with others. A time capsule is, in most respects, an imaginary 'thing' imbued with some power to affect future generations. Importantly, it is also, in a Baradian sense, a process of research-creation that is always an ongoing intra-action rather than a method of capturing experience 'in' time and space:

> Intra-actions are nonarbitrary, nondeterministic causal enactments through which matter-in-the-process-of-becoming is iteratively enfolded into its

> ongoing differential materialization. Such a dynamic is not marked by and exterior parameter called time, nor does it take place in a container called space. Rather, *iterative intra-actions are the dynamics through which temporality and spatiality are produced and iteratively reconfigured in the materialization of phenomena and the (re)making of material-discursive boundaries and their constitutive exclusions* (Barad, 2007, p. 179)

Put differently, the time capsule method has the potential to offer material, affective and embodied insights into timespacemattering during and beyond the pandemic.

Conceiving (and doing) the Time Capsule Methodology as a Feminist Research-Creation

As part of a larger project on the gendered relations of the return to sport during and beyond COVID, the time capsule workshops with girls were conducted after a piloting process and a series of one-on-one (online) interviews with sport administrators. Interviews are a productive and useful method, but in many ways struggle to connect with the 'affective dissonance' necessary for transformation (Hemmings, 2012). The development of the time capsule methodology was a way to question the processes of knowledge production. The open-ended nature of the research creation foregrounds the embodied and intra-active nature of subjectivity orienting the time capsule towards an activity that is at once individual and collective. Such a method orients the research encounter towards relationality while destabilising boundaries between past/future, individual/collective, researcher/researched. While it is inherently difficult to research the intangible, the potential of this method does not reside in its ability to 'capture' but rather to illuminate the instability of the boundaries between gender performance and affective memory, and importantly how these might be reconfigured otherwise. As Hemmings (2012, 151) writes, 'for feminist theorists this question of process is a political as well as methodological concern, in that it seeks to enhance knowledge and create the conditions for transformation through an engagement with others across difference'.

Towards the end of the first year of the pandemic, we gathered as a team online to think the recovery of sport in a COVID world. The notion of a time capsule was suggested by the first author as a way of materialising and opening up what the disruptions to sport did to participants and how they navigated this experience. We were granted ethics approval for our project from Griffith University (reference 2020/663). To begin experimenting with this approach and refining our methods, we undertook a pilot time capsule workshop with all authors (as well as Drs Nida Ahmad and Allison Jeffrey) via Zoom. Each person chose their desired medium for assembling objects for their own personal time capsule: including paper and pens, the Padlet platform and Pebble Pad. Run by the first author, she began the workshop with a brief preamble about time capsules which provided the following details:

> A time capsule is a container used to store a collection of present-day things and information that have been selected to represent a particular time period in history. It is then sealed until being opened at some time in the future. The objects in a time capsule can include letters, photos, art and craft work, newspaper or magazine articles, books, advertising material, videos, clothing and other everyday items. These are chosen to teach a future generation about what life was like during that historical period.

Some brief instructions were then given for the research team members to imagine they have been asked to contribute to a time capsule that the generation of Australians born today will open in 25 years' time (the year 2045). They were informed that the time capsule's contents would be objects and information that will demonstrate to this future generation what it was like to live during the COVID crisis of 2020 in Australia. We then asked: What would you put in your time capsule to demonstrate your experiences of living through the COVID crisis?

We all worked quietly on our own time capsule and once we were finished, we each shared our creation and discussed what we had chosen to 'put' 'inside'. Interestingly only a small majority of what we chose to put in were 'objects' but instead were experiences, or signifiers for feelings or sentiments we decided were important to share (words or images such as broken hearts, paths, places, scales, graphs). In some ways this may be expected due to the process used which was not really about physical objects but the creative rendering of our COVID lives through drawing, images and text. Nevertheless, it does point to the highly mediated nature of our experiences. Figure 10.1 shows some of the initial 'things' drawn/written into one of the research team's time capsules.

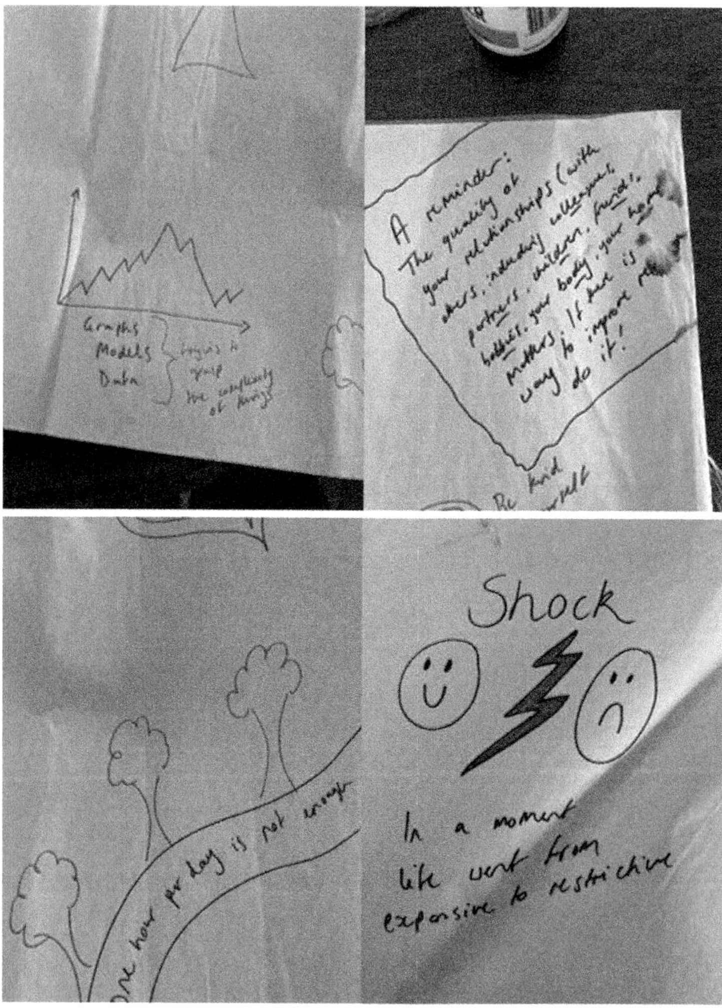

Fig. 10.1 Fragments of Adele's creative rendering of a COVID time capsule

This pilot with our research team was an important way for us to engage with the method and to see what it could 'do' to mobilise and surface different affects individually and collectively. For Simone, the time capsule was less about capturing the COVID experience for future generations in a decontextualised way, and it became more about making sense of the many, often competing affective intensities of the present. Words, photographs, fears, joys, people and non-human nature, sporting objects and places were enfolded into a Padlet gallery that evoked an affective dissonance in the face of (un)certainties (Fig. 10.2).

For Erin, although she found the method enjoyable and helpful in mapping out some of the affective dissonances she had been living through, she was notably struck by the depth of emotion it generated. Her grandmother had died during one of the lockdowns and strict restrictions in aged care meant that Erin and her family were limited in the care and presence they could provide. Erin writes,

> Tears welled up. I was embarrassed about this overwhelming display of emotion in front of scholars who I was excited to be meeting for the first time. However, it was an extremely supportive environment and this individual experience of being unable to 'make sense of it all' was made more bearable by not only having the space to 'process' but also the collective response of the group sharing similar affective dissonances.

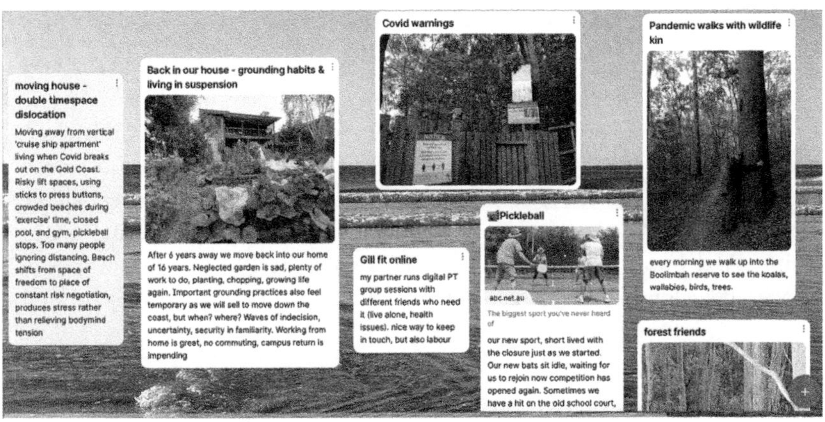
moving house - double timespace dislocation
Moving away from vertical 'cruise ship apartment' living when Covid breaks out on the Gold Coast. Risky lift spaces, using sticks to press buttons, crowded beaches during 'exercise' time, closed pool, and gym, pickleball stops. Too many people ignoring distancing. Beach shifts from space of freedom to place of constant risk negotiation, produces stress rather than relieving bodymind tension
Back in our house - grounding habits & living in suspension
After 6 years away we move back into our home of 16 years. Neglected garden is sad, plenty of work to do, planting, chopping, growing life again. Important grounding practices also feel temporary as we will sell to move down the coast, but when? where? Waves of indecision, uncertainty, security in familiarity. Working from home is great, no commuting, campus return is impending
Covid warnings
Gill fit online
my partner runs digital PT group sessions with different friends who need it (live alone, health issues). nice way to keep in touch, but also labour
Pickleball
abc.net.au
The biggest sport you've never heard of
our new sport, short lived with the closure just as we started. Our new bats sit idle, waiting for us to rejoin now competition has opened again. Sometimes we have a hit on the old school court,
Pandemic walks with wildlife kin
every morning we walk up into the Boolimbah reserve to see the koalas, wallabies, birds, trees.
forest friends

Fig. 10.2 Simone's Padlet

This struggle to 'make sense of it all' supported our desire to continue experimenting with methods that helped to surface these complex affects in a supportive process.

It was with such intentions in mind that we sought to recruit two groups of girls aged between 14 and 17, drawing on our own sporting networks in football/soccer and field hockey. We contacted the coaches/junior development officers for two clubs in Queensland with which we had networks and sent the informed consent form and information sheet which parents needed to sign. Dates were set and the clubs (one in Brisbane and one on the Gold Coast) agreed to let us use their club space. One time capsule workshop was held in December 2020 (football), and one in August 2021 (field hockey) with two members of the research team facilitating each. As with the academic pilot, the same brief information (as above) was given and then participants were given time to work on their creation. Materials included A2 sheets of white paper, and a range of coloured markers. They had between 30 to 45 minutes to work on their time capsule, after which time they each took turns at describing and explaining their work. Unlike the pilot, the workshops were held in person when many restrictions had eased and risk 'seemed' low and in-person (though social distanced) events were possible. In total eight girls aged between 14 and 17 participated: four from each sport.

Re-Turning to the Method

> So, at the start when school got cancelled, it was okay, but then as we got more through it and the end of term it started to get more stressful, and I missed schoolwork or doing something interesting, so that was quite stressful. And I was sad not to see my friends and family. But then, when school started again, I was excited to see my friends. We did a lot of social distancing. And I was sad when soccer events got cancelled but then when it started back up I was really happy. (Participant at soccer workshop)

This extended quote highlights the constant changes and adaptations the girls (and all of us) had to make over the course of 2020/2021. Lockdowns, restrictions, staged re-opening, risk management, hygiene requirements. Many sports cannot be adapted to social distancing requirements and often sport was the last community activity to reopen. As Barad (2007) writes, 'indeterminacy is never resolved once and for all' (p. 179). The time-capsule methodology materialised and made affective experiences speakable in tentative ways that included gaps and silences, what Barad (2007) calls the 'iterative differentiations of spacetimemattering' (p. 179).

In December 2020 Erin and Adele facilitated the soccer girls' workshop. Erin also plays soccer with some of the girls and brought along a soccer ball to 'get the ball rolling' and help the girls feel more comfortable. What we were asking them to do was experimental and we didn't know what the method would do. We were unsure and they were unsure. The blank page invited multiplicity, with no structure or order the girls navigated their uncertainty through some key objects—the ball, and sport, featured strongly in all their work (see example in Fig. 10.3).

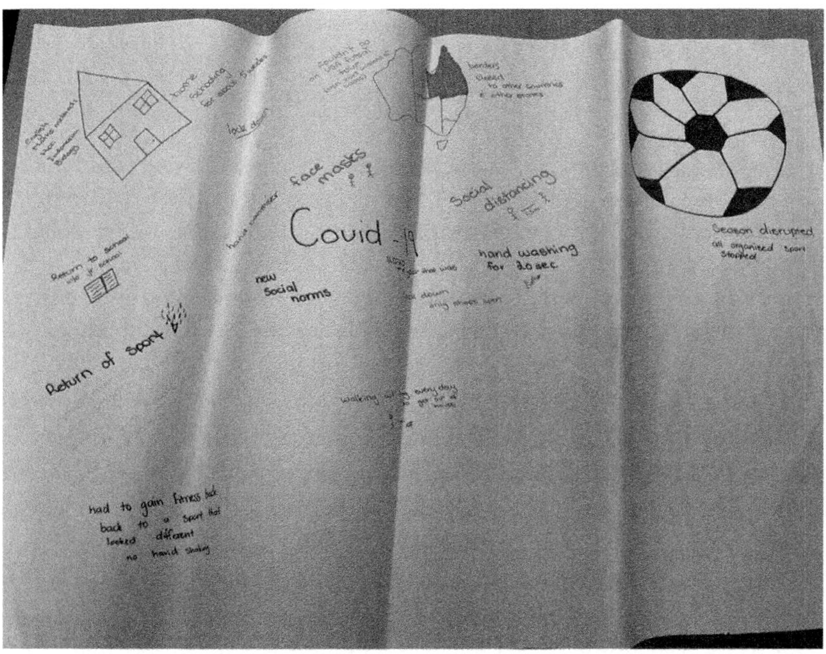

Fig. 10.3 A soccer player's time capsule

In each of the 'time capsules', the girls had drawn or written down key moments or experiences that they deemed important. As we went around the room afterwards the girls had the opportunity to explain and elaborate. School, sport and home were three locations that changed dramatically for the girls. Home was often described as a prison, being 'stuck', with a 'wall' up. Club sport was ceased or restricted, and of course school went online and was to be done at home. Returning to these spaces were often moments of affective dissonance: excitement but also feeling that things had changed, familiarity was disrupted. As one of the girls said about her return to school,

> We had like just an assembly and it was, like, you're not allowed to do any of this, you have to sit 1.5 metres away from everyone, and we all had hand sanitiser when we went into class and then when we left. So it was like a whole routine. But none of the kids followed the seating part. It was hard to do that because there's not many places to sit … You couldn't stand next to someone at the shops two minutes down the road but at school we were sitting on top of each other and they didn't even care, so it was really weird.

The same dissonance characterised the return to sport,

> It was like one person per family and stuff, so we were playing big important games and my mum was, "Oh, how did it go?" and I was like "But you were there." But she couldn't be there, obviously, because no one could come. And usually on a weekend there's thousands of people all in the same area because we all play at one place, and there was no one. It was really strange…there was none of the little kids around and it was really weird.

It was indeed a weird time that only became weirder. In August 2021, Adele and Simone facilitated the hockey girls' workshop. By this stage of the COVID-19 pandemic the Delta variant of SARS-CoV-2—a more contagious strain than the original coronavirus—had begun to spread through countries and communities, creating a new threat. Many countries had vaccinated large proportions of their population and were opening up after extended lockdowns. However, the Australian government had still not acquired anywhere near enough vaccines to inoculate large numbers of its citizens, and access to vaccines was restricted to high-risk groups only. Hence, at the time of the hockey workshops, the girls had experienced multiple short (often three days to one week) lockdowns and all different stages of restrictions with no clear path ahead. The situation was changing at a rapid pace, with weekly, sometimes daily, health advice updates and changes. At this stage, teenagers were not eligible to be vaccinated and so this was not a possibility for the girls at the time of the workshop.

Despite this uncertainty and the looming threat of lockdown and increased restrictions, the girls appeared happy—they were certainly happy to be at their club and back to training. These were 'can-do' girls (Harris, 2004).

After our initial introduction we left them to their creation, noticing an initial hesitancy with the girls glancing around at each other and holding pens in their hands and some asking, 'where to start?' Fig. 10.4 is an

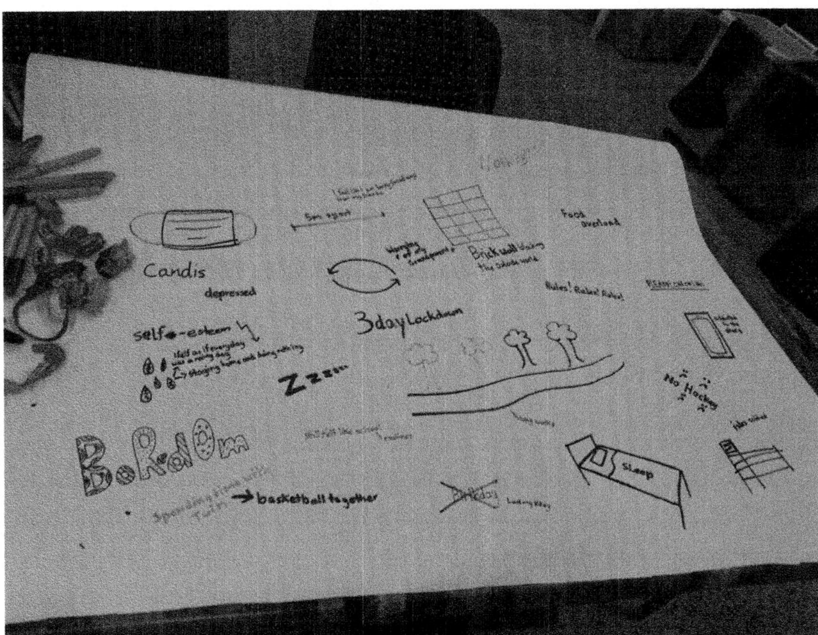

Fig. 10.4 A hockey time capsule

example of one of the hockey girls' creations. In this 'time capsule' we can see the seemingly random placement of 'things' and ideas. Larger features, such as the brick wall, or the word 'boredom' stand out. These expressions evoke affective intensities and entangled relations that characterise shifting experiences of home, study, sport and relationships, rather than a linear sense of time or bounded spatial order.

Talking about the interruptions to their hockey routine and everyday lives, a number of girls expressed a sense of affective dissonance when they began returning to the sport they loved—feeling the loss of skill, social uncertainty, a lack of embodied confidence and physical fitness. Returning to sport involved a more complex affective negotiation or transition that was able to be acknowledged through this method.

> It felt like I was free. Back into the—slowly I got back into the routine of hockey after this, hockey after that, but then after the lockdown and things were still like easing up a bit and then there was more cases, and then it went back to "Oh, we can't really do this, can't really do that." But coming back to hockey was—it felt so different because I hadn't been there, and it didn't feel like I'd been here before. And I don't know, I didn't know what to do. And then you just started getting used to things again and you had to learn everything all over again, because it felt like you didn't know anything".

Re-turning with the Time Capsule Method

Re-turning to our transcripts and images to write this chapter we noted that the girls (and us academics) were not that interested in creating a time capsule in the traditional sense, and many participants interpreted the task as a *timeline* of events rather than a time capsule. In this way, they were providing the future with a sense of what happened to them and what it was like. Interestingly, most of the girls (and the research team too) embraced non-linearity—time did not travel along a set path but shifted and changed. Moments merged together or appeared as random. Therefore, the creations made by the girls were neither a timeline per se, nor simply a list of things that happened. Instead, the time capsule process became a moment of individual and collective affective dissonance. A collection of objects, affects, entanglements and relations with humans and non-humans, including nature, siblings, places, and events. The temporal and spatial maps of living with COVID-19 were marked by affective intensities that ranged from fear, boredom, loneliness, to the pleasure of connection and anticipation of sport returning.

Words and images jarred with the happy dispositions of the girls in the moment as at times they (and even ourselves as academics entangled in these moments) struggled to articulate the negative affects of COVID lockdowns. Figure 10.5 shows Zarlee's time capsule where she tries to represent the uncertainly and non-linearity of time through a turn back on her timeline. Near the bottom of her picture she drew a simple jail cell with a person inside and the text reads, 'felt trapped inside behind the doors of my house'. Zarlee, like many others, noted that despite the 'bad impacts' of COVID, they gained better connections with their siblings and with nature.

The time capsule workshop process foregrounded the affective dissonances that participants navigated to make-sense of as they enfolded the world-changing events of 2020/2021 (at that time). The girls drew on a range of impressions, associations and imprints as they encountered the presence (and notably absence) of images, sounds, objects and people over this time.

In this way the time capsule workshops materialised the 'iterative differentiations of spacetimemattering' (Barad, 2007, p. 179). Their complex entanglements with their parents, their sport, their bodies, technology, nature, rules, and of course the virus, were visualised in their complexity. Causality was complicated and multiplicity erupted. If, as Barad (2007) argues, space, time and matter are mutually constituted, the time capsule process enabled participants to experience this in action—what mattered? When? Where? Rather than simply put in curious objects (though most did draw or write in masks and sanitiser) they took the opportunity to explore multiplicity and to express those moments of affective dissonance.

Many communicated (through images, text and words) feelings of loneliness, but found new connections. They experienced boredom, sadness, depression and even affects to their self-esteem. They wanted to get

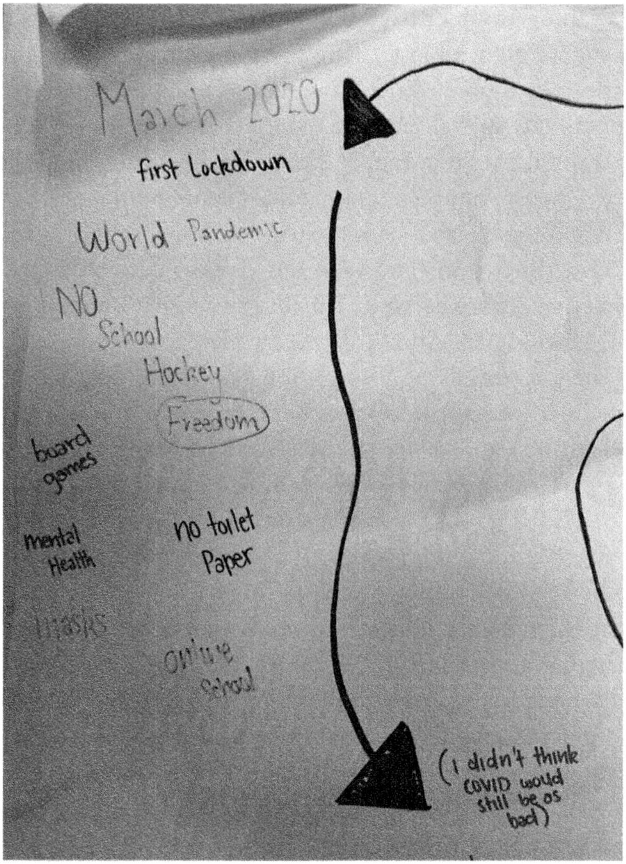

Fig. 10.5 fragment of Zarlee's hockey time capsule creative renderings

back to sport—to their bodies' feeling of flow and competencies. Sport was something they were good at and this was significantly disrupted. Feeling confident with hockey sticks and soccer balls was somewhat lost. Sport was the site of most of their friendships and a site of belonging too. This was also disrupted. As expressed in one of the soccer girls' ruminations about waiting for sport to return stating,

Because I was thinking that this was my last year of football and then I was just going to focus on school, but then I realised how important it was and how good of an outlet it is for me... The break helped me see how much I love football and how much it means to me.

The time capsule process provided an opportunity to map moments of affective dissonance. Hemmings (2012) argues that it is from moments of affective dissonance (rather than identity politics) that 'feminist politics necessarily begins from' (p. 148).

Learnings: What Can This Method *Do*

In this final re-turn to the time capsule method, we outline key learnings to consider the potential of this research creation approach for enabling more-than-human research practices and for addressing more-than-human research problems. The social contexts of COVID-19 and climate change, for example, are often framed through scientific discourses that rest upon positivist methods and quantitative representation of possible futures. Informed by feminist materialisms, research creation offers a methodological approach that moves away from these representational models that seek to measure and capture experience as a static object in time. Experimenting with the process of creating a time capsule, we have sought to develop a method that attunes us to the forces of affect that shape the complexity of experience within shifting spacetimemattering (see also Brice, 2021). This theory-method approach aims to surface the affective intensities that COVID-19 risk management guidelines largely ignore in relation to sport (non)participation.

Researching the impact of COVID-19 on girls' experience of sport called for dynamic methods to enable the exploration of how the future is continually unfolding through the past and present in ways that trouble linear notions of success and progress. We worked with the limitations and possibilities of what time capsules can 'do' as an anti-method rather than a prescribed set of steps to be imposed on a research context in the desire for neat, orderly meaning. We could not ignore the powerful affective relations—fears, sadness, joys, desires—that were implicated in the embodied learning process through which the girls and ourselves created visceral and discursive accounts of COVID impacts. As researchers, we moved with rhizomatic thinking to traversing human and more than human territories—girls' embodied lives, drawing, writing practices, sport clubs—without fixed assumptions about COVID-related sport experiences.

While we drew upon the tradition of arts-based inquiry to elicit thoughts and feelings through the time capsule approach, this was not simply a novel means of collecting 'data' to represent the inner worlds of human subjects (girls). Rather, the time capsule was a *process* for experimenting with 'making' practices that engaged girls as active producers of knowledge. Participants who engaged with the time capsule method were less interested in 'capturing' time through objects, instead they wanted to explore the multiplicity of their experience and articulate these through images and words that resonated with affect. In a similar way to the co-production of 'cellphilms' by the girls in Thompson and colleagues' study, these affective intensities included, isolation and connection, the moments of sadness and frustration, and the entangled timespace relations that also brought them some joy or reprieve from boredom or fear. As an embodied method, the time capsule became less about mapping the truth of living in COVID times for future generations and more about surfacing complex affects, moments of dissonance and difficult to articulate experiences that disrupt neoliberal notions of the progression of time, normality, identity and futurity. In both the hockey cohort and the soccer group, the girls were curious about the research process as they imagined their own future-selves. The opportunity to be part of research in a creative and supportive way opened possibilities beyond and through sport that were previously unknown to them. Specifically, they approached Adele (hockey) and Erin (soccer) after the workshops to ask questions and share how the process affected them and helped them gain clarity about the role of sport in their lives.

Working with a time capsule as a dynamic process is also a means of queering time in ways that materialise the social in the personal, as Misztal argues, 'while it is the individual who remembers, remembering is more than just a personal act' (Misztal, 2003, p. 6). Talking about and sharing time capsule drawings amongst the girls worked to materialise more than individual (and human) experiences as the transversal flows of affect produced recognisable intensities, dissonances and discomforts. As Hemmings notes, 'this may be a productive basis from which to seek solidarity with others, not based in a shared identity or on a presumption about how the other feels, but on also feeling the desire for transformation out of the experience of discomfort, and against the odds' (Hemmings, 2012, p. 158). The time capsule methodology presented in this chapter is simultaneously grounded in the lives of the individual (the girls in the study, us as academics) *and* connected to the pre-personal/transpersonal affects of the pandemic. In this way we can start to reveal the uncertainty and precariousness that has reverberated through and between subjects in diverse but similar ways.

The time capsule as a research-creation method moves beyond data collection to co-constitute new ways of learning about COVID-19 impacts through a pedagogical *relation* that emerged from a 'middle [milieu] from which it grows and which it overspills' (Deleuze & Guattari, 1987, p. 21). Rather than being a method for creating objects for a future audience, the process of making time capsules was valuable in terms of the shared and embodied production of meaning that occurred in the present, while acknowledging the entanglements with the past and future. These were moments of connection for both the sporting girls, and the academic women who engaged in this process. Moving beyond objects, they (and we) were able to begin to create something that was individual but also connected to others. It was in many ways a shared experience—we had all lived through COVID-19 isolation and lockdown and experienced disruption to our physically active lives—but our time capsules were our own interpretations of those experiences. This understanding of making-learning through the time capsule offers a method that can enable the exploration and expression of affective dissonance. Exploring dissonance through a research-creation approach respects how 'it is impossible to know in advance what apparently empty objects or insignificant tasks might generate later' (Huuki et al., 2021).

Engaging in this project has led us to consider the implications for research informed design processes that could contribute to more equitable and responsive sport policies and practices by recognising affective forces and more than human ways of knowing. Such design-oriented processes can include participatory action research that includes girls and nonbinary participants, co-creation and arts-based practices, as well as design activism to foster feminist collaborations for change. Lenskjold et al. (2015) draw upon DeluzoGuattarian ideas to articulate how design activism 'is a position in co-design engagements that strives to continuously maintain experimentation…a minor design activism challenges attempts to stabilize the initial design program around already unified agendas' (p. 67). Embracing experimentation in designing inclusive sporting futures also opens up more diverse understandings of sport participation beyond binary notions of winning and losing, success and failure, health and illness, past and future.

References

Australian Institute of Sport. (May 2020). The Australian Institute of Sport (AIS) framework for rebooting sport in a Covid-19 environment. AIS. https://www.ais.gov.au/__data/assets/pdf_file/0008/730376/35845_AIS-Framework-for-rebooting-sport_FA.pdf

Barad, K. (2007). *Meeting the universe halfway: Quantum physics and the entanglement of matter and meaning*. Duke University Press.

Bennett, J. (2009). *Vibrant Matter: A Political Ecology of Things*. Duke University Press.

Bowes, A., Lomax, L., & Piasecki, J. (2021). A losing battle? Women's sport pre- and post-COVID-19. *European Sport Management Quarterly, 21*(3), 443–461. http://ez.library.latrobe.edu.au/login?url=https://search.ebscohost.com/login.aspx?direct=true & db=s3h & AN=150936920 & site=ehost-live & scope=site

Brice, J. E. (2021). Women's bodies, femininity, and spacetimemattering: A Baradian analysis of the activewear phenomenon. *Sociology of Sport Journal, 1*(aop), 1–10.

Brice, J., & Thorpe, H. (2021). New materialisms, material methods, and the research process: A creative experiment in cutting together-apart. *Leisure Sciences*. doi:https://doi.org/10.1080/01490400.2021.1981504

Deleuze, G., & Guattari, F. (1987). *A Thousand Plateaus: Capitalism and Schizophrenia.* (B. Massumi, Trans.). Athlone Press.

Drummond, M., Elliott, S., Drummon, C., & Prichard, I. (2020). Youth sport and COVID-19: A potential generation lost. *Emerald Open Access, 2*(27), 1. https://doi.org/10.35241/emeraldopenres.13661.1

Eime, R. M., & Harvey, J. T. (2018). Sport Participation Across the Lifespan: Australian Trends and Policy Implications. In R. A. Dionigi & M. Gard (Eds.), *Sport and Physical Activity across the Lifespan: Critical Perspectives* (pp. 23–43). Palgrave Macmillan UK. https://doi.org/10.1057/978-1-137-48562-5_2

Elliott, S., Drummond, M. J., Prichard, I., Eime, R., Drummond, C., & Mason, R. (2021). Understanding the impact of COVID-19 on youth sport in Australia and consequences for future participation and retention. *BMC Public Health, 21*(1), 448–448. https://doi.org/10.1186/s12889-021-10505-5

Fitzgerald, H., Stride, A., & Drury, S. (2020). COVID-19, lockdown and (dis-ability) sport. *Managing Sport and Leisure*. https://doi.org/10.1080/23750472.2020.1776950

Forsdike, K., & Fullagar, S. (2021). Addressing the Complexity of Violence Against Women in Sport: Using the World Café Method to Inform Organizational Response. *Journal of Sport Management.*. [in press]

Fullagar, S. (2020). Recovery and regeneration in community sport: What can we learn from pausing play in a pandemic? *The Machinery of Government*, May 6, https://medium.com/the-machinery-of-government/recovery-and-regeneration-in-community-sport-9a217bd70aef

Fullagar, S., & Pavlidis, A. (2021). Thinking through the disruptive effects and affects of the coronavirus with feminist new materialism. *Leisure Sciences, 43*(1-2, 152), –159.

Fullagar, S., Pavlidis, A., Hickey-Moody, A., & Coffey, J. (2021). Embodied movement as method: Attuning to affect as feminist experimentation. *Somatechnics, 11*(2), 174–190.

Goldstein, A., & Flicker, S. (2020). "Some things just won't go back": Teen girls' online dating relationships during COVID-10. *Girlhood Studies*, doi:https://doi.org/10.3167/ghs.2020.130306

Graupensperger, S., Benson, A., Kilmer, J., & Evans, B. (2020). Social (Un) distancing: Teammate Interactions, Athletic Identity, and Mental Health of Student-Athletes During the COVID-19 Pandemic. *Jounral of Adolescent Health, 67*, 662–670. https://doi.org/10.1016/j.jadohealth.2020.08.001

Harris, A. (2004). *Future Girl: Young Women in the Twenty-First Century*. Routledge.

Harris, S., Nichols, G., & Taylor, M. (2017). Bowling even more alone: trends towards individual participation in sport. *European Sport Management Quarterly, 17*(3), 290–311. https://doi.org/10.1080/16184742.2017.1282971

Hemmings, C. (2012). Affective solidarity: Feminist reflexivity and political transformation. *Feminist Theory, 13*(2), 147–161. https://doi.org/10.1177/1464700112442643

Herrington, O., Clayton, A., Benoit, L., Prins-Aardema, C., DiGiovanni, M., Weller, I., & Martin, A. (2021). Viral time capsule: A global photo-elicitation study of child and adolescent mental health professionals during COVID-19. *Child and Adolescent Psychiatry and Mental Health, 15*(5), 1–18. https://doi.org/10.1186/s13034-021-00359-5

Hughes, D., Saw, R., Perera, N. K. P., Mooney, M., Wallett, A., Cooke, J., Coatsworth, N., & Broderick, C. (2020). The Australian Institute of Sport framework for rebooting sport in a COVID-19 environment. *Journal of Science and Medicine in Sport, 23*(7), 639–663. https://doi.org/10.1016/j.jsams.2020.05.004

Huuki, T., Kyrola, K., & Pihkala, S. (2021). What else can a crush become: Working with arts-methods to address sexual harassment in pre-teen romantic relationship cultures. *Gender and Education.* Advance online publication. doi:https://doi.org/10.1080/09540253.2021.1989384

Jarvis, W. (2015). *Time Capsules: A Cultural History*. McFarland & Company Inc.

Lenskjold, T., Olander, S., & Halse, J. (2015). Minor Design Activism: Prompting Change from Within. *Design Issues, 31*(4), 67–78.

Mendolia, S., Suziedelyte, A., & Zhu, A. (2021). *Have girls been left behind during the COVID-19 pandemic? Gender differences in pandemic effects on children's mental wellbeing*. Institute of Labor Economics. https://ftp.iza.org/dp14665.pdf

Misztal, B. (2003). *Theories of Social Remembering*. McGraw-Hill Education.

Mitchell, C., & Reid-Walsh, J. (2009). Girl Method: Placing Girl-centered Research Methodologies on the Map of Girlhood Studies. In J. Klaehn (Ed.), *Roadblocks to Equality: Women Challenging Boundaries* (pp. 214–233). Black Rose Books.

Oravec, J. (2013). Not Now, Perhaps Later: Time Capsules as Communications with the Future. *Leonardo Electronic Almanac, 19*(2), 72–81.

Pavlidis, A., & Rowe, D. (2021). The Sporting Bubble as Gilded Cage: Gendered Professional Sport in Pandemic Times and Beyond. *M/C Journal, 24*(1), 1.

Renold, E., & Ringrose, J. (2017). Selfies, relfies and phallic tagging: Posthuman participations in teen digital sexuality assemblages. *Educational Philosophy and Theory, 49*(11), 1066–1079. https://doi.org/10.1080/00131857.2016.1185686

Sport Australia. (2020). *Return to sport*. Australian Sports Commission. https://www.sportaus.gov.au/return-to-sport

Springgay, S., & Truman, S. E. (2019). Walking research-creation: QTBIPOC temporalitiesand world makings. *MAI: Feminism & Visual Culture, 4*, 1–15.

Staley, K., Seal, E., Donaldson, A., Randle, E., Forsdike, K., Burnett, Donna, Thorn, L. & Nicholson, M. (2021a) Staying safe while staying together: The COVID-19 paradox for participants returning to community-based sport in Victoria, Australia. *Australia and New Zealand Journal of Public Health* [in press]

Staley, K., Randle, E., Donaldson, A., Seal, E., Burnett, D., Thorn, L., Forsdike, K. & Nicholson, M. (2021b). Returning to sport post a COVID-19 shutdown: Understanding the challenges facing community sport clubs. *Managing Sport and Leisure*. doi:https://doi.org/10.1080/23750472.2021.1991440 [in press]

Teare, G., & Taks, M. (2021). Exploring the impact of the COVID-19 pandemic on youth sport and physical activity participation trends. *Sustainability, 13*(4), 1–15. https://doi.org/10.3390/su13041744

Thompson, J., Fraser, S., Perez, R. M., Paquette, C., & Frohlich, K. (2020). Girls and young women negotiate wellbeing during COVID-19 in Quebec. *Girlhood Studies, 13*(3), 1.

Thorpe, H., Brice, J., & Clark, M. (2021). Physical activity and bodily boundaries in times of pandemic. In D. Lupton & K. Willis (Eds.), *The Coronavirus Crisis: Social Perspectives* (pp. 39–52). Routledge.

United Nations. (9 April 2020). *Policy Brief: The Impact of COVID-19 on Women*. United Nations. https://www.unwomen.org/-/media/headquarters/attachments/sections/library/publications/2020/policy-brief-the-impact-of-covid-19-on-women-en.pdf

Victorian Health Promotion Foundation. (2020). VicHealth Coronavirus Victorian Wellbeing Impact Study. VicHealth. https://www.vichealth.vic.gov.au/-/media/ResearchandEvidence/VicHealthResearchFellows_2011/20200914_VicHealthVictorian_Coronavirus_Wellbeing_Impact_Study_Report.pdf?la=en & hash=27CB25E7BAAB7D673A81ED5CF46C5E75FB98B288

Woodward, S. (2019). *Material Methods: Researching and Thinking with Things*. University of Manchester.

11

Access & Crisis: Disrupting Ableist Definitions of Physical Activity & Culture

Sara H. Olsen, Stephanie J. Cork, Mollie M. Greenberg, and Erica Gavel

composed primarily
of water and light
this is my body
I am its light
a mere shadow remains
so that, the body is erased
excepting movement
I am all motion and
this motion is neither weak nor hideous
this motion is simply my own
—Jennifer Bartlett from *Beauty is a Verb*

S. H. Olsen (✉)
University of Maryland, College Park, MD, USA
e-mail: solsen@umd.edu

S. J. Cork • E. Gavel
Ontario Tech University, Oshawa, ON, Canada

M. M. Greenberg
University of Wisconsin, Superior, WI, USA

D. L. Andrews et al. (eds.), *Sport and Physical Culture in Global Pandemic Times*, Global Culture and Sport Series, https://doi.org/10.1007/978-3-031-14387-8_11

Jennifer Bartlett (2011), in the opening poem, presents an unnamed disability defined by movement, denying her disabled body as unwell, unruly, hideous, or weak. These perceptions of disability, throughout human history, however, have shaped the social and physical world that continues to inhibit disabled movement. Barriers that prevent disabled people from social and physical access, as understood by the social model of disability, include oppression, exclusion, neglect, and stereotyping that prevent physical and social access (Drum et al., 2009; Smeltzer, 2007). These denials of access permeate so deeply, they have become part of the social structure, a living ableism which construes disabled bodies as unwanted and even disposable. The social model of disability explains, in part, the ease in which the COVID-19 pandemic was described as *only* affecting the elderly, high risk, and disabled people. In this chapter, we describe how ableism is normalized; how it affects and exists within physical cultural arenas including sport and physical activity; the disruption of COVID-19 to physical fitness and wellness norms; how the COVID-19 pandemic highlighted the disabled body as disposable; and the ways in which COVID-19 disruptions to norms might be leveraged to support the disabled body now and in the future.

Ableism as Cultural Norm

Discrimination of individuals based solely on the presence of ability (either explicit or perceived) is called ableism (Linton, 1998). This form of discrimination toward those with disabilities also hinges on how other aspects of identity intersect with impairment, including race, class, gender, and origin, as well as characteristics and type of disability. This exclusion, though universal, is always largely dependent on culture and how disability is being defined and othered in a given space and time. Just as the global North and global South perceive and engage disability differently (Grech & Soldatic, 2016), the impact of COVID-19 on disability and cultural norms differ by region. How we address physical activity, ableism, and their intersection amid the COVID-19 pandemic in this chapter is centered in the global North (Western Europe, North America, Australia and New Zealand).

We (in the Global North) are most familiar with explicit forms of ableism. These are easy to pinpoint as examples of unequal treatment based on perceived ability level. Explicit ableism includes everything from inadequate physical access for those with mobility disabilities (lack of ramps and curb-cuts, stair-only buildings, etc.) to actively denying equal opportunities for people with all types of disabilities in education, healthcare, employment, sport, and other social institutions.

What is sometimes harder to identify is implicit ableism. While this type of discrimination is just as harmful to those with disabilities, it can be difficult to recognize and is often perpetrated without thought or bad faith. Instead of clear prejudicial acts, implicit ableism manifests in interactions with those with disabilities, particularly in the language used to describe disability and those with such conditions. Rather than being outwardly hateful in nature, some ableist rhetoric, paradoxically, most commonly comes from language used to describe our physical bodies and how they are 'meant' to function. Labeling certain bodies 'normal' and others 'disabled' for example represents a clear delineation.

Interestingly, some of the most ableist language comes from policy and directives designed to aid those with disabilities. The Americans with Disabilities Act (ADA), which influenced similar global disability policies, historically defined 'disability' as "an inherent loss or lack of function" (ADA, 1990). This definition implies not that people with disabilities may function differently than those without disabilities, but that they simply do not function as well or at all in comparison. In addition, the ADA defines the needs of disabled students and employees as separate 'accommodations,' which must be made by administration rather than putting these needs in the same category as other employee or student requirements. The stated intent of policies like the ADA is to help those with disabilities more fairly and equitably navigate the world. But use of language in these policies exceptionalizes people with disabilities. This categorizes disabled individuals as less than normal perpetuates and sustains both the explicit *and* implicit ableism. The history of ableist rhetoric is integrated in the history of physical culture, and more specifically how leisure time physical activity (LTPA) opportunities have evolved and continue to perpetuate historic expectations of physical fitness and wellness.

Ableism in Physical Culture

Physical culture encompasses all aspects of movement and activity, such as amateur and professional sport, leisure, and other forms of movement. Critical Disability Studies scholars have pointed to the ways in which ableism is embedded within normalized perceptions of health, wellness, and fitness (Cherney, 2019; Howe & Silva, 2017; Kirchner, 2010). The ongoing impacts of the global COVID-19 pandemic have put further strain on the needs and desires for physical activity, and increased pressure on performing 'good health' through conforming to public health guidelines and the pursuit of individual care and fitness. Through isolation during the pandemic, there is an expectation of self-management and regulation (care of the self). This individualization is not a new narrative, but instead has become exaggerated in the current moment, as access to communities of care and support have drastically changed. However, for many disabled individuals who live interdependent lives, this individual, neoliberal narrative excludes the reality of their lived experiences. This expectation has a long history in physical culture including sport, leisure, and rehabilitation. Disabled individuals have been excluded from such activities, unless they fit into a narrow parameter of high performance athleticism or acquired disability through combat.

Leisure time physical activities (LTPA) are those physical activities performed by choice and not related to occupational activities or activities of daily living. LTPA communities and cultures have traditionally excluded people with disabilities through pervasive structural ableism and classism and often continue to do so today. Leisure time itself has always belonged to the wealthy-- those not concerned with the toil of work for survival and whose environment and resources provided protection from disease. Social reforms and the emergence of a middle class tied to the industrial revolution at the end of the nineteenth century brought increased leisure time for middle and lower class workers (Grover, 1992). Seeking ways to spend newfound spare time, sport and recreation grew in popularity for those with traditionally less economic resources. Team sport offered new opportunities for both participation and spectatorship; and community fitness facilities (gyms, recreation centers) introduced physical activities in urban environments.

The advent of the industrial revolution clearly brought with it new opportunities for women, children, and men across a broader range of socioeconomic classes to be active. Despite the expansion of opportunities and the understanding of benefits, what kinds of bodies were expected to participate had not changed. LTPA was centered explicitly about how the body is able (Cherney, 2019). Bodies that demonstrated strength, speed, accuracy, or balance were historically elevated through LTPA. The government encouraged able-bodied men to use physical activity to maintain healthy bodies capable of waging war if called (DeOca, 2005). The disabled, and disabled men in particular, were not just excluded from this proverbial call to arms. They were not even considered.

This disconnect between policies concerning physical activity and health continued. War did come, and able-bodied men were called to defend their country multiple times throughout the twentieth century. However, many of these men did not return with the bodies with which they left. National governments were forced to reckon with the needs of men disabled through their service, who had sacrificed their bodies for their country and had earned compensation (Longmore & Umansky, 2001). As policy evolved to support wounded veterans, the benefits of physical activity for health were leveraged for the disabled, but for the specific purpose of rehabilitation. Sport and recreation became a medical tool to 'fix' disabled bodies while at the same time remaining a leisure time activity to be enjoyed by the able-bodied. Such policy allowed for the expansion of definitions of physical activity to include disabled bodies. However, given the diverging focuses, even as LTPA was redefined to account for the presence of wounded soldiers, most people with disabilities were still excluded from physical activity not based in rehabilitation (Batts & Andrews, 2011). This ableism organic to the exclusion of disabled people into sport, recreation, and fitness remains today.

Recreational spaces continue to be designed in ways that exclude those with disabilities (Corazon et al., 2019). Many parks and green spaces lack paved access. Gyms rarely invest in fitness equipment universally designed for all bodies, nor do they place the equipment to enable those with mobility-related disabilities to navigate the space in a safe manner

(Richardson et al., 2017). Personal trainers and other fitness professionals are not trained to work with bodies that don't fit their predetermined definition of 'normal.' So, when LTPA is an option for disabled people, it often keeps them out of sight. Their opportunities are relegated to segregated realms such as parasport clubs and rehabilitative settings.

Without designing LTPA spaces with accessibility in mind, the level of engagement and opportunity for engagement is limited (Sharon-David et al., 2021). It is further limited by ableist rhetoric reinforced during the COVID-19 pandemic that described the disabled body as disposable. The pandemic itself did nothing to alleviate the burdens of access from the shoulders of the disability community, instead it has exaggerated and exacerbated existing inequities, as scarce resources were reallocated and individual responsibility heightened. In fact, renowned Disability Justice activist Alice Wong has created a "High Risk Pandemic Stories: A Syllabus" which explores the myriad ways in which disability communities have been forced to reckon with the barrage of medical ableism as part of pandemic discourse and (in)action.

COVID-19 Reinforces Ableist Constructs

Beginning in 2020, the impacts of COVID-19 were heavily felt by the disabled community. Resources that were typically gained through in-person contact (such as physical therapy and medical supports) were extremely limited. COVID-19 restrictions caused a great decrease in the services that could be procured under strict social distancing guidelines around the world. Restrictions causing lack of access to traditional means of fitness and wellness also had an impact on physical activity and health for those who managed chronic pain as part of their physical disability or chronic illness (Lesser & Nienhuis, 2020). Those with learning, developmental, and other disabilities which impact learning and employment were left without the necessary support to fully participate in their classroom or workplace. The decreased availability and increased demand of virtual or remote support often amplified the existing access and procurement challenges for many individuals with disability, leading to worsening health outcomes (Dalise et al., 2021).

Access improved as nondisabled individuals increasingly required remote support. But isolation also increased. While this sense of isolation was not new for many within the disabled community, it became challenging for those who had not experienced the burdens of social distancing, medically necessary personal protective equipment, or risks associated with interaction, namely nondisabled people. The physical environment for disabled people changed and further shrunk for those already concerned with conditions secondary to their disability. The impact of restrictions has been recognized as an additional barrier for disabled people as understood through the social model of disability.

COVID-19 vs. the Social Model of Disability

The social model of disability focuses on the environmental and societal factors which cause barriers, instead of locating the deficit in the individual themselves–the latter is often referred to as the medical model of disability (Drum et al., 2009; Smeltzer, 2007). Throughout the COVID-19 pandemic, the experience of access being determined by social, cultural and public health factors has been co-opted to include nondisabled individuals. This is exemplified by nondisabled conversations around the challenges of social distancing and isolation, and other new-to-them pandemic experiences. As restrictions were lifted, nondisabled individuals return to 'normal,' but these facets of disabled life and survival will remain. While this enables the nondisabled community to perhaps better understand the struggles of people with disabilities heightened by COVID-19, it also presents a problem: equating disabled and nondisabled experiences. This false equivalency compounds with other ableist rhetoric which implies that disabled lives did not matter under these circumstances compared to nondisabled persons. Conversations continue to center on risk, normalcy and the very practical issues around medical access including personal protective equipment, vaccines, and hospitalization.

One of the most pervasive (and false) narratives that began in early 2020 was that 'only high-risk people need to worry.' This, though nonspecific in the risk discourse, pointed to the fact that only certain subsets of the population were going to contract and die from the COVID-19 virus. Older individuals and people with disabilities were simultaneously seen as the primary and only groups that would suffer. This created a sense of security in younger and 'healthy' people who often actively refused to see themselves as impacted by the threat of the pandemic. In this risk discourse (Olsen et al., 2022; Lupton, 1993), disabled bodies were negatively construed relative to the public perceptions of health.

Such discourse leads to a misunderstanding and misrepresentation of disability, sickness, and health, wherein disabled bodies are seen as inherently unwell and thus inferior, requiring increased scrutiny and surveillance as well as control to maintain their health. This is not only patronizing but severely ableist in implementation. The burden of care was not seen as necessary for the collective public health, but individualized responsibility. Adding to this confusion was the disparate labeling of certain disabilities as 'high risk' in some American states, while these conditions did not appear in other guidelines (CDC, 2021). While respiratory conditions were immediately understood to be within the high risk category, in almost all areas, other chronic health conditions as well as certain disabilities, such as Cerebral Palsy, were not considered as uniformly.

This ableist conflation of disability and health was furthered by the perception that, if only disabled individuals were controlled, everything would be 'back to normal' in no time. Financial impacts of the pandemic were seen as paramount, undermining the very real health risks for the entire population regardless of health status. These rhetorical shifts had material impacts in the dissemination of resources and prioritization of 'high risk' populations in care. Major outbreaks seen in long term care facilities throughout Canada and the United States brought these issues into stark relief (Mialkowski, 2020). Conditions for older and disabled individuals who were living in these spaces were abhorrent. Neglect led to major outbreaks and many unnecessary deaths. In this way it was made clear which lives were valued and which were seen as disposable (Lesser & Nienhuis, 2020).

Unfortunately, these trends continued as things like personal protective equipment, triage protocols, and eventually vaccine rollout, were not prioritized based on the high risk categories originally identified. Instead, rollouts were intimately tied to relationships to work and productivity. While it was clearly necessary to vaccinate and support the health and wellness of front line and essential workers, the confusing recommendations and implementation is troubling. This is especially surprising considering the ways in which disabled (and older) individuals were seen as the highest risk, but were not given the medical supplies necessary to prevent virus spread and death. This gap in policy and consideration reflects generations of gaps in understanding, and the social devaluing of, disability.

This initial inequality has led to continued confusion and misunderstanding of how the disabled communities are affected by the short and long term impacts of the global pandemic. While some disabled people are seen as a 'high risk' in terms of their capacity to contract and survive COVID-19, little assistance or attention has been paid to their unique needs (CDC, 2021; Clegg, 2021; Rodriguez, 2021). As restrictions loosen (and tighten, and loosen again) there is increased fear among people in the disabled community. Given that people with disabilities were already a neglected demographic in terms of research, support, and access, there is a very real worry that the risks many people with disabilities face with COVID-19 will no longer be taken into consideration at all. The implicit ableism that historically excluded disabled individuals from the equation of community health, wellness, and safety has again reared its head as disabled people are continually ignored or forgotten for the sake of national health needs. Considering the existing, preventable, health disparities for disabled bodies relative to able-bodied ones, it is clear that continued exclusion from medical, social, and physical cultural practices can mean life or death.

COVID-19 Disruptions to Activity Norms

The COVID-19 pandemic disrupted regular physical activity from several perspectives including regular activities in traditional gym environments connected to motivation, daily routines, and communal activities and opportunities. The disruption to routine and physical activity norms resulted in a global 27.3% decrease in average steps per day with maximal national decreases as high as 48.7% for example (Tison et al., 2020). When stratified by pre-pandemic activity level, all groups also increased sedentary behavior–behavior in a reclining, seated, or lying position requiring very low energy expenditure.

Disruptions to physical activity opportunities also meant disruptions to communities and social networks tied to those activities. As recommendations and requirements for social distancing increased, so did feelings of anxiety, loneliness and social isolation (Hwang et al., 2020; Pietrabissa & Simpson, 2020). Outlets that bolstered mental and physical health through community, fitness, and camaraderie associated with sport and LTPA were shuttered and no longer available or safe.

Fitness centers across the global North were closed for months. Whether beginning a physical activity routine for the first time or attempting to return to routine as the pandemic's timeline extended to the foreseeable future, people looked for ways to be active without putting themselves in danger associated with physical proximity to others. For example, interest in home fitness equipment increased by 547% in the months immediately following the first lockdown in the US, contributing to the shortage in the supply chain (Fitt Insider, n.d.).

Gyms and other fitness venues were required to adapt to and invest in virtual fitness, a previously niche or boutique market. Expanding social media presence, on-demand home workouts, and instructor led virtual classes enabled gyms to maintain their member base despite locking their doors. The market also responded to needs in other ways. Sales of fitness equipment that combined the ability to be active at home with the virtual presence of a trainer for example (e.g. Peloton, Tonal, and MIRROR) spiked dramatically.

Virtual training and fitness platforms had lower overhead and therefore low price barriers to participation. Fitness professionals were no longer geographically constrained in their marketing either. Acknowledging most people did not have home gyms, and to increase paid followership through apps and social media, the fitness activities being promoted changed. Fitness professionals were innovating ways to include more people—more options for body weight activities or fitness routines with minimal equipment needs; finding ways to promote and model activities with minimal space requirements; communicating health and healthy activities differently. Concepts of LTPA, with health as the prime motivator, were expanded. Fitness apps became wellness apps with opportunities for yoga, mindfulness, meditation, community, and fitness. While in quarantine, 74% of Americans said they used a fitness app with mental wellness app downloads increasing 24.4% between January and April 2020 (SensorTower, 2020). Suddenly, LTPA was—accidentally—more accessible to disabled people in terms of cost and availability. However, as COVID-19 disrupted the LTPA of those deemed able-bodied, spaces shifted to virtual realms that could be accessed while physically distanced from others. In this shift, we propose an opportunity to provide long-term, similar resources for the disabled community.

Using COVID-19 to Disrupt Ableist Norms in Physical Culture

The gap between disabled and nondisabled people that report achieving recommended or even regular physical activity has always been wide. In 2017, the Centers for Disease Control and Prevention released a study showing 42% of disabled people in the United States were sedentary, a much higher proportion than the 24.3% of those without disabilities (CDC, 2017). During the pandemic, that gap widened. Fears of contracting COVID-19, lack of information directed toward them about how to be active during the pandemic, chronic illness, and a cycle of social isolation were all voiced as reasons for inactivity (Kamyuka et al., 2020; Sepúlveda-Loyola et al., 2020; Turk & McDermott, 2020). Given the rules and policies surrounding capacity limits and available resources, many disabled people were left with less support and fewer resources.

In many cases the safest decision to prevent contagion was self-isolation, which dramatically reduced already low activity levels. Pre-pandemic, the path to activity for disabled populations was parasport gyms and clubs that mirrored Paralympic opportunities. Both were only available in select locations, in which expensive sport-specific equipment was accessible, and trained parasport coaches were engaged in the organization and training of athletes. Even if otherwise available, the more ubiquitous LTPA enjoyed by nondisabled people, such as local green spaces (rarely designed to include disabled people) and neighborhood gyms or recreation centers (both with accessibility limits and cost prohibitive fees) were closed. During the pandemic, LTPA had to be reimagined if disabled people were to be supported more broadly and beyond parochial parasport.

Several non-profit organizations have made headway in providing accessible LTPA options. In the United Kingdom, Activity Alliance has taken the lead on consolidating opportunities for easy messaging as well as communicating ways to take advantage of home workouts and Get Yourself Active, another UK nonprofit leader, has taken additional steps to bring activity to the disabled community. Activity Alliance is a national charity in England, established to be a voice for disabled people wanting to be active. They are partnered with multiple other organizations and nonprofits which allows them to be a sort of clearing house for inclusion best practices and sporting opportunities. Activity Alliance conducts an annual nationwide survey on disability and activity. During the pandemic, this survey provided data to inform evidence-based recommendations for inclusion that address physical and psychological needs as well as reduce the inequality in activity that has widened with the advent of the pandemic (Activity Alliance, 2021). The organization is active on social media, sharing home and virtual workouts and outdoor community activities sponsored by partner organizations. They have also developed a guide on how to become active or increase activity for disabled people and demonstrate some of these options through a library of examples.

Get Yourself Active is active on social media and offers articles and videos to support sport and activity opportunities for the disabled community. This organization recognized the increase in fitness videos and adapted fitness videos at the start of the pandemic but also recognized the wide range in quality of training being presented. They developed their Active at Home program in response. The first step they took was to survey and interview the disabled community to better understand needs and wants. Then they ensured all videos they developed or collated both met the stated needs and were accessible for a wide variety of disabilities. Finally, they developed a micro-grant program to provide funding to localized, user-led activity programs. These grants were intended to remove barriers to being active, such as hourly wages for additional support workers for activities and mini-buses to allow organizations to support transportation during a time when public transport was dangerous for immunocompromised individuals.

While focus on accessible and adaptive LTPA geared toward disabled people is important, some of these organizations also target their communications toward fitness professionals and policy makers. Activity Alliance, for example, offers training opportunities and easy to understand principles of inclusion, encouraging flexibility, integration of disabled perspectives in technology innovations, and accessibility considerations as regions begin to lift COVID-19 restrictions. The transition of so many gyms and leisure facilities to virtual activity classes and training has opened the door for more inclusive fitness environments that Activity Alliance has not only taken advantage of in their own programming but is using this as an opportunity to teach inclusion that can and should be sustained post-pandemic. The organization published guidelines, videos, and fact sheets for community sport and leisure providers on including disabled people and people with long-term health conditions.

In Canada, many organizations have also sought to provide more accessible LTPA. In particular, parasport organizations adapted quickly to COVID-19. The pandemic may have permanently altered the parasport landscape in an unexpected beneficial manner. Given that Canada is a very geographically spread country and suffers from a lack of parasport coaches and instructors, COVID-19 has encouraged and forced programs to happen virtually—this provided people in remote parts of the country programs previously only offered in more urban areas. Although COVID-19 has caused a lot of stress and anxiety, it may have contributed to a more accessible Canadian parasport environment. For example, the Canadian Paralympic men's and women's wheelchair basketball teams organized individual practices over Zoom. With that, coaches from around the world could coach their athletes without leaving their hometown. Moving forward, the organization plans to keep this tactic as it is effective and both cost and time efficient.

In the US, the National Center on Health, Physical Activity and Disability (NCHPAD) responded to the COVID-19 pandemic and associated extended periods at home with numerous inclusive resources including mindfulness videos, at-home fitness routines, and assistance for parents in helping their disabled children stay active without available school or community resources. NCHPAD works with partners to maintain an updated and extensive list of virtual or at home activity resources in a wide variety of interests from hip-hop dancing to kids yoga and group classes for older adults.

Along with nonprofits, for profit companies have also started to expand to serve more people. BurnAlong is a wellness app that offers pre-recorded video classes with the option to live stream a friend during the recording to add a social component to the activities. In early 2020, BurnAlong, a commercial wellness app developer, partnered with the nonprofit Crossroads Adaptive Athletic Alliance to include adaptive videos filmed and taught by certified trainers with physical disabilities. The intent through this partnership was to allow disabled users of the app to see themselves in the pre-recorded offerings and be able to adapt movements by observing trainers like them. This initiative is about providing the activity opportunity but also being aware of the social needs and developing activity that feels relevant, not just an afterthought. Preliminary research by the first author suggests BurnAlong's unique approach to physical activity decreased motivation related to physical activity and was strongly correlated with feelings of relatedness among amputees. Expanding app-based fitness offering to disabled people by disabled trainers disrupted the previously limited parasport opportunities to be active by offering peer and near-peer role models.

While there can be barriers to use based on the cost and issues with the accessibility of technology, the potential of reaching a wider audience outside of exclusive and inaccessible built environments is promising. In contrast to in-person physical activity spaces, which do not have the trainers or the equipment, virtual spaces can protect the health and safety of disabled individuals and align them with attentive trainers and on-demand training. However, this type of technology is just one form of engagement, as community-based physical cultural practices continue to emerge, and critiques of traditional physical cultural norms come under further scrutiny.

Every-body Is Welcome Here

While traditional informal and high performance movements can offer individuals with disabilities a variety of opportunities for positive health outcomes, there are limitations to these sport or rehabilitative models of movement (Howe & Silva, 2017). Physical cultural shifts which center the diverse voices and needs of othered bodies include disability as well as fat activism and body positivity. In contrast to traditional high performance and fitness aesthetics, these spaces cultivate more communal and inclusive practices, which focus on intuitive movement, nutrition and fitness.

The World Health Organization (WHO) has begun to redefine health in general as holistic experience through the development of a Social Determinants of Health model (Krahn et al., 2015). This means that physical activity and fitness are becoming recognized as a lesser part of a fulfilling and healthy life. This includes those with disabilities, who may not conform to traditional aesthetics of health. This recognition by larger health-focused institutions that healthy bodies come in a variety of shapes and sizes facilitates a better understanding of what types of physical cultural practices can affirm health. Instead of disciplining all disabled bodies which do not conform to a particular set of corporeal capacities, the model recognizes all disabled people regardless of the 'severity' of their disability are inherently valuable. Critical public health scholars have been able to shift historic understandings of disability as infirmity towards a more nuanced understanding of disability as part of a healthy life (Krahn et al., 2015). In short, using the model allows scholars to demonstrate that being disabled does not equal being sick or unhealthy.

Similarly to the scholarship and praxis of Critical Disability Studies, fat activism also proposes an alternative to mainstream health rhetoric which relies on outdated medicalized versions of physical fitness and ehealth (Justin & Jette, 2021; Lupton, 2013). This not only perpetuates ableism, but other intersections of oppression (Siebers, 2010). Critical disability scholars have linked normative expectations of aesthetic and function of bodies to colonialism, and in particular the oppressive standards of Euro-centric beauty which linked whiteness and 'good' health to wealth and status. This also has a moral valence, wherein those who are able to maintain their bodies 'properly' are good moral citizens, while those unable to conform to these ideals are seen as wounded, monstrous, or abject (Hughes, 2009; Lupton, 2013). Fat activism looks to push away from this history and instead brings forward a more inclusive view of bodies and health (Siebers, 2010).

The social isolation resulting from the COVID-19 pandemic has enabled even greater flexibility in where and how individuals are able to participate in physical activity. For example, online exercise spaces remove the gaze of instructors and other gym goers. This has increased motivation to be active—not needing to be 'beach ready' when attempting to follow a health and exercise routine—replacing traditional expectations of an able-bodied physique with the idea that movement is important, pleasurable, and can be followed at one's own pace. Many are electing to keep their online exercise regimens in lieu of the corporeal surveillance in public physical activity spaces. This privacy allows for individuals with disabled bodies to avoid the stigma, and the inaccessibility, of many fitness spaces (Kirchner, 2010). Therefore, understanding the ways in which disabled people themselves *want* to move is most important, rather than enforcing 'normalcy' (Davis, 1995).

The recentering of disabled needs and wants when it comes to physical cultural practices is not only an individualized desire but a reflection of the larger shift in discourse around what constitutes a healthy body. This shift is reflected in other public health renderings such as the Health At Every Size (HAES) model. HAES takes into account that not all bodies will have the same aesthetic when they are healthy. Thinness in particular, historically fetishized as the paramount reflection of good health, has been revealed to be less a function of individual health achievement, and more a reflection of other intersecting privileges, including whiteness and wealth (Justin & Jette, 2021). Through the lens of such understandings, there can be a reclamation of the ways in which all bodies, movements and physical cultural practices are inherently valuable. This can be linked to the larger body positivity movement, which foregrounds value in all bodies, regardless of perceived value, function or conformance to a particular aesthetic.

Body Positivity too, pushes back against traditional white, cis, heteronormative, racist, colonial and ableist ideals of physical fitness and beauty (Justin & Jette, 2021; Siebers, 2010). Historically the eugenic philosophy and entanglement of physical fitness with moral goodness precluded many from being seen as part of a 'healthy' population (Howe & Silva, 2017). This is especially true for those with disabilities, who are seen as inherently sick or unwell regardless of their actual health status. Body positivity itself has moved from generalized messaging of 'everybody is beautiful,' to messaging that says 'my body is not something for your consumption.' This shift poses resistance to traditional perceptions of fitness, beauty and wellness (Gibson, 2020). In contrast to formalized and professional physical activity and sporting spaces, much of the 'body posi' focus is community-based online and offline physical activity spaces such as Fat Girls Hiking (https://fatgirlshiking.com), Yoga for Everyone (https://www.yogaforeveryone.tv), No BS (Body Shaming) Active (https://www.nobsactive.com), Decolonizing Fitness (https://decolonizingfitness.com) and Black Girls Camping Trip (https://www.blackgirlscampingtrip.com) to name a few. Further, while these are all physical activity focused body projects, there are many that emphasize artistic or mental health outlets for those with comorbidities or complex health needs. In short, disabled individuals benefit from a more diverse understanding of what constitutes 'health' and 'physical activity' and this movement can look quite different from able-bodied and normative expectations of health, fitness and wellness. Inclusive physical cultural practices are those that bring together these ideas, and are the ways in which disabled individuals can be more fully included in all activity, improving health and wellness through more universal and equitable practice.

Progress is Important but Not Enough—Using Inertia to Motivate Change

Over the years, the global North has made significant improvements regarding inclusion and physical activity. Existing frameworks which include disability, such as fat activism and body positivity, further push the agenda for disabled bodies to be seen as more than sites of productivity, but as inherently valuable. While the number of opportunities has increased, there is still a lack of parity in all aspects of physical activity when comparing disabled people with their nondisabled counterparts. In the past, physical activity for people with disabilities was merely a means to rehabilitate from injury, with less emphasis on lifestyle, enjoyment, and recreation. Over time, physical activity programs which cater to, and even emphasize inclusion of, disabled people have become more prevalent. Moreover, technological advances in adaptive equipment have provided a wider variety of options for LTPA engagement across more and more disability types. With that, it is important to acknowledge that discrepancies remain, and LTPA is still not equitable.

Sport is an example of this need for continued improvement. While organizations expanded specific parasport programming pre-pandemic, these offerings were typically separate from the nondisabled environments and programming options. Additionally, outdoor spaces for recreation, such as parks, were not often created using universal design, and most physical education teachers currently do not have the background to successfully integrate children with disabilities into their activities. If schools do not provide a safe place or the resources for all children to become physically literate, how are they supposed to develop the skills to incorporate these habits into their daily life? Moreover, how are they supposed to pursue opportunities the same way nondisabled individuals can—socially, emotionally, and physically?

The rise of social media and the recent transition to virtual fitness has made disabled people more seen in the fitness world (French & Le Clair, 2018). Disabled athletes can follow the careers and training regimes of world-class Paralympians through social media. Athletes like Tatyana McFadden, Jonnie Peacock, and Patrick Anderson have taken the opportunity to showcase their athletic prowess and acquire sponsorships through social media. That said, top tier athletes do not provide peer models for newly disabled or newly active disabled people (Schantz & Gilbert, 2012).

A recent phenomenological study with amputees by the first author has revealed a level of intimidation or 'imposter syndrome' when Paralympians are invited to introductory sport and fitness clinics (Olsen et al., 2022). Participants were not inspired by the elite athletes and preferred to learn from peers, either in person or through online forums. The amputees in this study were in awe of and respected the Paralympians for their skills and accomplishments but were not motivated by them. Participants were more responsive to peer groups in which they were able to relate to the struggles of others and celebrate small successes. Apps like BurnAlong are attempting to provide peer modeling in a virtual environment through recruitment of certified trainers with disabilities, but their library is small and they are without brand recognition of more prevalent fitness and wellness apps. Through personal trainer education programs, Get Yourself Active, Crossroads Adaptive Athletic Alliance and NCHPAD are striving to increase the number of disabled people with certifications to train, but more often than not, they are teaching nondisabled people.

During the global pandemic much of the activity and interaction of business, education, and governance moved online. These universal in-person restrictions and online transitions offered a level of accessibility not previously available to the 15% of the global disabled population regularly forgotten, overlooked and underserved (Cork et al., 2019; Ouellette, 2019; Richards, 2008). Many individuals and entities embraced videoconferencing and web-based collaboration platforms not as an accommodation for disabled people but as a key means for continuation of work (Shew, 2020). As such, these changes have been implemented as organizational accommodations and not a means to make work and learning more accessible for disabled individuals who have been advocating for these changes for decades (Olsen et al., 2022).

Conclusion: Building Back Better?

The historic legacies of ableism continue to push the most marginalized individuals to the sidelines. As the pandemic continues to shift and change there is a clear need to pay greater attention to the needs of those who are most 'high risk,' especially disabled communities. Much of the global North has focused on a 'return' to a 'normal,' as the US, Canada, Britain, Australia and many other countries have clamored to push forward, regardless of the human cost. While new variants of COVID-19 have proven to be less severe for vaccinated individuals, the flippant approach taken by cities and countries who focus more on the economy instead of public health is deeply distressing. This desire to 'snap back' (Olsen et al., 2022) reveals the reality that ableism is still deeply embedded within our culture.

Even while being deemed disposable, disabled communities continue to push for greater recognition of the potential long term (long-haul) impacts of COVID-19. These individuals bring expertise and lived experience to the need for continued efforts towards distance, online and asynchronous education, working from home and access to physical activity and health practices through online fitness spaces and communities. Each of these shifts towards accessibility benefits disabled people, but also other marginalized groups including English language learners, immigrants and internationals abroad, and even the average employee or student who benefits from universal design for inclusion. There is an increased demand from many individuals outside the disabled community surrounding the benefits wrought by this crisis, towards greater access for all (Jenkins & Smith, 2021). Informal economies of mutual aid and collective care have proven indispensable during this time, and therefore it is the disabled community leading the way towards more inclusive physical cultural practice, both within and beyond fitness communities.

In the United States, one of the cornerstones of the current presidential administration is the Build Back Better plan. In this plan, the Administration lays the blueprint for ambitious economic relief and growth as well as improvement in infrastructure, education, housing and healthcare (The White House, n.d.). President Biden has continually stated his intent to build the United States back 'better' than it was or has been in these areas for the American people. However, given the historical lack of attention paid to accessibility concerns when the primary complainants are those with disabilities, there is real and valid concern that many of the strides in accessibility that have been made will simply disappear in this so-called post COVID-19 era and that the US will not be built back better for those with disabilities.

As disability-rights activist and author Emily Ladau stated in an interview, "… policymakers need to remember that we need to build back better because [these] systems were not accessible before the pandemic… if we're not focused on making infrastructure accessible moving forward, it's only going to be to the detriment of everybody" (Ladau, 2021). The question remains, can we truly 'build back better' if we are unable to attend to the needs of those most marginalized or impacted by the pandemic? How instead can we prevent a snapback and carry forward lessons learned to ensure that no one is left behind? Instead of a return to normal, which historically excluded and ostracized, we need to rebuild a foundation for greater support of disability communities in policies and physical cultural practices.

References

Activity Alliance (2021). *The impact of COVID 19 on disabled people* Retrieved August 2021 from https://www.activityalliance.org.uk/how-we-help/research/5854-covid19-and-disabled-people-snapshot-march-2021

Americans With Disabilities Act of 1990, Pub. L. No. 101-336, 104 Stat. 328 (1990).

Bartlett, J., Black, S. F., & Northen, M. (Eds.). (2011). *Beauty is a verb: The new poetry of disability*. Cinco Puntos Press.

Batts, C., & Andrews, D. L. (2011). 'Tactical athletes': The United States Paralympic Military Program and the mobilization of the disabled soldier/athlete. *Sport in Society, 14*(5), 553–568.

Centers for Disease Control and Prevention (CDC). (2021, June 21). *People with Disabilities*. Centers for Disease Control and Prevention. Retrieved August, 2021, from https://www.cdc.gov/coronavirus/2019-ncov/need-extra-precautions/people-with-disabilities.html.

Centers for Disease Control and Prevention (CDC), National Center on Birth Defects and Developmental Disabilities, Division of Human Development and Disability. (2017). Disability and Health Data System (DHDS) Data [online]. [accessed Oct 14, 2019]. URL: https://dhds.cdc.gov

Cherney, J. L. (2019). *Ableist rhetoric: How we know, value, and see disability (Vol. 11)*. Penn State Press.

Clegg, R. (2021, June 30) *Disabled people forgotten during Covid, BBC research reveals*. BBC News. Retrieved August 2021 from https://www.bbc.com/news/uk-57652173

Corazon, S. S., Gramkov, M. C., Poulsen, D. V., Lygum, V. L., Zhang, G., & Stigsdotter, U. K. (2019). I would really like to visit the forest, but it is just too difficult: A qualitative study on mobility disability and green spaces. *Scandinavian Journal of Disability Research, 21*(1), 1.

Cork, S. J., Douthirt-Cohen, B., Hoffman, K. M., Jaeger, P. T., & Strausser, A. (2019). Beyond Random Acts of Diversity: Ableism, academia and institutional sites of resistance. In *The Routledge Handbook of Disability Activism* (pp. 299-314). Routledge.

Dalise, S., Tramonti, F., Armienti, E., Niccolini, V., Caniglia-Tenaglia, M., Morganti, R., & Chisari, C. (2021). Psycho-social impact of social distancing and isolation due to the COVID-19 containment measures on patients with physical disabilities. *Eur J Phys Rehabil Med, 1*, 158–165.

Davis, L. J. (1995). *Enforcing normalcy: Disability, deafness, and the body*. Verso.

Deoca, J. M. (2005). "As Our Muscles Get Softer, Our Missile Race Becomes Harder": Cultural Citizenship and the "Muscle Gap". *Journal of Historical Sociology, 18*(3), 145–172.

Drum, C. E., Krahn, G. L., & Bersani, H., Jr. (2009). *Disability and public health*. American Public Health Association.

Fitt Insider (n.d.). *8 Charts That Explain COVID-19's Impact on the Fitness Industry*. Fitt Insider. Retrieved Aug 2021 from https://insider.fitt.co/covid-19-gym-fitness-app-downloads/

French, L., & Le Clair, J. M. (2018). Game Changer? Social Media, Representations of Disability and the Paralympic Games. In I. Brittain & A. Beacom (Eds.), *The Palgrave Handbook of Paralympic Studies*. Palgrave Macmillan. https://doi.org/10.1057/978-1-137-47901-3_6

Gibson, G. L. (2020). *Body Positive Babes: An Exploration of Contemporary Body Positivity Movement and the 'Acceptable' Fat Woman's Body*. PhD thesis, University of New York.

Grech, S., & Soldatic, K. (Eds.). (2016). *Disability in the Global South: The Critical Handbook*. Springer.

Grover, K. (Ed.). (1992). *Hard at Play: Leisure in America, 1840-1940*. University of Massachusetts Press.

Howe, P. D., & Silva, C. F. (2017). 'Challenging "Normalcy": Possibilities and pitfalls of Paralympic Bodies' in South African Journal for Research in Sport. *Physical Education and Recreation, 39*(1-2), 191–204.

Hughes, B. (2009). Wounded/ monstrous /abject: A critique of the disabled body in the sociological imaginary. *Disability & Society, 24*(4), 399–410.

Hwang, T. J., Rabheru, K., Peisah, C., Reichman, W., & Ikeda, M. (2020). Loneliness and social isolation during the COVID-19 pandemic. *International Psychogeriatrics, 32*(10), 1217–1220. https://doi.org/10.1017/S1041610220000988

Jenkins, F., & Smith, J. (2021). Work-from-home during COVID-19: Accounting for the care economy to build back better. *Econ. Labour Relat. Rev., 32*, 22–38. https://doi.org/10.1177/1035304620983608

Justin, T. A., & Jette, S. (2021). "That chart ain't for us": How Black women understand "obesity," health, and physical activity. *Health*. https://doi.org/10.1177/13634593211046844

Kamyuka, D., Carlin, L., McPherson, G., & Misener, L. (2020). Access to Physical Activity and Sport and the Effects of Isolation and Cordon Sanitaire During COVID-19 for People With Disabilities in Scotland and Canada. *Frontiers in Sports and Active Living, 2*, 183.

Kirchner, C. (2010). From "Survival of the Fittest" to "Fitness for All" to "Who defines fitness anyway?": 100 years of (US) sociological theory on disability. In *Disability as a fluid state*. Emerald Group Publishing Limited.

Krahn, G. L., Walker, D. K., & Correa-De-Araujo, R. (2015). Persons with disabilities as an unrecognized health disparity population. *Am J Publ Health, 105*(Suppl 2), S198–S206.

Ladau, E. (2021 March 21). Emily Ladau Interview by Johnson, H *Life After Lockdown: Experts answer viewer questions on pregnancy and parenting during the pandemic*. MSNBC. Retrieved August 2021 from https://www.msnbc.com/hallie-jackson/watch/life-after-lockdown-experts-answer-viewer-questions-on-pregnancy-and-parenting-during-the-pandemic-105026629681

Lesser, I. A., & Nienhuis, C. P. (2020). The Impact of COVID-19 on Physical Activity Behavior and Well-Being of Canadians. *Int. J. Environ. Res. Public Health, 17*, 3899.

Linton, S. (1998). *Claiming disability: Knowledge and identity*. New York University Press.

Longmore, P. K., & Umansky, L. (Eds.). (2001). *The new disability history: American perspectives (Vol. 6)*. NYU Press.

Lupton, D. (1993). Risk as moral danger: the social and political functions of risk discourse in public health. *International Journal of Health Services, 23*(3), 425–435.

Lupton, D. (2013). *Fat*. Routledge.

Mialkowski, C. J. J. (2020). *Long Term Care Facilities Ontario (3350-Op LASER 20-01 (COS))*. Joint Task Force Central.

Olsen, S. H., Cork, S. J., Anders, P., Padrón, R., Peterson, A., Strausser, A., & Jaeger, P. T. (2022). The Disability Tax and the Accessibility Tax: The Extra Intellectual, Emotional, and Technological Labor and Financial Expenditures Required of Disabled People in a World Gone Wrong...and Mostly Online.

Including Disability, 1, 51 – 86. https://ojs.scholarsportal.info/ontariotechu/index.php/id/article/view/170/78

Olsen, S. H., Aparicio, E. M., Jaeger, P. T., & Howard, D. E. (2023). Exploring Motivations to be Active among Amputees: a Phenomenological Approach. *International Journal of Qualitative Studies on Health and Well-being,* 18:1, DOI: 10.1080/17482631.2022.2143053

Ouellette, A. (2019). People with Disabilities in Human Subjects Research. In *Research Ethics.* doi:https://doi.org/10.1093/oxfordhb/9780190947750.013.50

Pietrabissa, G., & Simpson, S. G. (2020). Psychological consequences of social isolation during COVID-19 outbreak. *Frontiers in Psychology, 11,* 2201.

Richards, R. (2008). Writing the othered self: Autoethnography and the problem of objectification in writing about illness and disability. *Qualitative Health Research, 18*(12), 1717–1728.

Richardson, E. V., Smith, B., & Papathomas, A. (2017). Disability and the gym: Experiences, barriers and facilitators of gym use for individuals with physical disabilities. *Disability and Rehabilitation, 39*(19), 1950–1957.

Rodriguez, J. (2021 February 8). *'It's devastating' disabled people not prioritized in vaccine rollout, advocates say.* CTV New. Retrieved August 2021 from https://www.ctvnews.ca/health/coronavirus/it-s-devastating-disabled-people-not-prioritized-in-vaccine-rollout-advocates-say-1.5300728

Schantz, O. J., & Gilbert, K. (2012). The Paralympic Movement: Empowerment or Disempowerment for People with Disabilities? In H. J. Lenskyj & S. Wagg (Eds.), *The Palgrave Handbook of Olympic Studies.* Palgrave Macmillan. https://doi.org/10.1057/9780230367463_23

SensorTower. (2020 May 28). *Downloads of Top English-Language Mental Wellness Apps Surged by 2 Million in April Amid COVID-19 Pandemic.* SensorTower. Retrieved August 2021 https://sensortower.com/blog/top-mental-wellness-apps-april-2020-downloads

Sepúlveda-Loyola, W., Rodríguez-Sánchez, I., Pérez-Rodríguez, P., Ganz, F., Torralba, R., Oliveira, D. V., & Rodríguez-Mañas, L. (2020). Impact of social isolation due to COVID-19 on health in older people: mental and physical effects and recommendations. *The Journal of Nutrition, Health & Aging, 24*(9), 938–947.

Sharon-David, H., Siekanska, M., & Tenenbaum, G. (2021). Are gyms fit for all? A scoping review of the barriers and facilitators to gym-based exercise participation experienced by people with physical disabilities. *Performance Enhancement & Health, 9*(1), 100170.

Shew, A. (2020). Let COVID-19 expand awareness of disability tech. *Nature, 581*(7806), 9–10.

Siebers, T. (2010). *Disability Aesthetics*. University of Michigan Press.

Smeltzer, S. C. (2007). Improving the health and wellness of persons with disabilities: A call to action too important for nursing to ignore. *Nursing Outlook, 55*(4), 189–195.

The White House (n.d.) *The Build Back Better Agenda*. The White House. Retrieved August 2021 from https://www.whitehouse.gov/build-back-better/

Tison, G. H., Avram, R., Kuhar, P., Abreau, S., Marcus, G. M., Pletcher, M. J., & Olgin, J. E. (2020). Worldwide effect of COVID-19 on physical activity: A descriptive study. *Annals of Internal Medicine, 173*(9), 767–770.

Turk, M. A., & McDermott, S. (2020). The COVID-19 pandemic and people with disability. *Disability and Health Journal, 13*(3), 100944. https://doi.org/10.1016/j.dhjo.2020.100944

12

A Community of Athletic Pariahs?: Guilt, Shame, and Social Control in the COVID-19 Pandemic

Eileen Narcotta-Welp and Elizabeth S. Cavalier

Introduction

In the streets of Rome, a soothsayer warns Julius Caesar to "Beware the Ides of March." While Caesar does not take this prophecy lightly, he does ignore the warning and other omens of misfortune that eventually leads to his untimely death on the 15th of March and the collapse of the Roman Empire. Similarities can be found between this cautionary tale and the United States' response to the developing Sars-CoV-2, the potentially deadly virus that has led to the COVID-19 pandemic. Identified in early December of 2019 in Wuhan, China, the exponential growth of this novel coronavirus seemed to have no end point as it seeped beyond national borders and traveled across the globe. The soothsayer spoke this

E. Narcotta-Welp (✉)
University of Wisconsin-LaCrosse, LaCrosse, WI, USA
e-mail: enarcotta-welp@uwlax.edu

E. S. Cavalier
Georgia Gwinnett College, Lawrenceville, GA, USA

D. L. Andrews et al. (eds.), *Sport and Physical Culture in Global Pandemic Times*, Global Culture and Sport Series, https://doi.org/10.1007/978-3-031-14387-8_12

time to the world through the World Health organization (WHO) when they officially declared the COVID-19 outbreak a global pandemic. At this time, the U.S. government took little action to alert U.S. citizens to its severity; instead, taking a more dismissive approach, it minimized the virus and noted that it was no worse than the flu (Lewis, 2021).

As the U.S. government took little action to safeguard the public against COVID-19, corporations began to inconsistently and incongruously implement public health protocols as directed by WHO, national, regional, and local organizations. On March 11, 2020, the National Basketball Association (NBA) announced that it would limit access to the media because of the impending COVID-19 outbreak in the U.S. In response to the new policy, Utah Jazz center Rudy Gobert jokingly touched all of the microphones and recorders in front of him on a table at a post-workout media session minimizing the significance of the pandemic in sport and U.S. culture (ESPN, 2020). Consequently, two days later, Gobert became "patient zero" in American sports (Golliver, 2021). The positive test result sent shockwaves through the NBA, professional sport, and ultimately, American culture as "Gobert became the face of a deadly virus at a time when few people in the country knew much about it" (Golliver, 2021, para. 2). In response, the NBA suspended all play for the remainder of the 2020 season as the media painted Gobert a "pariah;" a cautionary tale of the U.S. government's ineffectual pandemic response. By March 13, 2020, all major U.S. professional leagues and the National Collegiate Athletic Association had cancelled or postponed play indefinitely. Sport, for the first time in over a century, ceased to exist.

Symbolically, March 11, 2020, can be considered the "Ides of March" for U.S. sport for this date "…tells the story of a day that started in one reality and ended in a new one" (ESPN.com, 2021). We do not want to imply a linear timeline of the impact of COVID-19 on global life, but rather, we merely want to suggest as feminist scholar Ann Kaplan (2003) did just after 9/11, that "there is an irrevocable line on both a conscious and unconscious level of 'before' and 'after'" (p. 54). As such, the past is written onto our present and inescapably connected to our future. Unlike the Roman Empire, however, U.S. sport did not crumble. Instead, sport, like the rest of civil society, had to genuflect to COVID-19 in order to stave off chaos and, ultimately, economic failure. In this current moment, the virus not only defines the rules and structures of when, how, and where organizations can compete safely, but also contextualizes the construction of dominant mediated narratives circulating through U.S. sport culture.

This is not the first pandemic in which contemporary U.S. sport has had to contend. In the late 1980s and early 1990s, three prominent athletes were diagnosed as HIV-positive—NBA basketball star Magic Johnson, Olympic Diving Champion Greg Louganis, and boxer Tommy Morrison. Dworkin and Wachs (1998) compare media coverage of Johnson and Morrision, both self-identified heterosexual men, with Louganis, a gay man, and argue that mediated surveillance of sexuality and the body reinforces hegemonic notions of masculinity and heterosexuality in professional sport spaces. Analyzing Johnson more deeply, Cole and Denny III (1994) contend that mediated narratives of heterosexual promiscuity and blackness circulated throughout U.S. sport culture after Johnson revealed his HIV status. These narratives worked to locate Acquired Immune Deficiency Syndrome (AIDS) outside of the dominant narrative of homosexuality (Nair, 2000), but contained the AIDS pandemic to the hypersexuality of heterosexual black men.

American literary scholar Susan Sontag has a different take on understanding the AIDS epidemic. Building upon her groundbreaking work in *Illness as a Metaphor* (1978), in which she analyzes the myths and metaphors surrounding cancer and how those narratives produce shame and guilt in the sick, Sontag tackled AIDS and its metaphorical constructions as a the "homosexual" disease in the U.S. While feminist scholar Paula Triechler (1987) was the first to to examine the linguistic signification of AIDS in an article titled, "AIDS, homophobia, and Biomedical Discourse," in this chapter we focus heavily on Sontag's work (1989) *AIDS and its Metaphors.* We do so as Sontag provides a broader analysis of AIDS that can be connected to our current COVID-19 pandemic well beyond the concept of "sexuality." Sontag's in-depth examination of AIDS allows us to map metaphorical conjunctures and disjunctures between AIDS and COVID-19.

In *AIDS and its Metaphors* (1989) Sontag defines metaphor through Aristotle in that a metaphor "'consists of giving the thing a name that belongs to something else'" (p. 93). She contends that one cannot think without metaphors for this linguistic apparatus is a basic form of comprehension and human expressiveness. Historically, scientific understanding and comprehension is inextricably linked to discourses containing medical metaphors. For example, the "plague" is the principal metaphor by which we understand the AIDS epidemic, and this linguistic connection reproduces feelings of paranoia, guilt, and shame. As such, AIDS and other sexually transmitted diseases are connected to morality: an individual choice between not contracting the disease (right and good) and getting the disease (wrong or evil) (Sontag, 1989).

We posit that there are parallels between the early days of the HIV-pandemic and the COVID-19 pandemic in the sports world. While COVID-19 does not carry the same stigma as sexually transmitted diseases, there are similarities between the ways in which HIV-positive and COVID-19 positive athletes were and are treated. First, we contextualize the COVID-19 pandemic. We reveal the similarities between the Reagan administration's and Trump administration's response (or lack thereof) to the HIV/AIDS epidemic and the COVID-19 pandemic, respectively. While the comparative actions of each administration to these independent crises are striking, the more significant revelation may be the ascendance of authoritarian neoliberalism. In 1981, President Reagan had a vision for the country: less government, a free market, and individualized medical care (Massih, 2016). Implementing this vision were Republican and Democratic neoliberals, alike, stripping the power of the federal government to maintain a democracy for and by the people. President Trump, as a mere vessel of this reproduced political and cultural ideology, continued to dismantle the levers of government and promote an authoritarian logic to the COVID-19 pandemic. Deep distrust for critical inquiry and the scientific community is combined with fear and misinformation leading to an "us versus them" binary that becomes impossible to bridge. Sport somehow continues to exist in this developing authoritarian neoliberal state.

Second, throughout the "pandemic year" of professional sports, there was a subtle narrative of stigma, shame, and guilt which shares remarkable similarities to those attached to the gay community through HIV/AIDS. The circulation of this narrative harkens back to the early days of the HIV-pandemic. The discourse of "deservedness" of infection, and the ways in which [mostly male] athletes were lauded for taking tournaments or seasons off to protect their [mostly female] partners and children helped reinforce the same type of hegemonic masculinity and heterosexuality that Dworkin and Wachs (1998) found in their study of HIV-positive athletes. As sports leagues rushed back to in-person competition, sport became a site of increasing medicalization. Leagues created "bubbles" and "wubbles," (some of which became the sites of "exclusive luxury camps that elevated the socio-cultural status" of athletes) (Pavlidis & Rowe, 2021), athletes were tested daily, and teams employed new technologies to enforce social distancing. With this increased medical surveillance, athletes who tested positive for COVID-19 were treated as pariahs, especially if they were doing something they "weren't supposed to" like violating the self-imposed bubble or quarantine protocols. Certain athletes (such as Rudy Gobert) were treated as though they "deserved" a COVID-19 diagnosis because they didn't take the pandemic seriously, and certain teams were punished for violations of "bubble" protocol (such as the Denver Broncos), while other teams were accommodated and treated as undeserving victims during an outbreak. This stigma was reinforced with "breaking news" about positive COVID-19 results scrolling along the bottom of 24-hour sport networks.

The majority of the chapter demonstrates the overlap in discourse between the AIDS epidemic and the COVID-19 pandemic in sport to underscore sites of cultural reproduction and power in conjunction with potential spaces of resistance in response to this global event. We want to note the slipperiness of discourses within shifting contexts. Sporting practices and the meanings it produces can only be understood when placed within the particular context in which they exist. However, this is not a one-way relationship. At the same time these sporting practices are constitutive of current social, economic, and political power relationships, sporting institutions also play a role in the constitution of the conditions and context from which they emerge (Andrews & Giardina, 2008). We elaborate on a major shift in the COVID-19 narrative: the development and distribution of the COVID-19 vaccine. This new pandemic context divided the nation, and thus, the U.S. sport world into a binary structure: vaccinated vs. unvaccinated. The narrative of stigma that so readily attached itself to those with COVID-19 shifted to, and seemingly with less empathy for, those who are unvaccinated.

A Growing Threat: Comparing Reagan and the AIDS Epidemic with Trump and the COVID-19 Pandemic

Susan Sontag (1989) points out that Stephen Gould, a historian of medical sciences, believes that AIDS should not be an event with "'a moral meaning'" for there should be "'…no message in its spread'" (p. 174). However, modern life does not allow for these phenomena to go unmediated. Language can be understood as one of the foremost approaches to understanding the contemporary social, political, and cultural milieu. Michel Foucault (1989), a poststructural theorist, argues that subjects are not only bound by language, but also part of a historical system of meaning making. Here, subjects are not able to make new meanings, but rather are simply recyclers of reconstituted meanings. The metaphors and cultural meanings of AIDS that Sontag so deftly reveals are, in fact, not new, but rather recycled forms of understanding that (re)produce power relationships in U.S. culture. The contemporary pandemic breathes new life into Songtag's work. COVID-19 allows us, once again, to recycle preconstituted meanings of disease and bifurcate reality into two distinct parts: the event and its image (Triechler, 1987).

In 1981, five young, previously healthy men from Los Angeles, California were treated for a rare lung condition. Doctors noted other unusual symptoms and that the immune systems of those afflicted were not "working." On June 5, the Center for Disease Control (CDC) reported in its *Morbidity and Mortality Weekly Report* the first case of AIDS. Moreover, on the very same day, the CDC confirmed that two of the five men had died from their symptoms (A Timeline, 2021). Misinformation and fear about those who were sick or feared to be sick were labelled as deadly "pariahs" (Casey, 2020). The virus was known to be highly transmittable through blood and "bodily fluids" from sexual acts, specifically among gay men. The neoconservative political culture of the Reagan administration flagrantly ignored the pandemic due to the uncouth and seemingly immoral implications for contracting the disease. Only after HIV/AIDS was mediated through Ryan White, a young, white, Indiana teenager, who contracted the disease through a blood transfusion for hemophilia and was refused access to an education, did President Reagan allow HIV/AIDS to slip publicly past his lips (A Timeline, 2021; Gibson, 2016).

The power of the U.S. government was peacefully transferred to the Reagan administration in January of 1981. Along with a new economic model that championed a free market and individual liberty, Reagan brought to Washington a new, conservative political ideology: the "New Right." The New Right combined religion, especially evangelical Protestantism, with an already conservative ideology undergirding U.S. culture (MacKinnon, 1992). Reaganites were obsessed with preserving the idea of the traditional family. As such, an individual only needs to be sexually prudent to reinforce American moralism through self-interest (Triechler, 1987). On the other hand, gay men, in particular, were identified as sexual deviants who threatened the sanctity of heterosexual family life and thus, individualism. These religious views clashed heavily with those held by the overwhelming secular and liberal community. Sontag (1989) argues that AIDS is seen as a disease of morality: a punishment or judgment on community. But what motivated neoconservatives was more than homophobia:

> Even more important is the utility of AIDS in pursuing one of the main activities of the so-called neoconservatives, the Kulturkampf against all that is called, for short (and inaccurately), the 1960s. A whole politics of 'the will'—of intolerance, of paranoia, of fear of political weakness—has fastened on this disease (p. 151).

The social movements of the 1960s and 1970s can be conceptualized as a strategy to redistribute cultural and economic wealth downward to the masses (Duggan, 2003). In response, the fiscal conservative bent of the Reagan administration did not seek to increase budgets for potential epidemics and actively sought to cut spending for social/medical research programs at the National Institutes of Health (NIH). Reagan's religious and economic ideology, regardless of whether it was targeted at the gay community or not, melded seamlessly into a narrative of vehement opposition to a Godless communism (Massih, 2016).

Almost forty years from the initial report on AIDS, the COVID-19 pandemic has altered global life. However, the context has shifted. In *The Terror of Neoliberalism: Authoritarianism and the Eclipse of Democracy,* Henry Giroux (2004) argues that the social contract of democracy—an emphasis on the public good and the expansion of social provisions—is under attack. He notes that democracy "has been replaced with a notion of national security based on fear, surveillance, and control rather than a culture of shared responsibility…(and) collective empowerment (has been) reduced to self-promotion and self-interest" (p. xv). Giroux makes clear the political path toward more authoritarian forms of neoliberalism was not an inevitable development, but rather a path of particular choices U.S. politicians made to national and global crises (Bruff, 2014). President Donald Trump, then, did not construct this context; instead, he captured a U.S. democracy weakened by neoliberal economic and cultural policies and used it to power his own self-interests. Along with defunding "the state," Trump employs proto-fascist strategies, such as narratives of traditionalism, nationalism, and a deep distrust of critical inquiry and media to enrich a selective popularism (Giroux, 2004). Self-identified as a "great unifer," Trump, in fact, has sowed more hate and discord into U.S culture than any other contemporary U.S. President (Diamond, 2015).

While AIDS and COVID-19 have vastly different epidemiologies, similarities can be found between the Reagan and Trump administrations in their responses to these pandemics. President Trump whole-heartedly ignored the seemingly undeniable signs of a coronavirus outbreak on U.S. shores. On February 29, 2020, John Casey (2020), a writer for the gay magazine, *The Advocate*, notes that Trump seems to have taken a page out of Reagan's epidemic playbook. Prior to the U.S. government instituting a national emergency on March 13, 2020, Trump and his administration "initially drags its feet, the president is dismissive of it, and experts fear that health…professionals and the administration are not prepared to deal with the consequences" (para. 4). Similar to Reagan's slow and anemic response to the AIDS virus in the 1980s, the United

States had another president who was disinterested, dismissive, and disoriented as to how to proceed. Linguistically, both administrations used unwieldy humor to downplay the crises. Ronald Reagan's press secretary called Lester Kinsolving, a White House correspondent and the first reporter to ask about the deadly AIDS epidemic, a "fairy" for his "interest" in the disease. On the other hand, Trump, himself, left no reporter or diplomat unscathed as he enlisted childish terms for Democrat House Representative, Nancy Peolsi (i.e. Crazy Nancy) and Democrat Senate Minority Leader, Chuck Shumer (i.e. Cryin' Chuck) or anyone who thoughtfully discussed the looming COVID-19 pandemic (Lopez, 2016).

In an attempt to further disempower the federal government apparatus and its "control" over U.S. citizens, the Trump Administration called for massive spending cuts on medical and scientific research, shrinking the NIH's annual budget from $31.8 billion to $26 billion in 2018. Most importantly, the National Institute of Allergy and Infectious Diseases (NIAID), the institute responsible for vaccine creation and the study of novel viruses, witnessed a $838 million cut from its annual budget (Collier, 2020). In conjunction with budget cuts, the Trump administration disbanded the Obama White House pandemic response team, created to track and contain the spread of Ebola and other infectious diseases in the U.S. According to Trump, private business and state governments, not the federal government, should individually oversee their own responses to a global pandemic (Tracy, 2020). Giroux (2004) argues that defunding "the state" or civil society, "...limits the vocabulary and imagery available to recognize anit-democratic forms of power, and reinforces narrow models of individual agency" (p. 49) resulting in a competition based society centered on supremacist ideology and supported by a sort of "moral" Darwinism. As the COVID-19 pandemic crossed U.S. borders, the moral implications of these decisions became clear: the federal government was not going to lead the charge against this invisible virus. This political context, instead, pitted state against state, and individual against individual leading to increased levels of cynicism and angst between those with differing opinions.

The divisions that lie within the social fabric of the United States run deep. In the twentieth century, according to Susan Sontag (1989) "...it has become almost impossible to moralize about epidemics—except those which are transmitted sexually" (p. 144). The fact that AIDS was a predominantly heterosexually transmitted disease in the African and Caribbean nations in which it emerged, but the dominant narrative continues to code it as a "gay" disease in the United States is telling. In U.S. culture, heterosexuality was deemed dominant and pure. Homosexuality was and considered to be the inverse to heterosexuality, and thus, a site of licentiousness (Triechler, 1987). As such, any subject who engages in homosexuality will be judged as "a source of pollution" and the cause of a moral plague (Sontag, 1989, p. 136). Described as the "gay plague," AIDS was initially termed GRID, the gay-related immunodeficiency disease, and those who were heterosexual and denied any same-sex sexual contact were assumed to be lying. In contrast, the media produced "innocent" victims, typically children and hemophiliacs, to underscore the immorality of the "guilty" (Fee & Krieger, 1993). Both the Reagan administration and the U.S. media interpreted the AIDS epidemic as a sign of moral laxity and political decline.

In the twenty-first century, the emergence of the COVID-19 pandemic could not be linguistically contained in a similar way to AIDS. There is no "at risk" group to blame for the downfall of a moral civil society (Lupton, 2021). Everyone is a potential victim if they inhale invisible and infected aerosol droplets. With a penchant for authoritarian and fascist power, Trump employs an old, but effective campaign of fear, otherness, and unruly xenophobia. Historically, the U.S. as an extension of colonial rule, is assumed to be "by right, free from disease" (Sontag, 1989, p.138). Disease is associated with the poor, and from the perspective of the most wealthy and powerful nation in the world, reinforces illness through the concept of the miasma. Miasma, or spontaneous generation of a disease, is associated with the dark, dirty city of a foreign, often exoticized space (Sontag, 1989; Triechler, 1987). For COVID-19, it's inauspicious beginning was first linked to the Wuhan wet market. Wet markets are where hundreds of exotic animals are housed, sold, and prepared into culinary delicacies. Lindsey Graham, U.S. Senator and fervent Trump supporter, described wet markets as "'absolutely disgusting'" reproducing longstanding narratives about Chinese hygiene, diseases, animal welfare, and food practices (Lucey, 2020, para. 1). Trump jumped on this narrative, constructing the coronavirus as the "China virus" or the "Chinese virus"

(Rogers et al., 2020). Moreover he "banned" travel from China to the United States, but only for non-U.S. citizens (Whitmore, 2020). Sontag (1989) correlates this rhetorical strategy with authoritarian ideology:

> Authoritarian political ideologies have a vested interest in promoting fear, a sense of imminence of takeover by aliens—and real diseases are useful material. Epidemic diseases usually elicit a call to ban the entry of foreigners, immigrants. And xenopobic propaganda has always depicted immigrants as bearers of disease (p. 149-150).

Trump uses an inflated sense of xenophobia to generalize the rising infection rates to an "us versus them" binary between "pure"—those of Global North, European, and white heritage—and "alien"—individuals with ties to Global South, Asian, non-white ancestry. Trump had seemingly done the impossible: he resurrected an exhausted xenophobic and fascist rhetorical strategy to moralize an invisible virus. COVID-19 became less of a battle over curing the physical symptoms of the disease, and more of a hyperbolic assault on its meaning.

U.S. sport is not exempt from this Trumpian authoritarian neoliberalism. In fact, COVID-19 in sport can serve as a site of production or reproduction of this ideology. The remainder of the chapter focuses on how sport reinforces a particular understanding of stigma and guilt surrounding illness and disease. Moreover, we explore how the medicalization of COVID-19 further stigmatize athletes and the reproduction of heterosexual norms. Finally, we articulate how the introduction of vaccines shifted the narrative of guilt and shame to the unvaccinated.

The Limits of Freedom: COVID-19, Stigma, and Social Control

Goffman (1963) explains that *stigma* is an "attribute that is deeply discrediting" (p. 3). In the early days of the COVID-19 pandemic, the disclosure of a positive COVID-19 test was both stigmatized and displayed for public consumption. As professional and collegiate sport leagues cancelled games, tournaments, and seasons entirely, athletes and celebrities represented larger cultural anxieties about the spread and potential dangers of this unknown virus. Superstar athletes (i.e.. Cristiano Ronaldo, Novak Djokavic, Tom Brady, Freddie Freeman, and Kevin Durant) and celebrities (i.e. Tom Hanks, Pink, and Idris Elba) disclosed positive COVID-19 tests reporting severe illness and in some cases hospitalization. In October 2020, the President of the United States, the First Lady, and several other members of the Trump circle, including Kelleyanne Conway and Rudy Giuliani, all tested positive for COVID-19. At the time of publication, there have been over 45 million reported positive cases, and over 720,000 deaths in the United States alone (New York Times, 2021), but athletes, entertainers, and politicians became unwelcome ambassadors for a virus that was dominating public discourse.

The stigma of a COVID-19 positive test correlates with the AIDS epidemic in regards to stigma and shame/guilt. For Sontag (1989), to contract a disease, like AIDS or COVID-19 "…is precisely to be revealed… as a member of…a community of pariahs" (p. 112). While some celebrities disclosed their positive COVID-19 status early in their infection, others waited weeks or sometimes months to disclose. Prince William tested positive for COVID-19 in April 2020, but did not discuss his positive test until November of the same year, in order to "avoid alarming the nation" (BBC, 2020, para. 4) NFL Quarterback Tom Brady tested positive in February 2021 shortly after winning the Super Bowl, but did not publicly report his diagnosis until September (Stroud, 2021). As the pandemic wore on, and as vaccines became available, the discrediting nature of the stigma was related to the public perception of the risky behaviors someone engaged in when they became exposed (Lupton, 2021). For example, when many members of the Trump inner circle tested positive after an unmasked large public gathering, the public schadenfreude was deafening. As Sontag (1989) notes, this "…unsafe behavior…is judged to be more than just a weakness. It is indulgence, delinquency" (p. 113) Other public figures who disclosed a diagnosis were spared the same treatment, especially if they followed public health measures regarding masks, social distancing, and vaccines. In contrast, some celebrities used their first-hand experience with COVID-19 to advocate for vaccinations. When disclosing his experience with COVID-19, comedian Chris Rock tweeted, "hey guys I just found out I have COVID. Trust me, you don't want this. Get vaccinated" (Yasharoff, 2021 para 2). While a stigma often accompanies a COVID-19 diagnosis, some were able to offset the discrediting nature of the diagnosis by using their celebrity platforms in order to share details of their ordeal with the public, thus, destigmatizing the disease.

While COVID-19 and HIV share little in common in terms of type of transmission, risk, or long-term effects, both share the experience of the stigma associated with contagion (Lupton, 2021). The stigma of a positive diagnosis quickly lent itself to social control. People who tested positive were directed to quarantine at home for two weeks, and the country quickly learned the language of "known exposures," "presumptive positives," and "close contacts." Workplaces, including professional sports leagues, quickly drafted policies for their employees, requiring a period of quarantine and/or multiple negative tests before returning to work. The NFL, for example, enacted a daily testing regimen for players and "essential football personnel whose job function requires direct access to players for more than 10 minutes at a time on a regular basis" (NFL.com, 2020). Land borders were closed, and countries enacted isolation, quarantine, and testing requirements prior to allowing visitors (Travel.gov, 2021). While these public health measures were necessary to try to reduce the spread and avoid burdening health care systems, some travelers resisted the efforts and attempted to skirt requirements. Most famously, a college student from the United States was sentenced to four months in prison for breaking quarantine restrictions in the Cayman Islands, later having her sentence reduced by two months (Gross & Eligon, 2020). After vaccines were widely distributed, many establishments began requiring proof of vaccination, and this again lended itself to efforts to avoid these restrictions (Smith & Chirbas, 2021).

Individual sports leagues enacted significant control measures. Both the NFL and the NBA utilized "SafeZone" tags in the 2020 season, which tracked violations of social distancing policies and also identified close contacts in the event someone tested positive for COVID-19, in addition to regular testing of all players and staff. As the NFL season began, the league scrambled to reschedule certain games when many players tested positive, but curiously required the Denver Broncos to play their scheduled game in November despite all of their quarterbacks being required to quarantine after one positive test and several close contacts (Reyes, 2021). It wasn't until a year later that the league revealed that the Broncos were punished not for testing positive for COVID-19, but for violations of the social distancing protocols. The four quarterbacks attended a video session together, but placed their tracking devices in the four corners of the room. The NFL's crackdown on the Broncos made it clear that violation of protocol, and not actual COVID-19 exposures themselves, were the impetus for punishment (Reyes, 2021).

As sports tentatively returned to competition in the late Spring of 2020, they created settings that closely resembled what Goffman (1961) referred to as "total institutions; a place of residence and work where a large number of like-situated individuals, cut off from the wider society for an appreciable period of time, together lead an enclosed, formally administered round of life" (p. xxi). In June, the WNBA began their season in a "wubble," an enclosed, totally controlled community in Bradenton, Florida, where all players, coaches, and staff quarantined and stayed isolated for 97 days as they successfully completed their season (without any COVID-19 outbreaks) (Cash, 2020). The NBA completed their regular season and the entire 2020 playoffs in a "bubble," and the NHL had a two-city bubble in Edmonton and Toronto for the entire playoffs. Both the MLS and the NWSL completed entire tournaments as a return to competition in a bubble. While these bubbles are widely cited as success stories, they also represented a shift in the dynamic between a player and his or her team. Much like with the Broncos, violation of protocol, if not actual exposure, merited punishment and suspension. Even players, who were injured in competition and had to leave the bubble to seek medical attention, were required to quarantine for several days before returning to the bubble (Hays, 2020). Like prisons, mental asylums, or army barracks, professional sport also became a total institution where every moment of an athlete's life was subject to surveillance and social control. The COVID-19 pandemic and AIDS epidemic demonstrate the "immediate *necessity* of limitation (emphasis original)" in order to curb the indulgence of certain appetites in the name of health and social well-being (Sontag, 1989, p. 166).

"I Got the Pfizer": Vaccines and Shifting Narratives of COVID-19

COVID-19, like HIV, did not affect every community in the same ways. Empirical data were clear in identifying racial and social class differences in mortality rates (see for example Bassett et al., 2020), exposure rates, test positivity, and case rates (see for example Reitsma et al., 2021). Early data suggest that members of the LGBTQ+ community were more likely to suffer negative effects of COVID-19 infection (Human Rights Campaign, 2021a). As such, the medical community must reassure "the general public," a segment of the population coded as white and heterosexual, that they are safe (Sontag, 1989; Triechler, 1987). Interestingly, public health studies confirm that LGBTQ Americans are more likely to be vaccinated than the general population (Human Rights Campaign, 2021b). Ninety-two percent of LGBTQ+ adults surveyed in the United States received at least one dose of a COVID-19 vaccination (compared to 78% of adults in the United States) (HRC2 2021, CDC, 2021).

Gay sports journalist, LZ Granderson, drew direct parallels between COVID-19 and HIV when noting high compliance with public safety measures in the gay community.

> In a community that had already been decimated once by a deadly virus, many of us in the LGBTQ community took very seriously the protocols from the Centers for Disease Control and Prevention. We had friends and loved ones who survived the AIDS epidemic but were now left at high risk because of a compromised immune system. So we wore masks. We used hand sanitizer. We did not compare life-saving measures to Nazi Germany or whatever else the party of Rep. Marjorie Taylor Greene was trying to tell us–because we knew better (Granderson, 2021, para 7).

Gay data scientist, Michael Donnelly, drew similar comparisons, "The norms of the gay community say: Share your medical history, share your risks with other people so that they can be responsible and take care of themselves as well…that came with years of practice within the community, particularly around HIV and AIDS." (Simmons-Duffin, 2021). Members of the LGBTQ+ community had seen a pandemic before that included both the stigma of the diagnosis and the public disclosures and behavior modification necessary to protect the public from a contagious disease (Lupton, 1993). Notably, the NIAID had the same director through both pandemics, Dr. Anthony Fauci, who was appointed to the position in 1984, and remains in the role nearly 40 years later.

As new experimental medications emerged to fight HIV/AIDS, Dr. Fauci and NIAID often found themselves in the crosshairs of political activists fighting to provide quicker and easier access to these lifesaving drugs. Under the name "AIDS Coalition to Unleash Power (ACT-UP), activists fought with the FDA and the NIAID to push for more clinical trials, and later, to make medications more affordable. Members of ACT-UP employed strategies such as "die-ins," and on at least one occasion, taking over the New York Stock Exchange in order to protest the cost of the lifesaving drug AZT (McGuill, 2020). As Dr. Fauci became a household name during the early days of the COVID-19 pandemic, AIDS activists remembered their mostly amiable relationship with him.

> [Fauci] dramatically loosened HIV-drug clinical trial requirements so that a far greater number of desperate patients could try new compounds (an approach called 'parallel tracking'), expanded research on HIV/AIDS and its treatment in underrepresented women and/or people of color, and gave activists and people living with HIV seats at the table of the planning committee of the AIDS Clinical Trials Group (ACTG)…[he] also played a key role in getting the federal research apparatus to incorporate those recommendations, in what amounted to perhaps the first time that federal health bureaucrats acceded almost fully to community and activist demands" (Murphy, 2020, para 9 -10).

In the early days of the COVID-19 pandemic, Dr. Fauci once again became a household name. He advocated for social distancing, hand washing, and mask wearing (once it became clear there were enough masks for medical workers). However, his common sense approach to combating the virus led to public clashes with President Trump, and he was sidelined in favor of Dr. Deborah Birx, who did not publicly intervene as the President mulled whether bleach injections or UV light could kill the virus instead (Gittleson, 2021). As Sontag (1989) notes, "The disparagement of effective, scientific medicine for offering treatments that are *merely* illness-specific, and likely to be toxic, is a recurrent misconjecture of opinion that regards itself as enlightened" (p. 124). While Trump spent much of his pre-pandemic Presidency engaged in public disagreements with professional athletes such as Lebron James and Megan Rapinoe, one of his early priorities was to return to a "normalcy" of live sporting events. He publicly complained that we "have to get our sports back," noting that he was "tired of watching baseball games that are 14 years old" (Lutz, 2020). Dissatisfied with the speed at which COVID-19 was "disappearing," Trump publicly threw all of his political capital behind "Operation Warp Speed," a public-private partnership between the federal government and pharmaceutical companies that incentivized clinical trials and the rapid development of vaccines to combat coronavirus (Lupkin, 2021). By August 2020, Pfizer and Moderna announced high success rates for their mRNA vaccines (along with other manufacturers including Johnson & Johnson and AstraZeneca) (Grady, 2020). Four decades earlier, ACT-Up activists pushed the medical bureaucracy to eliminate red tape to bring life saving medication to market quickly, and through the work of those activists, practices such as "Emergency Use Authorization" for new medications became possible, though the first federal usage was post-9/11 to approve the emergency use of a drug to fight anthrax (Gandhi, 2021). The country reaped the benefits of earlier political activism through the quick development and production of several effective COVID-19 vaccines, all of which were provided free of charge to the American public.

By the summer of 2021, the United States appeared to have turned a corner on the COVID-19 pandemic. Case numbers had declined, hospitalizations and deaths decreased dramatically, and the number of Americans getting at least one vaccine dose was continuing to increase (CDC, 2021). However, this proved to be a temporary decline, as the highly contagious Delta variant quickly took hold, case numbers skyrocketed (peaking in mid-September) (New York Times, 2021). The data regarding the Delta variant were clear—vaccinations had a significant impact on reducing serious disease, hospitalizations and death (CDC, 2021). Fully vaccinated adults were hospitalized at a rate of 4.5 per 100,000 in August, while unvaccinated adults were hospitalized at a rate of 83.6 per 100,000. By October 2021, more than 218 million Americans had received at least one dose of a vaccine (65.8% of the total population), and 77% of the population over age 12 had received at least one dose. Vaccines became the new flashpoint for disagreements regarding COVID-19.

Nearly two years' worth of partisanship and political disagreements about COVID-19 created deep divisions about vaccines. These divisions became political standoffs as the federal government, led by newly elected President Joe Biden, first incentivized and then mandated vaccines for federal employees and large companies, and Republican governors and business owners resisted such mandates (Healy & McCarthy, 2021). The emergence of widely-distributed, significantly effective vaccines proved to shift the stigma associated with COVID-19. Sport once again became the site of public discourse regarding vaccines and health. Initially, those who tested positive for COVID-19 were stigmatized, but it was the disease itself that carried the stigma. As teams returned to competition in 2021, many with full or fuller stadiums than the previous "bubble" season, every league created highly detailed testing and vaccine protocols. Once teams reached a certain vaccination threshold, many of the restrictions (such as mask wearing and social distancing) were reduced. While no league outright mandated a vaccine, they heavily incentivized it and planned to punish outbreaks or positive tests that were traced back to unvaccinated players (for example: NFL, 2021).

Many athletes did get vaccinated. By September 2021, vaccination rates in all major professional leagues exceeded 85%, and the WNBA led all leagues vaccinating 99% of their players (NBA.com, 2021; NFL.com, 2021; Poole, 2021). Those who refused to vaccinate themselves were painted as selfish and ignorant, as the cause of friction in their workplaces, and as deserving victims should they test positive for COVID-19. Despite representing a fraction of professional athletes, the narrative of resistance to vaccination circulated widely in U.S. sport culture. For example, NFL player Cole Beasley tweeted repeatedly throughout the summer about the NFL's restrictions on unvaccinated players, threatening to retire if he were forced to get vaccinated. When his team, the Buffalo Bills, began requiring vaccines in order to attend live games, he began offering to buy tickets for fans at away stadiums (Wolf, 2021).

Unvaccinated Brooklyn Nets star Kyrie Irving also participated in a public standoff about vaccines. New York City requires proof of vaccination to enter public buildings, including Barclays Center, and as such Irving is ineligible to play in home games for the Nets (Wimbish, 2021) Most recently, the NHL suspended superstar Evander Kane for violating of COVID-19 protocol as he reportedly faked a vaccination card to more easily travel between the United States and Canada. While Beasley, Irving and Kane represent both the numerical and ideological minority in professional sports, they received outsized public attention regarding their stance about the COVID-19 vaccine. Most of the attention was not positive–Irving was referred to as "top idiot in the country" by radio host Howard Stern (Mazza, 2021), and Beasley was booed by his own fans at a home game (Fierro, 2021).

Conclusion

Prior to COVID-19, modern medicine had made the potential reality of a pandemic a relic of the past. Ostensibly, the U.S. government was soundly prepared, but more importantly, vaccines and global health institutions had constructed a strong social safety net from disease. At the start of 2020, no one in the "general public" believed that a viral pandemic would travel across the globe and press pause on everyday life. Pandemics were considered subjects of science fiction, tailor made for dramas on the silver screen. But when that fiction became a reality, the "truth" seemed too much for our stripped down government to bear. The Trump administration's ahistorical approach and lack of engagement with scientific reason or public health precautions drove the 24-hour news cycle creating a culture of fear and uncertainty with this novel disease. Examining the present pandemic in relation to the most recent HIV/AIDS epidemic of the 1980s reveals the subtle, but shifting relationships of power in U.S. culture. The similarities between the "gay plague" and the "China virus" exposes how Reagan's economic and cultural policies not only laid the groundwork to hollow out government in the lives of U.S. citizens, but also set the stage for authoritarian ideals to be exploited during a time of crisis.

Sport is a site of pleasure, but that does not mean it is exempt from social, cultural, and political implications. During the COVID-19 pandemic, sport has become a vehicle in the (re)production and circulation of meanings about the virus, pandemics, and the need for appropriate measures of social control. No context remains fixed or consistent for the only constant in cultural spaces is change. The meaning of disease and pandemics, therefore, is never settled. Currently, the dialectical tension of power between agency and constraint seems fraught. The meaning of "plague" is polysemic. Plague may be a metaphor of disease, but in the current context, it may suggest an over-indulgent neoliberal ideology of self-interest. Let history be a guide for there is no inherent meaning to disease, just reconstituted meanings written into discourse.

References

A Timeline of HIV and AIDS. (2021). Retrieved on October 15, 2021, from https://www.hiv.gov/hiv-basics/overview/history/hiv-and-aids-timeline

Andrews, D. L., & Giardina, M. (2008). Sport Without Guarantees: Toward a Cultural Studies That Matters. *Cultural Studies—Critical Methodologies, 8*(4), 395–422.

Bassett, M. T., Chen, J. T., & Krieger, N. (2020). Variation in Racial/Ethnic Disparities in COVID-19 Mortality By Age in the United States: A Cross Sectional Study. *PLOS Medicine, 18*(2), e10003541. Retrieved from https://journals.plos.org/plosmedicine/article?id=10.1371/journal.pmed.1003402

BBC. (2020, November 2). Covid-19: Prince William 'tested positive in April'. Retrieved from https://www.bbc.com/news/uk-54774942

Bruff, I. (2014). The Rise of Authoritarian Neoliberalism. *Rethinking Marxism, 26*(1), 113–129.

Casey, J. (2020, February 29). Trump's Response to Coronavirus Recalls Reagan Ignoring AIDS. Retrieved from https://www.advocate.com/commentary/2020/2/29/trumps-response-coronavirus-recalls-reagan-ignoring-aids

Cash, M. (2020, October 30). How the Mastermind's Behind the WNBA's Bubble Successfully Avoided an Outbreak in the Heart of a COVID-19 Hotspot. Retrieved from https://www.insider.com/how-wnba-successfully-avoided-COVID-19-outbreak-in-florida-bubble-2020-10

Centers For Disease Control and Prevention. (2021). Retrieved from www.COVID.cdc.gov/COVID-data-tracker

Cole, C. L., & Denny, H., III. (1994). Visualizing Deviance in Post-Reagan America: Magic Johnson, AIDS, and the Promiscuous World of Professional Sport. *Critical Sociology, 20*(3), 123–147.

Collier, R. (2020). "Massive Cuts to Science and Medicine in Trump Budget." Retrieved from https://www.ncbi.nlm.nih.gov/pmc/articles/PMC5468112/

Diamond, J. (2015, October 26). Trump: 'I Will Be a Great Unifier. Retrieved from https://www.cnn.com/2015/10/25/politics/donald-trump-democrats-republicans-bipartisanship-great-unifier/index.html

Duggan, L. (2003). *The Twilight of Equality? Neoliberalism, Cultural Politics, and the Attack on American Democracy*. Beacon Press.

Dworkin, S. L., & Wachs, F. L. (1998). Disciplining the Body: HIV-positive Male Athletes, Media Surveillance, and the Policing of Sexuality. *Sociology of Sport Journal, 15*(1), 1–20.

ESPN. (2020, December 24). Jazz Center Rudy Gobert on Realizing He Had NBA Game, COVID-19, and the Infamous Mic-Touching Incident. Retrieved from https://www.espn.com/nba/story/_/id/30582683/jazz-center-rudy-gobert-loves-game-COVID-19-infamous-mic-touching-incident

ESPN.com. (2021, March 11). Visual Timeline of the Day that Changed Everything: March 11. Retrieved from https://www.espn.com/espn/story/_/id/30546338/visual-line-day-changed-everything-march-11

Fee, E., & Krieger, N. (1993). Understanding AIDS: Historical Interpretations and the Limits of Biomedical Individualism. *American Journal of Public Health, 83*(*10*), 1477–1486.

Fierro, N. (2021, October 4). Bills' Cole Beasley Missing Point Again on Booing Issue. Retrieved from https://www.si.com/nfl/bills/news/bills-cole-beasley-missing-point-again-on-booing-issue

Foucault, M. (1989). *Archeology of Knowledge*. Routledge.

Gandhi, M. (2021, April 15). Four Ways HIV Activists Have Saved Lives During Covid. Retrieved from https://www.medscape.com/viewarticle/949348

Gittleson, B. (2021, March 15). Birx on Trump's Disinfection "Injection" Moment: "I Still Think About it Every Day." Retrieved from https://abc-news.go.com/Politics/birx-trumps-disinfectant-injection-moment-day/story?id=76474960

Goffman, E. (1961). *Asylums: Essays on the Social Situation of Mental Patients and Other Inmates*. Anchor Books.

Goffman, E. (1963). *Stigma: Notes on the Management of Spoiled Identity*. Simon & Schuster.

Golliver, B. (2021, May 10). How American Sports' COVID Patient Zero Nearly Became a National Pariah. Retrieved from https://lithub.com/how-american-sports-COVID-patient-zero-nearly-became-a-national-pariah/

Grady, D. (2020, July 27). Moderna and Pfizer Begin Late-Stage Vaccine Trials." *New York Times*. Retrieved from https://www.nytimes.com/2020/07/27/health/moderna-vaccine-covid.html

Granderson, LZ. (2021, August 4). How the Delta Variant Shattered Provincetown's Brief Moment of Normalcy. *Los Angeles Times.*. Retrieved from https://www.latimes.com/opinion/story/2021-08-04/lessons-on-COVID-and-life-from-provincetowns-outbreak-of-normalcy

Gross, J., & Eligon, J. (2020, December 22). Sentence is Cut for U.S. Student Who Broke Quarantine. *The New York Times*. Retrieved from https://www.nytimes.com/2020/12/22/world/americas/skylar-mack-cayman-islands-COVID.html

Hays, G. (2020, July 20). The Mental Toll of Life in the NWSL Challenge Cup Bubble. Retrieved from https://www.espn.com/soccer/united-states-nwsl-challenge-cup/story/4141083/the-mental-toll-of-life-in-the-nwsl-challenge-cup-bubble

Healy, J. and McCarthy, L. (2021, September 10). See You in Court: G.O.P. Governors Express Outrage and Vow to Fight Biden's Vaccine Requirements. *New York Times*. Retrieved from https://www.nytimes.com/2021/09/10/us/republican-governors-mandate-reaction.html

Human Rights Campaign. (2021a, February 4). CDC Releases Report Confirming Lesbian, Gay and Bisexual People At Greater Risk of COVID-19 Illness, Calls for More Data Collection. Retrieved from https://www.hrc.org/press-releases/cdc-releases-report-confirming-lesbian-gay-and-bisexual-people-at-greater-risk-of-COVID-19-illness-calls-for-more-data-collection

Human Rights Campaign. (2021b, August 12). HRC Foundation Survey of U.S. LGBTQ+ Adults Shows 92% Have at Least One COVID-19 Shot. Retrieved from https://www.hrc.org/press-releases/hrc-foundation-survey-of-u-s-lgbtq-adults-shows-92-have-at-least-one-COVID-19-shot

Lewis, T. (2021, March 11). How the U.S. Pandemic Response Went Wrong—and What Went Right—During a Year of COVID. Retrieved from https://www.scientificamerican.com/article/how-the-u-s-pandemic-response-went-wrong-and-what-went-right-during-a-year-of-COVID/

Lopez, G. (2016, December 1). The Reagan Administration's Unbelievable Response to the HIV/AIDS epidemic. Retrieved from https://www.vox.com/2015/12/1/9828348/ronald-reagan-hiv-aids

Lucey, E. (2020, June 2). Absolutely Disgusting: Wet Markets, Stigma Theory, and Xenophobia. Retrieved from https://nursingclio.org/2020/06/02/absolutely-disgusting-wet-markets-stigma-theory-and-xenophobia/

Lupkin, S. (2021, August 25). The U.S. Paid Billions to Get Enough COVID Vaccines Last Fall. What Went Wrong? *National Public Radio.* Retrieved from https://www.npr.org/sections/health-shots/2021/08/25/1029715721/pfizer-vaccine-operation-warp-speed-delay

Lupton, P. (1993). Risk as Moral Danger: The Social and Political Functions of Risk Discourse in Public Health. *International Journal of Health Services, 23*(3), 425–435.

Lupton, P. (2021). Contextualizing COVID-19: Sociocultural Perspectives on Contagion. In P. Lupton & K. Willis (Eds.), *The COVID-19 Crisis: Social Perspectives* (pp. 14–24). Routledge.

Lutz, T. (2020). 'We Have to Get Our Sports Back': Trump Says He Is Sick of Watching Baseball Repeats. *The Guardian* April 15, 2020. https://www.theguardian.com/sport/2020/apr/15/donald-trump-sports-reopen-coronavirus-shutdown

MacKinnon, K. (1992). *The Politics of Popular Representation: Reagan, Thatcher, AIDS, and the Movies* (p. 1992). Fairleigh Dickinsin University Press.

Massih, J. (2016). Reagan and AIDS: A Complicated Legacy. In J. A. Pino & K. Karamanakis (Eds.), *Body Politics: What's the State Got to Do With It?* (pp. 141–150). Eagle Print Collegiate Press.

Mazza, E. (2021, October 19). Howard Stern Rips "Douchebag" Kyrie Irving Over Vaccine: Top Idiot in the Country. *Huffington Post.* Retrieved from https://www.huffpost.com/entry/howard-stern-kyrie-irving-covid-vaccine_n_616f7f63e4b00cb3cbd95488

McGuill, M. C. (2020, June 30). "What We Can Learn from the AIDS Crisis in the Race for a COVID-19 Vaccine." *WBUR.org.* Retrieved from https://www.wbur.org/cognoscenti/2020/06/30/larry-kramer-aids-act-up-coronavirus-vaccine-michael-caron-mcguill

Murphy, T. (2020, March 20). America, Meet Tony Fauci. HIV/AIDS Activists Have Known Him a Long Time. Retrieved from https://www.thebodypro.com/article/tony-fauci-md-coronavirus

Nair, Y. (2000). Dead Images, Live Transmissions: Greg Louganis and the Construction of AIDS on Television. *Discourse, 22*(1), 53–69.

NBA.com. (2021, September 30). Report: NBA Reaches 95% Vaccination Rate Among Players. Retrieved from https://www.nba.com/news/report-nba-reaches-95-vaccination-rate-among-players

New York Times. (2021). Coronavirus in the U.S.: Latest Map adn Case Count. *New York Times*. Retrieved from https://www.nytimes.com/interactive/2021/us/COVID-cases.html

NFL.com. (2020, August 31). NFL-NFLPA COVID-19 Testing & Treatment Protocols Fact Sheet (2020 Season). Retrieved from https://www.nfl.com/playerhealthandsafety/resources/fact-sheets/nfl-nflpa-covid-19-testing-treatment-protocols-fact-sheet

NFL.com (2021, September 23). NFL COVID-19 Testing Results and Vaccination Rates: Sept. 5-18, 2021. Retrieved from https://www.nfl.com/playerhealthandsafety/resources/press-releases/nfl-COVID-19-testing-results-and-vaccination-rates-sept-5-18-2021

Pavlidis, A., & Rowe, D. (2021). The Sporting Bubble as Gilded Cage: Gendered Professional Sport in Pandemic Times and Beyond. *M/C Journal, 24*(1), 1.

Poole, M. (2021, September 2). NFL, NBA, MLB players avoiding vaccines jeopardizing wins. Retrieved from https://www.nbcsports.com/bayarea/warriors/nfl-nba-mlb-players-avoiding-vaccines-jeopardize-wins-championships

Reitsma, M. B., Claypool, A. L., Vargo, J., Shete, P. B., & McCorvie, R. (2021). Racial/Ethnic Disparities in COVID-19 Exposure Risk, Testing, and Cases At the Subcounty Level in California. *Health Affairs, 40*(6), 1. https://www.healthaffairs.org/doi/10.1377/hlthaff.2021.00098

Reyes, L. (2021, September 7). "Denver Broncos QBs Who Became Ineligible As Close Contacts Tried to Cheat NFL's COVID-19 Protocols, Per Report." *USA Today.* Retrieved from https://www.usatoday.com/story/sports/nfl/2021/09/07/denver-broncos-qbs-tried-cheat-nfls-covid-19-protocols/5754961001/

Rogers, K., Jakes, L., & Swanson, A. (2020, March 18). Trump Defends Using "Chinese Virus" Label, Ignoring Growing Criticism. *New York Times.* Retrieved from https://www.nytimes.com/2020/03/18/us/politics/china-virus.html

Simmons-Duffin, S. (2021, August 6). How A Gay Community Helped the CDC Spot a COVID Outbreak–And Learn More About Delta. *National Public Radio.* Retrieved from https://www.npr.org/sections/health-shots/2021/08/06/1025553638/how-a-gay-community-helped-the-cdc-spot-a-COVID-outbreak-and-learn-more-about-de

Smith, P. and Chirbas, K. (2021, September 7). Carmine's Hostess Attacked After Asking Diners for Proof of Vaccination. *NBC News.* Retrieved from https://www.nbcnews.com/news/us-news/carmine-s-hostess-attacked-after-asking-diners-proof-vaccine-n1279410

Sontag, S. (1989). *AIDS and its Metaphors*. Farrar Straus and Giroux.

Stroud, R. (2021, September 4). Tom Brady had COVID-19, Believes Virus Will Be a Bigger Problem in 2021. *Tampa Bay Times.* Retrieved from https://www.tampabay.com/sports/bucs/2021/09/04/tom-brady-had-covid-19-is-vaccinated-and-believes-virus-could-be-a-bigger-problem-in-2021/

Tracy, A. (2020, May 1). How Trump Gutted Obama's Pandemic Preparedness Systems. *Vanity Fair.* Retrieved from https://www.vanityfair.com/news/2020/05/trump-obama-coronavirus-pandemic-response

Travel.gov (2021). COVID-19 Country Specific Information. Retrieved from https://travel.state.gov/content/travel/en/traveladvisories/COVID-19-Country-Specific-Information.html

Triechler, P. (1987). AIDS, Homophobia, and Biomedical Disourse: An Epidemic of Signification. *Cultural Studies, 1*(3), 263–305.

Whitmore, G. (2020, October 19). When Did President Trump Ban Travel From China? And Can you Travel to China Now? Retrieved from https://www.forbes.com/sites/geoffwhitmore/2020/10/19/when-did-president-trump-ban-travel-from-china-and-can-you-travel-to-china-now/?sh=1e8c49f74847

Wimbish, J. (2021, October 19). Kyrie Irving Vaccine Stance: Everything to Know, Including Fallout with Nets, New York Mandate, NBA Rules. *CBS News.* Retrieved from https://www.cbssports.com/nba/news/kyrie-irving-vaccine-stance-everything-to-know-including-fallout-with-nets-new-york-mandate-nba-rules/

Wolf, J. (2021, September 17). Bills' Cole Beasley, Reid Ferguson Buying Unvaccinated Fans Tickets to Road Games. *The Buffalo News.* Retrieved from https://buffalonews.com/sports/bills/bills-cole-beasley-reid-ferguson-buying-unvaccinated-fans-tickets-to-road-games/article_af01adb2-1730-11ec-9c5c-bb7090b42475.html

Yasharoff, H. (2021, September 19). Chris Rock Reveals he has COVID-19, Urges Vaccination: "Trust Me You Don't Want This.'" *USA Today.* Retrieved from https://www.usatoday.com/story/entertainment/celebrities/2021/09/19/chris-rock-covid-19-positive-comedian-urges-vaccine/8411020002/

13

On the Subject of Race and Sport: Covid-19, Zoom, and the Necessity of Antiracist Dialogic Pedagogy

Ronald L. Mower

Introduction: Covid-19, Sport, and Black Lives Matter

In March 2020, the world was upended by the imminent threat of the Covid-19 virus which has, at the time of writing, claimed more than 800,000 lives in the US, and over 5 million globally (https://www.cdc.gov/nchs/covid19/mortality-overview.htm). The human cost of the pandemic, revealing the vast chasms of inequitable political, economic, medical and technological capacities, has been swift and unforgiving, and new mutations such as the Delta/Omicron variants threaten to destabilize the hopeful, and preemptively assumed, return to normalcy. However, within a neoliberalizing late-capitalist econocracy (Earle et al., 2017), what really seemed to matter was the economic cost of the pandemic resulting from lockdown quarantine orders which shuttered businesses,

R. L. Mower (✉)
University of Maryland, College Park, MD, USA
e-mail: mower1@umd.edu

D. L. Andrews et al. (eds.), *Sport and Physical Culture in Global Pandemic Times*, Global Culture and Sport Series, https://doi.org/10.1007/978-3-031-14387-8_13

grinded global travel to a halt, and canceled the sport industry for months (Martinez, 2020; Nauright et al., 2020). The short-lived annulment of elite-level, commercialized sport exposed already existing inequalities within sporting structures, particularly for Women's professional basketball and soccer, various grassroots community sport leagues, and for thousands of low-wage seasonal stadium workers (Pape, 2020; Sheptak & Menaker, 2020).

Early reports indicated that Black, Indigenous, People of Color (BIPOC) were disproportionately impacted as a result of impoverished conditions, tighter living spaces, job losses, food scarcity, and lack of access to health resources and Personal Protective Equipment (Tsai, 2020). Emerging at a time of already heightened social anxieties and increasingly divisive and vitriolic political punditry surrounding Black Lives Matter (BLM), free speech and the right to protest, police brutality, the #defund movement, Black athletes kneeling for justice, the #MeToo movement, the executive banning of Critical Race Theory (CRT), the mixed messaging and subsequent politicization of masking, and the haphazard public enforcement of "social distancing" mandates, Covid-19 exacerbated confusion, anger, and frustration. As noted by David Rowe (2020), "During a pandemic when racist street attacks and Black Lives Matter protests were both in evidence, a sociological sensibility is well attuned to the dangerous implications of a language discourse that evokes an ideology of virus induced social segregation" (p. 710). It is precisely this condition of segregation—enacted through Jim Crow era policies, but maintained through precedence, discrimination, and the "color-blind" de-facto segregation of post-Civil-Rights America—that continues to prevent the kind of dialogic engagement required to combat the corrosive effects of white supremacy.

Amidst the chaos and uncertainty of Covid-19, this chapter speaks to the ways in which the circumstances (distrust, fear, mask mandates, lockdowns, misinformation) and timing of the pandemic (concurrent with BLM protests) were opportunistically seized by far-Right forces to politicize CRT as anti-American propaganda, sowing the seeds of separation and distrust alongside mask mandates and vaccinations. In the wake of appalling behavior at school board meetings and growing threats of violence and intimidation against teachers, staff, and administrators over these hot-button issues, US Attorney General Merrick Garland, on October 4th, 2021, empowered Justice Department prosecutors to investigate (Bella & Barrett, 2021). Akin to the social crisis over Brown v. Board of Education and subsequent integration efforts in the 1950's and 1960's, the violent backlash against CRT reprises the Anti-Civil-Rights argument—repurposed by the likes of Missouri Republican Sen. Josh Hawley—that racial integration is an infringement on white civil rights. Emerging as another heretical voice of the neo-fascist, Q'Anon, conservative Right, Hawley's attack on the Justice Department policy (Ujifusa, 2021) willfully ignores and downplays the violence and intimidation tactics of those protesting CRT and masking in public schools, condoning their repugnant actions much like those of the insurrectionist, capitol rioters of Jan. 6th.

Seeking to silence critical conversations, dialogue, and education about race and racism in America, the inter-assemblages of anti-CRT/anti-Black and anti-masking/anti-vax forces have revealed the fragility of, and desperate need for, an engaged politics of interracial, intercultural, collaborative civil discourse, particularly within spaces of education. Already working against the historical failures of post-Civil Rights integration efforts (busing, fair housing, equal opportunity, affirmative action, etc.), students today continue to be largely isolated along the same intersecting racial and socioeconomic lines of the not-too-distant past (Colby, 2012; Desmond, 2016). However, the structural underpinnings of those realities have been so effectively disguised under the political economic formation of meritocratic neoliberal colorblindness, that some students have great difficulty conceptualizing, let alone questioning, the structures and processes actually responsible for contemporary racial disparities in health, wealth, education, employment, housing, and rights of citizenship. This chapter draws these issues together within a pedagogical context where students were asked to confront the material outcomes of systemic racism within societal institutions, including sport as a powerfully instructive window into the American racial formation. Gleaned from the course *Hoop Dreams: Black Masculinity and Sport* (HDBMS), comments reflective of students' racial perceptions and attitudes between 2018 and 2021 appear herein, exposing how Covid-19 and the Right's politicization of the CRT "boogeyman" temporarily disrupted what had proven to be an effective model of critical self-reflexivity, interracial/intercultural classroom dialogue, and team-building activities designed to develop trust and cultural familiarity.

Centering Critical Race Pedagogy

> Antiracist pedagogy…requires educators to address not only racism, but also whiteness, and the discomfort that white people experience when faced with challenges to their (socially constructed) dominance and racial superiority (Galloway et al., 2019, p. 495).

While the implementation of terms such as "equity, diversity, and inclusion" or "social justice" in programs of higher education have become common, corroborating the establishment of EDI departments, programs, and committees, there remain significant questions concerning their actual pedagogical impact (Ishimaru & Galloway, 2014; Ladson-Billings, 2014; Paris & Alim, 2014). More specifically, Galloway et al. (2019, p. 486) note that the widespread use of such terms, "may center more on honoring difference, celebrating diversity, and ensuring representation, with less attention to racism, injustice, or the systems and structures that create disparate outcomes for students of color and other minoritized groups" (see also, Bensimon, 2005; Ladson-Billings, 2014). Despite significant changes to policy that evinces a commitment to equality and justice, the tendency for educators to employ "race avoidant" or "race-neutral" language continues to abound and has been shown to contribute to the persistence of student outcome gaps and reinforcement of the status quo (Carter et al., 2014; Dowd & Bensimon, 2015; Irby & Clark, 2018). For white students, the subtle reinforcement of race as a non-issue likewise teaches them how to employ "coded language" to avoid being labeled "racist" while continuing to reproduce and rationalize the normalcy of white privilege (Bonilla-Silva, 2002, 2018; Pollock, 2004; Rodriguez, 2011). As noted by Castagno (2008):

> Race is not part of the accepted or expected discourse within schools. The discourse that is prevalent in schools is instead one of culture, equality, and

> difference—constructs that are part of the contemporary culture of Whiteness and that merely serve to obscure race, racism, and inequities based on race (p. 315).

Furthermore, with a rise in EDI programs in education and the workplace, scholars warn that, "diversity ideology works by allowing whites to claim openness to and interest in people of color, but in severely delimited ways that avoid discussions of power, center whites' feelings, and ultimately uphold white supremacy. Diversity, in other words, is for white people" (Christian et al., 2019, p. 1737). Hence, in order to counter the familiar slide into colorblind racial politics and celebratory multiculturalism (Bonilla-Silva, 2002), scholars have long called for the explicit naming of antiracist pedagogy (Pollock, 2008) and critical race curriculum (Yosso, 2002) to directly confront the myriad ways in which white racial dominance has been reproduced throughout centuries of economic, political, and technological change (Delgado & Stefancic, 2017). Subsequently, a true commitment to antiracist practice and pedagogy must include embodied acts of dialogic engagement which openly addresses white privilege and Black oppression, facilitates a critique of systemic and structural inequalities, highlights students' own lived experience and recognition of the operation of race in their everyday lives, and explicitly calls out and addresses acts of racism and oppression (Galloway et al., 2019; Crenshaw, 2011; Delgado & Stefancic, 2017).

Facilitating Critical Thinking and Self-reflexivity

> It is not our role to speak to the people about our own view of the world, nor to attempt to impose that view on them, but rather to dialogue with the people about their view and ours. We must realize that their view of the world, manifested variously in their action, reflects their situation in the world (Freire, 2000, p. 96).

While those engaging his ideas occupy different lived conditions throughout distinct historical moments, the social action approach of

Paulo Freire has proven invaluable to emancipatory research, liberationist politics, and critical thought leading toward conscientization (Freire, 2000; Giroux, 2001; Kamberlies & Dimitriadis, 2005). Beneficial for Kinesiology students at a major research institution, Freire's critical pedagogy superbly complements C. Wright Mills' "sociological imagination" which encourages the recognition of "the vivid awareness of the relationship between personal experience and the wider society" (Mills, 1956, p. 6). Given the tools to begin thinking relationally and conceptually about the interconnections and interdependencies of sport and the broader society within which it is located, and of which it is a constitutive part, students learn to think reflexively about their own (sporting) lives. For scholar-pedagogue-activists teaching courses within the area of Physical Cultural Studies (PCS), including that which is the subject of this chapter (*HDBMS*), the underlying and articulating epistemological thread of radical contextualization informs how we seek to not only empower our students, but to help our students empower themselves (Freire, 2000; Denzin, 2014; Giroux, 2001). As Silk & Andrews (2011) note,

> The purpose, then, of PCS becomes a radical democratic practice that is equally theoretical, pedagogical, political, moral, and ethical, involving the enhancement of moral agency, the production of moral discernment, a commitment to praxis, change, justice, an ethic of resistance, and a performative pedagogy that resists oppression (p. 14).

In setting the foundation for generative classroom dialogue every semester, the presence of fresh faces and diverse backgrounds requires the establishment of points of intersection, empathy and understanding. As a young and naïve first-year college student, I remember being introduced to Mills' concept of the "sociological imagination" for the first time within a course called *Sport & American Society*. The professor, "ever-dedicated to the passionate pursuit of social justice and civil rights…turned 'sport' on its collective head, using it as a window through which to better understand the systemic operations of power and the politics of culture informing our late-capitalist moment" (Giardina, 2005, p. 12). Urging us to consider how our lived experience was historically interconnected to broader systems, processes, and conditions of the society in which we lived, we were invited to think reflexively about our varied social locations—particularly how those contexts not only shaped our lives, but how we embody and help constitute, those very structures of influence (Andrews, 2002; Andrews & Giardina, 2008). However disjointed and uninformed the product of my reflexive writing and conversational attempts may have been at the time, the exercise was nothing short of life altering for me. It was the planted seed that eventually blossomed into my decision to forgo an athletic-training career for graduate education in critical sport studies.

More than 15 years later, as a University Lecturer in PCS, I continue to draw upon those experiences to encourage self-reflexivity and empathic dialogic collaboration. To inspire my students to begin thinking in this way, I routinely present a self-reflexive reading of my own lived experience (a white cisgender heterosexual working-class male raised among young men of color who shared, and influenced, my near-obsessive love for basketball and hip-hop) to contextualize who I am, why I think the way I do, how I got to this point, and what it all means for my own anti-racist praxis, the research I conduct, and for the class more generally. Seeking to cultivate trust, genuineness, authenticity, and empathy, I choose not to alter my voice to sound more formal, professional, authoritative in the classroom, but instead allow my students to hear the local dialect and cadence of speech reflective of my regional upbringing in and around the Washington, D.C. area. My style of clothing, gait, gestures, non-conforming long hair, thick beard, and tattoos are likewise redolent of the formative influence that Black people and Black American culture have had on my 'cultural habitus' throughout my life (Bourdieu, 1984). While learning to necessarily disguise, code-switch, or diminish some accoutrements in certain spaces growing up, in my current role as PCS pedagogue, I allow my embodied performativity to speak as a disruptive text of decidedly pro-Black, neo-Marxist, radically-contextualist, feminist-communitarian politics.

It is through performative pedagogy that I aim to help my students learn that it is okay, indeed necessary, to acknowledge our forms of privilege and seek to be an ally for change; to understand that problems like racism are, in fact, systemic problems long embedded within institutional frameworks that benefit whites, reinforce "whiteness" as the standard American identity, and normalize the problematic manner in which whites have been taught to see ourselves within a supposedly fair and equal, "colorblind" society (Feagin, 2013; Lipsitz, 2006; Ware & Back, 2002; Wingfield & Feagin, 2012). The fact that I can feel safe and confident in a classroom of 100 students and ardently discuss such topics without having my credibility challenged is itself a product of this privilege (see, for example, "white-student backlash against minority teachers" in Rodriguez, 2009). While I wrestle with this actuality, my goal remains to consistently demonstrate and thereby encourage my students to imagine, being privileged with regard to race, gender, sexuality, nationality, ability, or social class while nonetheless choosing to "take sides" (Denzin, 2002, p. 487) with those marginalized and oppressed by the forces of neoliberal capitalism, white supremacy, systemic racism, patriarchal misogyny, gender violence, and homophobia (Denzin, 2004, 2014; Robinson, 2019).

While difficulties abound in creating "safe spaces" for discussion of topics like racism, sexism, inequality and injustice, Arao and Clemens (2013) suggest that instead we should be seeking to create "brave spaces" precisely because, "talking about race, oppression, power, and privilege requires the very qualities of risk, difficulty, and controversy that are defined as incompatible with safety" (p. 139, as cited in Galloway et al., 2019, p. 497). As such, challenging students to first think reflexively about their own lives helps establish (1) a baseline recognition of the complex interplay between historical structures and individual experience, and (2) relational-thinking, empathy, and awareness that is not only desperately needed in our anti-historical late-capitalist conjuncture, but represents the possibility for a more humane, equitable, and just future (Denzin, 2014).

Talking "race" and Sport in the Pre-Covid Classroom: Embodied Acts of Civil Dialogue and Trust

While HDBMS attracts a diverse sample of students in Kinesiology, the fact that it also counts toward General Education requirements draws students from a wide variety of majors across campus. No matter the background, HDBMS demands that students dig deeper in self-examining the role that race/racism plays in their daily lives, and/or how the invisibility and denials of it manifest in the reproduction of inequitable policies and practices across society and sport (Dowd & Bensimon, 2015; Irby & Clark, 2018). Prior to Covid-19 lockdowns, we facilitated these conversations to great effect, with students writing, and conversing, about the circumstances of their childhood; how socio-spatial location correlates with physical cultural practices and experiences, the experience of racialization in public/private spaces, and varied levels of familiarity with America's racial past and present. As can be imagined, and given the incredible failures of Civil Rights era integration efforts (Colby, 2012), such practices expose the oft-overlooked fact that most students are still growing up in extremely segregated, racially homogenous communities (Omi & Winant, 1994), far removed from the Civil Rights Act of 1964 or the Fair Housing Act of 1968. In fact, recent studies show that 81% of metropolitan areas across the US are actually *more* segregated as of 2019 than they were in 1990 (Menendian et al., 2021).

(Note: All markers of identity used herein are self-ascribed in students' own written responses):

> "I would say 90% of my community that I grew up with had the same racial background as me as my town had very little minorities"—White middle-class female
>
> "99%. When I got to high school there was one black family that moved into my neighborhood. Up until that point, everyone was white"—White upper-middle class male
>
> "When living in Baltimore 100% of the people I lived around were of the same background as me"—Black working-class male

> "I would say about 98% of people in my neighborhood growing up are from the same ethnic background as me…majority white"—White upper-middle class male
>
> "About 95%. I never had a white neighbor until I was 16 and was never friends with any white kids until I was 14"—Black working-class female
>
> "This assignment just made me realize I really don't blend in anywhere. I've grown up with mostly white people; I played sports with white people and was always the only minority on my team."—Mexican American middle-class female
>
> "Growing up from the South/West side of Memphis in the projects, I'd say 99% of the people living in my neighborhood shared my ethnic background.—Black working-class American male

Importantly, in light of these confessions, we discussed how post-Civil Rights de-facto segregation and racial inequity was not simply an unfortunate accident of a supposedly post-racist meritocratic society, which we are urged to believe, but the result of failed policies, flawed enforcement, and the residuals of government sanctioned discrimination in housing, education, and employment development (Alexander, 2020; Colby, 2012; Desmond, 2016; Rothstein, 2017; Omi & Winant, 1994). More specifically, the racial disparities of the GI bill, redlining and blockbusting, employment and educational discrimination, environmental racism, and neoliberal public retrenchment have all coalesced to reproduce the hierarchically racialized spatial arrangements of American society (Menendian et al., 2021; Rothstein, 2017; Pietila, 2010; Wacquant, 2007, 2009). Countering the "colorblind" euphemizing of racism as the discriminatory actions of "a few bad apples", we work to collectively expose the systemic embeddedness of racism within societal institutions, and our own implicit biases and ways of seeing (Bonilla-Silva, 2002; Feagin, 2013; Feagin & Vera, 1995). This requires asking questions to facilitate reflexive thinking and shared understanding. For example, one discussion-based activity begins by giving students a survey asking them to self-identify and comment on the question, "what do you perceive to be the most salient aspect of your stated identity?" Open-ended to allow any explanation of what they deem to be most important and defining about their lived experience, the question draws to the surface immensely different perceptions about the significance of race:

> "The most important, essential part to my identity I believe is that I am an American because of the patriotism that I feel is important to have in my country.—White American male
>
> "My skin color. Because before I am anything else, I'm Black, rather I want to be or not. I've learned it doesn't matter what I do, how I sound, the way I walk, nor education level; my baseline starts at the color of my skin.—Black male
>
> "I find my most important aspect of my identity that I am a young respectful, diverse woman who is very easy to talk to. I am open to anyone, I am strong, and hopeful.—White Caucasian American middle-class female
>
> "I feel as if being African-American plays the biggest part in my identity. From a societal perspective, the color of my skin is always the first thing people notice about me and assumptions follow that primary image in others' minds.—Black American middle-class male
>
> "I enjoy my freedom to pursue adventure and new experiences in life.—White American male
>
> "I am a Black African American woman in the middle-class. When I was younger on my blue card…I would check the other box and put brown because I didn't believe in people telling me what I was, or associate my color with negative things people tied to blackness. But now I embrace the term and combat the negativity people associate with it"

The six responses shown above (3 Black and 3 White) were chosen for being representative of general trends (i.e., white students answering much more succinctly, never once citing race as an important factor, and highlighting their personal qualities and beliefs, while students of color wrote significantly more, almost always highlighted skin color as a determining factor, and expressed much deeper reflexivity about the burdens of race). By collecting and codifying the responses according to their own self-reported identifications, students became aware of their own perceptions about themselves, and their racial counterparts, and could engage in critical dialogue about their self-assessments. White students, for example, when confronted with the realization that none of their peers cited 'race/ethnicity/whiteness' as an important aspect of their identity were challenged to think about why, and what exactly that means? As one example of several reflexive thinking prompts, this is particularly revealing because it organically brings to light that which is most often hidden, ignored, and exorcised under the "colorblind" social development of the self within white American culture—the recognition of the centrality of race underpinning material outcomes and the invisibility of white privilege which protects and sustains it (Bonilla-Silva, 2018; Feagin, 2013; Feagin & Vera, 1995; Ware & Back, 2002).

The desire to consistently downplay the material impact of race has, as a result of the pervasive dominance of colorblind racial politics, become so fluidly mobilized that most white students significantly lack awareness of how they have been taught "not to see" race, or rather, how they have been "raised to experience their racially based advantages as fair and normal" (Marty, 1999, p. 51). Nobody is made to feel guilty or ashamed for (un)knowingly being the recipient of white privilege—indeed, I consistently draw upon variations of the Marxist dictum we "make our own history, but not in the conditions of our own choosing" to highlight the reproduction of oppressive systems that, while we did not take part in creating, continue to reproduce inequality—but, by becoming aware, we can choose to change our thinking and participate in movements for a more equitable future (Denzin, 2014). Difficult and uncomfortable as it may be, and amidst GOP efforts to ban educational discussions about race that might make some white people *feel* uncomfortable, HDBMS students are reminded that in the struggle for justice and equality, we must not be willing to prioritize the protection of white *feelings* over the protection of Black *lives*.

> What I've realized is there is something fundamentally wrong with the way our country and our society treats Black Americans and the number of opportunities available for them to succeed in life is often very little compared to white people. This fact also suggests to me that this statistic will most likely remain true for many years to come if we don't start helping minority families achieve the same level of success—Black Mexican cisgender middle-class American female

In many ways, the field of sport and the college classroom represent key points of contact for young people who otherwise live incredibly disparate social, cultural, and economic lives in relative isolation from one another. They are generally aware of each other, but the knowledges are heavily mediated, with decades of persuasive messaging fueling a consumptive fascination with the athleticism and entertainment value of the Black body, whilst simultaneously reproducing an existential fear of the "savage" and "threatening" racial "other" (Hall, 1997; hooks, 1992; Runstedtler, 2018). In particular, the reproduction of the Athletic-Industrial-Complex (Smith, 2014; Runstedtler, 2018) and hyper-mediation of the Uber-sport spectacle (Andrews, 2019) produces an incessant surveillance of Black bodies, within which the "white gaze" can crudely determine, pace Wilson (1997), if those encountered in public space, or tele-visually, are "good Blacks" or "bad Blacks."

Drawing on Kitwana (2005), it has long been questioned how white youth's consumption of Black culture, specifically hip-hop and basketball, correlates with their racial awareness, political consciousness, and everyday engagement with people of color who are not athletes or entertainers (Yousman, 2003). Despite relatively low levels of sustained contact with people of color, white students' praise of athletes like Lebron James, Lamar Jackson, and Steph Curry were common. Representatives of "self-made success" and "overcoming the odds" to become the most "physically-gifted," "powerful," and "aspirational" models of "hard-work," and "perseverance," is how students generally described their respective "neoliberal" views of such athletes. The responses below (assessed early in the semester), when asked to explain why professional basketball and football are dominated by Black men, demonstrate some prevalent attitudes:

> "Black athletes are *naturally* more athletic. They work harder through racial adversity and have goals set in place."—White male
>
> "The fact that a majority of NBA and NFL athletes are African-American does not mean much to me. I think it is awesome that's a stat, but I think if *anyone of any race* puts their mind to something they can achieve it"—White middle-class male

> "African-Americans are *naturally* more talented in sports such as football and basketball and are also being more represented in those areas"—Middle-class White female
>
> "The black community tends to *focus more on sport* than education, for better or worse"—White female
>
> "Black Americans are being *pushed towards* sports. This often happens because from a young age we are made to believe that's the ticket out of our living situations"—Black working-class male
>
> "There is so much *emphasis on the abilities of Black bodies* in generating revenue than actual valuing of Black creativity, academic discovery, minds…"—Black Muslim Woman

The racial attitudes depicted here, while somewhat banal for critical sport scholars, are quite representative of prevailing race-based perceptual differences. More importantly, the pedagogical process of sharing and discussing the rationale behind these views, opens the door for counter-reification of two hegemonic ideas the course seeks to implode: (1) The dichotomous twin myths of *natural* Black athleticism and *natural* Black criminality. (2) The myth of a Black *sporting fixation* (hoop dreams) wherein the various assemblages of the Athletic-Industrial-Complex (AIC) are obscured in favor of the neoliberal view reflecting one's relative success or failure as nothing more than a composite of individual choices (Runstedtler, 2018; Smith, 2014). Using sport as a window to examine the history of racial hierarchy, power and oppression, and the contemporary state of race relations in America, students listen, share, and build trust with their peers in face-to-face scenarios. In effect, we practice the art of civil discourse around highly contentious, often misunderstood, and complexly multifaceted issues of racial inequity and oppression within a political, economic, social and legal system that subverts the continued impacts of racism under the fallacious ruse of colorblindness (Bonilla-Silva, 2002, 2018; Delgado & Stefancic, 2017; Ware & Back, 2002). For white students in particular, regular contact and collaboration across racial boundaries produced significant changes in perspective, self-awareness, and empathy:

"I don't know why I haven't ever really thought of it like that, but these leagues literally use black bodies for white entertainment"—White middle-class Jewish male

"Racism in this country is what privileges whites. I don't have to deal with the racism and hate that others deal with. I now view white supremacy as more of a terrorist/extremist idea"—White middle-class male

"I feel we have to listen to African-Americans in order to implement change, instead of fighting or arguing what BLM means..."—White middle-class female

Pre-Covid HDBMS students completed the course with a newfound confidence in themselves, and their ability to have more generative conversations about race. As a society, we take for granted how infrequent, fleeting, and superficial our interracial encounters have become under the "colorblind" neoliberal individualism of the post-Civil-Rights era. Representing our collective futures and hope of a multicultural democracy, young people desperately need more spaces of intercultural and interracial collaboration, beyond the sporting realm, where trust building and empathic concern can be fostered and normalized. Relatedly, a major concern with moving this heavily discussion-based course Online was the disembodied nature of virtual interaction, lack of intimacy, difficulty reading social cues/body language, and the degree to which intent gets "lost in [virtual] translation" when discussing sensitive topics. Prior to the pandemic, HDBMS had never been taught Online.

The Articulations of White Backlash Politics, Covid-19 Culture Wars, and the Shift to Zoom

In the months preceding Covid, there was no shortage of current news breaking on cases of police violence, BLM protests, athlete activism, and the controversial signing of executive order 13950 in September 2019. Within course topics about historical racial logics, mediated racial representation, and sporting nationalisms, Trump's ban on Critical Race Theory (CRT) offered a particularly ripe opportunity to discuss the interconnections of political power and systemic racism, particularly how the cultural politics of "patriotism" underpin white supremacist discourse, such as that flagrantly mobilized by the former president. For example, in the first (un)presidential debate of 2020, in response to Chris Wallace's question about 13950, Trump delivered "emotional goods for his majority white supporters" (Bonilla-Silva, 2019b, p. 1780), employing colorblind patriotism to grossly distort CRT as anti-American propaganda:

> I ended it because it's racist. I ended it because a lot of people were complaining that they were asked to do things that were absolutely insane, that it was a radical revolution taking place in our military, in our schools...We were paying people hundreds of thousands of dollars to teach very bad ideas and frankly, very sick ideas...they were teaching people to hate our country (Lang, 2020).

While an absurd mischaracterization of CRT, the statement connected with the racialized emotions of Trump's majority white base, suggesting "reverse-racism" and anti-white sentiment, and stoking anger towards "Others" made out to be against America (i.e., Blacks, Mexicans, Muslims, Immigrants, etc.). As noted by Bonilla-Silva (2019b), "the problems afflicting the white masses are not due to Blacks, immigrants, and Muslims, but the emotions whites feel—and their consequences, like race itself, are very real" (p. 1780), and they help to explain why so many working-class whites vote against their economic interests, support demeaning language about racial minorities, immigrants, and women, and are willing to believe unfounded conspiracy theories about white victimization (see also, Bonilla-Silva, 2019a). Even in the divisive wake of Trump, GOP lawmakers are pushing further than ever to outlaw CRT (Ray & Gibbons, 2021; Flaherty, 2021), redact Black historical figures from the teaching of American history (Impelli, 2021), and make it illegal to exercise one's first amendment right to protest oppression (Epstein & Mazzei, 2021; Zhang, 2021). As support for BLM and antiracism has increased, the opposition has likewise intensified efforts to brazenly whitewash American history and silence education about state-sanctioned segregation, institutionalized racism, and the re-tooling of slave economies under mass incarceration (Alexander, 2020; Rothstein, 2017). By engaging directly with news about 13950, Students in HDBMS in the

Fall 2019 and Spring 2020 were able to recognize the impulse of white supremacy within the reactionary politics of the proposed ban and decipher the purposefully deceptive language (crudely appropriating prominent Civil-Rights era discourse) used to justify anti-Black racial silencing campaigns.

However, something strange happened within the Fall 2020 and Spring 2021 semesters in which course instruction occurred 100% virtually via Zoom. This season of social isolation, public conflict, and anxiety-producing uncertainty had a profound impact on students' collaborative energies and stamina for racial dialogue. More specifically, in a time of heightened contestation over the CRT ban, George Floyd's murder, BLM protests, mask-mandate culture-wars, and the capitol-rioters, the once balanced racial composition of active student participation shifted noticeably. While white students have always been more reticent when it comes to open discussions about race—a byproduct of being socialized under the pedagogical auspices of a supposed "post-racial" colorblind meritocracy—the shared occupation of the classroom opened space for interracial collaboration and trust-building in which white students felt they could contribute meaningfully alongside their BIPOC peers. However, in the fully virtual environment, and without any prior in-person engagement and familiarity with their classmates, white students tended to indiscriminately police their own speech within larger class discussions (50 students on average) for fear of (a. "saying the wrong thing" (b. "upsetting someone else" or (c. being "wrongly accused of being racist"). The following comments, taken anonymously from course evaluations following the Spring 2021 semester, epitomize the general tone of detachment, and even the insinuation of favoritism on the part of myself and my Teaching Assistant (a bi-racial male graduate student):

> "This was a lot for a 200-level class. Yes, I did enjoy being educated on all the topics and enjoyed listening to discussions...Sometimes it's uncomfortable to speak out with the topics we discuss. As many times I wanted to participate, I never did because I didn't want to say something to upset another classmate. I'd get pure anxiety even sending something in the chat"
>
> "The conversation over zoom would lag sometimes. Some voices dominated and had more experience talking about race. I didn't feel confident

sometimes, but I liked the media text project…the course made me view the institution of sport in a different light"

"I really liked how our classes were based on our readings and discussion posts, but I often felt afraid of saying something in the wrong way and being unfairly labeled"

"I thought this class had a lot of potential to be a great experience. However, I felt sometimes the environment was hard to participate in. I realize this class was on zoom and made it harder for everyone, but *our professor and ta seemed as they favored some students than others*. We talked about important and hard topics and *as a white student I felt like it was not appropriate at times for me to express my opinion* and I feel like that will hurt my participation grade"

While not as troubling as some recent contestations and national backlash—for example, the swift reactionary decision of Boise State to suspend 52 diversity course sections after a report surfaced of a student being shamed and humiliated for being white, which an investigation later revealed to be wholly fabricated (Flaherty, 2021)—the feelings expressed by some white students are still concerning, particularly because this was not a sentiment expressed in HDBMS prior to Covid-19. Even within the Spring 2020 semester, the first six weeks of in-person engagement, and the familiarity that had been established, carried the collaborative precedent of trust and respect into our virtual discussions for the remainder of the term.

Amidst the kneejerk GOP-led legislative efforts to craft "dignity and nondiscrimination in public education" and "anti-divisive concepts" laws in more than 16 states (Flaherty, 2021), the drive to separate, silence, and prevent empathic engagement across racial boundaries represents a political weaponizing of moral panics; the individualizing of racism to deny systemic embeddedness, and the staunch resistance to having white supremacy and white privilege laid bare as enduring forces of structural racism. Microcosmic of the broader societal level failures to equitably integrate our communities, workplaces, educational institutions, and public spaces in the post-Civil-Rights era, the Covid-19 assemblage exacerbated the existential conditions of physical separation, anxiety, and fear, making it far more difficult to cultivate dialogic engagement, trust-building, and interracial collaboration.

Conclusion: Towards More Inclusive and Productive Dialogue on Race

Working at the intersection of people, pedagogies, politics, and performances, this chapter sought to articulate the role and function of antiracist pedagogy and dialogic discussion within HDBMS and how the disruptive impact of the Covid-19 pandemic jeopardized these efforts during two "locked-down" semesters of fully Online instruction. Establishing the baseline problematics of continued racial segregation in American society more broadly, HDBMS, and other courses rooted in an explicitly antiracist epistemology, represent some of the few spaces where young people are encouraged to collaborate, share, and discuss ideas and experiences pertaining to race, racism, and the intersections of gender, class, sexuality, and nationality. In both individual reflection exercises and collective small and large group discussions, students were challenged to think relationally and conceptually about the role that race plays within their daily lives. However, while classroom instruction, dialogue and collaboration proved effective in dismantling myths about Black athleticism and criminality and engendering greater familiarity and cultural competencies (reflected in student's collaborative works) across racial boundaries, the disruption of Covid-19 and shift to fully virtual Zoom classes produced a crisis of confidence. More specifically, white students were noticeably less active in group discussions and, as expressed through several anonymous course evaluations, felt constrained for fear of saying the wrong thing, being accused of racism, or the belief that they did not have anything meaningful to contribute amongst more vocal and engaged students of color. Following the Spring 2021 semester, and upon reading the aforementioned comments, and others like it, I began to reflect on:

1. What I recalled as being profoundly insightful Zoom discussions where students of color were in-fact more eager to make comments,

but never at the exclusion of white students. Why did some white students "feel" it was not "appropriate" for them to express their opinion? Was it to rationalize lack of participation, feeling constrained by the presence of people who wouldn't normally be privy to in-person classroom dialogue (family members, roommates, passers-by, etc.), or concern over being secretly recorded by another student? Note: To encourage participation, I made it a point to clarify that Zoom classes were never being recorded on the platform.
2. How disappointing it was to read that a student had perceived the cumulative interaction and engagement of my TA and myself with students of color as favoritism; interpreted from their viewpoint to be out-of-the-ordinary, preferential, and unfair (reverse-racism, perhaps).
3. How that accusation reflects invisible, normalized logics of white ethnocentrism. Whereas many classes treat race as a non-variable, HDBMS expressly centers the Black experience within societal and sporting structures. Were some white students frustrated by feeling less prepared and capable in critical conversations about the realities of race in America? White supremacy and systemic racism, in particular?
4. How, despite initial discomfort in learning about injustices and oppressions within society and sport, pre-Covid students worked through their fears, and with regular in-person contact, developed greater trust and respect leading to more fruitful conversations about race.
5. How two years of successful face-to-face dialogic engagement was so vastly ruptured with the onset of Covid-19 and the shift to virtual learning.
6. How more critical research is needed to examine the impact of students' home learning environments on virtual learning outcomes.
7. How could trust-building and collaborative engagement be better facilitated in fully-virtual environments?

Returning again to the basic premise of segregation, social separation, and lack of meaningful interracial contact, the late Critical Legal Studies scholar and founding contributor of CRT, Derrick Bell, citing economist Matthew Goldberg, argued that, "racial nepotism, rather than racial animus is the major motivation for much of the discrimination that Blacks experience" (Bell, 1992, p. 70). Written well before the debilitating Trump-era—"roll back the clock" and bring overt racial divisiveness back into the political fray—brand of politics, Bell's racial pragmatism highlights how the systemic nature of racism and the disguising of "colorblind" racial preference perpetuates division and inequity in the interests of the white elite (Bell, 1992; Mills; 1956). Inhibited, rather than prohibited, from developing interracial bonds and networks of association, our students today are faced with the very palpable and visceral realities of racial violence and oppression, divisive politics, and the technological forces of counter-intelligence, deception, and misinformation about the contemporary racial formation under neoliberalizing late-capitalist sprawl. The brief disruption of productive interracial cooperation within HDBMS during two virtual semesters serves as a reminder that 1) physical spaces of multiracial and multicultural collaboration are critical for trust building, empathy, and understanding in our increasingly divided society, and 2) sport, as a highly popular cultural product, serves as an effective pedagogical tool exposing inequity and injustice within our institutions, and our own ways of thinking. Through the chaos and liminal insecurities of global pandemics and racial oppressions, we must continue to bring our students together, to dialogue with one another, to recognize our common humanity, and to enable a commitment to antiracist, antisexist civil dialogue and collaborative action for justice, equity, and peace.

References

Alexander, M. (2020). *The new Jim Crow: Mass incarceration in the age of colorblindness*. 10th Anniversary edition. The New Press.

Andrews, D. L. (2002). Coming to terms with cultural studies. *Journal of Sport & Social Issues, 26*(1), 110–117.

Andrews, D. L. (2019). *Making sport great again: The uber-sport assemblage, neoliberalism, and the trump conjuncture*. Palgrave Pivot.

Andrews, D. L., & Giardina, M. D. (2008). Sport without guarantees: Toward a cultural studies that matters. *Cultural Studies <=> Critical Methodologies, 8*(4), 395–422.

Arao, B., & Clemens, K. (2013). From safe spaces to brave spaces: A new way to frame dialogue around diversity and social justice. In L. M. Landreman (Ed.), *The art of effective facilitation: Reflections from a social justice educator* (pp. 135–150). Stylus.

Bell, D. (1992). *Faces at the bottom of the well: The permanence of racism*. Basic Books.

Bella, T., & Barrett, D. (2021, October 5). Garland asks FBI to address recent 'disturbing spike' in threats against educators. *The Washington Post*. https://www.washingtonpost.com/education/2021/10/05/garland-educators-threats-masks-fbi/

Bensimon, E. M. (2005). Closing the achievement gap in higher education: An organizational learning perspective. In A. Kezar (Ed.), *Organizational learning in higher education* (Vol. 131, pp. 99–111). Jossey-Bass.

Bonilla-Silva, E. (2002). The linguistics of color blind racism: How to talk nasty about blacks without sounding "racist". *Critical Sociology, 28*(1–2), 41–64.

Bonilla-Silva, E. (2018). *Racism without racists: Color-blind racism and the persistence of racial inequality in America* (5th ed.). Rowman & Littlefield.

Bonilla-Silva, E. (2019a). Feeling race: Theorizing the racial economy of emotions. *American Sociological Review, 84*(1), 1–25.

Bonilla-Silva, E. (2019b). Toward a new political praxis for trumpamerica: New directions in critical race theory. *American Behavioral Scientist, 63*(13), 1776–1788.

Carter, P., Skiba, R., Arredondo, M., & Pollock, M. (2014). You can't fix what you don't look at: Acknowledging race in addressing racial discipline disparities. http://www.indiana.edu/~atlantic/wp-content/uploads/2014/12/Acknowledging-Race_121514.pdf

Castagno, A. (2008). "I don't want to hear that!": Legitimating whiteness through silence in schools. *Anthropology & Education Quarterly, 39*(3), 314–333.

Christian, M., Seamster, L., & Ray, V. (2019). New directions in critical race theory and sociology: Racism, white supremacy, and resistance. *American Behavioral Scientist, 63*(13), 1731–1740.

Colby, T. (2012). *Some of my best friends are black: The strange story of integration in America*. Penguin Books.

Crenshaw, K. W. (2011). Twenty years of critical race theory: Looking back to move forward. *Connecticut Law Review, 43*, 1253–1352.

Delgado, R., & Stefancic, J. (2017). *Critical race theory: An introduction*. New York University Press.

Denzin, N. K. (2002). Confronting ethnography's crisis of representation. *Journal of Con-temporary Ethnography, 31*(4), 482–490.
Denzin, N. K. (2004). The war on culture, the war on truth. *Cultural Studies Critical Methodologies, 4*(2), 137–142.
Denzin, N. K. (2014). *Interpretive autoethnography*. Sage.
Desmond, M. (2016). *Evicted: Poverty and profit in the American city*. Penguin Random House.
Dowd, A. C., & Bensimon, E. M. (2015). *Engaging the "race question": Accountability and equity in U.S. higher education*. Teachers College Press.
Earle, J., Moran, C., & Ward-Perkins, Z. (2017). *The econocracy: The perils of leaving economics to the experts*. Manchester University press.
Epstein & Mazzei. (2021). GOP bills target protestors (and absolve motorists who hit them). *The New York Times*. https://www.nytimes.com/2021/04/21/us/politics/republican-anti-protest-laws.html
Feagin, J. (2013). *The white racial frame: Centuries of racial framing and counter-framing* (2nd ed.). Routledge.
Feagin, J., & Vera, H. (1995). *White racism: The basics*. Routledge.
Flaherty, C. (2021, June 9). Legislating against critical race theory. https://www.insidehighered.com/news/2021/06/09/legislating-against-critical-race-theory-curricular-implications-some-states
Freire, P. (2000). *Pedagogy of the oppressed*. 30th Anniversary edn. Continuum.
Galloway, M., Callin, P., James, S., Vimegnon, H., & McCall, L. (2019). Culturally responsive, antiracist, or anti-oppressive? how language matters for school change efforts. *Equity & Excellence in Education, 52*(4), 485–501.
Giardina, M. D. (2005). Introduction: An ordinary citizen's guide to sport. In *Sporting pedagogies: Performing culture & identity in the global arena* (pp. 1–26). New York: Peter Lang.
Giroux, H. (2001). "Something's missing": Cultural studies, neoliberalism and the politics of hope. *Strategies: Journal of Theory, Culture & Politics, 14*(2), 227–252.
Hall, S. (1997). The spectacle of the 'other'. In S. Hall (Ed.), *Representation: Cultural representations and signifying practices* (pp. 223–290). Sage.
hooks, b. (1992). *Black looks: Race and representation*. South End Press.
Impelli, M. (2021, May 11). North Carolina seventh state set to ban critical race theory in schools. *Newsweek*. https://www.newsweek.com/north-carolina-seventh-state-set-ban-critical-race-theory-schools-1590620
Irby, D. J., & Clark, S. P. (2018). Talk it (Racism) out: Race talk and organizational learning. *Journal of Educational Administration, 56*, 504–518.

Ishimaru, A. M., & Galloway, M. K. (2014). Beyond individual effectiveness: Conceptualizing organizational leadership for equity. *Leadership and Policy in Schools, 13*, 93–146. https://doi.org/10.1080/15700763.2014.890733
Kamberlies, G., & Dimitriadis, G. (2005). Focus groups: Strategic articulations of pedagogy, politics and inquiry. In N. K. Denzin & Y. S. Lincoln (Eds.), *The Sage handbook of qualitative research* (3rd ed., pp. 875–895). Sage.
Kitwana, B. (2005). *Why white kids love hip-hop: Wanksta, wiggas, wannabees and the new reality of race in America*. Basic Civitas Books.
Ladson-Billings, G. (2014). Culturally relevant pedagogy 2.0: A.k.a. the remix. *Harvard Educational Review, 84*, 74–84. https://doi.org/10.17763/haer.84.1.p2rj131485484751
Lang, C. (2020, September 29). President Trump has attacked critical race theory. Here's what to know about the intellectual movement. *Time Magazine*. https://time.com/5891138/critical-race-theory-explained/
Lipsitz, G. (2006). *The possessive investment in Whiteness: How White people profit from identity politics*. Temple University Press.
Martinez, A. (2020, July 22). Can sports globalization survive a pandemic? *Globalsportmatters.com*. https://globalsportmatters.com/business/2020/07/22/can-sports-globalization-survive-a-pandemic/
Marty, D. (1999). White antiracist rhetoric as apologia: Wendell Berry's The Hidden Wound. In T. K. Nakayama & J. N. Martin (Eds.), *Whiteness: The communication of social identity* (pp. 51–68). Sage.
Menendian, S., Gambhir, S., & Gailes, A. (2021, June 30). The roots of structural racism project: Twenty-first century racial residential segregation in the United States. https://belonging.berkeley.edu/roots-structural-racism
Mills, C. W. (1956). *The power elite*. Oxford University Press.
Naurighr, J., Zipp, S., & Kim, Y. H. (2020). The sports world in the era of Covid-19. *Sport in Society, 23*(11), 1703–1706.
Omi, M., & Winant, H. (1994). *Racial formation in the United States from the 1960's to the 1990's* (2nd ed.). Routledge.
Pape, M. (2020, March 19). Rapid rise of women's sport at risk of being halted by Covid-19 outbreak. *The Guardian*. https://www.the-guardian.com/sport/2020/mar/19/rapid-rise-of-womens-sport-at-risk-of-being-halted-by-covid-19-outbreak
Paris, D., & Alim, H. S. (2014). What are we seeking to sustain through culturally sustaining pedagogy? A loving critique forward. *Harvard Educational Review, 84*, 85–100.

Pietila, A. (2010). *Not in my neighborhood: How bigotry shaped a great American city*. Ivan Dee.
Pollock, M. (2004). *Colormute: Race Talk Dilemmas in an American School*. Princeton University Press.
Pollock, M. (2008). *Everyday antiracism: Getting real about race in school*. The New Press.
Ray, R., & Gibbons, A. (2021). Why are states banning critical race theory? *The Brookings Institute*. https://www.brookings.edu/blog/fixgov/2021/07/02/why-are-states-banning-critical-race-theory/
Robinson, C. (2019). *On racial capitalism, black internationalism, and cultures of resistance*. Pluto Press.
Rodriguez, D. (2009). The usual suspect: Negotiating white student resistance and teacher authority in a predominantly white classroom. *Cultural Studies—Critical Methodologies, 9*(4), 483–508.
Rodriguez, D. (2011). Silence as speech: Meanings of silence for students of color in predominantly white classrooms. *International Review of Qualitative Research, 4*(1), 111–144.
Rothstein, R. (2017). *The color of law: A forgotten history of how our government segregated America*. Liveright.
Rowe, D. (2020). Subjecting pandemic sport to a sociological procedure. *Journal of Sociology, 56*(4), 704–713.
Runstedtler, T. (2018). More than just play: Unmasking Black child labor in the athletic industrial complex. *Journal of Sport & Social Issues, 42(30*, 152–169.
Sheptak, R., & Menaker, B. (2020). When sport event work stopped: Exposure of sport event labor precarity by the Covid-19 pandemic. *International Journal of Sport Communication, 13*, 427–435.
Silk, M., & Andrews, D. (2011). Toward a physical cultural studies. *Sociology of Sport Journal, 28*, 4–35.
Smith, E. (2014). *Race, sport and the American dream* (3rd ed.). Carolina Academic Press.
Tsai, J. (2020, September 8). Covid-19's disparate impacts are not a story about race. They're a story about racism. *Scientific American*. https://www.scientificamerican.com/article/covid-19s-disparate-impacts-are-not-a-story-about-race/
Ujifusa, A. (2021, October, 11). Is the Justice Department silencing parents or stepping up to protect educators. *Education Week*. https://www.edweek.org/policy-politics/is-the-justice-dept-silencing-parents-or-stepping-up-to-protect-educators/2021/10

Wacquant, L. J. D. (2007). *Urban outcasts: A comparative sociology of advanced marginality*. Polity Press.

Wacquant, L. J. D. (2009). *Punishing the poor: The neoliberal government of social insecurity*. Duke University Press.

Ware, V., & Back, L. (2002). *Out of whiteness: Color, politics, and culture*. Chicago University Press.

Wilson, B. (1997). 'Good Blacks' and 'bad Blacks': Media constructions of African-American athletes in Canadian basketball. *International Review for the Sociology of Sport, 32*(2), 177–189.

Wingfield, A. H., & Feagin, J. (2012). The racial dialectic: President Barack Obama and the white racial frame. *Qualitative Sociology*, first published online March 6, 2012.

Yosso, T. J. (2002). Critical race media literacy: Challenging deficit discourse about Chicanas/os. *Journal of Popular Film and Television, 30*(1), 52–62.

Yousman, B. (2003). Blackophilia and Blackophobia: White youth, the consumption of rap music, and white supremacy. *Communication Theory, 13*(4), 366–391.

Zhang, S. (2021, April 21). Republicans have introduced 81 anti-protest laws in 34 states just this year. *Truthout.org*. https://truthout.org/articles/republicans-have-introduced-81-anti-protest-laws-in-34-states-just-this-year/

14

Sport-for-Development and Peace and COVID-19: Technologies, the Body, and Virtual Forms of Programming

Mitchell McSweeney and Lyndsay Hayhurst

The COVID-19 pandemic has, like many other areas of life, disrupted the sport-for-development (SDP) sector. The onset of COVID-19 and physical distancing guidelines led to many organizations within the SDP field pivoting and altering program operations. This included SDP organizations innovatively adapting programs to online forms of delivery; for example, by using web-applications such as Zoom to facilitate SDP activities in a virtual space. However, shifting to online and virtual forms of SDP delivery resulted in program participants experiencing SDP in different spaces and through technological means. In other words, SDP program activities now took place through bodily movements intertwined

M. McSweeney (✉)
School of Kinesiology, University of Minnesota,
Minneapolis, MN, USA
e-mail: mcsweenm@yorku.ca

L. Hayhurst
School of Kinesiology and Health Science, York University,
Toronto, ON, Canada

D. L. Andrews et al. (eds.), *Sport and Physical Culture in Global Pandemic Times*,
Global Culture and Sport Series, https://doi.org/10.1007/978-3-031-14387-8_14

with and constituted by a range of economic, environmental, and technological assemblages and relations. Thus, in this chapter, we first discuss the impact of COVID-19 on SDP, in particular the effects the pandemic has had on the implementation of programs. Second, we review work related to feminist new materialism approaches, including research within the field of the sociology of sport, leisure, and physical cultures to begin to recognize the relations and associations of the body and technology. Third, we analyze a report on the impact of COVID-19 on the SDP sector, and discuss how both humans and nonhumans mediate and produce social and political life. In conclusion, we discuss how the COVID-19 pandemic has influenced new ways to implement SDP, and argue that feminist new materialism approaches present a timely and significant way to analyze the ways in which the material body in SDP intersects with technology, politics, and culture.

Introduction

> Sport for development must engage with technology as it can supplement the mission to get more people active.
>
> —Dame Louise Martin, President of the Commonwealth Games Federation

The quote above by Dame Louise Martin, the judge of a virtual debate (which concluded in a draw) during the Fifth Annual Commonwealth Debate (The Commonwealth, 2021) on whether investment in technology is the key to rebuilding the sport sector post-COVID-19, signifies how, like many other areas of social, economic, political, and cultural life, the global coronavirus pandemic has impacted the sport-for-development and peace (SDP) sector. SDP is the *intentional use* of sport to contribute to development aims and challenge social inequalities, such as social inclusion, gender rights, and conflict resolution (Kidd, 2008, 2011). The SDP field has grown tremendously since the early 2000s, becoming institutionalized and perhaps even professionalized (McSweeney et al., 2022) to the point where it is a recognizable subsector of international development, evidenced by its integration within the Millennium Development

Goals and Sustainable Development Goals (Lindsey & Chapman, 2017; Lindsey & Darby, 2019). Certainly, before the COVID-19 pandemic SDP organizations experienced a number of challenges related to resource-constraints, financial insecurity, and for many programs, a reliance on Global North donors (Clutterbuck & Doherty, 2019; McSweeney et al., 2019; Svensson et al., 2020); the COVID-19 pandemic has further perpetuated such issues at the same time as impacting the ability for organizations to implement SDP programs.

Indeed, it is perhaps unsurprising that—given the national and regional lockdowns and physical distancing guidelines legislated by governments around the world—that sport (and by extension SDP) experienced challenges operating. Such challenges were exacerbated by the fact that sport and physical activity often involve bodily contact and/or are pursued with bodies in close proximity to one another (depending on the type of sport played), making physical distancing requirements near impossible. Global sporting events were cancelled and/or rescheduled, youth sport leagues were halted, and sport and physical activities occurring in a team environment mostly disbanded for the foreseeable future (UN, 2020). Though the world has been living with COVID-19 since as early as January 2020 (AJMC, 2021), with vaccination rates rising (mostly in the Global North as the Global South has been faced with inequitable access and distribution of vaccines; UN, 2021), pandemic restrictions and guidelines continue to rapidly change and affect social life in different ways and in different locations, not least of which is influenced by COVID-19 variants such as Omicron.

The SDP field has thus—since the beginning of the pandemic in early 2020 to the present—been impacted in similar ways of other forms of sport noted above. In fact, given that many SDP organizations and networks depend on external funding, the pandemic has forced many SDP organizations to pivot program implementation from in-person, face-to-face activities, to virtual and/or online forms of program delivery to fulfill their social mission (Donnelly et al., 2020; SFDC, 2020; Sportanddev, 2021a). At the same time, such litheness is essential for demonstrating to future funders or partners that a given SDP organization has creative solutions to continue operating when faced with extenuating circumstances (i.e., global pandemics).

SDP organizations have innovated their program strategies in a number of key ways. For instance, Maple Leaf Sports and Entertainment Launchpad, in Toronto, Ontario, shifted their in-person programs to virtual programming for youth ages 6 to 29. These programs included prerecorded at-home workouts by Launchpad coaches (e.g., dance, soccer drills, volleyball drills, conditioning) as well as workshops focused on healthy eating, careers in mental health and wellness in sport, and virtual sport for development workshops for practitioners and other organizations (MLSE LP, 2021). Other initiatives, such as ChildFund Sport for Development, adapted by creating a Reconnect program where children can attend drop-in activities in safe and structured settings, following public health guidelines, and engage in skills development to cope with the uncertainty of the pandemic as a group and maintain hygiene practices (Sportanddev, 2021b).

Yet, at the same time as innovation and creativity in the SDP field has occurred via the alteration of program implementation strategies, there have also been noticeable limitations of changing to online, remote, and virtual programs in the SDP sector. For instance, Dixon et al. (2020), who highlighted how girls in SDP experienced some positive outcomes (e.g., family time, rest, better hygiene) from shifts in programs by Highway of Hope in Kenya, also raised notable challenges for participants based on the organization's innovative response to COVID. Specifically, salient challenges included restrictions around physical activity and difficulties at home for participants such as boredom. While the organizations were innovative by adapting to the core needs of the participants, Dixon et al. (2020) also noted that the experiences of the young women in relation to SDP and COVID-19 are likely gendered.

In addition, the World Health Organization, along with other large international governing bodies and networks such as The Commonwealth and United Nations, have highlighted how the move to utilizing technology in the SDP sector is often inequitable. Furthermore, technologies used for virtual SDP programs (e.g., phones, laptops, Ipads, internet access, screens, etc.), while offering potential ways to engage SDP participants in new ways not confined to a specific 'sport' setting (i.e., a court, field), vary widely in accessibility. While some participants may have the required technological instruments to engage in virtual or remote SDP activities, other participants, especially individuals living in rural areas without access to internet connection, may be further marginalized due to inaccessibility.

Thus, while Though here are no doubt various SDP organizations that have innovated due to the pandemic (as highlighted above), and there may be potential opportunities for the use of technologies moving forward in the SDP sector (see McSweeney et al., 2021b; Svensson & McSweeney, in press), the use of such technologies must be critically examined and assessed. This includes a more critical understanding of the ways technologies are not simply instruments utilized for the continuation of SDP in virtual forms, but instead considering how technologies are relational—as having ontological status and meaning through relationships with bodies, things, and ideas (Haraway, 1991). These relations (i.e., between bodies, technologies, and other social, material and abstract entities) make up an *assemblage*, which is a process made up of different "machines that link elements together to do something, to produce something" (Fox & Alldred, 2015a, p. 403).

Thus, the move to virtual and remote programming in SDP using technologies does not simply involve the use of objects (i.e., computers, Ipads, fitbits, phones) that already occupy distinct and delimited spaces in society. Rather, technologies both constitute and are constituted by relations in which they are embedded (e.g., bodies, emotions, things, ideas, places), whereby technologies have 'agential' capacities to *affect*. An affect "is a 'becoming' that represents a change of state or capacities of an entity—this change may be physical, psychological, emotional or social" (Fox & Alldred, 2015b, p. 3, see also Deleuze & Guattari, 1988). Indeed, a number of SDP scholars have underlined how the assemblage of SDP is shaped in a variety of ways by nonhuman actants, including: environmental degradation (Hayhurst & del Socorro Cruz Centeno, 2019), indicator culture (Henne, 2017), water (Bunds, 2017), and policies (Darnell et al., 2018). Given these assemblages, the purpose of this chapter is to serve as a departure point for further investigating the complex human and nonhuman relations that are invoked through a feminist new materialist approach to SDP. Specifically, the goal of our chapter is to explore the relations and associations of the body and technologies in

SDP, based on the innovative adaptations by SDP organizations in times of COVID-19.

In the section that follows, we provide a brief overview of feminist new materialism approaches, including research within the field of the sociology of sport, leisure, and physical culture. Second, we analyze a report, the *Impact of COVID-19 on the Sport for Development Sector* (SFDC, 2020), and think through the relations of SDP, COVID-19, and technology using a feminist new materialist approach. Importantly, the report provides insights into the adaptations of programming by SDP organizations as well as the challenges and inequalities for particular groups due to the global pandemic. In conclusion, we discuss how the COVID-19 pandemic has influenced new ways to implement SDP, and argue that feminist new materialism approaches present a timely and significant way to analyze the ways in which the material body in SDP intersects with technology, politics, and culture.

Feminist New Materialisms

New materialisms research "share a critique and focus on interrogating the nature of the 'human', including acknowledgement of the actors (including those normatively considered to be 'nonhuman') that come together to configure more-than-human worlds" (Lupton, 2019, p. 1999). New materialisms research acknowledges the role of humans *and* nonhumans as integral parts of knowledge production and power relations (Ulmer, 2017). Informed by, but also moving beyond, paradigms such as poststructural, postmodern, postcolonial, and other posts-, new materialism seeks to critically examine and further understand social life beyond lived experience by considering the "material-discursive relations that make the life of the body and its movement (im)possible" (Fullagar, 2017, p. 248). Approaches within new materialism seek to disrupt micro- and macro- divisions and recognize that the world and its materiality are produced by a wide array of material forces, including practices, doings, actions, and matter, and other biological, psychological, social, cultural, and physical entities (Barad, 2003). In bringing together mind and matter and nature and culture, traditional concerns within social sciences and humanities such as structural and macro-levels of social life are moved beyond, to instead address issues that are often considered as 'micro-sociological', "because of their association with how thoughts, desires, feelings and abstract concepts contribute to social production" (Fox & Alldred, 2015b, p. 3). When applied to sport, Markula (2019) notes how

> A new materialist perspective—without challenging the humanist narratives of social justice through emancipation, empowerment, and individual agency—can add the material world to sport sociological analyses by accounting for the agency of material objects around us. This type of new materialist research might examine how material objects and conditions in different sport and physical activity environments impact how the humans construct their selves and their worlds. (p. 5)

Lupton (2019) has discussed how seminal feminist scholars (such as Donna Haraway, Karen Barad, and Rosi Braidotti) have been influential for advancing *feminist* new materialism approaches that critically explore how human and nonhuman assemblages are gendered, nuanced, complex, and political. Rather than focus on language exclusively—practices, doings, actions, and matter—are all part and parcel of the assemblages that influence the social and political world (e.g., Bastian, 2017). For instance, matter, which is considered as things, objects, bodies, spaces, and places (Lupton, 2019) is "an active participant in the world's becoming" (Barad, 2003, p. 802). Intercorporeality (Merleau-Ponty, 1962), which is the distribution of embodiment beyond the individual both to other humans and nonhumans (Lupton, 2019), contests the view that the embodiment of the individual body is solely experienced by the self.

The key difference between other new materialism approaches and feminist new materialisms is how the latter takes an overt political and ethical stance: "Because of their feminist standpoint, these [feminist new materialism] scholars work to uncover the gendered dimensions of the more-than-human world" (Lupton, 2019, p. 1999). As we are interested in this chapter to provide insights into the way in which feminist new materialisms can be applied to understanding the relations of SDP, COVID-19, and virtual programs, we follow Lupton's (2019) propositions on how to engage with feminist new materialism. While not a fulsome review of the many methods and approaches of feminist new materialism theory, in what follows we attempt to 'think with theory' by taking a more-than-human approach to critically investigate SDP, COVID-19, and virtual programming. Sport, and more specifically SDP, has been recognized by numerous scholars as gendered, based on the ways in which men and boys' experiences, events, and programs often are privileged compared to women and girls (Hayhurst et al., 2021; Saavedra, 2009). Further, despite the intentions of SDP programs to contribute to gender equality, the contexts where SDP is implemented in possess existing structural gender inequalities (e.g., gendered divisions of labour) that maintain gender norms related to women and girls' participation in sport, their roles in their community, and the expected responsibilities that women and girls take on (Chawansky, 2011; Hayhurst & del Socorro Cruz Centeno, 2019). Such gender norms shape and are influenced by the material nature of SDP across local to global flows, from bodily practices (both related to sport and, for example, domestic work), the flow of money from SDP funders, appropriate sportwear, to the actual environment in which SDP takes place. Hence, a feminist new materialism approach is useful for thinking through the gendered nature of SDP and the human and non-human actors that play a role in the sector. We attempt to put our work in conversation with other sociology of sport and physical cultural scholars who are increasingly engaging with the posthuman, more-than-human, feminist materialist and multispecies approaches to better understand the intricate and vital relations between human and nonhuman agents (see Thorpe et al., 2021). To do so, we use research materials or research assemblages, which we as researchers are a part of (Lupton, 2019), to analyze the relations and assemblages in SDP made up by both humans and non-humans in relation to COVID-19. First, however, in the next section, we discuss the work of scholars using feminist new materialism in the sociology of sport, leisure, and physical culture.

New Materialism in the Sociology of Sport, Leisure, and Physical Culture

Inspired by the ontological and epistemological turn in the broader sociological and qualitative research disciplines (Giardina, 2017), sociologists of sport, leisure, and physical cultures have increasingly turned to the use of postqualitative and/or postinterpretive approaches that emphasize a decentering of the 'human' body (Fullagar, 2017; Millington & Wilson, 2015). Fullager (2017, p. 248) suggests that,

> Pushing our thinking beyond 'human experience' are ontological questions about how 'matter' is thought and constituted through entanglements of human and non-human bodies, affects, objects and cultural practices. Such a shift reorients thinking around relational questions about the material-discursive forces that are co-implicated in what bodies can 'do' and how matter 'acts'.

For instance, the use of Actor Network Theory (ANT), is a new materialist theory that seeks to understand the mechanics of power in the world and society, and "is a way of suggesting that society, organizations, agents and machines are all effects generated in patterned networks of diverse (not simply human) materials" (Law, 1992, p. 2). ANT has been utilized for several studies in the realm of sport and physical cultures (e.g., Weedon, 2015). Two specific studies relative to this chapter, however, are by Darnell et al. (2018) who use ANT to explore SDP (see also Webb & Richelieu, 2016) and McSweeney et al. (2021a) who apply ANT to the related field of bicycles for development (BFD) (i.e., the use of bicycles to achieve international, regional, and community development goals). Henne (2017) concurs that an ANT approach is useful for better understanding how various actants (human and nonhuman) influence the assemblage of SDP. That is, SDP is not simply socially constructed, but that other nonhuman elements such as technical support, the environment, money, etc., end up shaping the overall deployment of SDP (Henne, 2017).

In the abovementioned articles, attention is mostly paid to the nonhuman objects (e.g., bicycles, handlebars, tax and import laws, money, best practices) in SDP and BFD, and how these non-human objects play a significant role in forming assemblages that shape and influence the dynamic fields. Furthermore, this scholarship illustrates how non-human objects have agential capabilities that mediate and produce how human actors (e.g., SDP and BFD participants, organizations, nongovernmental organizations executives) experience social and political life. In their work centering non-human objects as paramount to the ANT approach utilized, McSweeney et al. (2021a) highlight how non-humans cause 'frictions' that unsettle, divert, and also contribute to the actions of BFD organizations—via the agency of both humans and non-humans. However, while the two studies shed light on how new materialism approaches are useful in studies of SDP, they follow other approaches that are not as overtly political as *feminist* new materialism by minimizing analysis related to "gendered dimensions of material processes, power relations, the environment and the Anthropocene" (Thorpe et al., 2020, p. 7).

Feminist New Materialism and Studies of Sport, Leisure, and Physical Cultures

Feminist new materialism approaches expand the exploration of 'more-than-human' worlds by uncovering the gendered dimensions of human and non-human life. An abundance of recent scholarly commentary and research in sociological studies of sport, leisure, and physical cultures has been conducted utilizing feminist new materialism approaches (e.g., Brice et al., 2021; Evers, 2019; Thorpe et al., 2021). Feminist new materialism seeks to understand matter in relation to gender—including for instance bodies (the affective, fleshy, sensory elements of human beings), the environment, and nonhuman entities, that are influential and actively shape and are shaped by social phenomena and human lived experience "in unpredictable ways" (Thorpe et al., 2020). For example, Markula (2019) draws attention to how the body—as matter—and its everyday practices and movements in physical spaces and places is important for the purposes of challenging the boundaries between mind and body and human and non-human, as well as uncovering the power relations in which materiality (human and nonhuman) are embedded.

The work of feminist new materialism in sociological studies of sport, leisure, and physical cultures has also brought to the fore the idea of 'embodied research' (Thorpe & Marfell, 2019). Fullagar, Pavlidis, and Francombe-Webb (2018, p. 1) note how, "new materialist thinking takes questions about the 'personal as political' as serious embodied and conceptual matters, while also urging feminists to engage with ideas critically, creatively, and hopefully, even playfully." Embodied research involves accounting for the 'fleshy' and material politics of sport and/or physical cultures: meaning that researchers 'live' physical culture (Giardina & Newman, 2011) such as engaging in observation (e.g., watching sport events or games), listening, conversing, feeling the actual aspects of sport or physical cultures (e.g., getting wet by rain and cold or hot), feeling pleasure, joys, frustrations, and challenges (Thorpe & Marfell, 2019) and overall embodying "the operations and effects of gendered power and agency" (Pavlidis & Olive, 2014, p. 220). This shift to embodied research moves away from 'meaning' (e.g., what is gender) to consider how gendered power relations actually materialize more fulsomely through "bodies, patriarchal institutions, objects, and nonhuman nature in multiple ways: regulating, normalizing, and opening up trajectories of becoming" (Fullagar et al., 2018, p. 9; see also Fullagar, 2017).

Other work using feminist new materialism approaches have been concerned with health, fitness, sport, and physical cultures and the technologies in which are "tethered to bodies and, through habitualization, designed to add value to everyday life in the form of physical wellbeing" (Gilmore, 2016, p. 2). Yet, as Fullagar et al. (2019a) say, while digital and physical culture leisure practices have begun to be studied more in leisure studies, feminist analysis is only starting to emerge (e.g., Fullagar et al., 2019b; Rich, 2018). This work has sought to consider the complexities, practices, and affective relationalities between technologies and the gendered body (Rich, 2018), such as examination of the gendered dynamics of Strava (Barrie et al., 2019). Other studies have included examination of social media (i.e., digital environments) and digital technologies to bring the nonhuman in to view (e.g., Brice & Andrews, 2019; King & Weedon, 2021). Many of these studies use new materialism approaches creatively and in ways of theory-method and, using a relational approach, "understand these practices as entangled, and as such, integral to the process of emerging meanings and practices that produce embodiment" (Fullagar et al., 2019, p. 9).

While growing work using feminist new materialism approaches in relation to sport, leisure, and physical cultures has been conducted, less work has utilized feminist new materialism approaches in the specific field of SDP and/or sport, gender, and development (although Thorpe and colleagues, as seen above, place some of their work related to sport and physical cultures in the context of development, however may not refer explicitly to 'SDP'). There remains a need to bring feminist perspectives into the study of SDP using new materialism approaches (see Hayhurst & del Socorro Cruz Centeno, 2019; Hayhurst et al., 2021). In particular, as noted above, embodied research which brings to the fore gendered inequalities, body politics, and reflexivity would advance feminist new materialism approaches. Further, scholars have called for research that brings specific nonhumans (e.g., animals, plants, the elements) into the research process (Fullagar et al., 2019; Thorpe et al., 2021). Such an approach to research will provide important empirical investigation and connections between the human and non-human in SDP and sport, gender, and development. In the following sections, we seek to modestly contribute to this growing literature through an analysis of the *Impact of COVID-19 on the Sport for Development Sector* (SFDC, 2020) report. In doing so, we echo the call by feminist scholars to engage with feminist new materialism approaches by investigating the interrelationships of humans and nonhumans related to SDP, COVID-19, and the innovations (particularly virtual programming) undertaken by organizations.

SDP in Times of COVID-19: Online and Virtual Forms of Delivery

In a recent article, Fullagar and Pavlidis (2021) used a feminist new materialism perspective to outline the disruptive effects of the COVID-19 pandemic. In this work, the authors critically explore the ramifications of the COVID-19 pandemic in terms of changes and leisure choices that are complex and emerging. Specifically, they focus attention on "multiple affects and (digitally mediated) interrelationships that produce expanded or limited agentic capacities, rather than atomistic agents" (p. 155). In doing so, they illustrate the multi-scalar phenomenon of leisure that is made up of assemblages between and within global and local relations, humans and nonhumans, and the gendered micropolitics of everyday life, which produce affects that plug into, for example, un/paid work, care, and community. Fullagar and Pavlidis' (2021) article provides insight into the way in which the COVID-19 pandemic has disrupted leisure practices and how "affective relations are transforming gendered experiences, environments and social institutions in the COVID-19 world" (p. 157).

Their article informs our analysis in the next section to explore the *assemblages* and *affects* that such assemblages produce in times of COVID-19. Specifically, by taking a more-than-human approach to critically analyze SDP, COVID-19, and the innovations taking place by organizations to move to virtual forms, we utilize a specific research material (Lupton, 2019), a report. We explore the report by the Sport for Development Coalition, the *Impact of COVID-19 on the Sport for Development Sector*, to think through the COVID-19 pandemic and SDP, in relation to both humans (bodies, practices, movements, spaces) and non-humans (technologies, spaces, places, equipment) that produce affective relations of gendered experiences.

Of note is that the following analysis focuses on the discursive portrayal of SDP and gender in times of COVID-19, and how SDP has been positioned by certain actors and for certain audiences through the report. We acknowledge that the 'material' of the report is thus examined through its words and how this material affects other human and non-human actors within the SDP field. Given that the authors did not write the report, nor have investigated the actual effects of the document on actors, we use this analysis as a departure point for probing more deeply into the ways that feminist new materialist approaches may provide new ways to consider how the materiality of the text may create assemblages and effects on other actors in the SDP field. Further research is needed to better understand how documents, such as policies and reports, 'come to life'—for example—with reference to the amount of copies made, in what ways the report was distributed and where, how SDP actors responded (if at all) to the report, and how documents take up space or place in offices, program locations, and SDP contexts. For now, while recognizing that the authors are unable to focus explicitly on this materiality of the report, we direct attention to how the report has capacity to potentially effect SDP programs and action strategies in times of COVID-19, and how the framing of SDP and gender produces affects that are relevant for both humans and non-humans. We do not intend for this to be a comprehensive analysis, but rather hope to provide a starting point for exploring how feminist new materialism can be applied to SDP in relation to COVID-19.

Impact of COVID-19 on the Sport for Development Sector Report

The *Impact of COVID-19 on the Sport for Development Sector* report was produced for The Sport for Development Coalition (SFDC), with a specific focus on the United Kingdom (UK). The SFDC is "a movement of organizations who believe and use the power of sport as an effective intervention tool" (SFDC, 2020, p. 2). These organizations, or actors, include a range of charities, governing bodies, funders, networks, and SDP implementation organizations who make up the SFDC. In a similar vein to Lupton's (2019) analysis of a digital health policy document, this report is a material object that is a part of—and made up by—heterogenous and dynamic assemblages. The report was configured by various human actors and agencies—indeed, the SFDC as noted above is made up of a number of organizations within the SDP field. Thus, the report is premised on information that was collected from numerous organizations and participants from the SDP sector, including program reports, social media, anecdotal evidence, news sources, and national data. The report is written for specific purposes; as a report by the SFDC, it has a political purpose that presents the SFDC to the public as a significant figure in the SDP sector, with an authoritative presence, particularly in the UK. The report thus draws on the SFDC's ideologies and ideas around SDP. The author,

Rose Chilton (Insight Manager at Sported) speaks with an institutional voice (see Lupton, 2019), i.e. on behalf of the SFDC, and has positioned this report as an "agential cut" (p. 2003) to make meaning of the SDP sector and COVID-19 impact from a wide range of possible meanings in the political environment in which the SFDC has created it. There are many potential audiences for the report, including other SDP networks, organizations, and practitioners, government agencies (particularly in the UK), SDP funders and donors, participants of SDP programs, and researchers (such as ourselves). Already then, the report is constituted by and constituted of a number of different actors, with certain political influences, and is a material object that seeks to make meaning of the COVID-19 impact on SDP.

Reading the document following Lupton (2019, p. 2003) to "identify the relational connections, affective forces, and agential capacities" that exist in the words and phrases the report deploys, we sought to investigate how the impact of COVID-19 on SDP is discursively portrayed in its text. The language used in the report positions SFDC as a leader and an institutional expert in SDP and an actor that can provide relevant insight into COVID-19 and SDP. Language and words that are employed to create SDP as an impactful, transformative way to achieve development goals is used throughout (SFDC, 2020):

> SFD [sport for development] is the intentional use of sport and physical activity to bring about positive changes in the lives of people and communities. (p. 2)

> SFD organization[s] work across outcomes and deliver valuable support targeted at certain demographics. They have built up trust over several years and are well placed to provide this support. (p. 24)

Throughout the report, the document positions SDP as impactful, lively, transformative, and (mostly) positive, working on people's lives (e.g., SDP participants, staff within organizations) and changing them, making connections with the people the report is intended to influence (SDP stakeholders). The document represents SDP as an ontologically-prior essence (Fox & Alldred, 2015b), ascribing power to the potential of SDP to contribute development goals. However, by doing so, the report downplays how SDP is relational, made up via its relationship to bodies, things, and ideas (such as the ideas above of SDP as positive and transformative). SDP participants in this document are situated as the 'end-users' or target beneficiaries of SDP and those who may benefit from SDP—but also, as individuals and groups who have faced challenges due to COVID-19 and in some cases further marginalization due to the pandemic and alternative forms of SDP implementation. The report then not only represents SFDC as a promoter of SDP and its associated development programs, but also as a protector of the participants and organizations who have been implicated by COVID-19, and an actor who takes on a role to ensure that SDP is inclusive, critical, and ready to take on the challenges of COVID-19.

The report not only positions SFDC as an agent and SDP as having agential capacity to transform people's lives, but also highlights the various non-human actors that are intertwined and make up the assemblages of SDP, COVID-19, and virtual programming. Highlighting various challenges of SDP due to pandemic restrictions and guidelines, particularly for systematically disadvantaged groups in society (e.g., mental wellbeing of young people, social isolation, decreased physical activity levels, reinforcement of gender roles, inequitable disparities for different ethnicities, financial loss for SDP organizations), the report brings into conversation the innovations that SDP organizations have undergone to continue SDP programming in new virtual and online ways, as well as raises issues with virtual delivery of SDP (SFDC, 2020):

> Organizations are developing online content and seeing this as an opportunity to make resources more accessible online, and potentially reach more beneficiaries in the future. (p. 18)

> Through virtual delivery which has included interactive creative tasks and activities such as online football gaming tournaments and a zoom youth clubs, individuals have maintained regular connection with positive role models. However, coaches report in this virtual world it is harder to subtly check in with vulnerable people and pick up on subtle clue as to the wellbeing and the most vulnerable might not access support at all. (p. 18)

The report positions the use of technology (e.g., computers to create online resources, Zoom to deliver SDP programs) as a novel way to respond to the challenges of COVID-19. But also, the report recognizes how virtual delivery is intermeshed with humans and non-humans—how virtual delivery may not allow for thoughts and feelings of young people to be identified and responded to. The report also overlooks how the use of computers (potentially) allows for a wider range of participants; how the required technological infrastructure is needed for successful online delivery; and how virtual delivery has resulted in the development of safeguarding policies for online engagement. Most organizations have ceased in-person delivery and moved to adapted forms of virtual implementation during the pandemic. Others have innovated by setting up safety nets for participants (e.g., frequent check-ins, support helplines, wellbeing packs, providing phones to keep participants updated about the changing situation of COVID, delivering food and COVID-19 support leaflets, data vouchers for internet usage, assisting with social services).

While there is no data in the report on the lived experiences of SDP participants in relation to these innovative strategies deployed by organizations (though the report does include quotes and insights from SDP staff), it is important, in analyzing more-than-human-life, to draw attention to the assemblages and affects that the report reveals. That is, while the report provides significant insights into both the possibilities of SDP and challenges that have arisen due to COVID-19, using a feminist new materialism perspective brings a focus onto the relations in which SDP and COVID-19 constitute and are constituted by. We thus briefly investigate these relations, both in terms of human and non-human assemblages which have agential capacities.

COVID-19 itself is a "non-living agent that halts the flow of capital, people, and commodities" (Fullagar & Pavlidis, 2021, p. 155). In SDP, this non-human agent has affected the ability of SDP organizations to continue programming in its usual ways. Innovations, such as virtual programming, have been positioned as a novel way to maintain SDP implementation; and yet, the *spaces* and *places*, in which these new types of SDP program take shape are intertwined with the micro-politics of space (Fullagar & Pavlidis, 2021). Women and girls take on the bulk of unpaid work during COVID-19, including childcare, whilst also being more likely to be exposed to COVID-19 as they are in higher-risk work roles (SFDC, 2020). The pandemic has also revealed significant increases in domestic, sexual and gender-based violence (GBV), with access to in-person support services significantly reduced as COVID-19 response has been prioritized. The mental health challenges of women and girls has also been reported as higher than men and boys (SFDC, 2020). The turn to virtual or online forms of SDP have thus produced multiple affects and are complex and emerging—mediated by digital technologies and interrelationships that, based on the report, limit agentic capacities. Home during COVID-19, as said by Fullagar and Pavlidis (2021) is a "intense site of practically everything" (p. 155).

Thinking through the report by applying feminist new materialism provides further insights into the human and nonhuman interrelationships that produce agential capacities (Fullagar & Pavlidis, 2021). Nonhuman agents, such as computers, reports, Zoom technologies, online videos, Ipads, and phones, produce meanings of SDP in new ways. Technologies such as Zoom constitute new forms of digital physical activity, within spaces and places in homes and local communities that often have not been associated with SDP programming. SDP and leisure practices are constituted by the global affects of the pandemic, which influence the way in which individuals think about SDP and its activities. The global flows of the COVID-19 pandemic, including lockdown restrictions, constitute micropolitics within homes that affect the way SDP is experienced and engaged with. Nonhuman objects form part of the assemblages in which SDP distributes agency; and yet, these generative affects of technology are also constituted by humans via the interrelationship humans have with matter. Internet connections relationally distribute agential capacity of humans to engage with SDP; Zoom quality constitutes the ability of humans to actually see and feel physical activity and leisure practices through screens and online videos; the visual and hearing ability required to engage in SDP virtually emerges via the global affect of COVID-19 and generate affects for individuals living with disabilities.

Home, a place with historical gender inequalities (Fullagar & Pavlidis, 2021) is reconstituted with new meanings—becoming a space, and time, for not only work, care, sustenance, and education, but also for SDP. Virtual forms and digital communication of SDP transform the relations of physical activity, sport, and leisure, making people feel (sometimes simultaneously) apart from others when engaging with SDP in their homes, and yet together via the distributive agency of virtual forms of delivery. The spaces and places affect the way in which people participate in SDP—or even be able to engage with SDP. Smaller homes, condominiums, apartments, and townhouses limit SDP participation or the space needed for physical activity, while larger places and homes allows for more access to activity. SDP participants (and staff) working from home must navigate income loss, gendered divisions of labour that have been exacerbated by the pandemic, unpaid care work (the majority of which is carried out by women and girls), and encounter anxiety, stress, and mental health challenges due to the pandemic. Humans and nonhumans configure assemblages which produce affects of agential capacities for different people to engage with SDP. Relations of home, SDP, and technologies for virtual programming are gendered configurations, with home, as Fullagar and Pavlidis (2021, pp. 156–157) say,

> [...] experienced as safe (from the virus and contagion) and dangerous (from domestic violence, coercive control); stressful (juggling care of young children with domestic work, paid work, self-care and more) and comforting (to be close with those you love during this crisis). These multiple affects shape agentic capacities for different women with respect to their material and discursive conditions.

Hence, while the report offers significant insights on the impact of COVID-19 on the SDP sector, the role of non-humans and how they mediate social and political life for humans, particularly women and girls, remains underplayed. As the focus in this analysis was on how the written words of the report produce affects and assemblages in the field of SDP, more research is required to move beyond examination of texts and its agential capacities to look more closely at the very materiality of reports, policy documents, tweets, and other textual materials in SDP. How non-humans make up assemblages and produce different agential capacities, especially now as technologies become ever more integrated into SDP programs, requires further investigation and discussion as well. For us, the key takeaway here is to illustrate the agency of such a report and the multiple, diverse ways it shapes and influences other humans and non-human actors in SDP—that is, how a report may be produced by and influence assemblages. Further, how such documents create agential cuts and material affects on SDP offers an opportunity to begin thinking about more-than-human life in SDP.

Conclusion: Feminist New Materialism, SDP, and COVID-19

In this chapter, we have demonstrated how the (dis)connections between SDP, COVID-19, and technologies are constituted through affective relations, and configured by humans (SDP participants, organizations, family members, funders) and nonhumans (technologies, food, sporting equipment, spaces, places). Our analysis highlights how multiple affects of SDP are produced and underline that innovative adaptations have been made by SDP organizations (as discussed in the report). While the challenges of virtual programming and the use of technologies, as well as inequalities of the COVID-19 pandemic are emphasized in the report, we contend that the *assemblages, relations* and *affects* of SDP and COVID-19 must be critically analyzed from a feminist new materialist perspective in order to reveal the gendered dimensions of power relations (for example). This contention aligns with a growing body of research in SDP that underlines the importance of understanding both humans and nonhumans as powerful agents not manifesting their capacities *on* other agents, but rather *with* them. Our goal in writing this chapter is to emphasize the SDP/technology/COVID-19 nexus as a site that might extend and build upon the momentum of feminist new materialist understandings of how "bodies [are] socially and culturally produced entities, always 'enmeshed' in broader material-discursive arrangements" (Thorpe et al., 2021, p. 14).

Though the above analysis—given limitations of the researchers to investigate how the report has been taken up, resisted, and utilized by actors within the SDP field—focuses more on the potential effects of the material documents and its agential capacities, it can be speculated that the report, with further research to confirm, influences assemblages and relations of SDP. Indeed, the report was informed by more than 20 actors within the SDP field as seen in its 'references' page. In addition, the report has been shared online with a wide audience by the SFDC, the Commonwealth, as well as other SDP actors such as Sports Think Tank—not to mention various SDP international and non-governmental organizations. Such actors play significant roles in the field of SDP, and through the sharing of the report and the relational effects the report produces, it is likely that the report has made up assemblages within the SDP field through its agency. Thus, the report potentially acts as an 'agential node' that is bringing about transformations and change to the SDP field. Although this has yet to be verified through further investigation, which is required, the involvement of various organizations and individuals—as well as non-humans in the report as seen by the above analysis—in the production of the report indicates the agency of the document for SDP.

Despite the limitations of our chapter focusing on one document, the work outlined here may be used as a departure point for better understanding how a feminist new material lens may be useful for exploring SDP and technology in the current (post-)pandemic moment. These are indeed entangled matters and knowledge lacunas that the chapter has aimed to discuss. Much work remains to be done to get at a deeper understanding of the (dis-)connections between humans, nonhumans, and SDP; and to better identify and account for the agentic capacities of nonhuman actors as they influence the work of SDP and technology in the broader context of COVID-19. We suggest this line of inquiry is, in fact, particularly crucial in the (post-)COVID moment, where a reliance on technology in SDP—and its gendered implications for shaping experiences of SDP—remain important to establish in order to unravel this complex entanglement.

References

AJMC. (2021). A timeline of COVID-19 developments in 2020. https://www.ajmc.com/view/a-timeline-of-covid19-developments-in-2020

Barad, K. (2003). Performativity: Toward an understanding of how matter comes to matter. *Signs, 28*(3), 801–831.

Barrie, L., Waitt, G., & Brennan-Horley, C. (2019). Cycling assemblages, self-tracking digital technologies and negotiating gendered subjectivities of road cyclists on-the-move. *Leisure Sciences, 41*(1–2), 108–126.

Bastian, M. (2017). Towards a more-than-human participatory research. In M. Bastian, O. Jones, N. Moore, & E. Roe (Eds.), *Participatory research in more-than-human worlds* (pp. 19–37). Routledge.

Brice, J., & Andrews, D. L. (2019). She believes, but does she? Complicating white women's understandings of the postfeminist-neoliberal empowerment discourse. *Leisure Sciences, 41*(1–2), 127–144.

Brice, J., Clark, M., & Thorpe, H. (2021). Feminist collaborative becomings: An entangled process of knowing through fitness objects. *Qualitative Research in Sport, Exercise and Health, 13*(5), 763–780.

Bunds, K. S. (2017). *Sport, politics, and the charity industry: Running for water.* Routledge.

Clutterbuck, R., & Doherty, A. (2019). Organizational capacity for domestic sport for development. *Journal of Sport for Development, 7*(12), 16–32.

Chawansky, M. (2011). New social movements, old gender games? Locating girls in the sport for development and peace movement. In A. Snyder & S. Stobbe (Eds.) *Critical aspects of gender in conflict resolution, peace building, and social movement* (pp. 121–134). Emerald Group Publishing Limited.

Darnell, S. C., Giulianotti, R., Howe, P. D., & Collison, H. (2018). Re-assembling sport for development and peace through actor network theory: Insights from Kingston, Jamaica. *Sociology of Sport Journal, 35*(2), 89–97.

Deleuze, G., & Guattari, F. (1988). *A thousand plateaus.* Athlone.

Dixon, M. A., Hardie, A., Warner, S. M., Owiro, E. A., & Orek, D. (2020). Sport for development and COVID-19: Responding to change and participant needs. *Frontiers in Sports and Active Living, 203.* https://doi.org/10.3389/fspor.2020.590151

Donnelly, P., Darnell, S., & Kidd, B. (2020). *The implications of COVID-19 for community Sport and sport for development.* Commonwealth Moves, Commonwealth Secretariat, London. https://thecommonwealth.org/sites/default/files/inline/D17145_Sport_Covid_Series_PaperOne_ V5.pdf

Evers, C. W. (2019). Polluted leisure. *Leisure Sciences, 41*(5), 423–440.
Fox, N. J., & Alldred, P. (2015a). New materialist social inquiry: Designs, methods and the research-assemblage. *International Journal of Social Research Methodology, 18*(4), 399–414.
Fox, N. J., & Alldred, P. (2015b). Inside the research-assemblage: New materialism and the micropolitics of social inquiry. *Sociological Research Online, 20*(2), 122–140.
Fullagar, S. (2017). Post-qualitative inquiry and the new materialist turn: Implications for sport, health and physical culture research. *Qualitative Research in Sport, Exercise and Health, 9*(2), 247–257.
Fullagar, S., Parry, D. C., & Johnson, C. W. (2019b). Digital dilemmas through networked assemblages: Reshaping the gendered contours of our future. In D. Parry, C. Johnson, & S. Fullagar (Eds.), *Digital dilemmas: Transforming gender identities and power relations in everyday life* (pp. 225–244). Palgrave Macmillan.
Fullagar, S., & Pavlidis, A. (2021). Thinking through the disruptive effects and affects of the coronavirus with feminist new materialism. *Leisure Sciences, 43*(1–2, 152), –159.
Fullagar, S., Pavlidis, A., & Francombe-Webb, J. (2018). Feminist theories after the post-structuralist turn. In D. Parry (Ed.), *Feminisms in leisure studies: Advancing a fourth wave* (pp. 34–57). Routledge.
Fullagar, S., Rich, E., Pavlidis, A., & Van Ingen, C. (2019a). Feminist knowledges as interventions in physical cultures. *Leisure Sciences, 41*(1–2), 1–16.
Giardina, M. D. (2017). (Post?) qualitative inquiry in sport, exercise, and health: Notes on a methodologically contested present. *Qualitative Research in Sport, Exercise and Health, 9*(2), 258–270.
Giardina, M. D., & Newman, J. I. (2011). Physical cultural studies and embodied research acts. *Cultural Studies? Critical Methodologies, 11*(6), 523–534.
Gilmore, J. N. (2016). Everywear: The quantified self and wearable fitness technologies. *New Media & Society, 18*(11), 2524–2539.
Haraway, D. (1991). *Simians, cyborgs and women: The reinvention of nature.* Routledge.
Hayhurst, L., & del Socorro Cruz Centeno, L. (2019). "We are prisoners in our own homes": Connecting the environment, gender-based violence and sexual and reproductive health rights to sport for development and peace in Nicaragua. *Sustainability, 11*(16), 4485.
Hayhurst, L. M. C., Thorpe, H., & Chawansky, M. (2021). *Sport, gender and development: Intersections, innovations and future trajectories.* Emerald Publishing.

Henne, K. (2017). Indicator culture in sport for development and peace: A transnational analysis of governance networks. *Third World Thematics: A TWQ Journal, 2*(1), 69–86.

Kidd, B. (2008). A new social movement: Sport for development and peace. *Sport in Society, 11*(4), 370–380.

Kidd, B. (2011). Cautions, questions and opportunities in sport for development and peace. *Third World Quarterly, 32*(3), 603–609.

King, S., & Weedon, G. (2021). The nature of the body in sport and physical culture: From bodies and environments to ecological embodiment. *Sociology of Sport Journal, 38*(2), 131–139.

Law, J. (1992). Notes on the theory of the actor-network: Ordering, strategy, and heterogeneity. *Systems Practice, 5*(4), 379–393.

Lindsey, I., & Chapman, T. (2017). *Enhancing the contribution of sport to the sustainable development goals*. Commonwealth Secretariat.

Lindsey, I., & Darby, P. (2019). Sport and the sustainable development goals: Where is the policy coherence? *International Review for the Sociology of Sport, 54*(7), 793–812.

Lupton, D. (2019). Toward a more-than-human analysis of digital health: Inspirations from feminist new materialism. *Qualitative Health Research, 29*(14), 1998–2009.

Markula, P. (2019). What is new about new materialism for sport sociology? Reflections on body, movement, and culture. *Sociology of Sport Journal, 36*(1), 1–11.

McSweeney, M., Kikulis, L., Thibault, L., Hayhurst, L., & van Ingen, C. (2019). Maintaining and disrupting global-North hegemony/global-South dependence in a local African sport for development organisation: The role of institutional work. *International Journal of Sport Policy and Politics, 11*(3), 521–537.

McSweeney, M., Millington, B., Hayhurst, L., Wilson, B., Ardizzi, M., & Otte, J. (2021a). 'The bike breaks down. What are they going to do?' Actor-networks and the Bicycles for Development movement. *International Review for the Sociology of Sport, 56*(2), 194–211.

McSweeney, M., Svensson, P. G., & Naraine, M. L. (2021b). Sport4Change: Adapting to COVID-19 through innovation. *Case Studies in Sport Management, 10*(S1), S6–S13.

McSweeney, M., Millington, R., Hayhurst, L. M., & Darnell, S. (2022). Becoming an occupation? A research agenda into the professionalization of the sport for development and peace sector. *Journal of Sport Management, 36*(5), 500–512.

Merleau-Ponty, M. (1962). *Phenomenology of perception* (C. Smith, Trans.). Routledge & Kegan Paul.
Millington, B., & Wilson, B. (2015). Golf and the environmental politics of modernization. *Geoforum, 66*, 37–40.
MLSE LP [Maple Leaf Sports & Entertainment Launchpad]. (2021). Virtual sport for development programming workshop series: Design, transference & engagement. https://www.mlselaunchpad.online/calendar-1/virtual-sport-for-development-programming-workshop-series-design-transference-engagement
Pavlidis, A., & Olive, R. (2014). On the track/in the bleachers: Authenticity and feminist ethnographic research in sport and physical cultural studies. *Sport in Society, 17*(2), 218–232.
Rich, E. (2018). Gender, health and physical activity in the digital age: Between postfeminism and pedagogical possibilities. *Sport, Education and Society, 23*(8), 736–747.
Saavedra, M. (2009). Dilemmas and opportunities in gender and sport-in-development." In R. Levermore & A. Beacom (Eds.), *Sport and International Development* (pp. 124–155). Palgrave Macmillan.
SFDC [Sport for Development Coalition]. (2020). Impact of COVID19 on the sport for development sector. https://sportfordevelopmentcoalition.org/sites/default/files/user/Impact%20of%20Covid%2019%20on%20the%20Sport%20for%20Development%20Sector.pdf
Sportanddev. (2021a). COVID-19. https://www.sportanddev.org/en/news-and-views/article-series/covid-19
Sportanddev. (2021b). Reconnect: Keeping children safe and connected through sport. https://www.sportanddev.org/en/article/news/reconnect-keeping-children-safe-and-connected-through-sport
Svensson, P., & McSweeney, M. J. (in press). Technology and sport for development: The past, present, and future. In M. Naraine, T. M. Hayduk, & J. P. Doyle (Eds.), *Routledge handbook of digital sport management*. Routledge.
Svensson, P. G., Andersson, F. O., Mahoney, T. Q., & Ha, J. P. (2020). Antecedents and outcomes of social innovation: A global study of sport for development and peace organizations. *Sport Management Review, 23*(4), 657–670.
The Commonwealth. (2021). https://thecommonwealth.org/news/investment-technology-however-useful-not-solution-sport-recovery-say-debaters
Thorpe, H., Brice, J., & Clark, M. (2020). *Feminist new materialisms, sport and fitness: A lively entanglement*. Springer Nature.

Thorpe, H., Brice, J., & Clark, M. (2021). New materialisms, sport and the environment: Imagining new lines of flight. *Sport, Education and Society, 26*(4), 363–377.

Thorpe, H., & Marfell, A. (2019). Feminism and the physical cultural studies assemblage: Revisiting debates and imagining new directions. *Leisure Sciences, 41*(1–2), 17–35.

Ulmer, J. B. (2017). Posthumanism as research methodology: Inquiry in the Anthropocene. *International Journal of Qualitative Studies in Education, 30*, 832–848.

UN [United Nations]. (2020). The impact of COVID-19 on sport, physical activity and well-being and its effects on social development. https://www.un.org/development/desa/dspd/2020/05/covid-19-sport/

UN [United Nations]. (2021). Unequal vaccine distribution self-defeating, world health organization chief tells economic and social council's special ministerial meeting. https://www.un.org/press/en/2021/ecosoc7039.doc.htm

Webb, A., & Richelieu, A. (2016). Sport for development and peace in action: Building facts for funding. *Journal of Sport & Social Issues, 40*(5), 432–456.

Weedon, G. (2015). Camaraderie reincorporated: Tough Mudder and the extended distribution of the social. *Journal of Sport and Social Issues, 39*(6), 431–454.

15

Reorienting the Cartography of Coaching to Pandemic Times

Jordan Maclean

This chapter reorients the cartography of coaching developed during my doctorate studies to pandemic times. Drawing inspiration from actor-network theory, I *follow the actors* of a national governing body of sport during the COVID-19 pandemic. Then, in the *translation* of restrictions (e.g., lockdown, social distancing, and mask wearing) to the cartography, there were significant differences between coaching before and during the pandemic. Governing the return of sport in pandemic times became a public health concern, where the Field of Play was a site of contagion among potentially parasitic players. With that said, there is an even greater risk that coaches will return to be seen as only facilitating participation in sport. This calls for more creative ways of reimagining coaching in post-COVID times.

The COVID crisis has caused a significant disruption to participation in sport for millions of children and young people across the world

J. Maclean (✉)
Institute for Social Marketing and Health, University of Stirling, Stirling, UK
e-mail: jordan.maclean1@stir.ac.uk

D. L. Andrews et al. (eds.), *Sport and Physical Culture in Global Pandemic Times*, Global Culture and Sport Series, https://doi.org/10.1007/978-3-031-14387-8_15

(Drummond et al., 2020; Giardina, 2021; Parnell et al., 2020). Participation in sport, which is usually recorded as *matter of fact* by numbers in government policy making (Department of Culture, Media, & Sport, 2015; Rowe, 2019), has now become a *matter of concern* (Latour, 2004).[1] The porous and perspiring body (Thorpe et al., 2021) is a matter of concern for how governing bodies of sport have governed the body of sport during a global pandemic. A matter of concern for coaches who are responsible for participation of children and young people at a time of increased sedentariness (Clark & Lupton, 2021). And a matter of concern for what coaching practices look like in lockdown and what they will become in post-COVID times.

Places of once moving bodies, now unmoving, and spaces once filled with materials, now immaterial. As illustrated in Fig. 15.1, the goal posts are out of the ordinary due to the absence of play organised around bodies, spaces, and materials. Where is the ball? Lines of cones? And, what about the players? There is no sign of play on this overgrown field. The Field of Play is usually well maintained, with netted goalposts and white lines clearly marking the pristinely cut eleven-a-side pitch. But this pitch has been left unattended for quite some time, like so many others across the world. Perhaps, this figure epitomises what Clevenger et al. (2020, p. 564) call 'nonanthropocentric sport', given that players (and coaches) have been decentred from the Field of Play. Making the familiar unfamiliar in this way can prompt us 'to engage with these entities anew' (Michael, 2016, p. 95). This form of 'defamiliarisation' can be a useful pedagogical tool for assessing how dominant identity formations become disrupted, leading to dis-identification or 'a break with established patterns of thought' (Braidotti, 2019, pp. 139–140). COVID has rendered the once familiar Field of Play, unfamiliar.

If the pandemic had occurred one year earlier, then it would have directly interfered with the fieldwork of my doctoral project: an eight-month actor-network theory (ANT) ethnography of two children/youth community football teams' coaching practices in Scotland. Inspired by Latourian ANT, I developed a cartography or a map for orienting to

[1] Latour (2004) described matters of concern where 'suddenly, in a stroke, an object had become a thing, a matter of fact was considered as a matter of great concern' (p. 235).

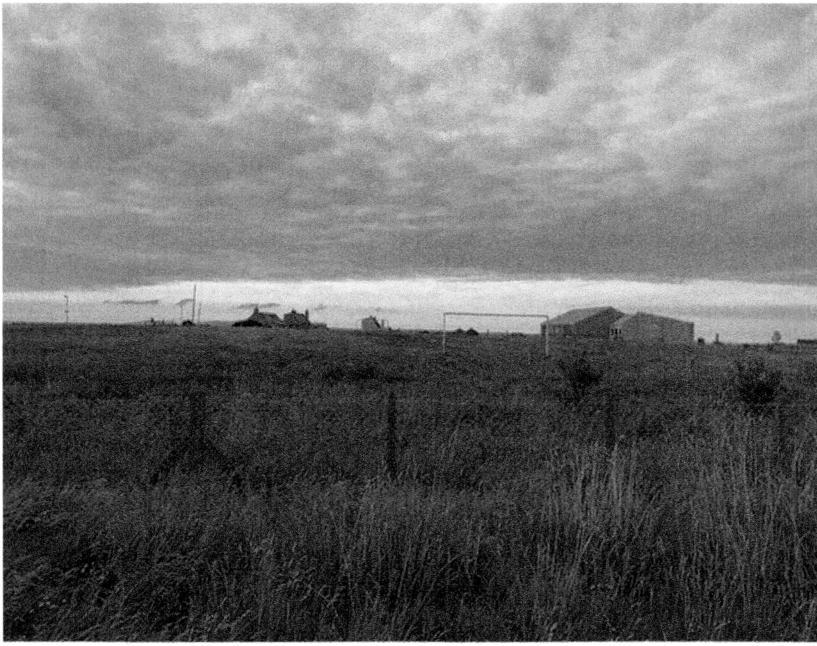

Fig. 15.1 Idle goalposts. (Figure 15.1 was taken by Jordan in August 2020 when lockdown restrictions on sport were easing in Scotland)

coaching practices. Maps are not *a priori* because they do not have meaning on their own but gain reality through their relations with people, discursive processes, and material things (Kitchen et al., 2009). However, it now seems more important than ever to 'reorient' (Latour, 2018) the cartography in order to understand the effects of the pandemic on coaching practices. In this chapter, first I introduce the sociology of associations of ANT. ANT is useful in pandemic times because it considers how 'a virus could once proceed perfectly well from mouth to mouth and from hand to hand and whizz round the world several times in a few months' (Latour, 2021, p. 107). I then follow the actors of a governing body of sport during pandemic times. Then, I translate how the cartography of coaching might have been assembled differently in pandemic times. Finally, I conclude by encouraging more creative ways of reimagining coaching in post-COVID times.

Actor-Network Theory

Actor-network theory (ANT) can be traced back to the early 1980s in Science and Technology Studies (Law, 1999, 2007). Although 'ANT' was not formally introduced until the following decade, its focus on the relations between humans and nonhumans in practices was very much present in some of the earlier works. For example, Callon (1986a) analysed the use of electric vehicles in response to increasing levels of air pollution in municipalities of France. Latour (1988) reframed the 'greatness' of Pasteur who developed an anthrax vaccine, as not solely a human achievement, but equally associated with nonhuman actants, such as microbes. And Law (1987) argued that nonhuman actants, such as devices and documents, were essential for enabling successful voyages to India during Portuguese Imperialism. The naming of ANT as a distinctive approach to social theory occurred around the 1990s. However, ANT has also been met with some antagonisms. For example, Latour (1999a) denounced ANT on four grounds: 'actor, network, theory, and the hyphen!', but then later accepted it because it was 'so awkward, so confusing, so meaningless that it deserves to be kept' (Latour, 2005, p. 9). With the increasing uptake of ANT studies in the late twentieth century outside of Science and Technology Studies and in different places across the world, it has come to be known as 'After ANT' (Law & Hassard, 1999). The 'After' epitomises the 'diasporic character' of its network (Law, 2006).

If ANT were to have a forefather, then it would be Gabriel Tarde whose sociology at the start of the twentieth century shared two major arguments that are now put forth by ANT: 1. there is no distinction between macro and micro for understanding society; and 2. the artificial divide between nature and culture limits our understanding of human interactions (Latour, 2002). The first argument of ANT is its adage 'follow the actors themselves' (Latour, 2005), which entails the '"art of describing" everything and the possibility of going from one type of visual trace to another' (Latour, 2012, p. 10). To follow an association of actors, Latour (2005, p. 108) returns to the oldest etymology of the word 'social', derived from the Latin word *socius*, for following someone else, a follower, an associate. Latour (2003) refers to this inquiry as the 'sociology of associations' because it focuses on the translation of forming an equivalence between an actor and its relations. This is opposed to the 'sociology of the social' which replaces translations with social explanations and subsequently sees nothing of the circulation between an actor and network. For this reason, ANT's network contrasts with macro-social entities, such as 'society'. A macro actor like society becomes meaningless, as it does not have the means of circulation. As a result of the dissatisfaction in coming to realise the inertia of macro entities, the inquirer is forced to move back to micro level interactions. But they soon feel the same sense of dissatisfaction and return to structure. The infinite regress of moving from micro to macro, however, is not to be confused with actor and network. Importantly, one does not focus on either micro or macro in ANT. Rather, the usefulness of the concept 'actor-network' derives from focusing on what lies *in-between* (hence, the hyphen!); the very means of circulation from actor to network (Latour, 1999b, p. 310). We do not end up with bigger and smaller networks, as the micro and macro scale would indicate, but rather with stronger or weaker networks depending on the alliances. The sociology of associations become visible through the circulation of the actor-network, while the extremes, micro and macro, disappear (ibid).

The second argument lies at the essence of ANT's relationist ontology, which was described as an epiphany moment when Latour (1988):

> taught at Gray in the French provinces for a year. At the end of the winter of 1972, on the road from Dijon to Gray, I was forced to stop, brought to my senses after an overdose of reductionism. ... Tired and weary, suddenly I felt that everything was still left out. ... I decided to make space and allow the things which I spoke about the room that they needed to "stand at arm's length". I know nothing, then, of what I am writing now but simply repeated to myself: "Nothing can be reduced to anything else, nothing can be deduced from anything else, everything may be allied to everything else". (pp. 162–163)

In this relationist ontology, 'subjects, culture and nonhumans are placed on equal footing' (Bryant, 2011, p. 225). In other words, nonhumans are no longer treated as subordinate to humans. This democracy of relations has been eloquently put by Harman (2009), where 'a mosquito is just as real as Napoleon, and plastic in a garbage dump is no less an actant than a nuclear warhead' (p. 34).

Governing the Body of Sport during the COVID Crisis

Before the COVID-19 pandemic, governing the body of sport was devolved to an association of football that operated like what Latour (1987, p. 131) calls a black box, where 'many elements are made to act as one'. In keeping with Tarde's first argument taken up by ANT, I *follow the actors* of the Scottish Football Association[2] during the COVID crisis. The timeline starts from the first COVID related 'News' item reported on their website in March 2020 until July 2021 and metamorphoses along the UK Government's (Department of Health & Social Care, 2020) staged approach for combatting the virus: contain, delay, research, and mitigate.

Contain Phase

The contain phase prioritised the detection of early cases, tracing people in proximity with those infected, and preventing the disease from taking hold in the country (ibid). COVID-19 was declared a pandemic by the World Health Organisation (2020) in March 2020, with many countries mandating tight government lockdowns. In this phase, the virus was not fully contained, but the Scottish Government (2020a) still allowed non-contact outdoor activities to continue (i.e., golf, hiking, canoeing, outdoors swimming, and angling). Consequently, all domestic professional and grassroots football was suspended (Scottish Football Association, 2020a). The governing body of sport was under threat, with spoken and written phrases on their website like 'fast-moving and unprecedented

[2] The governing body of sport for football in Scotland (Scottish Football Association) was chosen for consistency with my doctoral project (completed in 2020).

situation', 'survival of clubs', and 'existential crisis of our game' (Scottish Football Association, 2020a, 2020b, 2020c). The virus had un-black-boxed the body of sport beyond an association of football, as governing became contingent upon the COVID policies and guidance of the Scottish and UK Governments. This is consistent with sporting mega-events that were rescheduled during the pandemic, where decision-making and planning were informed by health experts *outside* the sphere of sport (Lee Ludvigsen, 2021).

Delay Phase

The delay phase prioritised 'slowing the spread of the virus' (Department of Health & Social Care, 2020). Lockdown measures set out in the Coronavirus Act included restricting public gatherings, self-isolation for seven-days if COVID-19 was contracted, working from home, and avoiding non-essential travel (UK Government, 2020). For sport, leisure, and culture there was a reopening of playgrounds and sport courts with social distancing, and the resumption of professional sport in line with public health guidance. The Scottish Government (2020b) introduced "test, trace, isolate, support", which aimed to reduce the risk of transmission until a vaccination programme for COVID-19 was established. The virus meant a delay in the day-to-day running of Scottish football, affecting all levels of the game. It was now an offence to train or play a game of football. Financial support from the UK Government was put in place for clubs due to the closure of their premises, and clubs were advised to review their insurance policies, sponsors, and broadcasters. Coach development also moved online, with the traditional delivery model of face-to-face coach education adapting to accommodate a blended learning approach (Callary et al., 2020). But even with mandatory restrictions, some 'dissident' (Callon, 1986b) clubs resisted the delay and continued to train. Unsworth and Tummons (2020) detail the 'resistance' from some teachers who 'continually disassembled and reassembled into new material representations' the localisation of a new government initiative called the 'mastery approach' for educating pupils on mathematics (pp. 12–13). With such a resistance against the virus, governing the body of sport had become a public health concern tasked to a *Joint Response Group* of medical and political actors.

Research Phase

The research phase prioritised learning from and responding to the virus by using 'research-informed evidence' to develop a vaccine and inform models of care (Department of Health & Social Care, 2020). The Scottish Government (2020c) updated their decision-making framework for assessing whether public health guidelines should be eased, maintained, or (re)introduced. For sport, leisure, and culture this permitted live events with restricted numbers and social distancing guidance (ibid). The Scottish Football Association (2020d) developed a three stage 'Return to Football' strategy: Return to Training, Return to Playing, and Return to Supporting. Returning to Training saw clubs returning pitch side to a 'restricted programme of football training and activity' (Scottish Football Association, 2020e). Return to Play for youth and adults lifted the suspension on contact training. Return to Supporting would allow for spectators, such as parents, to return to the sidelines. However, after professional clubs returned several positive cases, the pilot of supporters back in stadiums was abandoned until the 'national outlook for COVID-19 improve[d] significantly' (Scottish Football Association, 2020f). The existential threat of COVID loomed large once again.

With the resurgence of the virus in September 2020, results now appeared to be measured by how many COVID-19 tests were conducted in clubs. The Scottish Government (2020d) announced that they did not yet meet the criteria for the mitigate phase, as the virus was still considered a significant threat to public health in Scotland. Although there were exemptions for professional sport (Rowe, 2020), the new strain of the virus meant that over-18s football activity and travel was not permitted in high-risk areas. In December 2020, Scotland remained at the highest level of alert. Then, there was another temporary suspension to sport in January 2021 due to the 'escalating COVID-19 situation across the country' (Scottish Football Association, 2021a). The Scottish Government (2021) set out a new strategic framework to suppress the virus, notably as the vaccination programme was rolled out across the UK, with pop up centres located in football stadiums (Scottish Football Association, 2021b). Lockdown restrictions were reinstated: maintaining working from home arrangements, non-essential click and collect retail services, non-entry in takeaways, and barring the consumption of alcohol in public places. The collective effort to eradicate the virus was emphasised when the Scottish Football Association (2021c) said, 'football will play its part to support the collective effort to reduce the spread of the new variants of the COVID-19 virus'. Yet paradoxically, football must remain in lockdown to play its part (Black, 2021).

Mitigate Phase

Only when the virus is suppressed and no longer a threat can Scotland move into the mitigate phase (Scottish Government, 2020b). The mitigate phase prioritises minimising the overall impact of the disease on society, public services, and on the economy (Department of Health & Social Care, 2020). As we learn to 'live with the virus' (Delanty, 2021, p. 14), governing the body of sport will be like a black box once again, devolved back to an association of football.

Reorienting the Cartography of Coaching

In keeping with Tarde's second major argument that is shared by ANT, I *translate* the pandemic policies and guidance on governing the body of sport to the five parts of the cartography of coaching—(1) Moving from the game towards a field of practice, (2) Delegation, (3) Quasi-object, (4) Interruptions, and (5) Manufacturing—that I developed during my doctorate studies before the pandemic (Maclean, 2020). So long as the work of translation is done to show how actors enter into a relation, any relation can be made manifest. In the translation model, there is '*no transportation without transformation*', which means that the extent to which each part of coaching becomes transformed by the spread of the virus will be a 'little, a lot, excessively, or not at all' (Latour, 2002, pp. 118–119).

Moving from the Game towards a Field of Practice

During my PhD fieldwork, coaching practices took place on a third of a Field of Play but did not resemble it in any shape or form. Yet, the coaches often spoke about "the (eleven-a-side) game" when coaching. But whilst moving around on the Field of Play, I realised, with some disconcertment (Verran, 1999), that the eleven-a-side game was ontologically different to coaching. For what was usually only eleven-a-side consisting of two teams with one ball and a referee had now become split into three thirds with up to 80 players and just as many balls, bibs, and cones. I would have been forbidden to move as freely as I did on the Field of Play if it was an eleven-a-side game. Coaches arranged practices in areas that were conventional (e.g., using an eleven-a-side goal) or convenient (e.g, using the eighteen-yard box). Unlike the eleven-a-side game, coaching has no laws but rather unwritten rules that were created by the coaches themselves. In a field of practice, officials were absent and other actors present, like lines of cones which marked different practice areas. The focus on both social *and* material relations, the latter of which has often been overlooked in coaching research (Kerr, 2014), became crucial for conceptualising coaching as a field of practice.

The first lockdown in March 2020 led to a 'fundamental restructuring' of coaching practices. With the closure of the Field of Play (Adams et al., 2020), children and young people were forced to find alternative spaces, such as in the home or garden. This restructuring was recognised by the governing body of sport, 'training venues for footballers across the country have changed significantly' (Scottish Football Association, 2020g). Non-football related skill training and home learning packs were produced for clubs. Consequently, people were turning away from team sports to more individual leisure activities (Griffin et al., 2021).

When the second lockdown eased in March 2021, the Scottish Football Association (2021d) introduced 'field of play bubbles' for limiting the number of children, youth, and adults on the eleven-a-side pitch. Although the use of the word "play" connotes the eleven-a-side game, they do visually represent training areas in halves, thirds, and quarters.

Importantly, these pandemic "bubbles" reinforce coaching as a field of practice that is ontologically different to the eleven-a-side game.

Delegation

Prior to the pandemic, coaches delegated authority to humans and non-humans in a field of practice 'composed' (Latour, 2010) of cones, seven or eleven-a-side goals, balls, bibs, and players in different positions. Once positioned, coaches added conditions which became 'obligatory' for players to pass through (Callon, 1986b), and could be made progressively more challenging if needed. In Lopéz et al. (2021) study, the sacred nature of examinations was the obligatory point of passage for students to pass through in universities, despite being significantly disrupted and radically altered by the pandemic. But during the first and second lockdowns (March 2020 and January 2021, respectively), coaches no longer delegated authority to these 'familiar' (Michael, 2016) actors (i.e., cones, bibs, seven or eleven-a-side goals, and players) on the Field of Play. According to Kelly et al. (2020), practices moved pedagogically away from the more traditional practice-based (coach-led) to play-based (youth-led) activities.

When restrictions eased after the first lockdown in July 2020, coaches and players had to grapple with 'unfamiliar' actors (Michael, 2016). For example, COVID-19 coordinators ensured that clubs were risk assessed and followed public health guidance of mask wearing, applying hand sanitisers, and maintaining social distancing. Another 'partial lifting' of restrictions allowed outdoor contact small-sided games for children and youth, with two coaches socially distanced from a group of no more than ten players (Scottish Football Association, 2020h). However, a second lockdown in January 2021 led to further restrictions, with children only allowed to participate in 'non-contact group activity' and youth returning to individual leisure activities (Scottish Football Association, 2021e). Here, the restrictions became new conditions that limited the types of practices coaches could do (i.e., limit on number of players) and the interaction (i.e., non-contact) between the players. Consequently, coaches have had to be more creative, adaptable, and flexible in their training design in trying out new modes of delivery, media, and technologies (Koerner & Staller, 2020).

After the second lockdown eased in March 2021, club specific guidance specified several new restrictions: one-way systems at training venues, no mixing between different clubs, and parents/caregivers were not allowed to spectate at any time (Scottish Football Association, 2021e). There were also differences between coaching children and youth. For children, non-contact practices were allowed on a quarter of a pitch, while contact activity was allowed on a third of a pitch for youth. With a further relaxation in April 2021, contact activity was allowed for both children and youth, but the latter were still required to train using a quarter of a pitch (ibid). By the end of April 2021, coaching practices could take place both indoors and outdoors in different sized 'bubbles', with one parent/caregiver allowed to observe so long as they were socially distanced from their child (Scottish Football Association, 2021f). The pandemic's disruption to delegation foregrounds the changing material arrangement of practices.

The Quasi-Object

During my doctorate studies, I gave the ball agency by following its passage in practices. Consequently, I noticed that players were either seduced (i.e., led away) from their position by the player on the ball (quasi-object), or they were not seduced from their position, yet still failed to become the subject of the ball (quasi-subject) (Maclean, 2021a). When seduced, the middle of practices became 'crowded [with players] like bees around a honey pot hacking at the ball' (Light, 2012, p. 96). The ball in this instance became an object that seduced most players away from their positions. When players were not seduced in other practices, the ball crossed in became an object of force often avoided by players. Indeed, some players even ducked to avoid contact with the ball on their head. These examples brought to attention the often-overlooked material agency of the ball in practices.

In both lockdowns in March 2020 and January 2021, however, the quasi-object became something like what Serres ([1980] 2007) calls a 'parasite', where players avoid becoming the subject of the ball in case physical contact with another player leads to transmission of the virus. This is consistent with public health guidance, as players and coaches were expected to be socially distanced from each other (Scottish Football Association, 2020i, 2021d). But social distancing directly contradicts the essence of contact in *football*, where the ball was an object that seduced players from their positions. Rather, the ball becomes something unwanted, like when it was an object of force. If practices continued as they did before the pandemic, the ball would become an object of risk among potentially parasitic players, because they constantly move in all directions.

As practices resumed after both lockdowns, there were several relaxations in public health guidance that gradually allowed contact between players in practices. Thus, the player on the ball becomes less of a risk to others. When we learn to live with the virus, players, however, might return to be seduced from their positions. But the lesson of the ball as an object of risk in pandemic times gives impetus for players to remain in position.

Interruptions

In my previous phases of fieldwork, interruptions signaled a discontinuity when, for example, the ball went beyond practice areas. Players, assistant coaches, or other nearby teams would then retrieve the ball and initiate the next passage by either passing or throwing the ball back into the practice. But if an interruption warranted an intervention, coaches would intervene by either recreating, giving an alternative, or starting the passage anew. Coaches recreated by reviewing a passage up to the point of an interruption and/or giving an alternative passage from the point of the interruption. Starting the passage anew happened more spontaneously as they did not necessarily take place after a discontinuity had occurred.

But in pandemic times, players were required to wash their hands before and after every activity (Scottish Football Association, 2020h). This raises uncertainty over whether players should touch the ball with their hands when retrieving it after an interruption in a passage. Social distancing requirements between coaches and players also changed the way that coaches intervene, where they might be less inclined to become directly involved in a recreated or alternative passage. Facemasks were also mandatory for coaches when coaching indoors and before and after activities for players, but were not advisable during practices (sportscotland, 2021). Masks hide expression of emotion (e.g., a smile or grimace) and muffle voices (Lupton et al., 2021), which might make coaches even less likely to intervene in practices.

Manufacturing

The fifth part of the cartography was inspired by one of the coaches who described a practice during fieldwork as "manufactured". Manufacturing infers a duality that coaching was constructed and at the same time fabricated (Online Etymology, 2021). Coaching was constructed by assembling, disassembling, and reassembling the Field of Play. Fabrication was an intervention by coaches who invented passages that would not have otherwise occurred if it was during an eleven-a-side game. Thus, the cartography of coaching consisted of moving through all five parts in practices.

In both lockdowns in March 2020 and January 2021, the field of practice was no longer constructed on an eleven-a-side pitch. In other words, there was not one privileged structure that governed all practices like the eleven-a-side pitch which acts to govern the game. The eleven-a-side pitch has a relatively stable topology given its shape holds the network of actors together well. For example, the dimensions of the pitch are consistent with the Laws of The Game. However, as the pandemic has shown, coaching practices have no such limit to the possible rules and spaces that can be created, nor, at the very least, are they confined to the shape of the eleven-a-side pitch. Consequently, the pitch in Fig. 15.1 has lost its 'shape-continuity [and a] loss of identity' (Law, 2002, p. 99). In coaching practices, no shape is necessarily privileged given that materials give shape to, and materiality shapes, practices in many ways (Maclean, 2021b). The pandemic emphasises the many constructions of coaching from the 'mobile boundaries' (Law, 2002) of its practices.

Yet, the Scottish Football Association repeatedly called for a return to business-as-usual post-COVID. This longing to return took many iterations: 'return of football', 'return to training', 'return to competition', 'return to supporting', 'return to play', 'return to matches', and 'return to pitch' (Scottish Football Association, 2020b, 2020e, 2020h, 2020j, 2021c). However, Fullagar and Pavlidis (2021) argue that such a return fails to grasp how COVID-19 has transformed our lives. They instead propose a 're-turn' where one turns repeatedly to the changing circumstances of the pandemic. Such a re-turn emphasises the fabrication of coaching, for how coaches intervene and invent new passages after the pandemic's interruption to their practices.

Conclusion

This chapter has shown how a global pandemic's disruption to participation in sport became a matter of concern (Latour, 2010). By *following the actors* (Latour, 2005), we came to see how governing the body of sport during the COVID crisis extended beyond an association of football. Coinciding with each of the UK Government's phases for combatting the virus (Department of Health & Social Care, 2020), sport was contained through suspension, then delayed as new legislation and support schemes were put in place for clubs, followed by a research phase dedicated to the return of sport, and finally the mitigate phase where sport is no longer a possible site of contagion.

The *translation* (Latour, 1987) of the cartography of coaching—moving from the game towards a field of practice, delegation, quasi-object, interruptions, and manufacturing—to pandemic times revealed a longing to return to the all too familiar Field of Play. In comparison to my doctorate studies where coaching took place on an eleven-a-side Field of Play, the field of practice in lockdown moved into the home or garden. Consequently, the authority of delegation moved pedagogically away from the coach to players. And even as both lockdowns eased, social distancing had an adverse effect on the quasi-object (Serres, [1980] 2007), or the player on the ball, who became potentially parasitic to other players. Indeed, some restrictions such as social distancing and mask wearing seemed to discourage coaches from intervening and subsequently fabricating new passages in practices. This is problematic because intervening is what distinguishes participation in sport, like in the eleven-a-side game (non-intervening context), from coaching practices (intervening context). Coaching was constantly under construction during the pandemic, but how coaches intervened and fabricated practices was less clear. Therefore, matter of fact rates of participation in sport might be seen as only coaching in a limited sense. Yet, despite restrictions easing, there is a risk that coaches will return to be seen as only facilitating participation in sport.

There is an ever-greater need for new 'meaning and direction' (Latour, 2018, p. 98) for coaching action than before the COVID crisis. By moving through the five parts of the cartography, we can begin to map other field of practices. Ultimately, the parts of this map give crucial insight into the actor-network of coaching practices. The cartography recognises how the map is described and interpreted will be different for every coach because practices are mobile, messy, and never the same. With that said, the parts might be different across other sports and contexts, giving impetus for future research in this area. A limitation of the quasi-object is its focus on the ball, limiting its applicability to other sports. Nonetheless, by putting the cartography into practice similar problems can be brought to attention. By making explicit how coaches intervene and fabricate to overcome such problems in practices will be crucial for reimagining coaching in post-COVID times.

References

Adams, E. B., Blackwell, J., Dolan, P., Fahlén, J., Hoekman, R., Lenneis., V., ..., & Wilcock, L. (2020). Sports in the face of the COVID-19 pandemic: Towards an agenda for research in the sociology of sport. *European Journal for Sport and Society, 17*(2), 85–95.

Black, J. (2021). Football is "the most important of the least important things": The illusion of sport and COVID-19. *Leisure Sciences, 43*(1–2), 97–103.

Braidotti, R. (2019). *Posthuman knowledge*. Polity.

Bryant, L. R. (2011). *The democracy of objects*. Open Humanities Press.

Callary, B., Brady, A., Kiosoglous, C., Clewer, P., Resende, R., Mehrtens, T., ..., & Horvath, R. (2020). Making sense of coach development worldwide during the COVID-19 pandemic. *International Journal of Sport Communication, 13*, 575–585.

Callon, M. (1986a). The sociology of an actor-network: The case of the electric vehicle. In M. Callon, J. Law, & A. Rip (Eds.), *Mapping the dynamics of science and technology* (pp. 19–34). Palgrave Macmillan.

Callon, M. (1986b). Some elements of a sociology of translation: Domestication of the scallops and the fishermen of St Brieuc Bay. *The Sociological Review, 32*(1), 196–233.

Clark, M., & Lupton, D. (2021). Pandemic fitness assemblage: The sociomaterialities and affective dimensions of exercising at home during the COVID-19 crisis. *Convergence, 27*(5), 1222–1237.

Clevenger, S. M., Rick, O., & Bustad, J. (2020). Critiquing anthropocentric media coverage of the COVID-19 sport "Hiatus". *International Journal of Sport Communication, 13*, 559–565.

Delanty, G. (2021). Introduction: The pandemic in historical and global context. In G. Delanty (Ed.), *Pandemics, politics, and society* (pp. 1–25). De Gruyter.

Department of Culture, Media, & Sport. (2015). *Sporting future: A new strategy for an active nation.* https://www.gov.uk/government/publications/sporting-future-a-new-strategy-for-an-active-nation

Department of Health & Social Care. (2020). *Policy paper. Coronavirus: Action plan. A guide to what you can expect across the UK.* https://www.gov.uk/government/publications/coronavirus-action-plan/coronavirus-action-plan-a-guide-to-what-you-can-expect-across-the-uk

Drummond, M., Elliot, S., Drummond, C., & Prichard, I. (2020). Youth sport and COVID-19: A potential generation lost. *Emerald Open Research, 2*(27), 1–7.

Fullagar, S., & Pavlidis, A. (2021). Thinking through the disruptive effects and affects of the coronavirus with feminist new materialism. *Leisure Sciences, 43*(1–2), 152–159.

Giardina, M. (2021). "Daddy, help me; I forgot how to make a new friend": Emotional geographies of youth sport in pandemic times. *Cultural Studies ↔ Critical Methodologies, 21*, 1–7.

Griffin, S. A., Mendham, A., Krustrup, P., Murray, A., Peirce, N., Larkin, J., ..., & Kemp, S. Pt. (2021). Team sport in a COVID-19 world. A catastrophe in waiting, or an opportunity for community sport to evolve and further enhance population health? *British Journal of Sports Medicine, 55*(3), 130–131.

Harman, G. (2009). *Prince of networks: Bruno Latour and metaphysics*. re.press.
Kelly, A. L., Erickson, K., & Turnnidge, J. (2020). Your sport in the time of COVID-19: Considerations for researchers and practitioners. *Managing Sport and Leisure, 27*, 1–11.
Kerr, R. (2014). From Foucault to Latour: Gymnastics training as socio-technical network. *Sociology of Sport Journal, 31*, 85–101.
Kitchen, R., Perkins, C., & Dodge, M. (2009). Thinking about maps. In M. Dodge, R. Kitchen, & C. Perkins (Eds.), *Rethinking maps: New frontiers in cartographic theory* (pp. 1–25). Routledge.
Koerner, S., & Staller, M. S. (2020). Coaching self-defense under COVID-19: Challenges and solutions in the police and civilian domain. *Security Journal*, 1–15. https://doi.org/10.1057/s41284-020-00269-9
Latour, B. (1987). *Science in action: How to follow scientists and engineers through society*. Harvard University Press.
Latour, B. (1988). *The pasteurization of France*. Harvard University Press.
Latour, B. (1999a). On recalling ANT. *The Sociological Review, 47*(1), 15–25.
Latour, B. (1999b). *Pandora's hope: Essays on the reality of science studies*. Harvard University Press.
Latour, B. (2002). Gabriel Tarde and the end of the social. The social in question: New bearings in history and the social sciences. In P. Joyce (Ed.), *The social in question. New bearings in history and the social sciences* (pp. 117–132). Routledge.
Latour, B. (2003). What if we talked politics a little? *Contemporary Political Theory, 2*(2), 143–164.
Latour, B. (2004). Why has critique run out of steam? From matters of fact to matters of concern. *Critical Inquiry, 30*(2), 225–248.
Latour, B. (2005). *Reassembling the social: An introduction to actor-network-theory*. Oxford University Press.
Latour, B. (2010). An attempt at a "compositionist manifesto". *New Literary History, 41*(3), 471–490.
Latour, B. (2012). Visualisation and cognition: Drawing things together. *AVANT, 3*, 207–257.
Latour, B. (2018). *Down to earth. Politics in the new climatic regime*. Polity.
Latour, B. (2021). *After lockdown. A metamorphosis*. Polity.
Law, J. (1987). Technology and heterogeneous engineering: The case of Portuguese expansion. In *The social construction of technological systems: New directions in the sociology and history of technology* (Vol. 1, pp. 1–134). MIT Press.
Law, J. (1999). After ANT: Complexity, naming and topology. In J. Law & J. Hassard (Eds.), *Actor-network theory and after* (pp. 1–14). Blackwell.

Law, J. (2002). Objects and space. *Theory, Culture & Society, 19*(5/6), 91–105.
Law, J. (2006). Traduction/Trahison: Notes on ANT. *Convergencia: Revista De Ciencias Sociales, 13*(42), 47–72.
Law, J. (2007). Pinboards and books: Juxtaposing, learning and materiality. In D. W. Kritt & L. T. Winegar (Eds.), *Education and technology: Critical perspectives, possible futures* (pp. 125–150). Lexington Books.
Law, J., & Hassard, J. (1999). *Actor network theory and after.* Blackwell Publishing.
Lee Ludvigsen, J. A. (2021). When 'the show' cannot go on: An investigation into sports mega-events and responses during the pandemic crisis. *International Review for the Sociology of Sport, 57*, 1–18.
Light, R. L. (2012). Game Sense pedagogy in youth sport: An applied ethics perspective. Ethics in youth sport. In S. Harvey & R. L. Light (Eds.), *Youth sport: Pedagogy and policy applications* (pp. 106–120). Routledge.
Lopéz, C. A., Decuypere, M., Dey, J., Gorur, R., Hamilton., M., Lundahl, C., & Sjödin, E. S. (2021). Dancing with Covid: Choreographing examinations in pandemic times. *European Educational Research Journal, 20*, 1–20.
Lupton, D., Southerton, C., Clark, M., & Watson, A. (2021). *The Face-Mask in COVID times.* De Gruyter.
Maclean, J. (2020). *Coaching with Latour: An ontological manifesto for the socio-materiality of sport.* https://www.storre.stir.ac.uk/handle/1893/32982#.YeQAoS2l3rA
Maclean, J. (2021a). Coaching the beautiful game: An actor-network theory study of sport coaching. *Studies in Continuing Education, 43*(3), 328–342.
Maclean, J. (2021b). The 'lieutenants' of coaching: How materiality shapes coach developers' practices. *Somatechnics, 11*(2), 265–282.
Michael, M. (2016). Notes toward a speculative methodology of everyday life. *Qualitative Research, 16*, 1–15.
Online Etymology Dictionary. (2021). *Manufacture.* https://www.etymonline.com/search?q=manufacture
Parnell, D., Widdop, P., Bond, A., & Wilson, R. (2020). COVID-19, networks and sport. *Managing Sport and Leisure, 27*, 1–8.
Rowe, D. (2020). Subjecting pandemic sport to a sociological procedure. *Journal of Sociology, 56*(4), 704–713.
Rowe, N. F. (2019). *Sports participation in Scotland: Trends and future prospects. A report commissioned by the Observatory for Sport in Scotland.* https://oss.scot/wp-content/uploads/2019/06/Final-Revised-participation-report-for-publication28-05-2019.pdf

Scottish Football Association. (2020a). *Coronavirus—Joint Response Group Update 13 March*. https://www.scottishfa.co.uk/news/coronavirus-joint-response-group-update-13-march/?rid=13929

Scottish Football Association. (2020b). *Coronavirus—Joint Response Group Update 19 March*. https://www.scottishfa.co.uk/news/coronavirus-joint-response-group-update-19-march/?rid=13929

Scottish Football Association. (2020c). *Coronavirus—Joint Response Group Update 5 May*. https://www.scottishfa.co.uk/news/coronavirus-joint-response-group-update-5-may/?rid=13929

Scottish Football Association. (2020d). *Coronavirus—Joint Response Group Update 14 May 2020*. https://www.scottishfa.co.uk/news/coronavirus-joint-response-group-update-14-may-2020/?rid=13929

Scottish Football Association. (2020e). *Grassroots Football Update 29 July. COVID-19*. https://www.scottishfa.co.uk/news/grassroots-football-update-29-july-covid-19/?rid=13929

Scottish Football Association. (2020f). *Coronavirus Joint Response Group Update—23 September*. https://www.scottishfa.co.uk/news/coronavirus-joint-response-group-update-23-september/?rid=13929

Scottish Football Association. (2020g). *Football Community Clubs together to keep Scotland active*. https://www.scottishfa.co.uk/news/football-community-clubs-together-to-keep-scotland-active/?rid=13929

Scottish Football Association. (2020h). *Scottish FA Board approve partial lifting of training restrictions*. https://www.scottishfa.co.uk/news/scottish-fa-board-approve-partial-lifting-of-training-restrictions/?rid=13929

Scottish Football Association. (2020i). *Coronavirus Joint Response Group Update 23 December*. https://www.scottishfa.co.uk/news/coronavirus-joint-response-group-update-23-december/?rid=13929

Scottish Football Association. (2020j). *JRG presents its Return to Football strategy to Scottish Government*. https://www.scottishfa.co.uk/news/jrg-presents-its-return-to-football-strategy-to-scottish-government/?rid=13929

Scottish Football Association. (2021a). *Scottish FA Board confirms three-week suspension of professional football beneath SPFL Championship*. https://www.scottishfa.co.uk/news/scottish-fa-board-confirms-three-week-suspension-of-professional-football-beneath-spfl-championship/?rid=13929

Scottish Football Association. (2021b). *Grassroots Football—19 March*. https://www.scottishfa.co.uk/news/grassroots-football-19-march/?rid=13929

Scottish Football Association. (2021c). *Suspension of Football update 29 January*. https://www.scottishfa.co.uk/news/suspension-of-football-update-29-january/?rid=13929

Scottish Football Association. (2021d). *Updated guidance for Grassroots Football—11March2021*.https://www.scottishfa.co.uk/news/updated-guidance-for-grassroots-football-11-march-2021/?rid=13929

Scottish Football Association. (2021e). *Grassroots Football update—April 2021*. https://www.scottishfa.co.uk/news/grassroots-football-update-april-2021/?rid=13929

Scottish Football Association. (2021f). *Grassroots Football update—23 April 2021*. https://www.scottishfa.co.uk/news/grassroots-football-update-23-april-2021/?rid=13929

Scottish Government. (2020a). *COVID-19—Framework for decision making. Scotland's route map through and out of the crisis*. https://www.gov.scot/publications/coronavirus-covid-19-framework-decision-making-scotlands-route-map-through-out-crisis/documents/

Scottish Government. (2020b). *COVID-19—Test, Trace, Isolate, Support. A public health approach to maintaining low levels of community transmission of COVID-19 in Scotland*. https://www.gov.scot/publications/coronavirus-covid-19-test-trace-isolate-support/

Scottish Government. (2020c). *COVID-19—Framework for decision making. Scotland's route map through and out of the crisis*. https://www.gov.scot/publications/coronavirus-covid-19-framework-decision-making-scotlands-route-map-through-out-crisis-phase-3-update/documents/

Scottish Government. (2020d). *COVID-19—Framework for decision making. Scotland's route map through and out of the crisis*. https://www.gov.scot/publications/coronavirus-covid-19-phase-3-scotlands-route-map-update-10th-september-2020/

Scottish Government. (2021). *COVID-19. Scotland's Strategic Framework Update*. https://www.gov.scot/publications/coronavirus-covid-19-strategic-framework-update-february-2021/

Serres, M. ([1980] 2007). *The Parasite* (L. R. Schehr, Trans.). The John Hopkins Press.

sportscotland. (2021). Getting your facilities fit for sport. https://sportscotland.org.uk/media/6537/gettingyourfacilitiesfitforsportapril21-final.pdf

Thorpe, H., Brice, J., & Clark, M. (2021). Physical activity and bodily boundaries in times of pandemic. In D. Lupton & K. Willis (Eds.), *The COVID-19 crisis. Social perspectives* (pp. 39–53). Routledge.

UK Government. (2020). *Guidance. Our plan to rebuild: The UK Government's COVID-19 recovery strategy*. https://www.gov.uk/government/publications/our-plan-to-rebuild-the-uk-governments-covid-19-recovery-strategy

Unsworth, R., & Tummons, J. (2020). Reassembling teachers' professional practice: An ethnography of intertextual hierarchies in primary mathematics. *Ethnography and Education*, 1–18. https://doi.org/10.1080/17457823.2020.1788405

Verran, H. (1999). Staying true to the laughter in Nigerian classrooms. *The Sociological Review, 47*(1), 136–155.

World Health Organisation. (2020). *WHO Director-General's opening remarks at the media briefing on COVID-19—11 March 2020*. https://www.who.int/director-general/speeches/detail/who-director-general-s-opening-remarks-at-the-media-briefing-on-covid-19%2D%2D-11-march-2020

16

Virat over Virus, Cricket over Covid: IPL during a Global Pandemic

Kailash Koushik and M. M. Padmakumar

Introduction

On April 30, 2021, *The Hindu* reported that India became the first country in the world to register over four lakh infections in a single day with 408,323 new COVID-19 cases (Special Correspondent, 2021). Three days before that, the Indian Premier League (IPL from here on) cricket players received a persuasive email from Hemang Amin—the interim chief executive of the Board of Control for Cricket in India (BCCI from here on)—stating that their contributions on the field were bringing a positive distraction to a nation in the grip of the pandemic. "When you all walk out onto the field, you are bringing hope to millions of people who have tuned in. If, even for a minute, you can bring a smile to someone's face, then you have done well. While you are professionals and will play to win, this time you are also playing for something much more important-humanity" the email stated (Martin, 2021, para 11). Around

K. Koushik (✉) • M. M. Padmakumar
CHRIST University, Bangalore, India
e-mail: kailash.koushik@christuniversity.in

D. L. Andrews et al. (eds.), *Sport and Physical Culture in Global Pandemic Times*, Global Culture and Sport Series, https://doi.org/10.1007/978-3-031-14387-8_16

May 4, seven IPL players and a host of other administrative and supporting staff had contacted COVID-19 (Cricketnext, 2021). Finally, the BCCI, the organizer of IPL, had to announce that they were postponing the event. Their press statement remarked "…we have tried to bring in some positivity and cheer, however, it is imperative that the tournament is now suspended and everyone goes back to their families and loved ones in these trying times." (Iplt20, 2021, para 3). The pending matches of IPL 2021 were played after a four month break, in September and October, not in India, but in UAE.

The extraordinary conduct of a spectacle such as the IPL when India was witnessing COVID-19 casualty numbers crossing the four hundred thousand mark requires critical attention. The second wave of COVID-19, broke India's healthcare system, and spiraled into the worst medical crisis the country has ever witnessed. Overworked doctors battled hard to access fast depleting medical resources and provide medical care to the burgeoning number of patients; the affected scurried for medicines and health support and some of those who lost their family members to COVID-19 had to burn the deceased in open crematoriums as the system was not equipped to handle so many dead people. Amidst all this horror was the glitz and glamor, of the IPL 2021. Cricket, as stated by the BCCI, was used as a means of positive distraction and gliding over unpleasant realities.

Before progressing to critically unpack the incredible reception that IPL 2021 received, it is necessary for us to understand how cricket as a mass sport has operated as a "…sphere of activity that expresses, in concentrated form, the values, prejudices, divisions and unifying symbols" of Indian society. (Guha, 1998). Nandy (2002) famously observed that cricket was an Indian sport accidentally invented by the English. Cricket transcends the sporting terrain of India and commands an intimate space in the popular culture fabric of the nation, primarily because of the generous reception given by the media. What Kidambi (2011) cites to be one of the reasons for Sachin Tendulkar being celebrated as the supreme sporting idol of India—"…the intensified relationship between cricket, television and money…"—is indeed the central reason for the meteoric rise of cricket's popularity in India.

By promoting sport watching as a worthy leisure engagement and in turn strategically presenting the sports watching audience to advertisers, the media has indeed exploited the nexus with sports and boosted commercial prospects. Mediatization of sports in the twentieth and twenty-first centuries has at once benefitted spectator sports and the media to gain a global audience and thereby expand their profiteering. This global sports-media cultural complex that many theorists such as Jhally (1984), Rowe (2008), Horne (2007) and Schirato (2007), have often theorised about has a visceral demonstration in the context of the IPL.

IPL is tailored for primetime television, it is highly explosive, fast paced, and allows for a mix of sports and entertainment (Rasul & Proffitt, 2011). Despite being panned as "slam-bang cricket" (Kumar, 2009, para 2), "baseballisation of cricket," (Trivedi & Chaudhuri, 2015, p. 39) and as "Smash and grab crony league" (Guha, 2012) by the purists of the game, the T20 format and the IPL have consistently grown in popularity. Additionally, persuasive business strategies have made T20 the most popular format of cricket today.

This chapter aims to critically view the conduct of the IPL at a time when the country was witnessening roughly 3000 daily COVID-19 deaths. The obvious question that arises is why was this allowed? How was the BCCI able to organise it? As we peel the layers, we find that historically the BCCI has always been governed by the influential elite, but cricket is consumed by the masses. Its political power and cultural capital continue to be supplemented by its financial strength which it acquired through the sale of broadcast rights, culminating in BCCI assuming the role of a media company with the IPL. The chapter argues that the organization of a sport spectacle by BCCI during the pandemic illustrates the next step in the maturation of the BCCI-led sports-media complex into a quasi-governmental institution, capable of disregarding the democratic institutions of India. Before heading there, the chapter looks at the evolution of BCCI into the powerhouse that it is today.

BCCI: From A Board To A Behemoth

To understand the enormous power of BCCI, it necessitates revisiting two historical aspects which guaranteed and bolstered the power of the Board, leading to its extraordinary control over cricket (and Indian media) globally. One, the continued control of BCCI by the ruling elite, and two, its ability to sell broadcast rights, making BCCI the initiator of the sports-media complex in India.

Virats Before Kholi

One of the meanings of the name 'Virat' is a ruler, a monarch. Much before Virat Kholi—the former captain of the Indian men's Test cricket—made his presence on the cricket field, the administration of cricket was already brimming with '*Virat(s)*'.The BCCI was established (provisionally) in 1928 (BCCI, 2021). The board was established by British businessman Grant Gover and Anthony D'Mello (BCCI, 2021). During the pre-independence years, the Board and cricket in India were dominated by local princes, and the British administration (Majumdar, 2006; Bose, 2006).

An examination of who has held the helm at BCCI since its inception does reveal a very close proximity to politics, royalty and big business. While former Australian Cricket captain Ian Chappell complained that the BCCI had way too many politicians (PTI, 2015b), former BCCI secretary Ajay Shirke argued in the contrary stating that "if the players are being paid in millions, it is because of the politicians effort to fill the coffers of the board…the game has benefitted from its political contacts" (Tagore, 2019). These insights are true today, and have been so since the BCCI's inception. Cricket in India has always been in the hands of the ruling elite as seen in Table 16.1.

The association of politicians with sport is one of the strategies of smart power (Nye, 2013) used by politicians (and the elite) to attain and sustain power. Further the extensive media coverage of these sports is deftly exploited by opportunistic politicians to their advantage. Be it Hitler using the 1936 Berlin Olympics, Mandela using sport to shore up the international image of South Africa, or a poll-conscious French PM Emmanuel Macron choosing to indulge in wild celebrations after France's 2018 football World Cup win, one can see how sport has been used as a platform for gaining some form of political legitimacy. The Indian cricket media complex as well lends itself to such manufacturing of political

Table 16.1 Categorization of BCCI presidents

POLITICIANS	Sikander Hayat Khan; P Subbarayan; Maharajakumar of Vizianagaram; Surjith Singh Majithia; Fatehsignghrao Gaekwad; S K Wankhade; N K P Salve; Madhavrao Scindia; I S Bindra; R S Mahendra; Sharad Pawar; Anurag Thakur
ROYALTY	Nawab Hamidullah Khan; Maharajkumar of Vizianagaram; Maharaja Fatehsignghrao Gaekwad; Madhavrao Scindia; Raj Singh Dungarpur; M A Chidambaram; A C Muthiah
BUSINESSMAN/ INDUSTRIALIST	Grant Grover; Sikander Hayat Khan; M A Chidambaram; Z R Irani; S K Wankhade; B N Dutt; A C Muthiah; Jagmohan Dalmiya; N Srinivasan
CRICKET PLAYERS	R K Patel; Ramprakash Mehra; Shivlal Yadav; Sunil Gavaskar; Sourav Ganguly

consent amongst the masses, especially with the unpretentious trend BCCI has continued to exhibit. Be it the economic, political and cultural capital accumulated by royalty, or the economic and financial power of industrialists and businessman, or politicians [often backed by business, as in the case of Sharad Pawar (Stoddart, 2017)], BCCI has since its inception been controlled by individuals with significant power and influence.

The connection to cricket administration and the ruling disposition[1] has been more strikingly clear since 2014. Arun Jaitley, Rohan Jaitley, Narendra Modi, Amit Shah, Jay Shah, Anurag Thakur, and Arun Dhumal, are all directly or indirectly associated with the Bharatiya Janata Party (BJP), and have served/currently serving in the top management of the BCCI. So blatant is the political control of cricket in India that *Deccan Herald* published an article titled 'BCCI, where BJP plays family politics', stating:

> The BCCI will continue to be under political control, with only a change in the nature of the politics and the personalities who will dominate it. Whoever is in power and is in government at the central or state levels controls the administration of cricket also. (DHNS, 2019)

[1] Modi's party the BJP won the election in 2014 and 2019.

The presence of BCCI management who are close to the ruling party enables mutual support as and when required. This political power is supplemented with BCCI's financial might which it acquires through the sale of broadcasting rights.

Where is the Money?

BCCI's financial strength increased once the Board started selling the broadcasting rights of cricket matches to private companies and moved away from the government broadcaster. This initiated a symbiotic relationship between Indian cricket (read BCCI) and the media. It is this relationship, between the BCCI and private broadcasters, that fueled the phenomenal growth of BCCI, culminating in the IPL, which further made the board the richest sporting body in the world. The ability to sell broadcast rights had two effects. One, facilitating the BCCI to dominate international cricket administration; two, by commanding the 'attention' of a billion cricket frenzy fans, and owning the rights to their attention, it was able to not only select the highest bidders, but also push global cricket in a way ensuring India was always in the limelight. The transition from government broadcasts to selling of broadcast rights by BCCI was not a smooth transition.[2] However, BCCI persisted and, as shown in Table 16.2, it was able to profit so greatly through the sale of rights, that by the conclusion of the first IPL, BCCI had become wealthier and more influential than the ICC. ICC recorded a loss of $6.6 million in 2008, while the BCCI amassed $2.1 billion (Stoddart, 2017).

For Indian sports, this was the moment of birth of the sports-media complex that would change how sports would be organized, played and consumed in India.

The takeover of the broadcasting rights of Indian cricket matches by the BCCI is in contrast to the model often referred to as the Murdochization of the sports media. (Cashmore, 2000) The buying of sports clubs and thereby expanding a media company's sphere of influence in the sports culture context is a strategy Rupert Murdoch had worked with around

[2] Refer to Wilson (2020) for details about BCCI and its negotiations with broadcasting rights.

Table 16.2 Income received by BCCI through sale of broadcast rights

Year	Tournament/Media company	Broadcast rights (US$)
1993	Hero Cup/TransWorld International	$ 600,000
1996	World Cup/WorldTel	$ 10,000,000
2000–2004	Overall Rights/Doordarshan	$ 54,000,000
2006–2011	Overall Rights/Nimbus Media	$ 549,000,000
2012–2018	Overall Rights/Star Group	$ 750,000,000[a]
2018–2022	International Cricket/Star Group	$ 944,000,000
	IPL/Star Group	$ 2.55 Billion[b]

[a]From 1993–2018 Majumdar (2012)
[b]Gollapudi (2018)

the world. However, in the Indian cricket context, the BCCI has exercised supreme control and has gone on to establish their hold over the media. This phase of BCCI capable of calling the shots in telecast deals could be marked as the maturation of Indian cricket into a sports-media complex, with BCCI snatching the rights from the State broadcaster (*Doordarshan*).

A Media Company Called BCCI

The next transformation of BCCI is from a sports body into a media corporation. This is not a legal change of corporate identity, but has become evident in the views/decisions of the BCCI management. Two instances support this transformation. First, the BCCI's official website has the top-level domain identifier as '.tv' (bcci.tv). This identifier, similar to other identifiers such as .edu, .gov, .org etc., allows people to recognise that the website is associated with a specific kind of industry: in this case, the television industry (Merrill, 2016). The choice of the domain name, along with the use of the website for providing match highlights and live streams, allows us to perceive BCCI as a media corporation. Second, IPL has ordained the BCCI with tremendous ability to control television advertising revenue, subsequently controlling the television industry. A quote from the former CEO of BCCI Rahul Johri corroborates the transformation:

> If you look at television again, there is no property which gets the kind of audiences across demographics year-on-year that the IPL gets… I have been a television executive in my earlier avatar and all our schedules would go haywire… That is how disruptive the IPL is… That is why I do not hesitate in saying that the BCCI is the biggest media company in the country. (Amin & Sabherwal, 2017)

The control BCCI has is not just over advertising and media scheduling but it enforces its power to stifle news media too, morphing into what Ugra (2013) calls Big Brother BCCI! As mentioned in the quote above, IPL continues to be sacrosanct, to an extent where general television scheduling is adjusted based on the league, film releases are avoided during that time, and local stand-up comedians stop shows due to low turnouts.

The change in perception points to the fact that cricket as a sport has become secondary, while IPL and its media presence has become primary. This illustrates a second phase of maturation, moving from a sports-media complex consisting of BCCI and media companies to BCCI which perceives itself as a media company. We also need to understand the BCCI's supremacy over the Indian media by juxtaposing it to the fact that India is a cinema-crazy nation that continues to produce the largest number of films almost every year, in the entire world. What is even more unique is that the BCCI as a media company acquires its wealth through a single sport! However, how did this power manifest during the pandemic? While the entire nation was hit by the pandemic, IPL continued, as if it was happening in an alternate universe and a portal (in this case the television) had opened up to make this alternate universe visible to the masses!

IPL, Not Cricket

As highlighted in the beginning of the chapter, one of the cited reasons for continuation of IPL during the pandemic was that it would give a reprieve for all the cricket fans at least for a few hours everyday. Although on the surface this reasoning is sound, what needs to be questioned is BCCI's decision to offer only IPL, and not just any other form of cricket. If the BCCI is committed to promoting cricket, any form of cricket (international matches, highlights of famous matches) would have as well provided the fans relief. Strangely, domestic cricket and domestic cricket players were disregarded by the BCCI during the pandemic, whilst the IPL carried on in the name of providing hope.

BCCI, the richest cricket body in the world had not paid the salaries of domestic cricket players for almost two years, as most of the domestic competitions including Ranji Trophy, Vijay Hazare and Syed Mustaq Ali Trophy were canceled due to the pandemic (Krishna, 2021). How did the BCCI end up in such a state? Why was it keen on furthering the IPL, while its domestic players were looking elsewhere to put a meal on the table? One of the reasons domestic cricketers faced this situation is because the BCCI distributes its gross revenues every year, based on decisions taken in the general body meeting which has not happened since 2018 and players were forced to depend only on match incomes. With the pandemic putting a hold on matches, players were left without any source of income (Krishna, 2021). Some cricketers requested State associations to give annual contracts to players, a format followed by BCCI for the India A, B and C teams (Business Standard, 2021). However, these contracts also do not guarantee income. It is only recently did the BCCI decide to pay 50% match compensation for matches missed during the covid-hit phase. (Kishore, 2022) All these further corroborate that the BCCI is concerned more about the IPL and the fans (read audience commodity) than the sport cricket, or the domestic cricket players who are the lifeblood and future of the sport.

This perspective supports the previously mentioned argument that BCCI is a media company, as its priorities lie in ensuring the continuation of its most popular event, rather than focus on the sport and sports persons. The logic of accumulation that drives the BCCI lies bare in this illustration, neither caring for the domestic players, nor about the pandemic context.

It is surprising that while State associations canceled cricket matches even before the Government imposed any restrictions (ESPNcricinfo, 2021), BCCI was still receiving permissions from both State and Central governments for the IPL. This leads one to obvious questions: Why were State and Central governments lenient to the BCCI? Or is the BCCI so powerful that it acts like the State?

Public Resources, Pandemic, & Private Spectacle

Three cities—Mumbai, Ahmedabad and New Delhi—were shortlisted for the April-May IPL 2021 games to be conducted within a secure bio-bubble. Before we go into the details of the use of public resources in facilitating this bio-bubble, a brief account of the stadium in Ahmedabad is necessary to understand the nexus between the BCCI, the ruling party and big business of India.

The President of India Ram Nath Kovind, inaugurated the world's largest cricket stadium at Ahmedabad, Gujarat on 24 February 2021, with Amit Shah and Jay Shah, in attendance. The stadium with a seating capacity of 132,000, was named after the sitting PM, as Narendra Modi stadium. One of the two pavilion ends of the stadium was named after Reliance—the company owned by the richest Indian—Mukesh Ambani (an IPL team owner), and the other after the second richest Indian, Adani. The coming together of the ones holding the highest positions in the Indian Government, Indian business and Indian cricket is no coincidence. This culmination of politicians and businessmen, the christening of the place after Modi, involvement of Adani and Ambani, all reaffirm the historical trend of the ruling elite running the BCCI. The stadium, it was decided, would host 12 IPL matches including the playoffs and the final. As the IPL matches began in a secure bio-bubble, Ahmedabad was transforming into a COVID hotspot, a microcosm of the country that was witnessing 3000 deaths a day! (Yasir & Bengali, 2021)

The bio bubble and the stadiums required public resources which were ensured (with permissions from the government) for the safety of the cricket players and the staff. The government of Maharashtra permitted the IPL even when cases in Mumbai were skyrocketing (Pandey, 2021). The rationale behind the permission of IPL by the State government was that people would stay indoors watching cricket and thereby preventing the spread of the virus! At the same time the State government imposed a complete lockdown during weekends, and closed all public places such as educational institutions, places of worship, malls, markets and cinema theaters, while also restricting the congregation of five or more people outdoors. The BCCI on the other hand reasoned that shifting the IPL from Mumbai would be a 'logistical nightmare'(ibid), completely disregarding the medical logistical nightmare that India was already going through.

The bio-bubble became the BCCI's answer to conducting the IPL during the pandemic. Each city hosting required a completely secure cricket stadium and a secure accommodation that could house around 40 players and staff members from each franchisee, and a further 100 rooms within the bubble to accommodate the television crew (Pandey, 2021). The hotels in which the players were put up had sections sealed off for the purpose. The hotel staff who were attending to the teams had to undergo isolation and testing to ensure that the bubble stays secure.

The Arun Jaitley Cricket stadium in Delhi and the surrounding area of Kotla were sealed off a week before the first match. State police were to guard the stadium to ensure the bubble was secure on non-match days. On match days, the police force was increased to 200 personnel. Only required BCCI officials and teams were to be allowed in the biobubble, with the stadium having three secure zones within it: Zone 1 consisting of the participating teams and their staff, Zone 2 having the broadcast crew and staff and Zone 3 consisting of stadium ground staff and BCCI officials. All three sets of people were to have separate entry points. (AFP, 2021; More, 2021) At the same time, the capital was witnessing the most virulent spread of the virus. The argument that the IPL is funded by private investors and the conduct of the same did not deplete or divert government funds fails in this context. The police were not only put at risk, but also had to guard a private cricket tournament. The police, however, were not part of the bio-bubble. The bubbles also had 'Bubble Integrity Managers' who would accompany the team to ensure absence of breaches. In the previous edition of the IPL in 2020 held in UAE (Venue was shifted due to the pandemic) BCCI used bluetooth and GPS trackers to help in managing the tracing. However, although plans were there to implement the same in India, many teams had reported that they had not received the devices. (Pandey, 2021)

For the players and the staff, separate check-in counters and security corridors had been created in all the airports of Delhi, Mumbai and Ahmedabd to avoid the crowds and ensure covid restrictions (Vasu,

2021). The broadcast crew also had strict guidelines for testing and contact tracing and where to travel in special chartered flights to the different locations (Mandani, 2021) This would have not only required permission from the Central Government but also staff to run these counters and corridors, who were again not part of any bio-bubble but were at risk.

In case a player or staff from the bubble had to visit a hospital, a bubble-window had to be created. The state had allowed BCCI to establish a 'green corridor' in which a player would be taken to the hospital in a vehicle present within the bubble, by a driver from the bubble in full PPE kit. Further, all people attending to the player had to be in full PPE kits and masks (Wisden Staff, 2021). Each stadium was provided with three ambulances which could have catered to medical issues that would require intensive care (The Wire, 2021). As the journalist Sharada Ugra argues, although nine ambulances in three cities seems like a small number, one needs to remember that at the time of a pandemic, each ambulance can ferry 60 to 70 patients a day but instead they were stationed in the cricket stadiums, awaiting emergency requirements (ibid). The indifference shown by the organizers of the IPL to the Covid19 realities made an exasperated Sharda Ugra to state "For such an important entity to be detached from what is happening in the country it belongs to and generates its wealth from is either deliberate omission or callous abandon. You choose." (Ugra, 2021, para 8)

While the country's medical infrastructure was experiencing intense pressure, the residents of the IPL bio bubble were being tested for COVID-19 every two days (The Wire, 2021). These were not normal tests but tests that would provide a result within hours. As with the case of ambulances, testing across the country was taking a hit due to shortage of testing kits and personnel. The bio-bubble had the privilege of tests being conducted for all residents once every two days!

It is common knowledge that testing, requirement of ambulances are necessary for maintaining a secure bio-bubble. What needs to be questioned is whether it was necessary when the country was going through its worst medical crisis exacerbated by a shortage of medical resources. Further, the same government which was struggling to provide medical infrastructure, somehow felt it was alright to not only permit IPL to continue, but also mobilize medical resources for the IPL, at the cost of public health.

IPL: Marker of Good Governance and Savior of Indian Economy

By the end of April, as the criticism against IPL increased, the BCCI assured that the bio bubble would be made more stringent with increased testing (Banerjee, 2021). Apart from advising the IPL consumers—through the commentators—to follow covid-appropriate protocols, the BCCI largely remained silent about the suffering of people. The IPL officials provided statements that the IPL was contributing to the Indian economy which was down due to the pandemic, and that people will watch IPL, avoid venturing out, and thereby avoid crowding in public.

Sports has often been used for prestige and goodwill as noted by Allison and Monnington (2005) and Alan Bairner (2005). In this case, it appears that the IPL would have served the interests of the ruling government and big business in two ways: one, it would act as evidence of good governance for the Modi government, and two in the guise of acting towards reviving the Indian economy, it would benefit the continuation of accumulation of capital for all the other stakeholders of IPL. A brief explanation on each of these follows.

"The league generates considerable money for the economy. It has to be seen from that context too. How does stopping IPL help?" an anonymous source mentioned to Reuters (Banerjee, 2021). In 2020, when the lockdown was announced and there was a possibility of IPL being canceled, the BCCI stood to lose around $530 million (DNA, 2020). Further, in IPL 2021 the sponsorships at stake were around $540 million (₹4000 crores) (Mandani, 2021). A KPMG report in 2015 had estimated that the IPL had contributed $115 million to the Indian GDP, stating that it not only had a significant economic impact but also "positive effect on employment generation across various sectors, tourism development, upliftment of the tier 2 cities through media exposure and development of cricket and other sport participation across India." (PTI, 2015a) The economic rationale was very prevalent in the public discourse, and it also influenced the political decisions.

Elected officials wanted the IPL to be organised in their respective cities as it was seen as a booster for the economy. The day after Maharashtra—the

State that has been the most Covid-affected in India—announced a strict weekend lockdown to curb COVID-19, Cabinet Minister Nawab Malik confirmed that the State government had given permission to BCCI to conduct the IPL in Mumbai.. The Minister also assured that the tournament matches would go on "without hurdles" (ANI, 2021). In the lower house of the Parliament (Lok Sabha), Dr Ranjith Reddy challenged the decision to drop Hyderabad and proceeded to state that dropping a venue like Hyderabad was a loss of revenue, and that he could assure that Hyderabad would be the safest venue in comparison to Delhi or Mumbai (Lok Sabha, 2021). Reports stated that Hyderabad, similar to Delhi, was severely impacted by the second wave (Vadlapatla, 2021).

This is not the first time the IPL is being criticized for continuing the tournament in the midst of a calamity. In 2016, a public interest litigation was filed by an NGO named *Loksatta*, questioning the need for conducting IPL in three cities of Maharashtra (Mumbai, Pune and Nagpur) while the State was experiencing one of the worst droughts of the century (Shah & Mathur, 2019). The primary concern here was water usage (read use of public resources amidst a crisis). The courts sided with *Loksatta* and ordered that 13 matches be shifted out of Maharashtra, while only seven would be played in Mumbai, Pune and Nagpur. The dependency on IPL by the State governments for revenue, was used as an argument not to shift the IPL, along with the assumption that as IPL was a private business, it would use water in the most efficient way. IPL's contribution to the economy is also the main argument put forth by BCCI and others, while supporting the continuation of IPL during the second wave of Covid 19. However, as with the Maharashtra water crisis, even during the pandemic, resources were diverted to the IPL, when the same could have been used for the general public. All these show the continued dependence of the cricket spectacle by local governments for revenue, whilst also showing the power IPL/BCCI has, not just in cricket, but also in ensuring the reallocation of public resources.

Apart from utilizing public resources during a pandemic, BCCI can also possibly serve to boost the image of the ruling government, especially as one that is known for good governance. Narendra Modi's election campaigns have always forefronted development, good governance and reduction of corruption. This is furthered by a constant comparison with previous governments, especially targeting the Congress government. PM Modi's campaign is in line with the discourse that the previous regimes were weak and his 'rule' has been one with stability. Mr Modi had criticized the previous government in his public campaigns, on its inability to allow the IPL and the country's general election to happen at the same time, both in 2009 and 2014. The ability to create the environment for the IPL to smoothly progress is seen as evidence for good governance. During the previous government, security issues were cited as the reason for the IPL to be shifted out of the country. In response to that in 2019, Modi consistently made the remark that both IPL and elections will happen together, and there would be no security concerns (India Today, 2019). In the same line, facilitating IPL during the covid pandemic also seems like a case for the Modi dispensation to show the people that even with a raging pandemic the government is able to allow IPL. The same narrative has become normalized with even State governments trying to ensure that they also assist in organizing IPL, as evidence of good governance.

The IPL is one of the most watched cricket events in the world (Stoddart, 2017), and in 2020 half of all television viewers in India had tuned in to the IPL (Mukherjee, 2021). The very telecast can portray to a large section of the citizens the ability and success of the ruling government. Such an image management, a characteristic of neoliberal governments, has the potential within the country to counter international media that have often criticized the Modi government of mishandling the pandemic with ill planned lockdowns, ignorance towards the migrants and failing medical support (Sodhi, 2021). This is further corroborated by the fact that the BCCI, until their own players started to get infected with the virus had neither acknowledged the pandemic nor provided any support to the community (Ugra, 2021). Around the same time, individual cricketers like Pat Cummins and Jaydev Unadkat started to make monetary donations for Covid relief work. Abhinav Bindra, the country's first individual Olympic gold medalist was understandably upset when he remarked "Cricketers and officials can't just live in their own bubble, and be totally deaf or blind to whatever is going outside. I can only imagine that while you're having these IPL games, outside the stadium you have ambulances going to hospitals." (Bindra, 2021, para 13). It is after many such developments, that the BCCI was forced to pause the IPL season and publicly acknowledge the pandemic!

In a democracy one would expect the news media to question the government's decision to allow the IPL amidst a raging pandemic. However, this was not the popular narrative in Indian mainstream news media. *The New Indian Express* took a stance against this popular supposition that IPL provided a distraction for citizens from the pandemic. On April 25, 2021 *The New Indian Express* published an editorial announcement, stating that they would stop coverage of the ongoing IPL. The announcement read

> In such a tragic time, we find it incongruous that the festival of cricket is on in India, with layers of bio bubbles creating protection. This is commercialism gone crass [...] Cricket, too, must accept that we are passing through an unprecedented crisis. In the circumstances, The Sunday Standard and The Morning Standard will suspend IPL coverage in the newspaper with immediate effect till a semblance of normalcy is restored. This is a small gesture towards keeping the nation's attention focused on life and death issues. We are sure that our readers will see the point. These are times when we must stand as one nation with one resolve. (News Minute, 2021)

This was quite unprecedented as the IPL coverage normally dominated the sports section in both print and broadcast media. This move by *The New Indian Express* was an act of defying the sports-media complex and ensuring that focus was on the pandemic. However, *The Indian Express* (*The Indian Express* and *The New Indian Express* split in 1995), wrote an editorial on April 27, 2021, titled 'Game must go on' and called the request to cancel the IPL as "misguided moral outrage" (Editorial, 2021). This is not surprising as *The Indian Express* has, like most mainstream media, provided favourable coverage of the current dispensation (Bal, 2020). In this context, the decision by *The New Indian Express* not to cover the IPL was an act to bring attention back to the pandemic, in contrast to the compliance of *The Indian Express* to side with the IPL and the government. Further the call taken by *The New Indian Express* serves as an example of the media's potential to shift the attention back to what is important.

Quasi-Governmental Institution

The evolution of BCCI has moved from a sports body managed by the elite to a sports-media-political nexus, its self perception as a media company, and finally based on the aspects discussed in the previous sections, it seems to have evolved into a quasi-governmental institution. This is the next stage of maturation of the BCCI. The BCCI in its website claims that it is the "the single national governing body for all cricket in India" (BCCI, 2021). But it is important to remember that the BCCI is a private body, with no obligation to the public nor any control by the government. It assumes a 'state like' authority that could possibly impinge on fundamental rights. It functions on an economy of a small nation, but has no independent oversight nor legislation to check abuses of power. (Sondhi, 2010). As described before, BCCI's authority emerges from its historically compounded influence of political and economic elite in its top management, and furthered by its financial strength that it acquired through the sale of media rights. The introduction of IPL furthered its power to influence people and people's behaviour, disrupt television schedules and advertising budget plans across the country. During the IPL season at least, the BCCI does have the attention of the whole country in its control! It is a private body that represents India in global cricket. This ability to represent the country allows it to stoke nationalist fervor in its audience (audience commodity), and subsequently disseminate the hegemonic ideology of neoliberalism. In this case, the BCCI (and IPL) becomes a conduit for a. political leaders and parties to indulge in sportswashing; and b. the commercial business logic of the corporate sponsors of cricket matches and owners of IPL franchises. This was evident in the general discourse of media in which IPL was seen as a cure to the pandemic-hit economy, and in publicity events, especially when PM Modi interviewed Virat Kholi, as part of the publicity for a government initiative (Narendra Modi, 2020).

As we have seen, BCCI has had the ability to use public resources during crises, receive permissions unavailable to most other sports, and carry out media spectacles 'without hurdles'. Further, the BCCI's reaction to the Kashmir Premier League[3] illustrates the power of BCCI, its ideological leanings too, and its ability to comment upon decisions about other nations, as a representative of India and its people.

BCCI's power has increased so significantly that the ICC has become a proxy council with it being dominated by the BCCI (Stoddart, 2017). The alarmed observation made by the Pakistani Cricket Board's (PCB) Chief Rameez Raja highlights the monumental power that the BCCI commands: "PCB is funded 50% by the ICC that is funded 90% by the BCCI or in a way, the Indian business houses are running Pakistan cricket. If tomorrow Indian Prime Minister Narendra Modi feels that we won't provide any funding to Pakistan, then this cricket board can collapse." (CricTracker, 2021) So, the ability to command the attention of a huge population, to foster connections and nexus with ruling governments and big businesses, to represent a nation, to utilize public resources, to avoid legislation and oversight, to come across as a potential threat to the very existence of another nation's cricket board, and to seamlessly continue its business even within a pandemic, drives us to one conclusion. The BCCI and IPL are not an alternate universe, but a quasi-governmental institution, functioning with its own rules and rulers, capable of taking decisions that ensure the accumulation of power, while sidelining the larger interests of the sport and the country.

References

AFP. (2021, April 29). Police protect empty stadium as IPL arrives in Covid-hit Delhi. *Deccan Herald*. Retrieved June 12, 2021, from https://www.deccanherald.com/cricket/ipl/police-protect-empty-stadium-as-ipl-arrives-in-covid-hit-delhi-980270.html

Allison, L., & Monnington, T. (2005). Sports prestige and international relations. In L. Allison (Ed.), *The global politics of sport* (pp. 5–23). Routledge.

Amin, R., & Sabherwal, S. (2017, October 31). BCCI is the biggest media company in the country: Rahul Johri. *Exchange 4 Media*. Retrieved May 17, 2021, from https://www.exchange4media.com/media-tv-news/bcci-is-the-biggest-media-company-in-the-countryrahul-johri-86962.html

[3] Refer to Sirur (2021) for a detailed account of the controversy around the Kashmir Premier League.

ANI. (2021, April 5). IPL 2021: Permission has been given for Mumbai matches, says Nawab Malik. *The Economic Times*. Retrieved June 3, 2021, from https://economictimes.indiatimes.com/news/sports/ipl-2021-permission-has-been-given-for-mumbai-matches-says-nawab-malik/articleshow/81909431.cms?utm_source=contentofinterest&utm_medium=text&utm_campaign=cppst

Bairner, A. (2005). Sport and the nation in the global era. In L. Allison (Ed.), *The global politics of sport* (pp. 79–90). Routledge.

Bal, H. S. (2020, December 1). Executive (and) Editor. *The Caravan*. Retrieved May 27, 2021, from https://caravanmagazine.in/media/media-becomes-government-modi-indian-express-republic

Banerjee, A. (2021, April 29). 'How does stopping IPL help?' BCCI official says amid COVID-19 surge in India. *Indiadotcom*. Retrieved May 15, 2021, from https://www.india.com/sports/how-does-stopping-ipl-help-bcci-official-says-amid-COVID-19-surge-in-india-4623962/

BCCI. (2021). About the BCCI. https://www.bcci.tv/about/history

Bindra, A. (2021, April 26). Abhinav Bindra writes: 'Cricketers can't be totally deaf or blind to whatever is going on outside'. *The Indian Express*. Retrieved August 30, 2021, from https://indianexpress.com/article/sports/sport-others/cricketers-cant-be-deaf-or-blind-covid-ipl-abhinav-bindra-7288662/

Bose, M. (2006). *The magic of Indian cricket: Cricket and society in India*. Routledge.

Business Standard. (2021, May 27). Rohan Gavaskar wants states to give contracts to domestic cricketers. *Business Standard*. Retrieved June 24, 2021, from https://www.business-standard.com/article/sports/rohan-gavaskar-wants-states-to-give-contracts-to-domestic-cricketers-121052601377_1.html

Cashmore, E. (2000). *Sports culture: An A–Z guide*. Routledge.

Cricketnext. (2021, May 4). IPL 2021: Full list of Covid19 positive players, support, ground staff & broadcast team. *News 18*. Retrieved June 24, 2021, from https://www.news18.com/cricketnext/news/ipl-2021-coronavirus-positive-players-ground-staff-broadcast-team-full-list-3616256.html

CricTracker. (2021, October 8). 'PCB is funded 50% by ICC, which is funded 90% by BCCI'—Ramiz Raja feels PM Modi has power to trigger Pakistan cricket's collapse. *CricTracker*. Retrieved November 29, 2021, from https://www.crictracker.com/pcb-is-funded-50-by-icc-which-is-funded-90-by-bcci-ramiz-raja-feels-pm-modi-has-power-to-trigger-pakistan-crickets-collapse/

DHNS. (2019, October 16). BCCI where BJP plays family politics. *The Deccan Herald*. Retrieved July 11, 2021, from https://www.deccanherald.com/opinion/first-edit/bcci-where-bjp-plays-family-politics-768929.html

DNA. (2020, May 12). COVID-19 crisis: Cancelling IPL 2020 could cost BCCI $500 million. DNA. Retrieved August 30, 2021 from https://www.dnaindia.com/cricket/report-covid-19-crisis-cancelling-ipl-2020-could-cost-bcci-500-million-2824550

Editorial. (2021, April 27). Game must go on. *The Indian Express*. Retrieved July 22, 2021, from https://indianexpress.com/article/opinion/editorials/indian-premier-league-bio-bubble-coronavirus-7290345/

ESPNcricinfo. (2021, April 3). IPL 2021: BCCI monitoring fresh COVID-19 spike in Mumbai, keeps Hyderabad in contingency plans. *ESPNcricinfo*. Retrieved July 20, 2021, from https://www.espncricinfo.com/story/ipl-2021-bcci-keeps-hyderabad-in-contingency-plans-because-of-COVID-19-surge-1257671

Gollapudi, N. (2018, April 5). Star India buys Indian cricket rights for USD 944 million. *ESPNCricinfo*. Retrieved July 19, 2021, from https://www.espncricinfo.com/story/star-india-buys-indian-cricket-rights-for-usd-944-million-1142530

Guha, R. (1998). Cricket and politics in colonial India. *Past & Present, 161*, 155–190.

Guha, R. (2012, May 25). Smash-and-grab corny league. *The Hindu*. Retrieved July 11, 2021, from https://www.thehindu.com/opinion/lead/Smash-and-grab-crony-league/article12831999.ece

Horne, J. (2007). *Sport in consumer culture*. Palgrave Macmillan.

India Today. (2019, May 3). UPA shifted IPL out of India, Modi can hold both IPL and elections together: PM Modi. *India Today*. Retrieved November 30, 2021, from https://www.indiatoday.in/elections/lok-sabha-2019/story/pm-narendra-modi-ipl-1516204-2019-05-03

Iplt20. (2021, May 4). Vivo Ipl 2021 postponed [Press release]. *Iplt20*. Retrieved April 25, 2021, from https://www.iplt20.com/news/238268/vivo-ipl-2021-postponed

Jhally, S. (1984). The spectacle of accumulation: Material and cultural factors in the evolution of the sports/media complex. *Insurgent Sociologist, 12*(3), 41–57. https://doi.org/10.1177/089692058401200304

Kidambi, P. (2011). Hero, celebrity and icon: Sachin Tendulkar and Indian public culture. In A. Bateman & J. Hill (Eds.), *The Cambridge companion to cricket*. Cambridge University Press.

Kishore, S. (2022, January 3). BCCI disburses long standing Covid compensation for domestic players. *ESPN CricInfo*. Retrieved November 28, 2021, from https://www.espncricinfo.com/story/bcci-disburses-longstanding-covid-compensation-for-domestic-players-1295156

Krishna, V. (2021, May 27). Surviving tactics. *The New Indian Express*. Retrieved June 24, 2021, from https://www.newindianexpress.com/sport/cricket/2021/may/27/surviving-tactics-2308136.html

Kumar, K. (2009, October 12). Regulate matches to save young cricketers. *Times of India*. Retrieved July 3, 2021, from https://timesofindia.indiatimes.com/edit-page/regulate-matches-to-save-young-cricketers/articleshow/5132028.cms

Lok Sabha. (2021). Request to reconsider the decision of not selecting Hyderabad as IPL venue. *Lok Sabha*. http://loksabhaph.nic.in/Debates/Result17.aspx?dbsl=6075

Majumdar, B. (2006). *Lost histories of Indian cricket: Battles off the pitch*. Routledge.

Majumdar, B. (2012, April 16). How cricket was sold in India. *Open Magazine*. Retrieved May 27, 2021, from https://openthemagazine.com/sports/how-cricket-was-sold-in-india/

Mandani, R. (2021, April 6). IPL's home test amid rising cases. *Hindustan Times*. Retrieved December 5, 2021, from https://www.hindustantimes.com/cricket/ipls-home-test-amid-rising-cases-101617676191810.html

Martin, A. (2021, April 27). IPL players told 'you are playing for humanity' in midst of Covid pandemic. *The Guardian*. Retrieved March 20, 2021, from https://www.theguardian.com/sport/2021/apr/27/indian-premier-league-cricket-players-told-you-are-playing-for-humanity-in-midst-of-india-covid-pandemic

Merrill, K. (2016). Domains of control: Governance of and by the domain name system. In *The turn to infrastructure in Internet governance* (pp. 89–106). Palgrave Macmillan.

More, S. (2021, April 15). IPL 2021: How will matches take place in Delhi? DDCA officials reveal plan for no hiccups. *Republic World*. Retrieved December 5, 2021, from https://www.republicworld.com/sports-news/cricket-news/ipl-2021-how-will-matches-take-place-in-delhi-ddca-officials-reveal-plan-for-no-hiccups.html

Mukherjee, B. (2021, April 26). India's premier cricket league is playing through its COVID crisis—But players worry about the repercussions. *Fortune*. Retrieved December 8, 2021, from https://fortune.com/2021/04/26/ipl-2021-indian-premier-league-cricket-india-covid-cases/

Nandy, A. (2002). *The tao of cricket: On games of destiny and the destiny of games*. Oxford University Press.

Narendra Modi. (2020, September 24). PM Modi asks Virat Kohli about Yo-Yo test at Fit India Dialogue…Watch their interaction! [Video]. *YouTube*. https://www.youtube.com/watch?v=UHEwKC-AMgA

News Minute. (2021, April 25). 'Problem not with game but its timing': The New Indian Express suspends IPL coverage. *The News Minute*. Retrieved April 30, 2021, from https://www.thenewsminute.com/article/problem-not-game-its-timing-new-indian-express-suspends-ipl-coverage-147802

Nye, J. S. (2013). *Hard, soft, and smart power*. Oxford Handbooks Online. https://doi.org/10.1093/oxfordhb/9780199588862.013.0031

Pandey, D. (2021, April 8). Why BCCI has ruled out shifting of IPL from Mumbai despite Covid19 surge. *The Indian Express*. Retrieved December 1, 2021, from https://indianexpress.com/article/explained/explained-why-bcci-has-ruled-out-shifting-of-ipl-from-mumbai-despite-covid-19-surge-7259933/

PTI. (2015a, October 30). IPL contributes ₹ 1,150 Crore to India's GDP: KPMG. *NDTV*. Retrieved December 6, 2021, from https://www.ndtv.com/business/ipl-contributes-rs-11-5-billion-to-indias-gdp-kpmg-1238234

PTI. (2015b, December 5). BCCI has got way too many politicians involved: Ian Chapple. *Mint*. Retrieved July 26, 2021, from https://www.livemint.com/Politics/KTOZsUKjWCXT9MbwsuwoGO/BCCI-has-too-many-politicians-Ian-Chappell.html

Rasul, A., & Proffitt, J. M. (2011). Bollywood and the Indian Premier League (IPL): The political economy of Bollywood's new blockbuster. *Asian Journal of Communication, 21*(4), 373–388.

Rowe, D. (2008). *Sport, culture and the media: The unruly trinity*. Open University Press.

Schirato, T. (2007). *Understanding sports culture*. Sage.

Shah, A., & Mathur, N. (2019). Contestations around water allocation during a climate crisis in India: The case of 'IPL vs. drought'. *Global Environmental Change, 57*, 101927.

Sirur, S. (2021, August 2). Kashmir Premier League vs BCCI is the new India-Pakistan cricket faceoff. *The Print*. Retrieved August 20, 2021, from https://theprint.in/go-to-pakistan/kashmir-premier-league-vs-bcci-is-the-new-india-pakistan-cricket-faceoff/707855/

Sodhi, T. (2021, May 11). Why is Modi getting such bad international press? *Newslaundry*. Retrieved June 29, 2021, from https://www.newslaundry.com/2021/05/11/why-is-modi-getting-such-bad-international-press

Sondhi, A. (2010). The legal status of BCCI: Unwarranted ad-hocism, constitutional hurdles and the pressing need for a cricket-legislation. *National Law School of India Review, 22*, 111.

Special Correspondent. (2021, May 23). Number of India's COVID19 deaths crosses 3 lakh. *The Hindu*. Retrieved June 1, 2021, from https://www.thehindu.com/news/national/coronavirus-number-of-indias-covid-19-deaths-crosses-3-lakh-on-may-23-2021/article34629084.ece

Stoddart, B. (2017). IPL the global game changer. In A. Athique, V. Parthasarathi, & S. V. Srinivas (Eds.), *The Indian media economy: Vol. I: Industrial dynamics and cultural adaptation*. Oxford University Press.

Tagore, V. (2019, October 15). Politics, cricket go hand-in-hand in BCCI administration. *Mumbai Mirror*. Retrieved November 29, 2021, from https://mumbaimirror.indiatimes.com/sport/cricket/politics-cricket-go-hand-in-hand/articleshow/71587055.cms?utm_source=contentofinterest& utm_medium=text & utm_campaign=cppst

The Wire. (2021, May 1). The IPL spectacle: Event now part of government propaganda machine, BCCI lost all sensitivity [Video]. *YouTube*. https://www.youtube.com/watch?v=y9F8SVIUlKo

Trivedi, P., & Chaudhuri, S. (2015). *Fields of play: Sport, literature and culture*. Orient Blackswan.

Ugra, S. (2013). Big Brother BCCI is watching. *Economic & Political Weekly*, 48(38). https://www.epw.in/journal/2013/38/postscript/big-brother-bccis-watching.html

Ugra, S. (2021, April 29). From India to the IPL: Do you read me? *The Quint*. Retrieved June 20, 2021, from https://www.thequint.com/indian-premier-league-ipl/sharda-ugra-the-quint-COVID-19-ipl-pandemic#read-more

Vadlapatla, S. (2021, June 21). Second Covid wave in Hyderabad similar to peak of 2020. *The Times of India*. Retrieved July 9, 2021, from http://timesofindia.indiatimes.com/articleshow/83247104.cms?utm_source=contentofinterest&utm_medium=text&utm_campaign=cppst

Vasu, A. (2021, April 26). PL plays on as BCCI's cash cow while India's COVID-19 crisis worsens. *The Guardian*. Retrieved May 11, 2021, from https://www.theguardian.com/sport/2021/apr/26/ipl-plays-on-as-bccis-cash-cow-while-indias-COVID-19-crisis-worsens

Wilson, J. (2020). Live broadcasting of cricket in India & Pakistan: Right to information, commercialization & competition issues. *Indian Law Review, 4*(3), 316–342.

Wisden Staff. (2021, May 3). Explained: How the IPL's bio-bubble burst. *Wisden India*. Retrieved November 30, 2021, from https://wisden.com/stories/global-t20-leagues/indian-premier-league-2021/explained-how-the-ipl-2021-bio-bubble-got-breached

Yasir, S., & Bengali, S. (2021, April 30). India outbreak worsens further, prompting fury at a remaining outpost of normalcy. *The New York Times*. Retrieved August 21, 2021, from https://www.nytimes.com/2021/04/30/world/india-covid-cases.html

17

From Football Nation to COVID 19-Land: Cultural Pedagogies and Political Protests during Syndemic Times in Brazil

Jorge Knijnik and Luiz Guilherme Burlamaqui

Brazil was by far one of the countries that presented the worst response to the syndemic crisis around the world. By mid-2021, the country accounted for more than 500,000 deaths caused by the SARS-COVID19, and millions of infected people spread across the country. Since the beginning of the crisis, then Brazil's President Jair Bolsonaro, has undertaken every single step to deserve to be called the 'Virus Man', or the 'Bolsovirus' (Tamara, 2020). He initially denied the existence of the disease, calling it a "little flu" and fired the Health minister as he refused to suggest to Brazilians 'alternate' treatments (such as hydroxychloroquine). Moreover, his government literally abandoned Brazil's people during the syndemic, offering little to no support to its most vulnerable populations (Da Silva & Da Silveira, 2020; Paiva et al., 2021).

J. Knijnik (✉)
Western Sydney University, Parramatta, NSW, Australia
e-mail: j.knijnik@westernsydney.edu.au

L. G. Burlamaqui
Instituto Federal de Brasilia, Brasília, Brasil

D. L. Andrews et al. (eds.), *Sport and Physical Culture in Global Pandemic Times*, Global Culture and Sport Series, https://doi.org/10.1007/978-3-031-14387-8_17

Nevertheless, at the peak of the first wave of the COVID-19 infection, several groups of self-proclaimed 'antifascist football supporters' marched in the country's main cities to protest the federal government's (lack of) response to the health crisis. Representing the largest active supporters' groups from the leading Brazilian football clubs, these protesters tried to call upon civil society to pressure Bolsonaro's government to look after the lower classes who were heavily hit by the syndemic. During the protests, these football fans organized groups marched side by side with a series of new social movements that emerged in Brazil during the syndemic. One of those social movements were the "Entregadores antifascistas"—antifascists delivery workers that are employed by the Gig Economy (Uber Eats, Ifood, Rappi amongst others).

This paper hence addresses key questions on cultural pedagogies and everyday political practices in the Brazilian sports realm during the COVID-19 syndemic. Applying Giroux's (2011) concept of *cultural pedagogies* as well as Edward Thompson (2003) analysis of *class and popular resistance* movements on social media sources, news articles and media interviews with leaders of these movements, we intend to create a diffraction that might show how football and the COVID-19 crisis were intertwined in Brazil. As both Giroux's cultural pedagogies and Thompson's class and popular resistance concepts are underlined by a deep understanding of bottom-to-top democratic world vision, our analysis is also underpinned by Paulo Freire, the world-known Brazilian educator, and his radical view of an expanded and substantive democracy, based on citizens social consciousness and participation (Freire, 1998)

In the early 1990s, while analysing the effects of the AIDS health crisis among impoverished urban populations, Singer (1994, p. 933) coined the concept of 'syndemic'. According to him, when a range of epidemic biologically diseases meet endemic social issues, such as "high rates of unemployment, poverty, substandard nutrition", they act to mutually heighten each other, creating a social health crisis, or a syndemic (Singer, 1994, 1996). According to Rocha (2021) in Brazil "the standardised COVID-19 death rate was highest in the North region, where some of the most vulnerable states are located." Moreover, even if these were not the states where the typical COVID-19-related health risks (older age groups and burden of chronic disease) were the greatest, they observed greater scarcity in hospital resources and social inequality (Fig. 17.1)

At the early stages of the COVID-19 crisis, Horton (2020) used Singer's syndemic expression to challenge the narrow approach to the current health crisis. In his comment in The Lancet, Horton argues that, whilst all data pointed out that socially vulnerable communities—minority ethnic groups such as Black or Asian, older and unpaid people—where by large the most affected by the COVID-19 infection, the world was yet to develop a holistic approach to deal with this crisis. He argues that only by understanding the COVID-19 crisis as a syndemic, will allow us to have a broad vision that includes in the analysis social issues such as paid work, housing, education, income and environment (Horton, 2020).

Adding to Horton's concerns, this chapter argues that political struggles must be included in the large view of the COVID-19 as a syndemic. As Brazil is unfortunately the 'poster child' of how social and biological issues interweaved to create the perfect storm to the development of a syndemic, we narrate the cultural pedagogies embedded in the popular political resistance of the lower classes to overcome the syndemic.

The Cultural Pedagogies of the *Torcidas Organizadas*

Active support groups (known in Brazil as *Torcidas Organizadas*) started to be formed in the country in the late 1930s (De Toledo, 1996). They were originally created to engage the fans of a football team to become united under the same flag, and to chant the same support songs (De Toledo, 1996). However, after a few decades and particularly during the military dictatorship (1964–1985), when most political associations were suppressed, these groups became much more politicized, using the football stands to propagate democratic political messages, and consequently coping heavy police repression (Alvito, 2013). In 2014, in a collective effort to overcome club rivalries and create a strong voice to influence football policies and the larger political arena, the National Association of

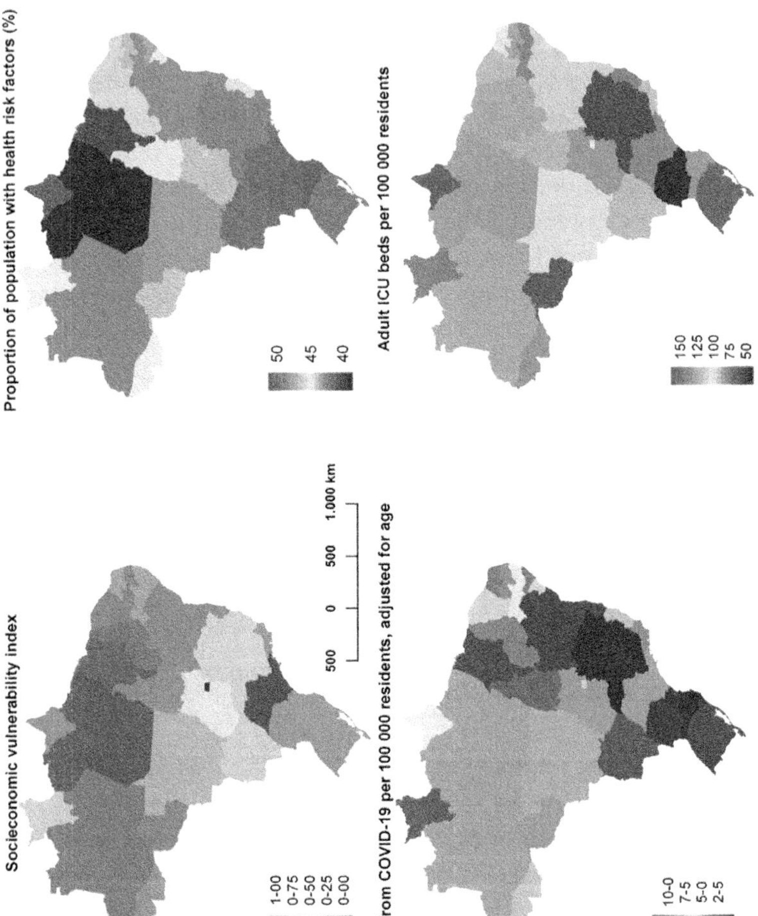

Fig. 17.1 Map on spacial inequality and COVID. (Source Rocha et al. (2021))

Torcidas Organizadas (Anatorg)[1] was created (Teixeira, 2018). The Anatorg is a typical example of a community organization that aims to educate, or create cultural pedagogies (Giroux, 2011) that can sustain a more fair and democratic life (Freire, 1998)

The *Torcidas Organizadas* (hereafter referred as TOs) currently are the Brazilian counterpart of a global social phenomenon called the football ultras. Originated in Europe, nowadays these groups of football fans exist in most continents (Doidge, 2013). They create not only a larger emotional connection between supporters and football teams; overtime, they lift the links among group fellows, leading to a robust feeling of social belonging (Knijnik & Newson, 2021), that invests aficionados to collective manifest their views on the rigid neoliberal forces that control football and their own lives. These signs of an enlarged social awareness within ultras can be seen in their talks, parades, hymns and manifestos (Kennedy & Kennedy, 2012).

According to Numerato (2018), the football terraces became one of the best spaces for young people to practice for social protests. More recently, one can note the growing number of antifascists supporter's collective. Those "antifascists supporters" act independently from the core of the TOs. While the TOs do not identify themselves with any specific political trend, these collective movements are identified with leftist politics.

It is worth noting that the TOs have always been seen by the hegemonic press as associate to violence and to depoliticization (Lopes & De Hollanda, 2018). In this paper, the effort will be to understand the role of the active fans in their *own political agency.* Others devalued the action of those groups because of the use of the violence in it. In contrast, E. P Thompson showed how the crowd organized itself behind complex cultural logics, which articulated values from popular culture, folklore, and everyday life. Edward Thompson's studies help us to reflect on the complex articulation between class struggle, culture and politics, showing the importance of cultural elements and everyday life in political resistance: "class happens when some men, as a result of common experiences ...feel and articulate the identity of their interests as between themselves, and as

[1] Disclosure: the first author of this paper is a board member of ANATORG.

against other men whose interests are different (and usually opposed to) theirs" (Thompson, 1963, p. 10).

With their wishes, values, banners, chants and battle cries, the TOs show in everyday life the complex cultural-social class link analysed by Thompson; furthermore, they are the prototype of what Giroux (2011) sees as organized cultural workers, who embed in their daily actions, instructions on how to set a common life (Giroux, 2011). The TOs also amplify their members' human agency, thus augmenting their participation and voice, hoping to enlarge the possibilities of an actual and participatory democracy that goes beyond the mere action to vote on a representative (Freire, 1998). By understanding the central importance of embodied emotions for any learning process (Freire, 1998), the TOs create specific and contextualized cultural pedagogies, which are practiced within a pulsating and partisan open domain. These are the *TOs' cultural pedagogies* (Giroux, 2011): they go past the ordinary diffusion of square knowledge, as they are sustained by the emotional investments that members carry to this social universe. Such pedagogies are not pre-given procedures, but results of past and present social struggles; they try to make "visible the operations of power and authority as part of its processes of disruption and unsettlement" (Giroux, 2011, 147).

Thus, the lived lessons, or cultural pedagogies, that led the TOs members to a social fight, aim to restore the modern football arena and its surrounds as public spaces occupied with much other goods than marketable products and shopping centres; they want to inhabit these spaces with their undisciplined bodies, songs and ways of life—by the TOs culture, embedded by their social class struggle. Eventually, the TOs' cultural pedagogies have the prospective to contest the repressive commodified environment of their everyday lives, in order to engender "the conditions of their own agency through dialogue, community participation, resistance and political struggle" (Giroux, 2011, p. 111).

Next, we describe the broad political context in Brazil that led to the grassroots revolts we discuss in this chapter. It is an intricate scenario where it becomes clear that, on the one hand, there was a federal government working to worsen the conditions of the virus' dissemination; on the other hand, there was a weak institutional opposition, too slow in their capacity to respond to the president's cabinet tactics. We then show

how and why the football fans from lower classes took on the streets, despite the elevated health risks, to fight for their lives.

The Syndemic Political Context in Brazil

The first cases of COVID-19 in Brazil appeared in February 2020. In March, the announcements of the first deaths began to occur (SP1, 2021). Firstly, the big cities were affected, but COVID-19 spread quickly to smaller cities, even reaching far-distant and isolated native Indigenous populations. Then Health Minister Luis Mandetta organized daily press conferences, in which he updated the population on what was happening, while encouraging social distancing and the use of face masks.

Despite the scientific-informed actions of the Minister of Health, President Jair Bolsonaro and his entourage seemed to go against the grain. Inspired by transnational far right-wing groups, Bolsonaro began to criticize the social distancing measures and advocate the use of the drug hydroxychloroquine as a magic cure for COVID. It wouldn't take long for Bolsonaro start attacking the vaccines (Estadão Conteúdo, 2020). It should be added that, till the end of his term in the presidential seat (December, 2022), Bolsonaro was one of the few international leaders that had not been vaccinated (Soares, 2021). In parallel, the president's supporters organized weekly demonstrations in his defense, mainly against a possible lockdown, but also contrary to everyday social distance measures. The situation between Mandetta and Bolsonaro became untenable; Mandetta was dismissed and the president appointed Nelson Teich as new Minister of Health (Schreiber, 2020).

The pandemic in Brazil spread considerably, with the number of cases and deaths getting out of control. Moreover, every weekend far right-wing movements, including racist and fascist groups, demonstrated in front of the presidential palace to support the president against the "dictatorship" of mask wearing and social distancing measures. Meanwhile, progressive and traditional leftist groups were afraid and reluctant to protest and, by doing so, helping to spread the virus and worsen the syndemic situation. At that moment, traditional social movements and the left political parties did not compromise in defense of the lockdown and limited themselves to social media protests.

It was then that two new social actors emerged in the public scene: the TOs and the "entregadores antifascistas" movements occupied the main streets of São Paulo (South America's largest city), challenging Bolsonaro`s government for the first time.

"History is Full of Contradictions": The TOs Initial Battle against Bolsonaro

On the eve of Jair Bolsonaro's successful election, Mano Brown—a well-known Brazilian rapper music, idol of the outskirts' black youth and political activist—performed a speech at Fernando Haddad's—former mayor of São Paulo and presidential candidate representing the Worker`s Party (PT)—electoral stage: "I don't like the party atmosphere. I don't like it. (…) If (the left) doesn't know what is going on, it is better go out to the streets once again". (Salgado, 2018) Mano Brown speech shocked the audience, which was expecting a cheerful and optimistic speech. In the past years, it has become a commonplace to say that the leaders of the traditional left—more associated with the Worker's Party, labor movements, and trade union centers—have distanced themselves from their own social base. This distancing would be felt in the years to come, when the traditional left struggled to oppose to Bolsonaro's government measures.

Latin-American sociologists, such as Felipe Paes Tavares Lopes and Bernardo Borges Buarque de Hollanda (2018) and Jose Garrica Zucal (2011) wrote about a *representativeness crisis*. For them, membership in more traditional and institutional spaces, as unions, political parties, traditional spaces for making politics, were losing their representativeness and their capacity to produce "belonging". In the same process, cultural associations, such as Escolas de Samba ("Samba Schools"), hip-hop movements, and the *Torcidas Organizadas* (TOs), acquire even deeper significance. In many ways, *Torcidas Organizadas* act as social networks. There, where the State is not able to provide basic care and welfare, the TOS create networks of affection and mutual economic aid. (De Toledo & Souza Junior, 2020). In times of economic crisis, the TOs carry out food drives, aid unemployed members and help each other in their daily lives. They also start to act in this "political vacuum" (Lopes & De Hollanda, 2018), occupying the political arena as well.

That said, it helps us to understand how football fans have taken the lead in opposing the Bolsonaro government. While the traditional left refused to go out to the streets to protest during the syndemic, football supporters took it upon themselves the responsibility of going out and demonstrate, even though they were aware of the health risks of their actions. This shows how football in the country is a social space full of paradoxes: controlled by every growing neoliberal forces, it also has the capacity to help civil society's organization (Alvito, 2013).

Daniel Passaro, leader of one of the country's largest and most traditional TOs, the *Gaviões da Fiel* ('the Hawks of the Faithful'), a Corinthians SC group of supporters, gave a thought-provoking statement.

> I don't understand why other social movements didn't start this struggle. (…) History is full (and made) of contradictions. I think is possible to defend the importance of social distancing measures and quarantine, while going to the streets for the struggle against fascism. (…) In our evaluation, this dispute of narratives in the Brazilian Society nowadays is also an *essential service.* (Daniel Passaro in Movdoc, 2020)

Passaro is refereeing here to the struggle against the government's lack of action to protect its people against COVID-19. It is relevant to point out that the TO *Gaviões da Fiel* has a history of being part of the democratic struggle in the country. In 1982 and 1983, they were a central part of the social movement known as the 'Corinthians Democracy', when relevant professional players such as Sócrates, and Casagrande, stood out for more democratic practices within Brazilian football—and also against the military dictatorship in the country (Florenzano, 2010; Knijnik, 2014). Thus, it was not a total surprise neither for the public nor for us when, in May 2020, in the midst of the country's severe health, political and economic crisis—the syndemic—, aggravated by the Bolsonaro misgovernment, a group of *Torcedores Organizados*—active supporters—mainly from the *Gaviões da Fiel*—held up a banner on Avenida Paulista: *We are Democracy* ('Somos Democracia'). The following week, members of other TOs groups, such as supporters of Santos Futebol Clube ('TO Jovem'), Sociedade Esportiva Palmeiras ('Mancha Verde TO'), Clube de Regatas do Flamengo ('Falange Rubro-Negra' TO) and other football clubs' supporter groups, hold massive demonstrations in the four major Brazilian cities: São Paulo, Rio de Janeiro, Belo Horizonte and Porto Alegre. They were part of a large football supporters' movement that called themselves as 'antifascist football supporters'; they carried banners with 'Bolsonaro out' and "in defense of democracy" slogans, as well as with antifascists mottos. Whilst the Bolsonaro's government have demonstrated since its inception its 'anti-working class character', the COVID-19 situation pushed these TOs to organize themselves to protest in a unified manner.

The Torcidas Organizadas met the Antifascists Delivery Workers

The TOS, however, counted on a new ally: the "entregadores antifascistas": *antifascist delivery workers.* In January 2020, when the syndemic hit the world economy, the job market was completely transformed. While jobs dwindled, the Gig Economy became a reality for an increasing number of families in South America (Howson et al., 2020). The large technology companies, the Gig Economy and the companies associated with e-commerce have seen their profits multiply, while the material situation of workers has deteriorated in the same proportion.

Like the TOs, the *antifascist delivery workers'* movement cannot be framed as a traditional union. This new universe of labor organization had started to force new forms of social, cultural and political association. Whilst we do not have specific demographic data about these movements, we could perfectly observe that the fluid and loose membership of both intertwine: TOs associates are from popular classes and, in order to feed their families, took jobs in the Gig Economy, including those of delivery workers. On the other hand, delivery workers, as many within the Brazilian working force, are very loyal fans of their football clubs.

Thus, both groups had many features in common to proceed with their political movement (Ghiraldelli, 2021).

Those demonstrations, that started in May/2020—thus just a few months after the COVID-19 hit the country with its disastrous effects in all aspects of Brazilians' lives—, went through the month of June and can definitely be considered a benchmark in the political/syndemic situation in Brazil. The movement grew quickly, driven by national contradictions but also due to a favorable international context—especially the *Black Lives Matter* that took place simultaneously in the United States after the murderer of George Floyd (Caetano & Gabriel, 2020). Some of the TOs sung antiracist chants as well, praising Brazilian Black leaders such as world known Marielle Franco, Rio de Janeiro popular leader and council woman who was brutally murdered in 2018 by local militia associated to Bolsonaro's family; as well as other songs in the memory of anonymous who were victims of police brutality in the recent past. The protest songs' central themes were interwoven—such as labor precarization, the struggle for human rights, the defense of democracy, demands for support against the syndemic and the fight against racism. More importantly, the TOs' protests were the first ones in the country to raise the hashtag #ImpeachmentBolsonaroNow (Ghiraldelli, 2021).

In São Paulo, right-wing groups went to the streets to protest the antifascist demonstrators, and to defend Bolsonaro's presidency; they were meeting not far from the main square where the TOs and gig economy workers were demonstrating, but no physical clashes were reported. For the first, time since the June 2013 massive street protests for better public transport in every single mega and medium Brazilian city (Knijnik, 2018; Jourdan, 2018), the left-wing protests outnumbered the demonstrations of the (far) right-wing supporters.

The TOs and the antifascists delivery workers' political movement created novel and unique cultural pedagogies for social movements (Giroux, 2011). In these unprecedented syndemic times, they were able to put together unparalleled modes or self-organization. This claim is supported not only because this new movement did not rely by any means on political parties, trade unions or other traditional left-wing civil societies; they were better off using their own social media and digital channels. In this sense, TO's and gig economy workers were clearly inspired by the anarchists and other popular collective groups from the June 2013 movements, which were then violently repressed by the State police (Jourdan, 2018).

However, this time they were brave enough to face not only the violent State police, but also the virus threat. From the inception, it was clear that the football stands were the perfect stage for the TOs to practice their collective embodied moves for years in the past (Numerato, 2018; Knijnik & Spaaij, 2017); their 'training' as active supporters was particularly handy in these political journey, and gave them the needed pedagogical support to create new cultural forms of protesting (Giroux, 2011). TOs were mindful of the virus' modus operandi, and keen to protect themselves as much as they could; they all used face masks and provided hand sanitizers to protest attendees; furthermore, they did not concentrate in a spot to listen to 'representative leaders' on the stage. They were pretty aware that large concentrations of demonstrators, crowding the same locations, without allowing any social distance, would be dangerous. Instead, they made the decision to perform walking demonstrations; the different TOs groups arrived in the agreed landmark, took some videos and photos, then went marching vigorously on the cities' streets (Nômade, 2020). Their stomping feet, antifascist banners and flags, chants and covered faces produced new visual performances that quickly gained momentum across the several social media platforms; those were powerful acts of popular resistance (Thompson, 2003),as well as manifestations of the cultural pedagogies (Giroux, 2011) uniquely developed to try and overcome the limit-situation they faced with the syndemic.

But the novelty of these protests went far away and had larger implications than their notable visual enactments; TOs and gig economy workers produced an innovative and democratic way of political assemblage (Giroux, 2011). Their movement was open and horizontal; for them, the representativeness crisis was clear (Lopes & De Hollanda, 2018); they were not there to praise any left-wing old school politician, neither to listen to them nor to cheer them after an institutional opposition leader's speech on a stage (Nômade, 2020). On the contrary, they were a collective movement that wanted their voices to be listened and their demands to be met; they did not want to be blind followers anymore; they wanted to lead, without mediation of traditional and, at that stage, past and unrepresentative leadership (Thompson, 2003).

The Middle Class Backlash

The TOs and gig economy workers' movement received the already expected violent police repression, accompanied by mainstream media reproach and right-wing politicians' condemnation. However, the most notable backlash came from non-expected sources: liberal and arguably democratic commentators as well as institutional left-wing political parties not only did not support these protests, but also dismissed them (Ghiraldelli, 2021). In order to suffocate this relevant grassroots political movement, and in a similar fashion described by Thompson (2003) when analysing the dismissal of the hunger riots in modern Europe by orthodox thinkers, these traditional Brazilian leaderships used the same argument across the board: due to the pandemic, 'it was not the time' to go to the streets and generate crowds to protest; there was 'no evidence' to support an impeachment process against Bolsonaro. A relevant social media influencer, connected to these progressive political parties, claimed in her YouTube channel that the TO's and the antifascist deliverers were 'genocidal', as they could not demonstrate during the COVID-19 syndemic (Ghiraldelli, 2021).

The TOs and antifascist deliverers alliance simply responded that all the 'pro-democracy' internet manifestos put together by middle-class liberal people, were just empty words with no real effect; after all, the TOs' members and their families were already on the streets on a daily basis, either delivering food or moving around within the cities' packed and inefficient public transport systems, to go to their workplaces, that did not close during the pandemic. They were also working for the same middle and high classes that were comfortably self-isolating in their homes. Why should they risk their lives to serve the middle-class during the weekdays, but could not protest against their terrible situation during the weekends? (Nômade, 2020).

This shock of world views becomes clearer as we next look at the ideas of the most visible representatives of the TOs and antifascist deliverers movement.

Emerson Osasco: The Voice of the TOs

Emerson is a member of the above mentioned Gaviões da Fiel, one of the largest TOs in Brazil, which has always been at the front of democratic movements on the stands and also on the streets. He is from Osasco, a peripheral city in São Paulo state, hence is known by his 'full name': Emerson Osasco. However, he became well-known by his appearances on street protests at 'Avenida Paulista', a core place where large political gatherings and demonstrations take place in São Paulo city.

Avenida Paulista serves as the pulse to assess the strength of a political protest: the amount of people there indicates the success, or failure, of a particular demonstration. Avenida Paulista is at the center of São Paulo City, a symbol of São Paulo economic and political power: looking from the top of its multiple skyscrapers that nowadays accommodate powerful investment banks and employers' associations, one still can see some of the preserved colonial mansions that once housed the elite of the eighteenth century country's farmers and their families.

After the demonstrations at the Avenida Paulista, Osasco became known in the City. Due to his online videos, explaining the protesters' social actions (Thompson, 2003), he started to gain some popularity across the grassroots social movements networks: "People look at me and recognize me as the 'Avenida Paulista guy'. But I have been fighting in other Avenidas Paulistas for a while". (Osasco, 2020) Emerson Osasco's *other Avenidas Paulistas* were on the outskirts of São Paulo, where he was born, and where he has learnt and developed the cultural pedagogies of protesting that he would later use on the larger stage of the Avenida Paulista (Giroux, 2011).

The day after the demonstrations, Emerson Osasco was fired: 'Around 4 pm I received an email from the company saying that I had been dismissed. One day after the act. I had just been promoted in the prior week…" Some voices complained in social media and tried to revert Emerson's dismissal, with no significant results. The complacency of

Brazilian companies with authoritarian governments is nothing new, but the level of political persecution had reached high levels under Bolsonaro regime. Henceforth, however, Emerson would opt for entry into traditional politics. He joined REDE (a left-wing Green-indigenous party), and then entered institutional politics, running as a candidate for councilor of Osasco. Emerson's strategy differed from Paulo Gallo, the leader of the anti-fascist deliverymen, who remain outside the institutional politics.

Emerson's entry into political activism came amid a teachers' strike. In Brazil, especially in the 1990s, *contracts*—rather than permanent positions—became the norm that neoliberal state governments started to use for hiring their teaching workforce. It was cheaper and with no formal bonds between the parties, forcing teachers to keep moving from one school to another, where they could find a new contract. Then, Emerson found that the teacher he liked the most at his High School, would no longer be there in the following school term. He was, in his own words, enraged. This trigged what Freire calls a *limit-situation* (Freire, 1998), which denotes happenings that are not restrictions but rather dares that move persons, groups and societies to see past events and, by undertaking limit-actions, to accomplish the conditions to achieve the utopia yet to be imagined, the Freirean *untested feasibility.* (Freire, 1998).

Thus, Emerson decided to act. It was the start of his political activism against the precarization of teachers' work in the State of São Paulo. It is significant that both Galo—the delivery antifascist leader—and Emerson, bring in their trajectory, the role of education and teachers as decisive for joining the political struggle.

Anyway, it was in the Torcida Gaviões da Fiel that Osasco learned politics. The conversations between members, and the different ways they create to support their teams, served as life lessons for Emerson to learn how to critically analyse his social context (Giroux, 2011), as well to develop new forms of political protest (Numerato, 2018). Like many TOs, the Gaviões da Fiel emerged in the 1960s, in the wake of the global movement of 1968. The defense of "young power", contestatory and rebellious against all traditional authority, was part of the lexicon of the TOs movement. In a national context, the Torcidas opposed to the Brazilian military dictatorship (Florenzano, 2010). In the case of the

Gaviões, members like to say that the fans were born from a double struggle—both against "dictators" of Corinthians, such as club's presidents Wadih Helu and Vicente Matheus, as well as the "dictators" of the central government. (Osasco, 2020; Knijnik, 2014) In rhetoric, the fans would have overthrown both, with a central role in the process of political reopening of Brazil: "our fight arose from the struggle against the dictatorship and in favor of democracy". (Osasco, 2020)

In the case of Brazil, a country marked by racialization, the mainstream mostly white press, usually associate blackness with violence. Sidney Chalhoub (1989) called this ideological process as "white fear", in producing a stigma of blacks as "a dangerous class". It was no different in the case of the TOs. In that, any episode of violence produced this immediate association between such acts, the skin color of their members to depoliticization and stigmatization. However, Emerson says that fans are uncomfortable with these stereotypes, not because of the race prejudice, but because it embeds social class discrimination: "the vast majority of fans are from the periphery, from the less favored classes. This causes revolt and annoyance". (Osasco, 2020) Nevertheless, Osasco preferred an alternative image, where he not only challenges the notion of lower classes being not politicized, but he also adds his dream of more fans acquiring political consciousness, hence achieving a more socially just society to everyone:

> The fans are the most politicized group of the inferior masses. That's why I always speak on the day when organized fans acquire political knowledge can change the country for the better. (Osasco, 2020)

This political knowledge came to fruition when the TOs started to organize side by side with the antifascist deliverers. It is interesting to understand how Osasco's political dreams match with the actions and imaginations of the Gig economy worker activist Paulo Gallo, who wants to spread political education and consciousness to his category. Next, we look at how one of the most conscious amidst among the Gig economy workers raised his voice among their social movement.

'I Want to be Paulo Freire': Protests and Street Cultural Pedagogies

Paulo Galo, one of the leaders of the *antifascist delivery workers'* social movement, and a fan of Corinthians SC, was one of the first deliverer worker to start organizing the category, and quickly he emerged as a leader of these invisible workers. Leading the demonstrations in 2020 alongside the TOs, Galo declared that his greatest pride was "being able to see workers again regarding themselves as workers, no longer as neoliberal entrepreneurs." (Rodrigues, 2020) In 2017, Paulo Roberto da Silva Lima, who presents himself as "Galo" (meaning Cock, the animal, with no other double meaning in Portuguese) lost his full time job in an electricity company; in need to raise some money to support his young family, he decided to get back to his former occupation as a motorised courier, known in Brazil as 'motoboy'. However, the job market landscape was already completely different from what it was when he worked as a 'motoboy'. The Gig Economy companies had taken control of the motoboys' market, completely restructuring the pre-existing labour relations. Galo realized soon that the job as a delivery worker was something completely different from what it used to be.

Paulo Galo was used to an old-fashion routine as a delivery worker, when he was thrown into the Gig Economy. In less than a decade, the Gig Economy reshaped the labour market as a whole. The so-called "uberization" (Slee, 2017) of labour relations is not a phenomenon restricted to the delivery market and the transportation services. Contrary to what is commonly advocated by the market, one of the consequences of precarization is more bureaucracy. Several issues that used to be solved quickly, are presented as insurmountable due to the technological barrier. Galo himself reports:

> Before, when the local pizzeria had an annoying customer, you already knew you were going to find an irritating patron. You already knew... (...) now, questions that were simple, take hours to be answered, you need to contact the application, everything takes much more time. (Rodrigues, 2020)

It was precisely one of these situations that made Paulo Galo enter the universe of politics. He was carrying an order when his motorcycle tire got flat. Paulo contacted the App saying that he would not be able to complete the order that night, and that he will have to go home. On the phone, the attendant assured that Galo would not be blocked. But the next day, when he returned to work, Galo was blocked for the third time, meaning he was out of the job. That's when he started to create the conditions of his own political liberation (Giroux, 2011); employing the same technology that was taking his job off, Galo recorded a video that went viral. In the film, he raises questions that laid the groundwork for the popular uprising that would follow (Thompson, 2003): "Do you know how hard it is to deliver food with an empty stomach? How hard it is to deliver food without having anything to eat?". (Rodrigues, 2020)

After that episode, Galo was then invited by *Exame*—a relevant Brazilian weekly magazine on Economics and Markets—to talk about the social situation of the delivery workers. He gave an unabashed interview, where he further extends the framework of his popular knowledge (Freire, 1998), discussing the precarious and exploitative environment of the sharing economy. Galo began immediately to be politically persecuted by the Gig Industry, suffering the so-called "bloqueio branco" (white block)—when you are blocked for political reasons. Gallo simply stopped receiving delivery requests in the Ifood App—even if he was not "technically blocked" by the digital systems. (Rodrigues, 2020)

In that interview and in a few follow-up internet videos, Galo explained that his political and social radical views were shaped during his youth years, by listening to the hip hop movement in São Paulo. This is the type of popular education that was accessible to lower income and marginalized youth, which created social consciousness among them (Giroux, 2011; Freire, 1998). Rap and hip-hop, and in particular the above mentioned rapper Mano Brown, were responsible for introducing Galo to the anti-racist and anti-capitalist struggle.

But it was the precarity of the labor relations in the Gig Economy that transformed him in a leader. Galo started to act as an educator, having long conversations and organizing the delivery workers' movement. It didn't take long for the Media to start to trace parallels between Galo and former President Lula, who, in the 1970s, was a workers' union leader who commanded the largest strikes in Brazil's recent history, confronting the wage cuts caused by the military dictatorship economic policies. Galo, however, refused to enter institutional politics: "I don't want to be like Lula, I want to be like Paulo Freire." (Rodrigues, 2020)

Freire's educational proposals and practices act to bring social consciousness to its participants. Thus, Galo's choice of Freire over Lula is symptomatic. As Freire, he also understands that teaching is a social action produced via dialogue within collective contexts (Knijnik, 2021). In doing so, he clearly aligns himself with the grassroots movements and the popular resistance (Thompson, 2003). He constantly refuses institutional politics as an exclusively arena, as he repeats in several interviews: "In the Parliament you can make a career, but on the streets, you can make history". (Rodrigues, 2020)

As discussed above, one of the key causes of the crisis of representation of the left, was the gap between the leaders of the social movements and the movements itself. By rather 'being Freire than Lula', Galo shows that the cultural pedagogies that the antifascist's delivery workers movement have been shaping to struggle for better work and life conditions, is the same fight of other relevant workers, as teachers and educators (Giroux, 2011).

Galo's alliance with the São Paulo TOs should be seen in the is lights of his philosophical choice. For an educator, which partnership could be more prolific than that with the "greatest mass social movement" in Brazil (Teixeira, 2018). If the traditional left did not see anything in TOS than depoliticization and violence, Galo saw a possibility in raising a common agenda with them. This political agenda would then create a multiplicity of grassroots political ways to act, in order to bring consciousness to the precariat which they belong to. According to Galo, though, this alliance's new forms of resistance (Thompson, 2003), would only be relevant if embedded and soaked in their own practice (Freire, 1998).

Hope and Courage: Lessons from the TOs Cultural Pedagogies

At the early stages of the COVID-19 syndemic, amidst the high levels of uncertainty and anxiety that it caused across the Earth, there were also some signs of hope. It appeared that the forced shutdown of entire countries and economies would push communities and global leaders to rethink the ways that we, as human beings, interact with each other and with the planet. The initial lessening of carbon emissions in the atmosphere; the sudden appearance of wild animals in empty but highly urbanized spaces in megacities, these looked like small lights of hope showing that 'another world is possible'.

The cooperation between TOs and delivery workers, that started in São Paulo and quickly disseminated across the main capital cities across Brazil, was part of this global beacon of hope. The Gig economy workers were living under extremely oppressive work conditions; the syndemic scenario further suffocated their voices; the representativeness crisis were adding to their hopeless. Then, they found, in the already consolidated communal space of football supporters in the country, the strength they needed to articulate their political protests, as well as the room they were seeking to voice their demands. Thus, it is important to acknowledge that, even under great oppression by the neoliberal forces that try to control any aspect of the sport, football is also a prominent social space for Brazilian communities to share and to shape their social lives. This is evidenced by the *ad hoc* grassroots unification that resulted from the joint antifascist political venture of the TOs and delivery workers.

The demonstration tactics of the TOs, on the other side, were revamped by the arrival of the delivery workers; together, they have created new forms of protest that were yet to be seen across Brazilian streets. Moreover, they came out of their invisibility to show to the upper classes that their work and their lives were essential, particularly during the syndemic. They were, in fact, the blood that kept the Brazilian cities alive during the forced lockdowns.

It seemed that their movement was ephemeral, as they were quickly smashed by every political side of the dominant powers, the mainstream media, and the traditional left-wing political parties, trade unions and influent internet voices. A superficial analysis would erase these movements from the history, claiming they had no impact whatsoever in the political opposition to Bolsonaro's presidency inefficient and corrupt response to the health crisis.

However, claiming that these movements did not achieve anything, would be a short-sighted analysis. Firstly, because in the short-term, a few of the Gig economy deliverers' main demands were attained. The Apps started to support them with hand sanitizers, some funding for meals during their breaks, water stations, gloves, face masks and other protective material. In the medium-term, the National Parliament, observing the vulnerability of the precariat, approved a much better governmental pandemic support package than the initial one planned by Bolsonaro's government.

Furthermore, it is in the long-term where we can see that, even if highly undermined by the powers that be, the seeds of the TOs and Gig economy deliverers' political movement beared relevant fruits. Far from being in vain, their cultural pedagogies, their new forms of protest and their revolutionary purposes, slowly spread thru other social groups. One year later, and following the lead of the TOs, several middle-class individuals started to organize themselves to go to the streets to demand #ImpeachmentBolsonaronow. Claims that early on were deemed as 'absurd' and 'out of purpose', gradually started to penetrate other social groups' minds and hearts; new middle-class organized communities started to gain the streets, the Avenida Paulista and other protest spaces across Brazilian cities. Mimicking the TOs' protest strategies, they kept marching while singing their revolutionary chants, targeting Bolsonaro and his lack of action to protect the nation from COVID-19.

Each day it is becoming clearer to more sectors of the country's population, that this health crisis is a syndemic, caused by a combination of bio, political and social issues; thus, it won't be eradicated only by sanitary measures; there is a need of a holistic approach that takes into account several dimensions in order to protect people's lives. Recently in Brazil, more people started to agree that the crisis' political dimension is the most urgent. Whilst the coronavirus exists in nature, SARS-COVID-19 is a syndemic caused by a sum of natural, political and social factors.

Thus, its elimination depends that the 'Virusman', who favours the conditions of the illness' dissemination, is also removed. The early political and brave actions of the football TOs finally made more and more people to realize that, just by ousting Bolsonaro from his presidential chair, the country would start to feel some relief from this terrible situation.

The cultural pedagogic lessons of the early protests by the TOs' and the Gig economy deliverers, showed how football in South America can be a relevant space for social transformation. They achieved one of the most important outcomes of any revolutionary process: an effective legacy of hope and courage to inspire people to struggle for their rights, even when facing terrible life-threatening prospects.

References

Alvito, M. (2013). Maçaranduba neles! Torcidas organizadas e policiamento no Brasil. *Tempo, 17*(34), 81–94.

Caetano, G., & Gabriel, R. S. (2020, May 31). Torcidas organizadas de clubes rivais saem às ruas em defesa da democracia em São Paulo, Minas e Rio. *O Globo*. https://oglobo.globo.com/brasil/torcidas-organizadas-de-clubes-rivais-saem-as-ruas-em-defesa-da-democracia-em-São-paulo-minas-rio-24455430?verSão=amp

Chalhoub, S. (1989). *Visões da liberdade: uma história das últimas décadas da escravidão na corte*. Cia das Letras.

Da Silva, E. F., & Da Silveira, E. S. (2020). A Pandemia de Covid-19 sob a benção de Bolsonaro e Evangélicos. *Revista Inter-Legere, 3*(29), c23426–c23426.

De Toledo, L. H. (1996). *Torcidas organizadas de futebol*. Autores Associados.

De Toledo, L. H., & Souza Junior, R. A. P. (2020). Redes populares de proteção: Torcidas Organizadas de futebol no contexto da pandemia da COVID-19. *Ponto Urbe, 26*, 1–20.

Doidge, M. (2013). 'The Birthplace of Italian Communism': Political Identity and Action Amongst Livorno Fans. *Soccer & Society, 14*(2), 246–261.

Estadão Conteúdo. (2020, December 25). Bolsonaro zomba de suposta baixa eficácia da Coronavac. *Exame*. https://exame.com/brasil/bolsonaro-zomba-de-suposta-baixa-eficacia-da-coronavac/

Florenzano, J. P. (2010). *A democracia corinthiana: práticas de liberdade no futebol brasileiro*. Educ/Fapesp.

Freire, P. (1998). *Pedagogy of freedom: Ethics, democracy and civic courage*. Rowman & Littlefield.

Ghiraldelli, P. (2021). *A democracia de Bolsonaro*.

Giroux, H. A. (2011). *On critical pedagogy*. Continuum.

Horton, R. (2020). Offline: COVID-19 is not a pandemic. *The Lancet, 396*(10255), 874.

Howson, K., Ustek-Spilda, F., Grohmann, R., Salem, N., Carelli, R., Abs, D., Salvagni, J., Graham, M., Balbornoz, M. B., Chavez, H., & Arriagada, A. (2020). 'Just because you don't see your boss, doesn't mean you don't have a boss': Covid-19 and Gig Worker Strikes across Latin America. *International Union Rights, 27*(3), 20–28.

Jourdan, C. (2018). *2013: Memorias e resistências*. Circuito.

Kennedy, P., & Kennedy, D. (2012). Football Supporters and the commercialisation of Football: Comparative responses across Europe. *Soccer & Society, 13*(3), 327–340.

Knijnik, J. (2014). Playing for freedom: Sócrates, *futebol-arte* and democratic struggle in Brazil. *Soccer & Society, 15*(5), 635–654.

Knijnik, J. (2018). *The world cup chronicles: 31 days that rocked Brazil*. Fair Play Publishing.

Knijnik, J. (2021). To Freire or not to Freire: educational freedom and the populist right wing '*Escola sem Partido*' movement in Brazil. *British Educational Research Journal, 47*(2), 355–371.

Knijnik, J., & Newson, M. (2021). 'Tribalism', identity fusion and football fandom in Australia: the case of Western Sydney. *Soccer & Society, 22*(3), 248–265.

Knijnik, J., & Spaaij, R. (2017). No harmony: Football fandom and everyday multiculturalism in Western Sydney. *Journal of Intercultural Studies, 38*(1), 36–53.

Lopes, F. T. P., & De Hollanda, B. B. B. (2018). "Ódio eterno ao futebol moderno": poder, dominação e resistência nas arquibancadas dos estádios da cidade de São Paulo. *Tempo, 24*(2), 206–232.

Movdoc. (2020, July 18). Protesto Futebol Clube: torcidas organizadas contra o Governo Bolsonaro [Video]. *YouTube*. https://www.youtube.com/watch?v=t5SVqEC0Ogc&ab_channel=MOVdoc

Nômade, U. (2020). Nas redes e nas ruas: pela democracia já, contra o golpe que está em curso. *Lugar Comum–Estudos de mídia, cultura e democracia, 1*(58), 5–12.

Numerato, D. (2018). *Football fans, activism and social change*. Routledge.
Osasco, E. (2020, October 31). #Conheça: Emerson Osasco—a periferia ocupando os espaços de poder em SP. *Mídia Ninja*. https://midianinja.org/vereadoresquequeremos/emersonosasco/
Paiva, V., Garcia, M. R. V., França-Jr, I., Silva, C. G. d., Galeão-Silva, L. G., Simões, J. A., Ayres, J. R., & Research Group on Youth's Health and Human Rights. (2021). Youth and the COVID-19 crisis: Lessons learned from a human rights-based prevention programme for youths in São Paulo. *Brazil. Global Public Health, 16*(8–9), 1454–1467.
Rocha, R., Atun, R., Massuda, A., Rache, B., Spinola, P., Nunes, L., Lago, M., & Castro, M. C. (2021). Effect of socioeconomic inequalities and vulnerabilities on health-system preparedness and response to COVID-19 in Brazil: a comprehensive analysis. *The Lancet Global Health, 9*(6), e782–e792.
Rodrigues, P. (2020, June 11). Galo de luta. *UOL*. https://www.uol.com.br/ecoa/reportagens-especiais/lider-dos-entregadores-antifascistas-paulo-galo-lima-quer-comida-e-melhores-condicoes-de-trabalho-para-o-grupo/
Salgado, D. (2018, October 25). Mano Brown acaba com clima festivo em ato do PT. *O Globo*. https://oglobo.globo.com/epoca/mano-brown-acaba-com-clima-festivo-em-ato-do-pt-23183740
Schreiber, M. (2020, May 15). Três temas que expuseram racha entre Nelson Teich e Jair Bolsonaro. *BBB News Brasil*. https://www.bbc.com/portuguese/brasil-52684841
Singer, M. (1994). AIDS and the health crisis of the US urban poor; the perspective of critical medical anthropology. *Social Science & Medicine, 39*(7), 931–948.
Singer, M. (1996). A dose of drugs, a touch of violence, a case of AIDS: Conceptualizing the SAVA syndemic. *Free Inquiry in Creative Sociology, 24*(2), 99–110.
Slee, T. (2017). *Uberização: a nova onda do trabalho precarizado*. Elefante.
Soares, I. (2021, August 04). Bolsonaro sobre CoronaVac: "Eu não posso tomar essa vacina lá de SP". *Correio Braziliense*. https://www.correiobraziliense.com.br/politica/2021/08/4941721-bolsonaro-sobre-coronavac-eu-nao-posso-tomar-essa-vacina-la-de-sp.html
SP1. (2021, March 17). Primeiro anúncio de uma morte por Covid-19 no Brasil completa um ano. *G1*. https://g1.globo.com/sp/São-paulo/noticia/2021/03/17/anuncio-da-primeira-morte-por-covid-19-no-brasil-completa-um-ano.ghtml

Tamara, K. (2020, April 23). The virus man: Bolsonaro's Further destruction of the Brazilian Republic. *The Globe Post*. https://theglobepost.com/2020/04/15/bolsonaro-coronavirus/

Teixeira, R. C. (2018). A Associação Nacional das Torcidas Organizadas do Brasil na arena pública: desafios de um movimento coletivo. *Antípoda. Revista de Antropología y Arqueología, 30*, 111–128.

Thompson, E. P. (1963). *The making of the English working class*. Victor Gollancz Ltd..

Thompson, E. P. (2003). *Costumes em comum: estudos sobre a cultura popular tradicional*. Cia das Letras.

Zucal, J. G. (2011). *"Nosotros nos peleamos": violencia e identidad de una hinchada de fútbol*. Prometeo Libros.

18

Parenting in Pandemic Times: Notes on the Emotional Geography of Youth Sport Culture

Ryan King-White and Michael D. Giardina

Proem

It was an odd sight—seeing professional and collegiate sport alike reduced to playing in empty arenas, Potemkin-like 'bubbles', or simply not being played at all. The beginning of the end of the normal operation of sport can be pinpointed to March 11, 2020, when Rudy Gobert—the three-time National Basketball Association (NBA) Defensive Player of the Year from the Utah Jazz—tested positive for the virus prior to a game with the Oklahoma City Thunder. The league paused the season immediately; no NBA games would be played for four months. Numerous other professional and amateur sports around the world followed suit the next day, as the National Hockey League, Major League Baseball, Major League

R. King-White (✉)
Towson University, Towson, MD, USA

M. D. Giardina
Florida State University, Tallahassee, FL, USA

D. L. Andrews et al. (eds.), *Sport and Physical Culture in Global Pandemic Times*, Global Culture and Sport Series, https://doi.org/10.1007/978-3-031-14387-8_18

Soccer, La Liga, and numerous NCAA conferences (e.g., ACC, SEC, Big 10, Pac-12) all suspended operations on March 12, 2020 (see Spain, 2020).

And while the lingering effects of COVID-19 on the world of commercial sport may have been frustrating for fans, workers, organizations, broadcasters, and the like, what has often been written out of the discussion is the impact of COVID-19 on *youth sport*. For youth sport programming—a cottage industry and seeming rite of passage for many children and their parents in the United States—was quite simply *devastated* (Drummond et al., 2020). Local community-run recreation programs were shuttered across the country, highly competitive travel teams, leagues, and training programs were temporarily paused, and, for a time, many public parks across the country were deemed off-limits by rule of law (Fang et al., 2021). With K-12 schools quickly shifting from in-person instruction to online distance learning over video conferencing platforms like Zoom in the late Spring of 2020, millions of children suddenly had no regular access to playground time, limited (or no) physical contact with other kids, and no sporting outlet to expend their considerable energy reserves anywhere but in their own homes. Outside of E-Sports, iPad games from the App Store, and massive multiplayer Internet platforms like Roblox (Thomas & Rogers, 2020) all was quiet, but it did not *quite* last forever.

* * *

As of this writing (late 2021), millions have been infected, perished, and/or had their lives forever altered by the pandemic in a variety of ways.[1] For much of March 2020 to March 2021, families of all types were forced to essentially shelter-in-place for extended periods of time as schools, restaurants, large gatherings, and other forms of external human group contact were reduced to a variety of pixelated, cellular, and electronic communications. Lockdowns, travel restrictions, and a whole host of other impediments were erected in an effort to slow the spread of the virus long enough for a vaccine to be developed. And while such policies (mostly) 'followed the science' and were in the best interest of all, the

[1] As of September 1, 2021, globally there have been 218 million cases, and 4.5 million deaths.

emotional and psychological strain experienced by children (and their parents) is one of the primary horrors of this still-ongoing pandemic.

In this chapter, we discuss through narrative vignettes and critical analyses the (still evolving) realities of youth sport in pandemic times, especially in terms of the emotional geographies (see Davidson et al., 2005; Tamas et al., 2021) of sport and physical culture we traversed with our children during this time. To that end, we engage with the un/ease with which we have negotiated fatherhood in the contemporary moment, essentially raising what Margaret Hagerman (2018) would characterize in her book *White Kids: Growing up with Privilege in a Racially Divided America* as children who are growing up "with upper-middle-class privilege in a society where private wealth shapes the experiences, opportunities, and outcomes that follow such childhoods of privilege" (p. 2). And while we additionally recognize that our positionality as white, cisgendered, heterosexual fathers (to four children—Ryan three; Michael one) within such a socio-economic dynamic—especially one in which we de facto benefit from whilst also trying to critique—will not mirror the experiences of everyone, there is a need for multiple (if competing) accounts of these pandemic times. As Hugo Ceron-Anaya (2019) has noted in his research on the intersection of sport and affluence, to engage with questions of class privilege can reveal the workings of power that operate on those without such privilege.

COVID-19, Neoliberalism, and Public Health in the United States

Debates about the best way to manage a nation's health system and policy have persisted for years (e.g., Benefield et al., 2000; Gawande, 2009; Herzlinger, 2006; Mintzberg, 1993; Porter & Teisberg, 2006). The U.S. health care system, enmeshed deeply in late capitalism and big-P politics, has long been celebrated both internally and externally for its ability to produce landmark advances in treatments for a variety of medical issues (Vogenberg & Santilli, 2018). However, the weaknesses in this approach have become quite clear during the often-catastrophic management of the COVID-19 pandemic (Walker, 2020). Oppel Jr. et al. (2020) state:

> Early numbers had shown that Black and Latino people were being harmed by the virus at higher rates. But the new federal data—made available after *The New York Times* sued the Centers for Disease Control and Prevention—reveals a clearer and more complete picture: Black and Latino people have been disproportionately affected by the coronavirus in a widespread manner that spans the country, throughout hundreds of counties in urban, suburban and rural areas, and across all age groups. (para. 5)

Thus, those feeling the brunt of the pandemic were and continue to come from racially and economically disadvantaged populations.

Using federal infection data accessed after successfully suing the *U.S. Centers for Disease Control*, Oppel Jr. et al. write in the *New York Times* that Black, Latinx, Native American, elderly, and poor populations are being disproportionately affected by the COVID-19 virus since they often work in jobs that require being present and/or have difficult living conditions (read: housing with multiple people who have contact with numerous others often with the inability to escape elsewhere). Put differently, though there exists some evidence that high blood pressure and obesity when contracting COVID-19 is a contributory factor to the severity of one's case,

> The focus on comorbidities "makes me angry, because this really is about who still has to leave their home to work, who has to leave a crowded apartment, get on crowded transport, and go to a crowded workplace, and we just haven't acknowledged that those of us who have the privilege of continuing to work from our homes aren't facing those risks," said Dr. Mary Bassett, the Director of the FXB Center for Health and Human Rights at Harvard University. (quoted in Oppel Jr. et al., 2020)

In sum, the COVID-19 pandemic has been instructive in shining a bright light on the systemic inequities in the American health care system.

Disparities in a population's access to a better quality of life do not begin and end with COVID-19, of course. Indeed, these differences are witnessed and experienced across numerous sites (health care, education, child care, and physical activity). Scholars often seek out ways to reach these "disadvantaged" populations in order to provide methods to inform and care for those who do not have readily available access in a system so entangled in late capitalist sensibilities. Such activist work is difficult for numerous reasons, but namely because systemic change requires both helping the underserved whilst also convincing the privileged to relinquish or at least share access to opportunity.

As noted at the outset, we have been working through our struggles with our place in this system—as individuals, fathers, husbands, and academics. Borrowing from extensive work on utilizing narrative as a form of inquiry with which to better understand contemporary socio-political questions (see, e.g., Denison, 2016; Markula & Denison, 2005; Pringle, 2001; Sparkes, 1996) we aim to make linkages between politics, socialization, and ourselves. Following Denison (2016), locating our struggles with (white) privilege and parenting is required,

> [o]therwise we will be left with texts, no matter how poignant or emotional, that are for the most part one-dimensional and apolitical: stories that fail to illuminate anything critical or captivating or tell us what lies behind and beyond the surface details (read description) the simple who, what, when and where of our lives. When what our research narratives really need to do is explore with depth the why's and how's around those details. (p. 8)

Both of us see and desire the overarching benefits to national health through some form of collective care and, in the case of this chapter, opportunities for young people to "play." However, this yearning creates a separate, but related, challenge for the both of us. Primarily, what to do as liberal-minded people whilst being fathers in the neoliberal moment—particularly when it comes to our relationship with the evermore *privatized* physical activity options available during COVID-19. To give some brief context, the private U.S. youth sport landscape is estimated to be a $15–$20 billion per year industry. In recent years it has come under increased criticism for its largely unregulated nature, its promise of future rewards (college scholarships, professional sport opportunities), and disparities in access due to its outsized costs relative to community-based leagues and programs. Writing in *Time* magazine, Gregory (2017) explained:

> Across the nation, kids of all skill levels, in virtually every team sport, are getting swept up by a youth-sports economy that increasingly resembles the pros at increasingly early ages. Neighborhood Little Leagues, town soccer associations and church basketball squads that bonded kids in a community–and didn't cost as much as a rent check–have largely lost their luster. Little League [baseball] participation, for example, is down 20% from its turn-of-the-century peak. These local leagues have been nudged aside by private club teams, a loosely governed constellation that includes everything from development academies affiliated with professional sports franchises to regional squads run by moonlighting coaches with little experience. The most competitive teams vie for talent and travel to national tournaments. Others are elite in name only, siphoning expensive participation fees from parents of kids with little hope of making the high school varsity, let alone the pros. (para. 4).

As parents of young children who participate in this space—largely out of necessity, given locality and geography—we are both wary and critical of it, which again speaks to a certain kind of privilege in not having to take it too seriously as the end-goal for our children is not college scholarships or professional careers, but rather enjoyment and fun.

Contextually speaking, we want to make clear that our behaviors as fathers during COVID weren't consciously feminist, but could be read that way. In the moment it would be fair to say that we were simply concerned with 'getting through the day' rather than debating gendered divisions of labor in the household. To wit, Michael's partner—a successful healthcare executive with far-reaching responsibilities—regularly worked 14-hour days with non-negotiable deadlines imposed by C-suite actors. Similarly, Ryan's partner works as a speech pathologist in the elementary school that their kids attend, meaning that she was required to be at work while the children had to log in during formal learning hours. There was neither heroism nor martyrdom in going to the park mid-afternoon or building LEGOs or making sure that at various times the kids followed a schedule for online instruction, completing learning modules, producing artwork and music, procuring and reading library books, and engaging in structured physical activity lessons instead of working on a journal article or book chapter. We acknowledge that this situation is an outlier in regard to national labor trends (see: Collins et al., 2021; Zamarro, 2020), and might suggest that some of the feminist or feminist-adjacent behavior we exhibited during the pandemic could be attributed to the fact that the groundwork for doing so had already been laid insofar as we had fallen in love with, supported, and encouraged our partners to achieve and maintain successes in their chosen professions.

Recent research would suggest that the pandemic typically impacted women who are parents (Brown et al., 2020; Gassman-Pines et al., 2020), and those who are low income (Bernstein et al., 2021) the hardest. According to Kerr et al. (2021), 76% of women reported being mostly responsible for childcare during the pandemic in 2020, whereas only 6.2% stated that men did more though these numbers were slightly more even in higher income families. Additionally, low-income families experienced more job loss (Kerr et al., 2021), had less access to online educational resources, struggled to eat (Gundersen et al., 2021), be physically active (Dunton et al., 2020), obtain health care and were more likely to be infected (Bibbins-Domingo, 2020). That our partners were not among these statistics does, in no way, suggest that they were not present or a major part of our children's experiences during COVID, but rather that we took the rather traditional and gendered role as male figureheads driving sport selection and participation when it came to play and physical activity in this particular instance (Fredricks & Eccles, 2004).

Perhaps our situations bespeaks the privilege with being tenured, and of our own privileged insouciance at pretending that work was more important than family in the face of a global pandemic that has killed millions. We get that, and we'll own that (and the anxiety that comes with it; see Bunds, 2021). We can complicate and overcomplicate the socio-economic imperatives embedded in navigating the pandemic, in dividing up our familial roles—that's what we do as academics—but navigating those emotional geographies throughout the past two years months were often just the mechanics of *survival.* And we were fortunate to be in a position to get through it. In what follows below, and with the privilege of self-reflection and reflexivity, attempt to look critically on our actions by providing two narratives detailing our experiences and locating them within the contemporary socio-political pandemic *conjuncture* (see Grossberg, 2010, p. 66).

Michael[2]

The COVID-enforced school closings didn't come as a surprise to my wife and me. She is a healthcare executive intimately involved with big data for a large hospital conglomerate—and could see the spikes in admissions, geographic hot spots, and C-suite concern over the emerging public health crisis. It was going to be all hands on-deck at work and home for a while. In March of 2020, our then-just-turned-four-year-old-son, who was in Pre-K at the time, saw his school and the rest in the district close well into the summer of 2020, and eventually reopen in the Fall as a virtual format in Pre-K4 (which we declined to participate in). As both my wife and I transitioned to working remotely—a privilege often cast as the 'new normal' across news reporting that focused only on a particular slice of Americans (see Thomas & Rogers, 2020)—we essentially home schooled him from March of 2020 to February of 2021.

The academic element was relatively easy to negotiate, as I turned off my professorial mannerisms (or at least attempted to) and took on the role of an early childhood educator during part of the daytime hours (though my son might disagree). Although many of my friends in academia—who were also in similar situations with their children—uneasily joked that our 4- and 5-year-olds would become easily bored with our teaching methods, or that our sons and daughters were less stubborn than our doctoral students—I genuinely enjoyed the year spending time with him on his educational journey through PreK and Kindergarten workbooks dutifully purchased on amazon.com or at the local Target, through various iPad apps such as Reading Eggs, and more LEGO sets than any one person should probably purchase in a given year (or two).

Yet the *sporting* gap was harder to fill, as youth soccer leagues went on hiatus (McAvoy, 2020), gymnastics and swimming programs offered through the city shuttered (WTXL, 2020), and even the public parks were locked down. As someone who has long written about sport and physical culture (e.g., Giardina, 2005; Giardina & Donnelly, 2007; Newman & Giardina, 2011)—and understands and largely accepts the critiques of for-profit youth sport programs—I was still troubled—or

[2] Portions of this section revisit and update arguments in Giardina (2021).

perhaps put better, *disappointed*—by the thought that my son was going to 'miss out' on a formative engagement with team sports, or, for a time, any sort of physical activity not contained within our small backyard. This mindset smacks of a particular biopolitics of privilege (see Bunds, 2014), of course, for large portions of the population were simply concerned with staying gainfully employed and keeping their families healthy.

After several cabin-fevered months of official city and state lockdowns, some restrictions were eventually loosened in terms of outdoor gathering and activities. Cautiously at first but then with greater gusto, we went on hikes in the Western North Carolina mountains—pretending the trails and eventual waterfalls at their endpoints were part of some training mission for the Avengers or the Power Rangers. We took up fishing in the intracoastal waterways near Hilton Head Island, South Carolina, where my son caught a nice 12-pound red fish on his first day out. And we fooled around on the practice green of the golf club in the community, which was still restricting hours for its members due to the pandemic. Further, he learned to swim at the HOA pool in our community, which had implemented a reservation system to keep the number of attendees at about a dozen at any given time. All of this was great fun—quality time we never would have spent together during the course of a 'normal' school year, and something I would never want to trade despite the circumstances under which it came into being. That is, until he confided in me one day when there were several other kids about his age also swimming with their parents that he "forgot how to make a new friend" (Giardina, 2021). The kids, to turn a phrase, weren't *really* okay—and no amount of 'safe' recreational activities could paper over that reality.

As the summer turned to Fall and the parks eased their restrictions, we went to the large park near our house, which had soccer fields, tennis courts, ball fields, and a playground. It was moderately populated, but one thing was abundantly clear—all the kids were starving for interaction with people their own size, and my son ran around and generally had a blast. Yet the specter of COVID-19 was never too far off the radar:

Masks.
  Hand Sanitizer.
  Long baths immediately after we returned home.

In other words, things that were difficult to obtain for some but were readily available in our community (and, dare I say, taken for granted aspects of the "hygiene theater" [Magary, 2020, para. 4] we took part in throughout the early days of the pandemic).[3]

The Phase II re-opening wouldn't last for too long, though. As the next wave of infections hit and folks once again receded to extreme caution, we spent almost every afternoon for about a month on the now-largely-empty-again soccer field at the park—just the two of us, taking turns as the goalkeeper—or just goofing around with the ball. It was good father-son bonding time, and he was developing some good ball-handling skills for his age, but he wanted to play on a team—or, perhaps more acutely, he wanted to play sports with kids his own age. But…that really wasn't possible. To compensate, I bought him a couple youth soccer jerseys online so he could at least imagine a different reality. (And, maybe, I could, too).

Fast forward to February of 2021. The local soccer leagues were opening back up, and schools had become fairly consistent in their in-person teaching and safety protocols that we felt he could safely re-enter the school system. Whether it was an empirically-sound decision or just COVID-fatigue, we signed our son up for one of the two local for-profit soccer academies—community-run public leagues having been essentially closed down by private youth sport companies and academies in the county we live in. On the first day of practice, the 5-year-olds ran around in their new branded soccer jerseys and Nike cleats, without a seeming care in the world as they listened to Coach B and Coach C give instructions. The parents, by contrast, kept socially distant and most wore masks even in the warm north Florida sun. He scored his first goal on a 1-on-1 drill, and I was about the happiest person on earth at that moment.

Looking critically and reflexively at the above, however, I'm struck by the relative ease with which our son was able to negotiate the pandemic and, more than that, the relative ease with which my wife and I were. Stable middle-class jobs that allowed us to work from home with relative ease; resources within our community that (eventually) allowed for more

[3] Case in point, a boy he became friends with saw both of his parents—who worked in the food industry—contract COVID-19 and have hospital stays, including his father being on a ventilator for nearly a week before responding to experimental drug therapy.

outdoor leisure activities; being able to forego online school experiences in favor of home-schooling for a year; and so forth. But there's another thing: looking around the soccer sidelines that day of his first practice, we were also struck by the decided lack of diversity on the pitch: Tallahassee, Florida, with a population of roughly 200,000, is 55% white, 35% black, 4% Asian, and 1% Latino. Yet it surprised no one that the make-up of the players that day did not nearly align with those numbers. Nor, looking around the other soccer fields that were filled with older kids, did it align there, either. Soccer, arguably the most international of all sports with supposed easy access to play (i.e., a ball and an open space to play on), had in our home community effectively become a *country club sport* like golf or tennis. A combination of pay-to-play fees and uniform costs,[4] and practice and game times (early afternoons after school, early weekend mornings, etc.), coupled with the aforementioned politics of class privilege, had clearly—and for the foreseeable future—widened the chasm between those who could return to sport and those who couldn't (at least in our community).

Yet this now folds into and cuts across the reflection of my white middle-class privilege, or at least a performance of it, for other than having to a wear a mask at school for a while, our son was largely shielded from the pandemic and experienced it very differently, wrapped in his own biopolitics of privilege.

Ryan

In the Spring of 2020, I was dealing with a personal health issue and, in some ways, well positioned to parent during the COVID shutdowns in terms of 'free' time. I had course releases for the semester, and had already met my annual scholarship goals. Yet, for someone working through a (mental) health condition both the idea and eventual reality of being

[4] The cost for an 8-week 'winter' season was roughly US$150 (which included one practice and one game per week); the adidas adizero soccer kits for games were roughly US$100; an additional weekly training session was US$50. There was also a yearly club fee to participate with the organization, which was roughly US$100. That 5- and 6-year-old kids were wearing adidas adizero tech jerseys (which retail for US$34.99) is a far cry from the community-run youth sport programs of yesteryear where the youth league was sponsored by the local pizza place or autobody shop.

stuck inside with three kids and my wife all day with no end in sight was psychologically daunting. Lost was any semblance of privacy or freedom, replaced with school scheduling, preparation and clean-up of breakfast, lunch, dinner and snack, and after school activities at a time when outdoor physical activities would be closed down by the state of Maryland from March to Early-May. All youth sports were also shuttered. Gone was a season of baseball, softball, and dance sessions. Summer swim team, camps, and soccer were eventually cancelled for the Fall, and for a time we turned to daily neighborhood bike rides as our sole reprieve from the day-to-day monotony of pandemic life—like Bill Murray's *Groundhog Day* but without the dry humor.

Complicating matters, my wife's and my own parents live out of state, and neither of us have close family members who live within an hour of our home (and, even then, they had their own health conditions that prevented visiting anyone outside of our household circle since COVID restrictions hit).[5] The only place we had the privilege of really going to in 2020–2021 and utilizing for "safe" physical activity was the country club that we were able to join at a steep discount as a perk for working at an institution where both the Women's and Men's NCAA teams practice and the former hosts an annual home event.

In Summer 2020, there were strict quotas on who could use the pool ("Member's Only") and for how long (two-, then three-hour time blocks), before the pool deck was disinfected for the next session. For a time, indoor dining was suspended, and the restaurant operated as carryout or poolside only. Still, we spent nearly every single non-rainy day during the Summer of COVID at the pool where the kids met up and swam with about 6 to 10 other kids ALL.SUMMER.LONG. This was all we had, and were fortunate enough to have that (realizing that complaining about access to a pool for a hot summer does not put me in the best of lights).

We tried the tennis courts a few times as a thing to do, but the one physical activity outside of the pool that really got us through this deeply insular period was golf. Years prior to joining the club our son (who at 10 is the oldest), Colin, demonstrated a strong interest in the game as I

[5] We saw her parents for the second time in a year on May 2021 and visited with my parents for the first time in June 2021.

would take him to the local municipal course to play on the putting green for free as we rotated through weekly activities like the zoo, science center, library, and story time at Trader Joe's grocery store in the summer. Having played the sport in some form since he was two-years-old, he has acquired a certain level of skill and interest in the sport and his younger sisters have followed suit.

Linked deeply with class division, particularly golf of the country club variety, this choice is one that I struggle with from a political, ethical, and moral standpoint (e.g., Geaman et al., 2021; see also Ceron-Anaya, 2019). However, my children, wife, and I have grown to love the game in spite of ourselves. The late comedian George Carlin (2001) once called golf 'an arrogant, elitist, racist game which takes up entirely too much room in this country'; and, Brad Millington and Brian Wilson (2019) remind us of the dizzying array of negative environmental impacts a typical golf course produces—both largely accurate arguments. Contextually, however, the pandemic reframed how golf was viewed; that is, it became looked at by many as a safe, outdoor, "lifetime" sport where an individual carrying their clubs can log 6–8 miles walked over 18-holes and could serve as a fill in and/or new passion in physical activity and competition lost at indoor sites of physical activity. Following a *CNN* report, we aren't the only ones to have turned to golf since as equipment sales, viewership (as other major sports have sputtered), rounds played, and, yes, country club memberships have soared in the last year (membership at our particular club increased from 330 to about 450 in 2020 and held in 2021).[6]

[6] Indeed, these participation, sales, use, and viewership numbers are being equated to the late-1990s era of *Tigermania* (Matuszewski, 2021). Something we suspect is in large part the marriage of parents of young children who came of age during that era now repeating that as a "thing to do" in conjunction with the aforementioned reasons others may have. To wit: even with a 7-week closure in 2020, no outside events, or tournaments from March-May, our club surpassed its average annual rounds played prior to Labor Day! Anecdotally, there was increased diversity along racial (though certainly not class) lines a tick, but not substantially, and, to my knowledge, the only publicly LGBTQ members (one of whom was a colleague and is the reason we found out about the discount as well as a male couple who were my golf skill level and frequent match play opponents) left for professional and travel considerations respectively. My current research on golf and COVID did find that mothers who previously only made use of the club for pool usage and dining with their families (re)engaged with sport, at first with their partners (colloquially referred to as "love golf"), then in same-sex groups more competitively (King-White et al., 2022).

This reemergent or exploding interest carried over to competitive youth golf as well: my children had previously played a few summers on the Baltimore City Golf Tour, held across five city-run courses; participation rates were low (four to six kids in each age bracket), and there was no groundswell of public support to expand the program. The city course that all three of our kids learned to play at, Pine Ridge, experienced significant growth in youth participation for skills development and on course play. Oddly, even though it is located in Baltimore County, the course is owned by the city of Baltimore and they had to follow the city's more restrictive COVID rules. This meant that Pine Ridge, as well as the other four city courses, could not host tournament events during 2020. As such, despite the growth in youth participation the city tour was shut down and eventually folded.

In contrast to the public youth golf tour, the for-profit *Under Armour (UA) Junior Tour*, where kids 6 through 18 years of age can play some of the finest public and private courses is the area, capitalized on pandemic conditions; registration for a six-round event series costing $395 per player sold out in 24–48 hours. Much different from the city tournaments that were mainly fun with a little competition sprinkled in (and certainly closer to my socio-political physical cultural worldview), the UA tournaments were populated by some of the best youth golfers in the country—and it showed. Our kids were badly outmatched as they had never received any formal individual lessons outside of camps or group offerings, and their equipment was the bottom-rung brands that we bought simply so they could play—but they got better. So much so that in Fall 2020, Colin and, Spring 2021, our daughter, Meredith, qualified to play in the national championship events at *IMG Academy* and *Disneyworld* in Florida.

This is the part where the needle skips and scratches the vinyl, putting a stop to the fun we were having with the sport. These kids hadn't seen family, just recently began to attend school in person, and we (almost out of sorrow for their lost summer) very seriously considered making the trip to Florida during a pre-vaccine time period. For on the one hand, they lost so much time being kids and having fun, and during this period they became good enough at golf to go represent their region to the rest of the nation. On the other hand, we were so fortunate to have had just the opportunity and access to a sport that many do not, both my wife and I remain gainfully employed, did not have anyone close fall *seriously* ill with COVID-19, and experienced progress in the classroom (whilst others basically lost a year of schooling). Our son, who suffers from extreme food allergies and learning challenges brought about by mixed dyslexia, benefitted from the one-on-one learning time at home, as did our two girls, who developed ahead of grade level in all standardized measurable learning areas. In the end, we decided not to go through with it though our kids did receive serious upgrades to their golf equipment (again at a discount[7]) through the sport's insular hand-me-down economy—we felt it was the least we could do (a sentiment expressed by many parents as they 'rewarded' their children for making it through the pandemic), though such a statement reads (fairly) like rationalizing our way out of having to confront the criticism levied against golf and 'rewards' through consumption in the first place.

Discussion

Nearly a year has passed from when we first conceived of this paper, and, our children are now vaccinated. Prior to and following that our (Ryan) girls (Meredith and Evelyn) resumed a robust outdoor sport schedule with spring golf, softball, summer swimming, Fall (travel) soccer and are scheduled to start dance class, while Colin played local and travel baseball, swam, and golf all year. They all attended outdoor summer camps despite our trepidation about sending them at once exercising privilege, their bodies, and not being entirely safe.

Yet, they did get to experience tears of frustration with a shot hit into a penalty area, the finality of a playoff loss in an evenly matched game,

[7] We got Meredith a used set of Cobra Junior Clubs that retail for $300–500USD brand new for $30USD through Facebook Marketplace the night before Christmas 2020. As she grows this set will be passed down to Evelyn, and eventually donated to the city. Colin is a lefty which makes things more challenging in attempting to find used youth clubs. In the end we purchased Ping Prodi G's that were $1000USD, but get free shaft lengthening as he grows meaning that he essentially gets a new set every few years. These clubs are designed for "tournament" players, and often resell for $300–500USD/set meaning that we are renting the clubs for a few years and then passing them on.

the pain associated with a bloody nose that resulted from a soccer ball to the face that was matched by the elation of game-deciding saves, runs through the opposing defense resulting in magisterial goals, clutch hits, selections to travel teams, a butterfly swim by Meredith that shattered a 31-year-old pool record, and, yes, an invitation back to Florida for Colin to compete in the 2022 national championship for which we will be attending (unless the pandemic decides otherwise).

Our (Michael) son, too, had a successful run in his youth soccer skills development program, so much so that he was invited up to the competitive Jr. Academy level 6U–8U program—pretty good for a five-year-old.[8] He also played loads of pickup basketball in the driveway of friends who live a few houses down, got the feel for tennis, and cheered on Florida State University football and the Los Angeles Kings hockey club. He could look the part and now play the part, which is also quite the loaded socioeconomic statement.

It all seems (new) normal again, or to borrow from David Roth (2021), "what it's supposed be like," but it really is not. Rather it is a conundrum emblematic of being an American parent with privilege, particularly for those of us who have been and remain deeply critical of the organized youth sport system, to so willingly support our children's interests in physical activity. Doing so while COVID-19 numbers spike and fall, family members and friends still fall ill with the disease as some continue to refuse vaccinations and others experience a breakthrough case (e.g., a vaccinated individual contracts COVID-19 or a variant thereof) feels even more irresponsible in a vacuum devoid the social pressures levied on our children to be like other kids and as parents to provide avenues for them to do so. A constant, mind-numbing, reminder that this pandemic and our engagement with the deeply problematic youth sport industry is not over—not by a long shot.

The pandemic was frequently referred to as 'a great equalizer' in that it did not discriminate who it infected. And whilst that may be true epidemiologically, it is not true socio-economically. Low-wage workers realized

[8] The cost of the "Winter Season" came out to about $150 in registration fees (which goes to procuring field time, paying coaches, equipment, and so forth); the cost for uniforms—home and away adidas adizero technology jerseys, shorts, and socks—was an additional $100.

higher pandemic job losses; COVID-19 death rates were higher for Black, Hispanic or Latino, and Indigenous people in the United States relative to White, and Asian people (CDC, 2021). The former are much less able to work from home, per the Bureau of Labor Statistics, and frontline workers were both overwhelmingly women, and women were more likely to be laid off than men during the height of the pandemic. And, as we have seen, global vaccine distribution has been starkly unequal (see Asundi et al., 2021). Compounding these issues research has shown that women have weathered the brunt of care and domestic work (Thornton, 2020), decreased physical and mental health (Sediri et al., 2020), received less support in economic relief (Madgavkar et al., 2020), and an alarming increase in domestic violence (Boserup et al., 2020).

Time and again local, state, and national representatives—as well as businesspeople and fellow citizens—have demonstrated an aversion to caring about the health of one another when life was reduced to getting through the day alive so that Americans, in general (and we include ourselves here) could watch *Tiger King* (Chaiklin & Goode, 2020) or binge seasons of *The Mandalorian* (Favreau, 2020) on Disney+. Caring for children during this period left us wanting for answers, as the general parenting experience is wont to do in relatively 'normal' times. Upon reflection, we ask what would have been considered best practices for raising children in a morally and ethically sound manner during the pandemic? Should we have been marching in the streets with other unvaccinated people for George Floyd and the numerous others who have been unfairly treated and/or murdered by the hypermilitarized police? Should we have taken some of our time set aside for the pool, fishing, soccer, and golf in a family unit to volunteer our services as unvaccinated people to unvaccinated others in desperate need of food, clothing, and shelter? Should we have never left our houses under any circumstances? None of the answers to these questions and numerous others really sit well with us, and yet they would likely yield disparate responses within our own critical physical cultural studies community without venturing across the aisle as it were to those with a more "get back to normal" socio-political outlook (see: the academic reaction to David Roth's contemplative *Defector* article "This is what it's supposed to be like" [2021] cited earlier).

Yet, handling things as parents the best we could does not feel entirely right either. And even dialoguing about them invokes a particular privilege—the privilege to be self-reflexive. Perhaps it is at this juncture that we must simply admit that the privilege to make these choices is in and of itself part of the disquiet that made simply getting through the pandemic even more difficult. There were no right choices other than the ones that ended with us coming out the other side with our children and family alive. What an awful place that was and is to be.

Coda

The previous two vignettes demonstrate some of the more "mundane practices of privilege" (see Silva, 2021) we encountered and performed—though dare we say they are instructive aspects for how inequality to basic physical culture came to be experienced during the height of the COVID-19 pandemic as well. One could argue that our experiences outlined above could be dismissed as the introspective musings of two 40-something semi-liberal white guys rationalizing their behaviors in the face of the pandemic. But at the same time, unmasking how power operated (and continues to operate) in the very uneven pandemic context—even in a youth sport context—is especially revelatory for it helps to understand the very uneven distribution of privilege in the United States. As noted by Jon Solomon of the U.S.-based think-tank Aspen Institute's Sport & Society Program, "Families have fewer options to play youth sports. Increasingly, kids and families are returning to sports, but some of them who are coming back or want to come back, are returning to diminished services" (quoted in Anzidel, 2021, para. 5). According to a study by the Aspen Institute titled *State of Play*, 44% of families said their community-based program either closed, merged, or returned with limited capacity; it is these community-based programs who generally service low-income populations. As Solomon chronicled, the pandemic "increased the haves versus the have nots and, really, the divide [of[who plays and who doesn't. Wealthier parents and kids have returned faster. They've been able to, and some of them continued to play, because the have the infrastructure" (quoted in Anzidel, 2021, para. 8). Importantly, a study investigative journalists associate with Marquette University that was published in the Milwaukee Journal-Sentinel in late-2020 conversely found that while community-based sports leagues shut down, private/for-profit youth leagues "the largely unregulated $19 billion youth sport industry...powered ahead" (Bannon, 2020, para. 6).

Moreover, in terms of K-12 education, scores of academic and popular press articles have highlighted how low-income students have been further disadvantaged due to a lack of stable (and fast) Internet connections, availability of devices to utilize Zoom or Microsoft Teams applications, and diminished if not eliminated opportunities for personalized attention or homework assistance (see, e.g., Tappe, 2021). The U.S. Department of Education's Office of Civil Rights also provided findings in a report titled *Education in a pandemic: The disparate impacts of COVID-19 on America's students* (2021) that listed eleven items across K-12 and postsecondary levels such as the widening of pre-existing disparities, deepening disparities in access and opportunity for students of color in public schools, a rise in new barriers of entry to postsecondary education for low-income and students of color, and unequal socio-economic disparities in terms of mental health challenges.

We likely did capitalize on Bunds's (2014) concept of the biopolitics of privilege—the socially conditioned advantages of whiteness, social class, sexual, and gender orientations—because there is no doubt that this is infused throughout the vignettes we presented—burned into the consequence of our actions. And although small in scale, our experiences with the American privatized youth sport system demonstrates the ways we—and many of our colleagues, we are sure—have uneasily, yet all-too-willingly, navigated this program of structural inequality in a style that would belie our global beliefs in order to benefit our children.

Upon reflection, we have come to the uneasy conclusion that there is not martyrdom in denying these privileges to our families by turning away from them; rather, there is a need to lean into it so much so that we work to make these privileges available to more people. This could be through fundraising or reducing costs to participate, but that seems to be only part of the issue. In some of my (Ryan) more recent research I have found that economic support for access to youth sport of most types exists ("growing the game" through youth participation is a consistent goal for many sport organizations like *First Tee*, *Baltimore Youth Hockey Club*, *Baltimore Youth Lacrosse Foundation*, *Baltimore Metropolitan Urban Tennis Organization* and *Baltimore Field Hockey Association*), but broader issues such as information this support is available, transportation, time, as well as a lack of familial and social circle encouragement plagues these efforts. Indeed, Colin often laments that his school friends do not care about his golf successes, and only his golf friends do. It also does not absolve us from utilizing a system that has been set up to our benefit, be it through white privilege or otherwise. To wit, this chapter is part of a larger project that looks at the intersection of familial privilege, health care, education, physical activity, and parenting in the contemporary moment. Moving forward, we aim to critically evaluate more aspects of the typical American life via our relationships with child care and rearing, education, and physical activity to further explicate and lay bare the stark disparities that have emerged from a neoliberal system—just as we come to terms with the fact that we have utilized it to our benefit. What we don't seek to do is invoke a politics that are contained within and limited solely to visibility, to the slogan, to the easy critique. Rather, as Sarah Banet-Weiser (2018) might say, the substantive politics contained within a critique of neoliberalism are too often short-circuited in favor the slogan or the publicly expressed political position, which has the correlative effect of anchoring neoliberalism and the challenges to it in a never-ending cycle; political action collapsed into personal identification. Grant Farred (2008) once wrote in a different context, "Absolute or careless fan, you always owe someone"; it's high time to own up to it.

References

Anzidel, M. (2021, February 8). COVID hit low-cost youth sports. So wealthier kids are reutnring to play at higher rates. *NorthJersey.com*. https://www.northjersey.com/story/sports/2021/11/08/covid-hit-low-cost-youth-sports-reducing-lower-income-kids-access/8549349002/

Asundi, A., O'Leary, C., & Bhadelia, N. (2021). Global COVID-19 vaccine inequity: The Scope, the impact, and the challenges. *Cell Host & Microbe, 29*(7), 1036–1039.

Banet-Weiser, S. (2018). *Empowered: Popular feminism and popular misogyny*. Duke University Press.

Bannon, T. (2020). 'I just want to play': $19 billion youth sports industry powers ahead through the pandemic largely unregulated. *Milwaukee Journal-Sentinel*. https://www.jsonline.com/in-depth/news/2020/09/11/youth-sports-industry-powers-through-pandemic-unregulated-covid-19-wisconsin-illinois-indiana/5764743002/

Benefield, L., Clifford, J., Cox, S., & Hagenow, N. (2000). Nursing leaders predict top trends for 2000. *Nursing Management, 31*(1), 21–23.

Bernstein, H., Gonzalez, D., & Karpman, M. (2021). Adults in low-income immigrant families were deeply affected by the COVID-19 crisis yet avoided safety net programs in 2020. *Urban Institute*, 1–22. Retrieved January 6, 2022, from https://www.urban.org/sites/default/files/publication/104280/adults-in-low-income-immigrant-families-deeply-affected-by-pandemic-yet-avoided-safety-net_0.pdf

Bibbins-Domingo, K. (2020). This Time must be different: Disparities during the COVID-19 pandemic. *Annals of Internal Medicine*. Retrieved January 6, 2022, from https://www.acpjournals.org/doi/full/10.7326/M20-2247

Boserup, B., McKenney, M., & Elkbuli, A. (2020). Alarming trends in US domestic violence during the COVID-19 pandemic. *The American Journal of Emergency Medicine, 38*(12), 2753–2755.

Brown, S., Doom, J., Lechuga-Pena, W., & Koppels, T. (2020). Stress and parenting during the global COVID-19 pandemic. *Child Abuse & Neglect, 110*, 1–14.

Bunds, K. (2014). The Biopolitics of privilege: Negotiating class, masculinity and relationships. *Cultural Studies↔Critical Methodologies, 14*(5), 517–525.

Bunds, K. (2021). "Please let it stop": Fear, anxiety, and uncertainty on the neoliberal tenure track. *Qualitative Inquiry, 27*(8–9), 1040–1047.

Carlin, G. (2001). *Napalm and silly putty*. Highbridge audiobooks.

Ceron-Anaya, H. (2019). *Privilege at play: Race, class, gender, and golf in Mexico*. Oxford University Press.

Chaiklin, R., & Goode, E. (2020). Tiger King [TV Series]. Universal Content Productions.

Collins, C., Landivar, L., Ruppanner, L., & Scarborough, W. (2021). COVID-19 and the gender gap in work hours. *Gender, Work & Organization, 28*(S1), 101–112.

Davidson, J., Bondi, L., & Smith, M. (Eds.). (2005). *Emotional geographies*. Routledge.

Denison, J. (2016). Social theory and narrative research: A Point of view. *Sport Education & Society, 21*(1), 7–10.

Drummond, M., Elliott, S., Drummond, C., & Prichard, I. (2020). Youth sport and COVID-19: A Potential generation lost. *Emerald Open Research, 2*(27), 1–10.

Dunton, G., Do, B., & Wang, S. (2020). Early effects of the COVID-19 pandemic on physical activity and sedentary behavior in children living in the U.S. *BMC Public Health, 20*, 1351–1364.

Fang, Y., Lijun, Z., Jiang, Y., & Wu, B. (2021). The Immediate and subsequent effects of public health interventions for COVID-19 on the leisure and recreation industry. *Tourism Management, 87*, 1–8.

Farred, G. (2008). Careless whispers: The doubleness of Spanish love. *Cultural Studies↔Critical Methodolgoies, 8*(4), 453–476.

Fredricks, J., & Eccles, J. (2004). Parental influences on youth involvement in sports. In M. R. Weiss (Ed.), *Developmental sport and exercise psychology: A lifespan perspective* (pp. 145–164). Fitness Information Techonology.

Gassman-Pines, A., Ananat, E., & Fitz-Henley, J., II. (2020). COVID-19 and parent-child psychological well-being. *Pediatrics, 146*(4), 1–9.

Gawande, A. (2009). The Cost conundrum: What a Texas town can teach us about health care. *The New Yorker*. Retrieved October 19, 2021, from https://cchs.ua.edu/wp-content/blogs.dir/24/files/2014/06/The-New-Yorker-2009-Gawande.pdf

Geaman, B., King-White, R., & Hawzen, M. (2021). The Counted outs: COVID-19, golf and disparities in public health. In *Bridges to Baccalaureate Conference*, July 21, 2021.

Giardina, M. (2005). *Sporting pedagogies: Performing culture & identity in the global arena*. Peter Lang Publishing.

Giardina, M. (2021). "Daddy, help me; I forgot how to make a new friend": Emotional geographies of youth sport in pandemic times. *Cultural Studies↔Critical Methodologies, 21*(5), 365–371.

Giardina, M., & Donnelly, M. (2007). *Youth culture and sport: Identity, power, and politics*. Routledge.

Gregory, S. (2017). How kids' sports became a $15 billion industry. *Time*. https://time.com/4913687/how-kids-sports-became-15-billion-industry/

Grossberg, L. (2010). *Cultural studies in the future tense*. Duke University Press.

Gundersen, C., Hake, M., Dewey, A., & Engelhard, E. (2021). Food insecurity during COVID-19. *Applied Economic Perspectives and Policy, 43*(1), 153–161.

Favreau, J. (Producer) (2020). *The Mandalorian.* [Television Series]. Lucas Film: Disney+.

Hagerman, M. (2018). *White kids: Growing up with privilege in a racially divided America.* New York University Press.

Herzlinger, R. (2006). Why innovation in health care is so hard. *Harvard Business review.* Retrieved October 19, 2021 from https://hbr.org/2006/05/why-innovation-in-health-care-is-so-hard

Kerr, M., Rasmussen, H., Fanning, K., & Braaten, S. (2021). Parenting during COVID-19. A Study of parents' experiences across gender and income levels. *Families Amidst Covid-19 Responses, 70*(5), 1327–1342.

King-White, R., Hawzen, M. & Geaman, B. (2022). 3 in a Hole: Golf, COVID, and Access to "Safe" Outdoor Physical Activity. *North American Society for the Sociology of Sport.* Las Vegas, NV.

Madgavkar, A., White, O., Krishnan, M., Mahajan, D., & Azcue, X. (2020). COVID-19 and gender equality: Countering the regressive effects. *McKinsey Global Institute.* Retrieved January 6, 2022, from https://www.mckinsey.com/featured-insights/future-of-work/covid-19-and-gender-equality-countering-the-regressive-effects

Magary, D. (2020). The National pastime is a national disgrace. *GEN.* Retrieved October 19, 2021, from https://gen.medium.com/the-national-pastime-is-a-national-disgrace-cbf01304df1f

Markula, P., & Denison, J. (2005). Sport and the personal narrative. In D. Andrews, D. Mason, & M. Silk (Eds.), *Qualitative methods in sport studies* (pp. 165–184). Berg.

Matuszewski, E. (2021). 6 of golf's top youth programs. *Links Magazine.* Retrieved October 19, 2021, from https://www.linksmagazine.com/6-of-golfs-top-youth-programs/

Mcavoy, E. (2020). Youth sports return with coronavirus distancing restrictions. *AP News.* Retrieved October 19, 2021, from https://apnews.com/article/fl-state-wire-tallahassee-virus-outbreak-health-baseball-0eb2b2610f95aced7a1638103c55bc62

Millington, B., & Wilson, B. (2019). *The greening of golf: Sport, globalization and the environment.* Manchester University Press.

Mintzberg, H. (1993). The Illusive strategy...25 years later. In A. Bedeian (Ed.), *Management Laureates: A Collection of autobiographical essays* (pp. 1–40). JAI Press.

Newman, J., & Giardina, M. (2011). *Sport, spectacle, and NASCAR nation: Consumption and the cultural politics of neoliberalism.* Palgrave Macmillan.

Oppel, R., Gebeloff, R., Lai, K.K., Wright, W., & Smith, M. (2020). The Fullest look yet at the racial inequity of coronavirus. *The New York Times*. Retrieved February 22, 2021, from https://www.nytimes.com/interactive/2020/07/05/us/coronavirus-latinos-african-americans-cdc-data.html

Porter, M., & Teisberg, E. (2006). *Redefining health care: Creating value-based competition on results*. Harvard Business School Press.

Pringle, R. (2001). Competing discourses: Narratives of a fragmented self, manliness and rugby union. *International Review for the Sociology of Sport, 36*(4), 425–439.

Roth, D. (2021). This is what it's supposed to be like. *Defector*. Retrieved November 12, 2021 from https://defector.com/this-is-what-its-supposed-to-be-like/

Silva, K. (2021). COVID-19 and the mundane practices of privilege. *Cultural Studies, 35*(2–3), 238–247.

Stewart, M. (2018). The 9.9 percent is the new American aristocracy. *The Atlantic*. Retrieved November 18, 2022 from https://www.theatlantic.com/magazine/archive/2018/06/the-birth-of-a-new-american-aristocracy/559130/

Sediri, S., Zgueb, Y., Ouanes, S., Ouali, U., Bourgou, S., Jomli, R., & Nacef, F. (2020). Women's mental health: Acute impact of COVID-19 pandemic on domestic violence. *Archives of Women's Mental Health, 23*, 749–756.

Spain, S. (2020, March 11). *That's What She Said Podcast*. Retrieved October 18, 2021 from http://www.espn.com/espnradio/podcast/archive/_/id/14603142

Sparkes, A. (1996). The Fatal flaw: A Narrative of the fragile body-self. *Qualitative Inquiry, 2*(4), 463–494.

Tamas, S., Georgaras, K., & Dabboussy, M. (2021). The Emotional geographies of academic writing: Writing as a method of survival. In N. K. Denzin & M. D. Giardina (Eds.), *Collaborative futures in qualitative inquiry: Research in a pandemic* (pp. 56–69). Routledge.

Tappe, A. (2021, June 29). The pandemic is making a vicious cycle even worse for low-income students. *CNN*. https://www.cnn.com/2021/06/29/economy/pandemic-inequality-children-education/index.html

Thomas, M., & Rogers, C. (2020). Education, the science of learning, and the COVID-19 crisis. *Prospects, 49*, 87–90.

Thornton, A. (2020). COVID-19: How Women are bearing the burden of unpaid work. *World Economic Forum*. Retrieved January 6, 2022, from https://www.weforum.org/agenda/2020/12/covid-women-workload-domestic-caring/

Vogenberg, F. R., & Santilli, J. (2018). Healthcare trends for 2018. *American Health & Drug Benefits, 11*(1), 48–54.

Walker, C. (2020). Trump's "lethal screwup" on COVID-19 led to 130,000 avoidable deaths. *Truthout*. Retrieved February 22, 2021 from https://truthout.org/articles/trumps-lethal-screwup-on-COVID-19-led-to-130000-avoidable-deaths-study-says/

WTXL. (2020). We're open, Tallahassee: Gym force gymnastics used shutdown to increase COVID-19 safety. *WTXL Tallahassee*. Retrieved October 19, 2021, from https://www.wtxl.com/open/were-open-tallahassee-gym-force-gymnastics-used-shutdown-to-increase-covid-19-safety

Zamarro, G. (2020). COVID-19: For Women it's one step forward, 30 steps back. *Ursuline College Institute for Women, Wellness & Work*. Retrieved January 6, 2022, from https://womenwellnesswork.ursuline.edu/covid-19-for-women-its-one-step-forward-30-steps-back/

19

Te Mana Whakahaere: COVID-19 And Resetting Sport in Aotearoa New Zealand

Jeremy Hapeta, Farah Palmer, Rochelle Stewart-Withers, and Haydn Morgan

Introduction

Globally, COVID-19 has impacted sports participation from the highest echelons (e.g. the Tokyo 2020 Olympics and Paralympics; the 36th America's Cup Regatta; the ICC Women's Cricket World Cup, the Women's Rugby World Cup 2021) right down to the 'grassroots' community-level. As an example, large parts of the local Play, Active Recreation and Sport (PARS) sector in Aotearoa New Zealand (NZ) were significantly impacted by COVID-19. On 25 March 2020, for instance, the NZ Government imposed a nationwide lockdown which meant that no public gatherings could take place, including participation in or

J. Hapeta (✉)
University of Otago, Dunedin, New Zealand

F. Palmer • R. Stewart-Withers
Massey University, Palmerston North, New Zealand

H. Morgan
University of Bath, Bath, UK

D. L. Andrews et al. (eds.), *Sport and Physical Culture in Global Pandemic Times*, Global Culture and Sport Series, https://doi.org/10.1007/978-3-031-14387-8_19

attendance at any sport matches and other active recreation events. From early March 2020, organised community-level PARS activities were progressively suspended, including the remaining summer sport season competitions and pre-season for winter sports codes (Sport New Zealand, June, 2020a).

On 11 May 2020, the NZ government's sport agency, Sport New Zealand—Ihi Aotearoa (hereafter 'Sport NZ'), announced an immediate $25m relief package to help support the wider PARS sector remain viable throughout the global pandemic. This initial 'relief' package included the Community Resilience Fund Phase One, Exceptional Systems Support Fund, and the Partner Support Fund. Later, the NZ Government announced an additional $264.6m investment into the sport and active recreation sector to encourage sporting organisations to respond to the disruptions caused by the COVID-19 pandemic. This became known as the 'Sport NZ Recovery Package' which aimed to support the PARS sector to respond to disruptions caused by the global pandemic and the challenges faced locally due to the associated lock down measures.

Primarily, the emphasis was to 'reset' and 'rebuild' community-level PARS organisations, but it also included funding for elite-level, Olympic and Paralympic sports. Sport NZ developed a funding framework to support the distribution of the $265m Recovery Package, over a four-year period, with these three key outcomes in mind, to:

- **Reset and Rebuild**: Short-term support to help sport and active recreation organisations at all levels get through the initial impact of COVID-19. ($82.6 million).
- **Strengthen and Adapt**: Support to help the sector rebuild in the medium term and make changes to operate successfully in the post-pandemic environment (e.g., new operating models and more collaboration). ($104 million).
- **Different and Better investment outcome**: Innovative approaches to delivering PARS into the future. ($78 million).

As noted above, the (short-term) aim to 're-set' and 're-build' the PARS system signalled a (mid-term) desire to 'strengthen and adapt' it in order to do things 'different and better' (long-term) into the future. In its role as kaitiaki (guardians) Sport NZ (2020a, June) is tasked with leading this work, not only to respond to immediate sector needs, but also drive transformation for the betterment of generations to come. Implicit in these outcomes is acknowledgment that, previously, Sport NZ (September, 2020c) was not necessarily delivering desired results in these areas. Indeed, within the 're-set' there appears to be an attempt to reconcile with their community-level partners, especially Māori (Indigenous) groups.

More explicitly, sitting underneath Sport NZ's overarching 'Recovery Package' lies their 'Kaupapa Māori Response Plan' (KMRP). According to Miskimmin (2020), the Chief Executive at that time, this represented Sport NZ's Māori-specific response to the COVID-19 pandemic and its subsequent impacts on Māori whānau (families), hapū (sub-tribes) and iwi (tribes). The KMRP is incorporated into recent Sport NZ policies such as 'Te Aho a Ihi Aotearoa' their Māori Activation Plan (MAP) and 'Te Pake o Ihi Aotearoa' their Māori Outcomes Framework (MOF). These Sport NZ (2022a, 2022b) strategies signalled their intent to engage with whānau, hapū, iwi, and Māori with the aim to deliver on its commitment towards different and better future outcomes.

As a government agency, Sport NZ's five leadership responsibilities include: Direction setting; Insights; Advocacy; Collaboration and Investments (Sport NZ, July, 2020b). In terms of this current chapter, we are interested in exploring these last three leadership responsibilities specifically, in an attempt to provide some insights back to the organisation to help them 'map out' equitable pathways for future direction setting. Thus, the focus of this chapter is to offer a critically informed, Kaupapa Māori, analysis of the past, present and future relationships between Māori National Sporting Organisations (NSOs) and Sport NZ. Therefore, we consider the perspectives, experiences and lived realities of Māori NSOs, past and present, alongside current policies (KMRP, MAP, MOF) and practices (i.e., PARS interventions) especially those targeted at vulnerable communities and/or highly deprived groups vis-a-vis the Government's responses to address social inequities and to re-engage these groups in PARS post-COVID-19.

Employing a critical, Kaupapa Māori prism and principled analytical approach, this chapter applies the whakatauki[1], '*ka mua, ka muri*', to explore the idea that in order to know the direction in which you are heading, you must know where you have been. Key to these understandings are past ***relationships,*** present ***resources***, and future ***resiliencies*** required, which will ultimately enable a 're-set' for PARS in the context of Sport NZ's 're-set and re-build' via the $265 million Covid-19 response package. Finally, we conclude this chapter by offering insights and commentary on the future opportunities and directions ahead for NZ's PARS organisations to realising their responsibilities sector-wide.

Background Context

The title of this chapter (Te Mana Whakahaere) is the idea of 'being able to go in, or determine, your own direction' (Durie, 1999). More recently, respected Māori scholar, Professor Sir Mason Durie, suggested that leadership means being able to identify what people are searching for and working with them to achieve that goal. It is not about one person "standing out and saying, 'this is the way we should go' but, it might be about one person being able to say, 'I've listened to everybody this is the way we want to go, now let's plot a path' to get there" (Durie, 2017). Historically, in the Aotearoa NZ context, notions of self-determination and autonomy (Te Mana Whakahaere) for Māori were aligned with principles of partnership, participation, and protection (McLeod et al., 2011) enshrined within Te Tiriti o Waitangi (The Treaty of Waitangi).[2] After signing the Treaty, however, successive NZ governments repeatedly failed to uphold their promises and as a result of enduring Māori activism, especially during the 1970s, the Waitangi Tribunal was eventually established in 1975. The Waitangi Tribunal is a permanent commission of

[1] Whakatauki are proverbs which draw on symbolism and metaphor to convey key messages. Moreover, they seek to convey the wisdom, wit, values and common-sense of tangata whenua (people of the land).

[2] On 6 February 1840, over 500 Māori chiefs signed Te Tiriti o Waitangi (the Treaty of Waitangi), which is Aotearoa New Zealand's founding document, on behalf of their people and representatives of Queen Victoria's British Crown (McLeod et al., 2011).

inquiry that makes recommendations to government on claims brought by Māori relating to Crown actions which breached Treaty promises (Waitangi Tribunal, n.d.). Despite the rhetoric, also witnessed in other settler colonial settings, that seek to reconcile and (re)build relationships, tensions remain in relation to Māori and their relationship with the state (Moewaka Barnes & McCreanor, 2019).

Over a decade ago, in 2011, as one of five 'champion agencies' within government, Sport NZ signed the "Kia Tūtahi Relationship Accord" and committed to engage more effectively with communities to achieve social, economic, environmental and cultural outcomes. Considered a paradigm shift for the sector, Sport NZ moved away from supporting the participation *of* Māori in sport to participating and leading "as Māori" in PARS. At that time, it was viewed as a deliberate intent by Sport NZ among other agencies, to be responsive to Māori needs. However, after the organisation's internal cultural capabilities were lost, Māori responsiveness rapidly eroded, as it no longer had champions to lead the work. The decline in Māori capabilities within this 'champion agency' had impacts upon the wider workforce, whereby staff felt ill equipped and unsure when engaging in Māori settings. This loss of cultural capability and capacity had additional effects, reducing the positive workforce experiences of those who had embraced elements of Māori culture that permeated the entire PARS sector (KTV Consulting, 2017).

As part of the $265m 'recovery package' Sport NZ (2020a, June) announced a new $7million investment over four years (2021-2024) targeted at improving wellbeing outcomes for Māori. This saw them invest in new organisations who contribute towards Māori physical activity outcomes as an acknowledgement and recognition of the adverse effect that COVID-19 has had on Māori wellbeing and physical activity levels. The newly released 'MAP' and 'MOF' policies take a unique Te Ao Māori (worldview) approach that focuses on culturally distinctive pathways to enable Māori to succeed *as Māori* through PARS activities. The investment into establishing new organisations is to contribute towards wellbeing outcomes that are *for, by and with* Māori. At that time the (former) Sport NZ Chief Executive (CE) said:

> This is an important and significant milestone. This is the first time Sport NZ will… engage whānau, hapū, iwi, Māori and build meaningful relationships in these communities…every week, 31% of Māori do not participate in [PARS] activities…We are seeking to enable and empower Māori communities to improve physical activity levels through Te Ao Māori and Mātauranga Māori approaches, and we believe this will make a significant difference…Sport NZ is on a journey to honour our commitment to Te Tiriti and are working hard to live up to our commitment to a bi-cultural future…We are excited to be taking the first step on this journey through these Kaupapa Māori initiatives that enable Māori to participate as Māori (Miskimmin, 2020).

Thus, the KMRP prioritises four initiatives that seek to engage whānau, hapū, iwi and Māori to improve their wellbeing through increased physical activity *as* Māori:

- **Māori National Sport Organisations**—enabling the network to continue their valued contribution to our sector. The intention of the fund is to support the re-engagement of their respective memberships, remove some of the barriers to participation, enable their unique way of being, *as* Māori, survive the current social and economic conditions and acknowledge their contribution to the PARS, some for over 100 years. ($0.35 million).
- **He Oranga Poutama Programme**—supporting Māori wellbeing by improving participation and increasing leadership through physical activity. Increased funding will enable a nationwide approach and focus on Māori communities that need it the most. ($4.45 million).
- **Marae Fit Aotearoa**—this is a new Marae-centric digital tool designed to increase Māori participation and create more opportunities for whānau to connect with their marae and community through physical activity. ($1.1 million).
- **Te Ihi Fund**—an activation fund to increase Māori participation by supporting existing culturally distinctive organisations and channels. ($1.1 million) (Sport NZ, June, 2020a).

Traditionally, Sport NZ has partnered with NSOs across the various codes who either enjoy, or otherwise, a relationship with their Māori NSO counterparts. This chapter shines light on the first initiative above, specifically Māori NSOs and their perceptions of any such relationships or partnerships with Sport NZ. Only recently has Sport NZ (Miskimmin, 2020) acknowledged the valuable contribution that Māori NSOs have made to the sector and to wider Aotearoa NZ society. Thus, Sport NZ has committed to a system re-set and rebuild, to strengthen and adapt the sector, to do things differently and better, realising a bi-cultural future that gives effect to Te Tiriti o Waitangi. Their view is that the dedicated Māori NSO funding ($350,000) is a starting point towards building stronger partnerships and relationships with that network. According to Sport NZ the intention of these funds is to "support the re-engagement of their [Māori NSO] membership, to remove some of the barriers to participation, enable their unique way of being to survive these trying times and go some way to acknowledging their insurmountable contribution to the sport and recreation sector for over 100 years" (2020, p.28). Herein we ask the question: what do Māori NSOs think about this new approach? Especially given the admission of their (former) CEO that they are only just setting out on this journey.

Kaupapa Māori Methodology

Generally described as research *by* Māori (although not exclusively) *with* Māori and *for* Māori, Kaupapa Māori research is an Indigenous and decolonising research methodology (Smith, 1999), founded upon a Kaupapa Māori theoretical perspective, which we employed in conceptualising this chapter. Kaupapa Māori Theory (KMT) refers to knowledge that was, is and always will be critical to the development of Māori epistemological and ontological constructions (Lee, 2009; Pihama et al., 2014). It infuses Māori-centred philosophies, theoretical frameworks and research practices, underpinned by the principle of 'tino rangatiratanga' (self-determination) (Hapeta, Palmer, et al., 2019a; Hapeta & Smith, 2021; Lee, 2009; G. H. Smith, 2000). Kaupapa Māori research is, therefore, typically critical of Pākehā (non-Māori) systems of knowledge creation and dissemination (G. H. Smith, 2000). Aligned with the notions of *by*, *with* and *for*, this chapter is authored *by* Māori researchers alongside a non-Indigenous accomplice (Whitinui, 2021) who worked *with* pūkenga Māori (Māori experts, knowledge holders) to critique past practices, present policies and future directions in order to reaffirm the mana of Māori (*for* Māori) to determine their priorities and define their desired outcomes.

Participant's Pūrākau: Māori National Sporting Organisations' Stories

Pūrākau are Māori narratives, involving a storytelling process of passing on mātauranga (knowledge) through key messages or 'lessons' embedded within stories. An ancient and valid pedagogical process, they should be understood as an anthology of knowledge still relevant today (Lee, 2009; Pihama et al., 2014). As a research strategy, employing pūrākau is a similar approach to narrative inquiry (Lee, 2009) insofar as honouring oral traditions and highlighting the core messages contained within these Indigenous forms of expression. A benefit of adopting a pūrākau (storytelling, narrative) approach, from an Indigenous research perspective, is that there is fluid use of the temporal tenses of past, present and future—*ka mua, ka muri*—walking backwards into the future.

The following results section of this chapter presents pūrākau from the perspectives of pūkenga (experts; Māori knowledge holders) in relation to their respective Māori NSO's past or present engagements with their 'partner' NSO counterparts, who receive funding directly from Sport NZ. Importantly, these key knowledge holders were either previously or are currently involved in governance or leadership positions within their respective Māori NSOs. The list of Māori NSOs, previously not acknowledged or directly funded by Sport NZ, were invited to participate in this research, including Aotearoa Māori Netball; Māori Tag Football; Māori Basketball; Māori Football; NZ Māori Rugby; Māori Rugby League; Māori Touch; Māori Golf; and Māori Hockey. Overall, seven pūkenga (pseudonyms Ataahua, Tumanako, Maia, Aroha, Manaaki, Awhina and

Waka) representing seven of these Māori NSOs accepted our invitation to participate in this study, which was evaluated by peer review and judged to be 'low risk'. Consequently, it was not fully reviewed by the University's Human Ethics Committees. However, in line with Kaupapa Māori axiology and ways of conducting culturally responsive and ethical research, we were informed by the cultural values as articulated by acclaimed Māori scholar, Professor Linda Tuhiwai Smith (1999, 2006).

Data Collection: Past Practices, Present Policies, Future Resiliencies

Typically, the kōrerorero (interviews) with Māori NSO representatives either opened with karakia (prayer) and/or whakawhanaungatanga (establishing a rapport) and lasted between one to one and a half hours. The semi-structured interview schedule included open-ended questions in relation to: (**a**) the reason why their Māori NSO exists and their role within it; (**b**) their main activities and how these events/practices reflect Indigenous (Māori) aspirations and outcomes; (**c**) historical and/or present issues in terms of their relationship (if any) with Sport NZ via their NSO and (**d**) the barriers that their Māori NSO faced and continues to face vis-a-vis the level of support received from Sport NZ or their 'parent' NSO. Once transcribed, their experiences and stories (pūrākau) were analysed employing an Indigenous approach to conducting thematic analysis (see Hapeta, Palmer, Kuroda & Hermansson, 2019a) and they are presented in the next section as authentically as possible (Stride et al., 2017) in terms of representing their collective views.

Data Analysis: A Principled Kaupapa Māori Prism

E hara taku toa i te toa takitahi, engari, he toa takitini (my strength is not mine alone, but that of many). Analytically, from a thematic stance, this whakataukī (proverb) can be interpreted to mean that there is 'strength in numbers' or that a single voice can still represent a multitude of perspectives. Briefly, while there are several key Kaupapa Māori principles, our Indigenous informed thematic analysis (see Hapeta, Palmer, et al., 2019a) applies this notion of the 'collective voice' by relating singular (i.e., an individual's) ideas with the thoughts of others that are considered closely related. The following section, therefore, presents quotes from individual participants, although these are representative of the collective views of the majority of participants in the Māori NSO group. Thus, this section is focused on the following three Kaupapa Māori principles combined, to collectively illuminate the focus areas of building relationships, distributing resources equitably, and pathways towards strengthening resiliency:

Ata—The Principle of Growing Respectful Relationships

Developed by Pohatu (2005) primarily the principle of āta is a transformative approach within the area of social services. It relates specifically to building and nurturing relationships. It acts as a guide to the understanding of relationships and wellbeing when engaging with Māori.

Whānau—The Principle of Extended Family Structure

The principle of Whānau acknowledges the relationships that Māori have to one another and the world around them. Whānau (akin to family) and the whakawhanaungatanga (process of creating and sustaining relationships) process are key elements of Māori society and culture. This principle also acknowledges the responsibility and obligations of the researcher to nurture and care for these relationships and also the intrinsic connection between the researcher, the researched and the research as kaupapa whānau (family with a purpose).

Kia piki ake i ngā raruraru o te kainga—The Principle of Socio-Economic Mediation

This principle asserts the need to mediate and assist in the alleviation of negative pressures and disadvantages experienced by Māori communities asserting a need for Kaupapa Māori research to be of positive benefit to Māori communities. It also acknowledges the relevance and success that Māori derived initiatives have as interventions for addressing inequity.

Results and findings

In terms of the results this section aligns findings them with the idea of 'ka mua, ka muri' walking backwards into the future. Briefly, Table 19.1 below outlines 12 key ideas that emerged within the interview dialogue, which are further explained according to the past, present and future.

Past relationships—Ata—and Growing Respectful Relationships with Māori NSOs

Despite receiving no direct funding or support, Māori NSOs have existed for many years, ranging from 20 to 100 years. Essentially, they are considered an anomaly within the sector, despite having existed—in the case of Aotearoa Māori Tennis—for over 100 years. "*If you went around and did a survey at all the Māori tournaments and asked them 'why did you come here' the answer will be because we get to see our relations and it is just awesome being together, that whanaungatanga, the mana of who we are as [Māori] people*" (Maia).

As a result of not being recognised, Māori NSOs have reignited discussions to develop a National Māori sport body and progress a collective, coordinated approach to seek support so that Māori NSOs can play a role of greater importance in terms of increasing participation and engaging as Māori in PARS activities. While Sport NZ could claim that NSOs are supposed to distribute resources on to them, it appears there were

Table 19.1 Summary of Results

The past	The present	The future
Māori NSOs had non-existent to poor **relationships** with the Crown / Sport NZ / NSOs.	Multiple hats: Māori NSO members are all volunteers, undertaking multiple roles.	Māori NSOs hope to rebuild **relationships** with partners and build both internal and external capabilities.
Māori NSOs expressed mamae (pain) as in the past promises to them had been broken by NSOs.	Layers of governance and suitable frameworks to guide practical applications need to be developed to reflect an Indigenous approach. A lack of females on boards.	An overarching National Māori Sport Organisation would help in realising Sport for Development outcomes and building collective relationships with each other and across the sector.
Māori NSOs distrust NSOs and the Crown due to, little funding, lack of personnel, false financial reporting from NSOs to provide Sport NZ funding and **resources** to Māori NSOs.	Align with reference to the setting of strategic plans, KPIs, shared services and tools rather than being siloed in their own (individual Māori NSO) and work.	Te toa takitini—the power of a unified authority- an overarching National Māori Sport Organisation is argued to be an important enabler and **resource** for Māori NSOs.
Behaviours felt transactional. That is Māori NSOs reported only being consulted when it suited NSOs with a lack of understanding of tikanga (protocols) or basic respect. Changes in NSO leadership resulted in starting over to build relationships with new CEs.	Well-being is intrinsically positioned as a strategic pillar to reflect a holistic governance and leadership approach that is fit for purpose and emulates a te ao Māori (worldview) perspective.	Sport NZ must play a more active part in educating the sport sector at large. Further, conceptions of '**resilience**' must be reimagined in a more uplifting and enhancing way.

insufficient checks or balances in place to ensure that funds earmarked for Māori NSOs actually ended up there. "*We used to get funding from [NSO] and then that just got cut straight away, no reasons or anything, we weren't told, we just got told it was cut. To find out [NSO] are getting a portion of that funding for Māori, you know, it's not getting to where it is supposed to be*" (Tumanako).

Majority of partcipants were resolute that their Māori NSOs will continue to operate into the future regardless of (a lack of) financial assistance or support. Although everyone we spoke with agreed that funding and support would be beneficial. For the reasons expressed above, majority of the Māori NSOs admitted that they have struggled to set up their governance structures, but, simultaneously, they suggested that this is a reflection that, overall, the current system is broken. Indeed, Māori NSOs were not supported or funded by Sport NZ, nor did many of them have functional relationships with Sport NZ. As a result of their status, Māori NSOs are volunteer-driven organisations that must source their own funds and develop their own infrastructure to survive. "*Funding is not the only thing Māori sport needs, they need lots of help with foundational stuff, entry processes, developing strategies, identifying their brand, all of that work needs to happen...one thing I know is if you look at anyone that's volunteering, especially if they are Māori, they'll be stretched*" (Ataahua).

Due to these barriers, among others, Māori NSOs generally are only able to deliver one major tournament each year. Ideally, Māori NSOs preferred to offer multiple initiatives throughout the year, but due to funding constraints they cannot. The underlying philosophy for majority of the Māori NSOs we interviewed was closely aligned with a 'plus-sport' approach (Hapeta, Stewart-Withers, & Palmer, 2019b) insofar as Māori NSOs use sports as catalysts to achieve wider social outcomes for participants. "*The kaupapa [purpose] hasn't changed, the core rules of a vehicle for wellness, a vehicle for Te Reo [language] and Tikanga [cultural protocols] you know, none of that has changed...our commitment to do this was always about iwi [tribal/people] development*" (Aroha).

Other outcomes identified include but are not limited to: Promoting health and wellbeing, e.g., alcohol free, drug free and smoke free sport; Connecting participants to Te Ao Māori and their whakapapa; Promoting the use of te reo (language); Promoting whānaungatanga (social cohesion); Encouraging intergenerational participation; Developing life and career skills; Promoting confidence; Leadership; Pride in being Māori and participation "as Māori". "*It's not just about [sporting code] to us, it's about whanaungatanga [relational/social cohesion], aroha [love], manaakitanga [hospitality/caring], kaitiakitanga [guardianship], kotahitanga [unity] bringing people together to enjoy each other's company"* (Waka).

Another key finding from Māori NSOs stories was not only the relational component of their sports, but also intergenerational participation (grandparents, parents, children). This supports previous findings in the 'Māori Participation in Community Sport review' (KTV Consulting, 2017) that found compared with all boys and girls, Māori boys and girls are more likely to watch family/friends play sport and vice versa: "*When we were young just about every marae [village] had a [sports] team…so we never hesitated, started supporting them straight away, our son plays [sport A] but our other children play Rugby and Netball*" (Manaaki).

Supporting Māori NSOs supports Māori boys and girls to remain connected to sport through their whānau and friends. Formal relationships with these organisations could provide further insights into how they have successfully maintained intergenerational participation despite limited annual events and no financial support. Further, Māori NSOs identified two priority needs: Recognition from the sector that they are an important part of Māori participation "as Māori"; and Functional support with infrastructure, administration, funding and sponsorship.

Present Policies: The 'MAP' and the 'MOF'

Sport NZ's (2022a) recently released 'MAP' acknowledged that it did not have in place "any Te Tiriti or investment partnerships with Māori" (p.12). Further, that Māori were under-represented in leadership and management positions both externally in terms of the wider sector and internally within their own organisation (Sport NZ, 2022a). There were, for instance, currently no Māori among the Senior Leadership Team and only five Māori staff who were in senior leadership or management roles within Sport NZ's priority partner groupings. Moreover, and perhaps just as alarmingly, any Māori relationships/initiatives were almost entirely dependent upon the Rautaki Māori team within Sport NZ which consists of three (3) people who are spread across a 1.4 full-time equivalent

(FTE) allocation. "*The [Sports] organisation only have one Māori staff member and needs to take responsibility for that*" (Ataahua).

Further, there were either no, or minimal at best, Te Tiriti partnerships with Māori by priority partners nationwide. "*None whatsoever, [CE of NSO] we're meant to have an annual catch-up, there's been sometimes he messages me, at the moment there's no inclusion…on our whenua [land] the treaty relationship is that we have the right to have equal participation*" (Aroha).

While Sport NZ (June, 2021) acknowledged that 'trust' is at the core of any partnership, there is much work to be done by them to re-build any sense of trust with Māori given their past experiences and a deep-seated distrust of the Crown due to its consistent failure to give effect to the principles of the Te Tiriti in over eight successive generations.

More optimistically, the newly released 'MAP' is grounded in a unique, holistic, Te Ao Māori (Māori Worldview) approach that focuses on culturally distinctive pathways to enable Māori to succeed *as* Māori through PARS. As acknowledged by their (former) Chief Executive, this was the first time Sport NZ will have a direct mechanism to engage whānau, hapū, iwi, Māori to build meaningful relationships and achieve better outcomes in these communities (Miskimmin, 2020). "*I want that to happen so that there is a generation of kids that don't have to dig these trenches, because we've dug the trenches and now, they can just go and build on the set foundations and build the [Māori] customs on top of it*" (Awhina).

Present Resourcing: Kia piki ake i ngā raruraru o te kainga—Socio-Economic Mediation

In Aotearoa NZ, COVID-19 continues to be challenging for the entire PARS sector, however, it has highlighted the inequities for Māori within that system. In attempt to help alleviate these challenges, Sport NZ's overall \$265m COVID-19 recovery package invested \$7m (2.6%) to develop and deliver on the KMRP. These funds (2.6%) were specifically allocated to support the implementation of initiatives which ultimately sought to empower Māori communities and improve their wellbeing through both Te Ao Māori (Māori worldview) and Mātauranga (knowledge) Māori approaches. Launched in December 2020, the KMRP's four main kaupapa (initiatives) were considered "a significant milestone in Sport NZ's cultural journey" (Sport NZ, November, 2020d, p.4) to enable and explore new relationships with Māori as well as to strengthen partnerships. In total, by June 2021, Sport NZ had delivered $201.8m to the PARS sector and during the four years 2021-2024, a further $62.8m will respond to the needs of the overall PARS system.

Additionally, to reflect their 2020/21 strategic priorities, Sport NZ July, 2020b attempted to ensure they focussed on 'priority groups': Māori, women and girls, disabled communities, tamariki (children) and rangatahi (youth) to raise their physical activity levels. Thus, signalling Sport NZ's intent to 'prioritise' these targeted groups when allocating investment. Overall, the intention of the $7m (2.6%) set aside for the KMRP was to support Māori, across the following four components: 1) Support for Māori NSOs (0.35million); 2) expand 'He Oranga Poutama' (Sport NZ's longest running and only Kaupapa Māori programme); 3) fund the 'MaraeFit Aotearoa' pilot programme—a marae-centric 'Everybody Active' initiative; and 4) provide funding for a Te Ihi activation fund.

This following section, however, critiques the KMRP specifically regarding the first component—Māori NSOs. From a Kaupapa Māori analytical perspective of socio-economic mediation, the new $350,000 (equating to 5% of the $7million) funding allocation provided by Sport NZ for Māori NSOs goes some way towards addressing the principle of—Kia piki ake i ngā raruraru o te kainga. In theory, though, this principle is about providing assistance to alleviate disadvantages or negative pressures experienced by Māori communities. Thus, the "key learning here is the need to 'level the playing field' in terms of resources available to Māori" (Hapeta, Evans & Smith, 2021, p.91). Our assessment is that 5% of the $7million is insufficient to 'level the playing field' and meet the principle of socio-economic mediation, especially in light of some of the issues that Māori NSOs face to secure funding: "*We've got no money, really, I got declined 9 times with funding applications, and the rigmaroles and circles of that just sent my head into a spin, so I said I'm not going to do another one ever again…the politics of this [grants] game are disgusting*" (Manaaki).

This Sport NZ funding (5%) allocation, therefore, attempts to align with the above principle. Although, while it is welcomed, in the overall context of the $265million 'Recovery Fund' $350,000 (0.13%) is a drop in the ocean. However, most Māori NSOs we spoke with run an annual operating budget of between $5-$25,000. In this respect, $350,000 could provide a certain 'level of support' for several different Māori NSOs over the next few years. From a Kaupapa Māori position, which reasserts the need for outcomes to be of positive benefit to Māori communities, we contend that this level of resourcing acknowledges the relevance and successes that Māori-led initiatives can have as targeted interventions for addressing Māori needs, yet it still does not prioritise enough funds towards addressing the past or present socio-economic inequities.

Strengthening Resilience—Back to the Future

In their own words, Sport NZ (July, 2020) stated the intention of the $350,000 funding was to help Māori NSOs to "survive the current social and economic conditions and acknowledge their contribution" (p.10). Yet, Indigenous peoples aspire to see beyond survival mode, because they have well and truly demonstrated resilience throughout historical struggles and socio-political agendas such as annihilation, assimilation, colonisation and appropriation. Rather what Indigenous peoples and their entities such as MNSOs are seeking is a position of self-determination (Durie, 2007) which from a Māori perspective is 'tino rangatiratanga'. "*One of the core values is that all Māori sports codes have their own mana Motuhake [autonomy / self-determination]...what's possible, is like, we could rule the world in our own way if we stick to who we are as Māori... and people do it in little ways or some in big ways, but I see some sport codes really get sucked into trying to emulate the national body*" [NSO] (Aroha).

Specifically in the ecological sense, resilience is understood as the capacity to survive threats, stress or damage and recover from these quickly. In terms of 'bouncing back' as an ecosystem, it is vital for Māori NSOs that Sport NZ reconsiders notions of resilience and that 'doing things differently and better' are understood beyond western framings; furthermore, that bouncing back does not simply mean returning to 'business as usual'. Rather, in the spirit of adapting, this is a real opportunity for authentic adjustment and transformation (Thomas et al., 2016); pivotal if the resources and the relationships of present and future, are to be more uplifting and mana enhancing for Māori NSOs and their communities. "*Some have never experienced the [Māori] cultural side of things, so with the juniors we're quite staunch…they have to learn their pepeha [introduction / ancestral recital] …they could do it in Māori, but some of them do it in English…it's been a real mind-blowing experience*" (Maia).

Dominant resiliency discourse tends to focus on the individual, but in this case the 'unit' that perhaps needs to be more resilient is the Sport NZ organisation itself. In consideration of their experiences, such as not being acknowledged, resourced or supported from their 'parent' NSOs nor from Sport NZ, Māori NSOs have arguably been incredibly resilient, some for over 100 years. Resilience, however, has also been criticised by some Indigenous scholars as "a polite expression of a Darwinian belief about the survival of the fittest" (Newhouse, 2006, p.2), and for failing to "acknowledge the political, social, economic and environmental realities of Indigenous communities"… misdirecting "the responsibility away from governments and colonial policies and onto the individuals themselves" (Thomas et al., 2016, p.116). How then, will this small gesture from Sport NZ help Māori NSOs to achieve their desired state of tino rangatiratanga and other rights as outlined in Te Tiriti o Waitangi? "*If we [Māori NSOs] turn to mainstream… [NSOs] need to have a commitment within strategies and organisations that honour the Treaty…they're still developing their Treaty response plan…so in time, you know, I was in a meeting 20years ago…still getting no support*" (Ataahua).

Discussion

Our findings from interviews with representatives of seven Māori NSOs revealed that they were faced with both negative and positive impacts within the context of the COVID-19 provoked Sport NZ system 're-set'. In terms of their not so favourable perceptions—presently, where established relationships do exist between Māori NSOs and their 'partner'

(Sport NZ funded) NSOs, they are somewhat strained. This present predicament, however, is primarily due to past instances of 'last minute' tokenistic and transactional practices that Māori NSOs have experienced in relation to their mainstream NSO parents. Although, some recent 'transactional requests' also indicate present and continuous issues too. "*I had 13 of my [Māori] kids get selected for National squads…so we started running holiday programmes. Then, I get a phone call from the [NSO] regional officer saying 'can you stop what you're doing', no I can't, there are people loving it in here, 'but we're meant to be running the programmes there', well I hadn't seen or heard from you since I asked you for help, so why are you coming to stop what is working for us?*" (Manaaki).

Consequently, due to examples such as that above, among many other instances, there remains a heightened element of distrust from the Māori NSO network who feel that their mana is neither enhanced nor uplifted by these NSOs (who are directly funded by Sport NZ) and many of those we spoke to have quite frankly had enough of these mana diminishing experiences.

On a more optimistic note, the present 're-set' and 're-build' phase has, perhaps, provided the platform to strengthen relationships and reimagine an alternative future to the pre-COVID-19 experience. Promisingly, Sport NZ are not ignorant to the challenges ahead, they acknowledge that the aim of enabling all New Zealanders to focus more on their wellbeing through PARS "is critical in both the current [Covid-19] environment and in the future. However, achieving inclusion, openness and redistribution of power through a wider network has profound implications. It requires deep structural and cultural changes, and not solely in the play, active recreation and sport sector" (Sport NZ, November, 2020d, p.20). It appears, based upon this acknowledgement, that such structural and systemic practices have (re)produced inequalities (Amis et al., 2020) and that the intention is for more equitable change and transformation within and beyond the sector in the future.

In turning the focus towards a different and better future, our recommendation is that a more deliberate, reconciliatory, approach is required from Sport NZ to re-establish trust and re-build positive, productive relationships with Māori NSOs. For example, other settler colonial settings have explicit bodies to address reconciliation efforts, such as the Truth and Reconciliation Commission (TRC) in Canada and in Australia the Council for Aboriginal Reconciliation (CAR). Reconciliation Australia's (2022) five dimensions upon which reconciliatory efforts are understood are: Historical Acceptance, Race Relations, Equality and Equity, Institutional Integrity, and Unity. These dimensions provide a framework to conceptualise reconciliatory efforts, progress and for identifying areas of need.

In terms of the title of this chapter, Te Mana Whakahaere, the aim was to contribute past and present insights from Māori voices to help inform future direction setting for Sport NZ and the wider sector. From a '*ka mua, ka muri*' viewpoint, poor past experiences raised by Māori NSOs must be acknowledged in relation to historical (race) 'relations' between respective NSOs and their counterparts. Our analysis has also highlighted ongoing issues of inequality and inequity in terms of (un)levelling 'the playing field'. Māori NSOs have also called into question some NSOs for their (lack of) institutional integrity, which has not necessarily led to unity and cohesion between these parties. In attempt to honour the Kaupapa Māori spirit, we have given rise to the visibility of Māori NSOs, so they know that their perspectives based on lived realities and intergenerational knowledge are being shared and their collective voices have the opportunity of being heard. It appears that all is not lost or falling on ears that do not listen and eyes that cannot see, as the excerpt below from Sport NZ (2020d) indicates:

> In our preferred future…an 'Agency of Movement' loosely coordinates a network of communities and participation providers. The agency [Sport NZ] is designed to serve as an enabler rather than a controller. It fosters an inclusive, collective and organic movement that enables a strong sense of intent and shared purpose. Communities and participation providers are well connected and work together in a collaborative way. The principles of Te Tiriti are ingrained in everyday practices and decision-making, with the agency ensuring our commitment to Te Tiriti o Waitangi is upheld (p.20).

Conclusions

Globally, almost all countries, communities, industries and sectors have been affected by the ongoing uncertainty surrounding the COVID-19 pandemic. The impact of COVID-19 on the PARS sector in Aotearoa NZ has been disruptive to say the least. This disruption, though, has also provided a unique opportunity to serve as a catalyst for change: to re-set, rebuild, strengthen, and adapt the system for a better and hopefully more equitable future. This chapter set out to offer a critically informed, Kaupapa Māori, analysis of the past, present and future relationships between Māori NSOs and Sport NZ via various NSOs.

In considering these past and present Māori NSOs perspectives and lived realities, we believe that, if indeed the aspirations underpinning current policies (KMRP, MAP, MOF) and practices (i.e., targeted PARS interventions) via an empowered 'Agency of Movement' can be realised, then the future will be different and better, especially if solutions are tailored towards whānau, hapū, iwi and Māori communities. Although the government's responses to address social inequities and to re-engage these priority groups in PARS post-COVID-19 are not perfect, the development and design of recent Sport NZ policies bodes well for realising an ideal future, but some key learnings that emerged from the pūkenga indicated that things will need to be done differently and poor practices ceased. New partnerships and old relationships need to be (re)built upon solid, trusting foundations.

Applying a critical, Kaupapa Māori theoretical lens alongside a principled analytical approach has enabled us to explore the idea that you must know where you have been in order to know which direction you should be heading. Key learnings about past ***relationships,*** the development of current policies, the present distribution of ***resources,*** and the type of ***resilience*** required to circumnavigate challenges on the journey ahead have been discussed. Ultimately, we do not want to see a repeat of situations in the PARS sector such as this, shared by one of the pūkenga: "*Basically, the social part of me, which included the [Māori] cultural element, it was very weak, yeah, I had a weak [Māori] cultural identity...I reflected back on my own upbringing and my lack of awareness of other*

Māori playing the game…there is actually a massive uptake of Māori wanting to play [sport code]…a growing generation of kids so…I've decided it's not good enough, it's not good enough that this is being done" (Awhina).

With those words in mind, we reassert a 're-set' is required for the PARS sector in terms of its relationships with Māori NSOs which was and is much needed and longer overdue. Essentially, the future opportunities and directions ahead for all of NZ's PARS organisations to realise these lofty aspirations will require unity and collaboration country-wide, across various government agencies and local communities that include tangata whenua (Māori people) and entities they align to.

References

Amis, J. M., Mair, J., & Munir, K. A. (2020). The organizational reproduction of inequality. Academy of Management Annals, 14Placeholder Text, 195-230.

Durie, M. (1999). 'Te Pae Māhutonga: a model for Māori health promotion', newsletter, Health Promotion Forum of New Zealand, 49: pp. 2-5.

Durie, M. (2007). Indigenous resilience: From disease and disadvantage to the realisation of potential. *Matariki. Te Mata o Te Tau Monograph Series No 1.* Retrieved https://www.massey.ac.nz/massey/fms/Te%20Mata%20O%20Te%20Tau/Publications%20%20Monograph/(2007)_%20Matariki,%20vol_%201,%20no_%201.pdf?BF8E62F90E1A8BF8017F312AC701E794

Durie, M. (2017). Sir Peter Blake Trust Leaders 2017 Sir Mason Durie. Retrieved (12/8/21) from https://www.youtube.com/watch?v=aSis9SHFfag

Hapeta, J., Evans, J.R, & Smith, G.H. (2021). Ako and Indigenous Athletes: Kaupapa Māori Principles and Game Sense Pedagogy. In Light & Curry (Eds.) *Game Sense for Coaching and Teaching: International Perspectives.* : Routledge.

Hapeta, J., Palmer, F., Kuroda, Y., & Hermansson, G. (2019a). A Kaupapa Māori, culturally progressive, narrative review of literature on sport, ethnicity and inclusion. *Kōtuitui: New Zealand Journal of Social Sciences Online, 14*Placeholder Text, 209-229.

Hapeta, J., Stewart-Withers, R., & Palmer, F. (2019b). Sport for Social Change With Aotearoa New Zealand Youth: Navigating the Theory–Practice Nexus Through Indigenous Principles. *Journal of Sport Management, 33*Placeholder Text, 481-492. doi: https://doi.org/10.1123/jsm.2018-0246

KTV Consulting. (2017). *Māori participation in community sportreview*. Sport New Zealand.

Lee, J. (2009). Decolonising Māori narratives: Pūrākau as a method. MAI Review, 2Placeholder Text, 1–12.

McLeod, J., Brown, S., & Hapeta, J. (2011). A bicultural model, partnering settlers and indigenous communities: Examining the relationship between the principles of the Treaty of Waitangi and health and physical education. In S. Brown (Ed.), *Issues and controversies in physical education: Policy, power, and pedagogy* (pp. 3–14). Pearson.

Miskimmin, P. (2020). Sport New Zealand: Kaupapa-Māori-response-fund Media Release. https://sportnz.org.nz/about/news-and-media/media-centre/kaupapa-Māori-response-fund-media-release/

Moewaka Barnes, H. & McCreanor, T. (2019). Colonisation, hauora and whenua in Aotearoa, Journal of the Royal Society of New Zealand, 49:Placeholder Text, 19-33, DOI: https://doi.org/10.1080/03036758.2019.1668439

Newhouse, D. (2006). From woundedness to resilience: Editorial. *Journal of Aboriginal Health, 3*Placeholder Text, 2-3.

Pihama, L., Tipene, J., & Skipper, H. (2014). *Ngā hua a tāne rore: The benefits of kapa haka—Scoping the research needs and options for developing a better understanding of the contribution that kapa haka makes to Aotearoa New Zealand society*. Manatū Taonga—Ministry for Cultural Heritage.

Pohatu, T. W. (2005). Āta: Growing respectful relationships. Retrieved from http://kaupapamaori.com/assets/ata.pdf

Reconciliation Australia. (2022). *The five dimensions of reconciliation*. Retrieved from https://www.reconciliation.org.au/reconciliation/what-is-reconciliation/

Smith, L. T. (1999). *Decolonizing methodologies: Research and indigenous peoples*. Zed Books.

Smith, G. H. (2000). Māori education: Revolution and transformative action. *Canadian Journal of Native Education, 24*Placeholder Text, 57.

Smith, L.T. (2006). Researching in the Margins Issues for Māori Researchers a Discussion Paper. *Alternative: An International Journal Of Indigenous Peoples, 2*Placeholder Text, 4-27. doi: https://doi.org/10.1177/117718010600200101

Sport New Zealand. (June, 2020a). Strategic foresight—Ensuring the Play, Active Recreation and Sport Sector is Fit for the Future. Wellington, NZ.

Sport New Zealand. (July, 2020b). 2020-2021 Strategic Priorities—Sport NZ's response to COVID-19. Wellington, NZ.

Sport New Zealand. (September, 2020c). Report 2: Māori perspectives on drivers and implications of change—the future of play, active recreation and Sport in New Zealand. Wellington, NZ.

Sport New Zealand. (November, 2020d). Report 3: Developing alternative futures—the future of play, active recreation and Sport in New Zealand. Wellington, NZ.

Sport New Zealand. (2022a). Te Aho a Ihi Aotearoa—Māori Activation Plan. Wellington, NZ.

Sport New Zealand. (2022b). Te Pākē o Ihi Aoteaora—Māori Outcomes Framework. Wellington, NZ.

Stride, A., Fitzgerald, H. F., & Allison, W. (2017). A narrative approach: The possibilities for sport management. *Sport Management Review*, *20*Placeholder Text, 33-42.

Thomas, D., Mitchell, T., & Arseneau, C. (2016). Re-evaluating resilience: From individual vulnerabilities to the strength of cultures and collectivities among indigenous communities. *Resilience, 4*Placeholder Text, 116-129.

Waitangi Tribunal. (n.d.). Retrieved August 12, 2021 from https://waitangitribunal.govt.nz/

Whitinui, P. (2021). Decolonizing sports sociology is a "verb not a noun": Indigenizing our way to reconciliation and inclusion in the 21st century? Alan Ingham memorial lecture. Sociology of Sport Journal, 38Placeholder Text, 3-15.

20

The Uptake of Modern Monetary Theory (MMT) and the COVID-19 Pandemic: Implications for Sport and Physical Culture

Andrew M. Hammond

Introduction

Sociologists of Sport and Physical cultural studies scholars have long critiqued and illuminated the impact of neoliberal rationalities of government on the enactment of sport and physical culture (Hammond et al., 2019; Newman, 2014; Newman & Giardina, 2010; Rowe, 2004, 2020; Silk & Andrews, 2012). Specifically, Silk and Andrews define the essence of neoliberalism as the:

> Morbidity of the social sphere, evidenced from the hegemony of a cynicism toward all things public and collective, the corollary of which has been the rise of a virulent content for the social welfare provision; an equally pernicious and questioning attitude towards its recipients; and a individualizing culture of surveillance, accountability, and resentment. (Silk & Andrews, 2012, p. 6)

A. M. Hammond (✉)
University of Essex, Colchester, UK

D. L. Andrews et al. (eds.), *Sport and Physical Culture in Global Pandemic Times*, Global Culture and Sport Series, https://doi.org/10.1007/978-3-031-14387-8_20

Of particular interest to the following chapter is how neoliberalism has led to the winding back of the welfare state by rich democracies such as the United States, the UK, Canada, and Australia.

The following chapter draws on and extends on a commentary I recently published in the journal Managing Sport and Leisure (e.g., Hammond, 2020). In my article, I highlighted how unprecedented deficit spending was being used by governments in an attempt to avoid economic, social, health, and political catastrophes during and following the COVID 19 pandemic (British Broadcasting Corporation, 2020; Smyth, 2020). Heterodox MMT economists argue that states that have sovereignty over their currency should run government budget deficits to increase consumption and capital investment to reach and maintain full employment. MMT is about making sure the economy is using its excess resources and capacity. It is not a blank check for governments, rather spending should be moderated by material constraints of the 'real' economy. Thus, inflation should provide the hand break, not just the politics of debt and deficit (i.e., debt is bad, immoral, and wrong) (Mitchell et al., 2016). The implementation of MMT provides a way forward through neoliberalism to resurrect social welfare policies in capitalist societies by naturalizing fears about debt and deficit.

The political economy, acceptance, proliferation of MMT is of interest to sport scholars as much of our research is focused on critiquing government intervention in sport (Green & Houlihan, 2006; Houlihan, 2014; Silk & Andrews, 2012; Stenling, 2013). In many areas of sport research, the amassing of public debt is a strawman argument used by scholars to be critical of spending on the Olympic games and other mega-sporting festivals (cf. Flyvbjerg et al., 2021; Macintosh & Bedecki, 1988; Rowe, 2020; Thibault & Harvey, 2013). Arguably, readers of this anthology believe that sport and physical culture adds value to our lives (and society and large) otherwise why would spend so much time writing and debating the subject area? Given that many of us cannot build our own private lap swimming pool, amass land to erect private hiking trails, or construct our own ski hills, we are to some extent reliant on government to provide leisure where entrepreneurs and the private market do not seek to enter. This is because many forms of sport and physical activity, especially those enabled by municipal/national parks, recreation and leisure centers is unlikely to pass the profit test without public assistance.

Sport and Debt

Scholars who write about sport often argue that sporting mega events such as the Olympic Games are bad because they are very likely to run over budget. In fact, every Olympic game since 1960 has run over budget and often costs on average 172% more than anticipated. For instance, some scholars such as Flyvbjerg et al. (2021) state that the "cost overrun and associated debt from the Athens 2004 Games weakened the Greek economy and contributed to the country's deep financial and economic crises," (p. 234).

At the same time, the publication of *The Deficit Myth* by Stony Brook University Professor Stephanie Kelton in 2020 has helped to question if deficit spending by governments is bad. The introduction of 'new' economic ideas such as Modern Monetary Theory (MMT) prompted me to question if austerity spending was ever needed to combat the perceived mounting debt crisis incurred by many nations who had to "fight" the existential threat of the global financial crisis of 2008. After all, no one wanted to end up like Greece (who had a sovereign debt crisis starting in 2010), thus many of us accepted the belt tightening proposed by politicians.

Kelton has previously argued that nation-states who issue their own currency cannot become insolvent in the same way a business or household can. This is because in contemporary times, most governments issue fiat money, that is a currency guaranteed as legal tender by government decree or fiat. Currencies that are convertible to other currencies issued by independent bodies (e.g., the Euro) or exchangeable for commodities (e.g., gold or silver) are not guaranteed the same flexibility. For fiat curacies (e.g., the British Pound, the Japanese Yen or the U.S. Dollar) Kelton argues that inflation, not debt, is the more important technical metric when it comes to curtailing government spending. Kelton goes on to argue that because currency issuing governments have these special powers, these nations do not need to raise taxes to fund government spending. Indeed, some MMT theorists have gone as far to say that in the MMT paradigm, taxes should be thought of as an extension (or branch) of social policy (e.g., Baker & Murphy, 2020; Murphy, 2019), that is to say stamp duty or other taxes on the sale of homes is more or less a mechanism for keeping some stability of price in the housing market rather than a tax that is needed to fund particular government programs.

It is true that some sporting practices have been used by governments to pork barrel (e.g., Smith, 1999) or certain sporting activities have engaged in rent seeking behavior to use public money to sustain their activities and increase their private profits (e.g., Rowe, 2020). Where this chapter extends on what is already published, is a more detailed discussion about rise of heterodox macroeconomic theories (i.e., Modern Monetary Theory) and how these 'alternative ideas' are displacing or augmenting the orthodox neoclassical (or neoliberal) doctrine of macroeconomics that has dominated public policy making in governments and central banks since the early 1980s (Mitchell et al., 2016).

In sum, MMT ideas that have become more popular through the COVID-19 pandemic have much to add to the conversations around political economy already circulating within sociology and physical cultural studies. Of particular interest to scholars of physical culture studies are policies such as the abolishment of student debt, tuition free college and a federal jobs guarantee that have implications for debates about the Mcdonaldization of the university (Hawzen et al., 2018; Silk et al., 2014; Silk & Andrews, 2012) and the political economy of college sports (Kalman-Lamb, 2019). Following Newman and Bunds (2016) scholars of political economy and physical culture share a concern for how to "best organize the State in relation to markets and exchange activities (and vice versa) so as to optimize the citizenry's well-being," (Newman & Bunds, 2016, p. 1),and given the salience of MMT ideas in the popular press and the Federal Reserve's desire and mandate to maximize full-employment it seems timely to think about how once fringe ideas are becoming more mainstream and contributing to policy debates in the United States and beyond.

The COVID 19 Recession

The COVID 19 recession is unique because while it may have been as deep as the great depression by some measures, it has also likely been the shortest (Wheelock, 2020). The reason why the recession was so short, was because governments, spent trillions of dollars on social welfare and other measures designed to stimulate the economy and to lift aggregate demand (Sharma et al., 2021). For instance, the OECD (2021) forecasted at one stage that the American Rescue Plan, passed in March 2021 would lift global growth by 1%. While such schemes (including Furlough in the UK and other increases to social welfare) have provided crucial lifelines to many individuals made vulnerable by the pandemic, there are concerns that if support is ended too prematurely the world and some economies could slide back into recession (Sharma et al., 2021).

Critics suggest the amount of debt governments are taking on to assist in the economic recovery is "unsustainable", and it is well documented that the effects of the last recession (i.e., the Great Recession or the Global Financial Crisis) lingered for some time because governments were too restrained in their recovery spending. In short, the cure to recession appears to be increased government spending (Keynes, 2007), but governments are generally unwilling to increase debt (for political reasons) (Kelton, 2015). Thus, policy makers appear to be caught in a 'catch 22'. For the Sport Sociologists unfamiliar with debates within Economic Sociology it may come as a surprise that government debt is more of a discursive construction than a real material constraint on government investment. The rising popularity of Modern Monetary Theory (MMT) shows how politics constrains government spending, not the materiality of debt.

Modern Monetary Theory (MMT)

> Let us never forget this fundamental truth: the State has no source of money other than money which people earn themselves. If the State wishes to spend more it can do so only by borrowing your savings or by taxing you more. It is no good thinking that someone else will pay—that "someone

> else" is you. There is no such thing as public money; there is only taxpayers' money. (Thatcher, 1983, p. 3)

The above remarks are some of the most influential comments made by a politician in the last three decades. In 1983, then Prime Minister Margert Thatcher argued in Blackpool in 1983 that the state's budget is analogous with a household budget. What Thatcher neglected to mention is that a household cannot invite more people to come and work in it (through immigration) nor can a household print its own currency, two very important distinctions between a household and the nation states budget (especially when the nation state has autonomy over its own currency). The metaphor of a household however helped Thatcher convince the public of the need for particular neoliberal economic reforms such as the privatization of railways, the Telecoms, and the state-owned airline British Airways.

President Barak Obama provides a key example of how under neoliberal rationalities of government (Brown, 2015; Dean, 2010; Hammond et al., 2019), debt rhetoric is not only a disease of the right but also the left. Echoing the remarks of Thatcher, Obama uses again the analogy of the household budget to help label national "debt" and "deficit" as being reckless and immoral in 2008:

> The problem is, is that the way Bush has done it over the last eight years is to take out a credit card from the Bank of China in the name of our children, driving up our national debt from $5 trillion for the first 42 presidents—#43 added $4 trillion by his lonesome, so that we now have over $9 trillion of debt that we are going to have to pay back—$30,000 for every man, woman and child. That's irresponsible. It's unpatriotic. (Obama cited in Toomey, 2012)

That is, taxes can be thought of as a mechanism of ensuring equity and social welfare in and of themselves (Baker & Murphy, 2020). For instance, Tobacco excise taxes are levied to discourage smoking through pricing. Stamp duty on housing transactions is arguably used to keep house prices at stable levels. In both these instances, under MMT, the government does not "need" money from tobacco to fund the treatment of smoking related diseases, nor does it need a cut of the money from the sale of a home to subsidies infrastructure, rather taxes are used to control consumption in asset prices to safeguard social welfare (Baker & Murphy, 2020).

To illustrate that government debt is political and not materially relevant, one just has to observe the differences in the politics around Greek debt in 2010 versus in 2020. For example, at the height of the Greek sovereign debt crisis, the Greek government had a Gross Domestic Product to debt ratio of 146%. On April 27, 2010, financial markets reacted, and the 10-year spread of yields between the 10-year Greek government bonds and German bunds peaked at 1000 basis points (or 10%) prompting ratings agencies to class Greek bonds as "Junk" assets. That meant, in simple terms, actors within financial markets decided that the Greek government was likely to default on its loans and had little confidence in their ability to pay back their debt. In the preceding years the Greeks eventually defaulted on their debt and were subject to austerity to shore up the state's finances. Austerity was responsible for unemployment of 23%, cuts to public services, and risked plunging record numbers of citizens into poverty. During the preceding years, it seems nations elsewhere became obsessed with tackling "national debt" and implementing austerity to not "end up like the Greeks".

Arguably, the Greek experience was politically weaponized to promote an austerity agendas that led to the election of governments obsessed with debt and deficit reduction. Politicians successfully convinced electorates to vote for governments with austere policy agendas in the U.K., the U.S., Canada, and Australia by comparing a governments budget with a household's budget. The corrosive effects of austerity on sport, recreation and leisure is well documented by several sport and leisure studies scholars (e.g., Parnell et al., 2018; Widdop et al., 2017), highlighting collectively that access has become more unequal and is leading to a decline in participation, such studies argue for the need for government spending in order to promote equity in terms of access. A decade later and at the time of writing in June 2021, Greek government debt is over 200% of GDP (Papadopoulos, 2021). And yet the 10-year spread of yields against German bunds has fallen to its narrowest level since 2008 (107 basis points) and that is despite government debt accelerating from

10 years ago (Arnold & Oliver, 2021). So, what's changed? The politics of debt temporarily shifted when governments were forced to be on a crisis footing. Therefore, MMT helps us to understand why governments can spend unlimited money at times (i.e., to prop up the banking system or in the face of a deadly virus) but uses debt politics selectively to, for example fund tax cuts, but not healthcare.

In the case of the United States, Australia, and the U.K.; MMT illuminates how debt is weaponized by both sides of politics to demonize policy choices mooted by rival political parties. By using MMT as a lens for understanding better the relationship between government spending and inflation, we can illuminate how most (if not all) government spending are calculated political choices, and that concerns about debt are quickly forgotten in the face of much larger political obstacles (such as global pandemic). Given this realization, MMT economists are quick to offer alternatives that are supported by many left-leaning politicians including Democratic congresswomen Alexandria Ocasio-Cortez and former democratic presidential candidate Senator Bernie Sanders.

MMT Policy Alternatives

In her own context of the US, Kelton (2020) argues for a federal job guarantee where the nation-state would employ anybody who is jobless for an agreed wage. The policy, she argues, would promote full employment while keeping inflation stable. She contends people with this wage could engage in health, social care, or other sectors that would enrich others' lives (Kelton, 2020). It is argued that graduates of physical cultural studies would benefit from such a policy, given the strong numbers of our graduates in sport and physical culture studies who seek work in the community sector after graduating. Moreover, many of us would agree that countless of our newly minted (and unemployed) sport studies graduates who are graduating with skills in health, wellbeing, and physical activity (especially at the grassroots and community level) would benefit from such a scheme and would make a substantive contribution to society. Another policy mooted by MMT theorists is cancelling college tuition and abolishing student debt, a policy we know would shift the relationship between collegiate sport and the academy, given that tuition is offered in exchange for student athlete labor.

As I have noted elsewhere, the main difference between MMT theorists and mainstream economists is the question of how much more should be spent without raising inflation. Mainstream economists such as Mankiw (2019) are extremely cautious, whereas Kelton (2020) points to how nations could be spending much more. For instance, at the height of the financial crisis 2008, many experts in the U.S. contended that the government needed to spend trillion more dollars than it did to adequately boost aggregate demand (Kelton, 2020). Instead, politics got in the way and Obama and his aides, worried a voter backlash, and instead delivered a much smaller stimulus (Kelton, 2020). The result of the Obama administrations caution was that and millions of people remained unemployed. Kelton (2020) argues that in the U.S., prudence towards debt and deficit is coming at the expense of social welfare, and is hurting those that depend on public services the most (i.e., the working class, female, the young, dis/abled etc.).

Given that debt is not bad and that public spending in and of itself is not reckless (or immoral) provides sport sociologists and those interested in inequality and social justice with an opportunity. As scholars invested in recreation and other life-enriching activities, we should collectively argue against increasing public spending in a recession and advocate for policies that would increase the public debt and aggregate demand in the sport and recreation sector. With policymakers currently considering spending more money to maximize social welfare, then we need to argue as a field for why sport and leisure should be part of the plan. However, to understand why some scholars might be uncomfortable with advocating for public spending on sport and recreation, it is crucial to examine how scholars have written about public debt and sport. Writing about the Montreal Olympics illustrates why some scholars might think spending on sport is wasteful (or even immoral).

The 1967 Canadian Montreal Olympics

I (Hammond, 2020) have previously pointed to how some scholars (e.g., Thibault and Harvey (2013)) have used the "financial disaster" (p.14) of the Montreal Olympics as the poster child for why governments (or 'the state) should not spend money on sport activities classed as 'special projects'. In the case of the Montreal Olympics, we can use MMT's analytical tools uncover why the Montreal Olympics was such a financial disaster.

A key problem with Thibault and Harvey's initial assessment of the Montreal games as "financial disaster" does not discuss who (i.e., what branch of government) financed the Montreal Olympics. They did not mention that the games were primarily financed by the City of Montreal and the Québec provincial government of Canada (both are currency users whose budgets are constrained by taxes and revenue). Thibault and Harvey's initial analysis thus did not mention that the Federal Government (the currency issuer not constrained by debt and deficit) did little to finance the games (apart from pointing out that they set up a lottery to fund the games). The federal (Canadian) government's commitment to underwrite the future Calgary and Vancouver Winter Olympics highlights how mega events can be potentially more problematic if the debt burden falls to a government who does not have sovereignty over its currency (such as a state or a city or a country that uses the Euro: e.g., Greece (Flyvbjerg et al., 2021).

As I have noted elsewhere (e.g., Hammond, 2020), the events that transpired after the Montreal Olympics prompt us to think more critically about the effects of debt, based on the type of governments that incur the debt (i.e., a currency issuer versus a currency user). To be very clear, I have argued here, and elsewhere that the debt accrued by the City of Montreal for hosting the Montreal Olympics did lead to a crisis and a decline in public services that is because Montreal and the Province of Québec must use federal government money and thus cannot spend any more of the federal government's money than they make through taxation (Kelton, 2011). We must then question if the Federal Government funded the Montreal Olympic games would the financial disaster for the city be avoided (like it had for Calgary and Vancouver).

In hindsight, we cannot speculate what might have happened if the Federal Government of Canada financed the Montreal Olympic Games. As I mentioned elsewhere (e.g., Hammond, 2020) because in the 1970s the oil crisis and other issues related to unemployment and inflation (i.e., 'stagflation') meant that the federal government might have struggled to make full use of the tools of MMT (remembering a handbrake on spending is inflation, not debt) to cushion the impact of hosting the games that were hampered by a myriad of issues (including industrial relation disputes). As I have mentioned elsewhere, we cannot move past the divisive politics of helping out Québec in a nation that was becoming deeply divided (Kidd, 1992; Whitson & Horne, 2006).

As I have shown elsewhere, Québécois were keen to differentiate themselves from English speaking Canada (Hammond, 2020; Whitson & Horne, 2006). It was only ten years earlier in 1967 when President Charles de Gaulle of France (a head of state of a foreign country), announced 'Vive le Québec libre!' at Expo 67 (an event underwritten by the Federal government). Canadian studies experts cite de Gaulle's remarks at Expo as one of the catalysts for the Québec nationalism movement that could have resulted in Canada's break-up in 1980 and 1995 (Hammond, 2020; Jedwab, 2017; Meren, 2012).

Following Kelton and others (Kelton, 2011; Sharpe & Watts, 2013) after 1970 Canada floated the dollar and therefore (to paraphrase Kelton, 2020) could never become insolvent and could never run out of Canadian dollars. Arguably, Québec separatism and politics related to provincial favoritism (as Pierre Elliot Trudeau was a Québécois) was more influential in the conditions that led to the Montreal Olympics debt crisis (Hammond, 2020). As Whitson and Horne (2006) point out the politics of the time and the pressure from Front du libération de Québec meant that the Canadian federal government was reluctant to provide unpopular financial support for an event that might have exacerbated existing political divisions in Canada (Hammond, 2020).

The Case of the NRL

The Liberal government of Pierre Elliot Trudeau did not finance the Montreal Olympics out of fear of stoking tensions between French and English-speaking Canadians. Arguably, if his government did, the city of Montreal may not have suffered as much. It might be tempting to think at this stage, why should we fund sport and recreation. Should the government be funding health care, education, or childcare instead of sport? In his recent article, Rowe paints sport in a trivial light when he argues that sport is an "essential industry in which athletes, audiences, and stadia were represented as the symbolic equivalents, respectively, of health professionals, patients, and hospitals" (Rowe, 2020, p. 5). Rowe argues that elite sport has special status through what he regards as exceptionalism, which can be inferred to suggest that he is skeptical of the public financing of elite sport in Australia and around the globe.

Rowe, in his article, rightly points out the of misappropriation of public money through sport. He is right to point out the atrocious rent-seeking behavior of the National Rugby League (NRL) who resisted the claw back A$800m dollars from a pre-COVID commitment of AU$2.3 billion by the New South Wales (NSW) government to fund the controversial demolition and rebuilding of three stadia for purposes unrelated to sport. Although the NRL's rent-seeking behavior is contentious, he rightly points out that NRL games are "undoubtedly prized by a substantial proportion of the population," (Rowe, 2020, p. 6) thus it is not unreasonable to suggest that public finances are used to fund sporting infrastructure and entertainment.

A potential problem however is that the State government of New South Wales is a currency user and must balance its budget while fighting the pandemic through the state's universal healthcare infostructure. A potential problem is that money and resources are diverted to sporting upgrades rather than health care, but if the federal government of Australia steps in (a currency issuer) and directs idle labor and materials towards the building of stadia then following Kelton's MMT logic that policy could be a net good for both he people of New South Wales and Australia as the state budget can be freed up for fighting covid in line with their constitutional obligations. I argue that the link between NRL and the organizers of the Montreal Olympics are rent seekers. They both want public money to put on sporting entertainment spectacles. The argument is that the politics of the day will dictate when spending on sport is okay and when it is not.

Discussion

Sociologists of Sport and Physical cultural studies scholars have long critiqued and illuminated the impact of neoliberal rationalities of government on the enactment of sport and physical culture (Hammond et al., 2019; Newman, 2014; Newman & Giardina, 2010; Rowe, 2004, 2020; Silk & Andrews, 2012). This chapter has sought to extend on previous debates on neoliberal ration in PCS and the sociology of sport by highlighting how concerns about the debt have led to a zero-sum game where critical sociologists of sport have argued that spending on sport under neoliberalism can erode social welfare provision and public goods (Chen, 2022; Giardina & Cole, 2012; Miller, 2012; Nauright & Schimmel, 2005). Giardina and Cole (2012), for example are right when they are critical of public spending on buildings such as the Superdome in New Orleans, Louisiana. In this article, I argued based on heterodox economic theories such as MMT while spending on stadia might not be the best use of public funds for currency users such as the Louisiana state, currency issuers (such as the United States federal government) can afford such debts since the US dollar is a fiat currency.

Therefore, I cautiously argue that new economic theories such as MMT can be used to highlight how it is possible to both promote policies that advance social welfare while still embracing cultural activities related to conspicuous consumption in sport and leisure. I have done this by highlighting how national debt is not the limiting constraint it is believed to be and that as part of the neoliberal project, we as a field, I cautiously suggest that maybe we have collectively internalized the neoliberal idea that the nation-state must balance its books like a business or a household as per Thatcher's remarks (see for example: Chen, 2022; Giardina & Cole, 2012; Miller, 2012; Nauright & Schimmel, 2005;

Newman, 2014; Thibault & Harvey, 2013). Indeed, new ideas promoted by heterodox economists show us that inflation, not national debt is the better metric for curtailing government spending. This means, that ultimately as a society we should focus on using monetary tools to increase social welfare and (re)imagine the role of leisure, physical culture, and sport in increasing social welfare.

While I have championed the case for financing sport and recreation as part of the recovery, there is a need to acknowledge recent research by Yoon (Yoon, 2019, 2020) and colleagues (Yoon & Wilson, 2019) who highlight the need to consider a myriad of ethical, social and governance issues in relation to sport spending. In her work Yoon (2019) highlights the disastrous environmental consequences and anti-democratic decisions made because of the 2018 PyeongChang Olympics hosted in South Korea. Yoon discusses in detail environmental consequences that occurred because of partially bulldozing Mount Gariwang in South Korea for a onetime event (the extension of a ski run for the Olympic games). Both Yoon's (2019) and Rowe's (2020) recent comments work highlight the need to balance environmental concerns to address climate change issues when thinking about what programs and activities should be publicly financed as part of COVID recovery strategies around the world (Hammond, 2020).

In trying to articulate how sport and recreation in the recovery I contend that we should return sport and recreation policies of the past (such as the Bloomfield report commissioned by the Whitlam government in Australia) to plan for the future recovery (Adair & Vamplew, 1997; Stewart et al., 2004). As sport scholars, as a field we should be arguing for responsible investment by government into sport and recreation. However, we should be using the power of currency-issuing governments to finance projects and programs at the local level, like Whitlam's social democratic agenda (Hammond et al., 2020).

While the implementation and expansion of social programs at the local level is not without challenges (such as pork barreling, vanity projects, and other forms of corruption) arguably the special powers of currency issuing governments is needed to fund ambitious projects that would otherwise hamper currency user governments that are reliant on taxation. Again, as I have stated above, we should not be playing the neoliberal game of declaring that all public debt is bad, instead we should be having a conversation as a field about what initiatives, policies, and programs should be funded and be raising the level of discussion to have a more informed discussion that balances commercial interests with social welfare and the costs of sport to the environment.

Moreover, there is a discussion needed about for whom public money should be spent. In the rebuilding of society conversations about how public money is allocated towards physical activity programs, the media sports cultural complex and physical education. Public money must be spent in the democratic interests of the society it serves, not just rent seekers or other special interests' groups who seem to have no problem eliciting public funding during debt and deficit disasters. Also, recent debate about inflation and overblown public spending should be met with caution as other exogenous shocks related to supply chain disruptions and the semi-conductor shortage, according to the OECD are leading to transitory inflation that should pass in coming months, thus based on my original article (Hammond, 2020) there still is a need for governments around the world to spend money to stimulate the economy. And if there are governments willing to spend money (either through tax cuts or through new projects) sport and physical culture scholars should be making arguments for sport and recreation to be part of social welfare and other forms of spending.

With regards to further research, it is clear there is a need for physical culture researchers to explore the implications of the adoption of MMT policies (such as cancelling student debt and a federal job guarantee) on sport and physical culture. It is unclear at this stage to what extent the Biden administration may adopt some of the more radical policies put forward by MMT proponents. Of a particular need is studies that model and explore the impact of cancelling student debt and free college on intercollegiate athletics. Also, scholars could look to explore the impact of the Olympic games on national debt in Japan from hosting the Tokyo games. Finally, there is a need to develop a more nation-specific or systematic approach to comparing the various aspects of different national systems with regards to the financing of sport and its relationship to broader fiscal and monetary approaches, beyond the general benchmarking published by De Bosscher et al. (2015) that focuses just on spending.

Given the over-arching concern in PCS and sport sociology for questions related to neoliberalism, social welfarism, etc. (hundreds of articles and books) it is important to systematically research how different financial systems and economies allocate resources to finance sport and physical cultural 'heterotopias of difference' to create "spaces of representation," (Cenzatti, 2008, p. 2) as part of recovery efforts.

Concluding Remarks

In sum, In articulating why and how sport and recreation can contribute to the recovery, I contend that we should return to sport and recreation policies of the past (such as the Bloomfield report commissioned by the Whitlam government in Australia) in planning our recovery (Adair & Vamplew, 1997; Stewart et al., 2004). Rather than avoiding debt, a conversation as a field is needed about what initiatives, policies, and programs should be funded and how sport impacts the environment. Moreover, there is a discussion needed about for whom public money should be spent. As I have highlighted elsewhere, I stand resolute in arguing that conversations about how public money is allocated towards physical activity programs, the media sports cultural complex, and physical education are essential if we are to truly 'build back better'. Public money must be spent in the democratic interests of the society it serves, not just rent seekers or other special interests' groups who elicit public funding easily during debt and deficit disasters.

References

Adair, D., & Vamplew, W. (1997). *Sport in Australian history*. Oxford University Press.

Arnold, M., & Oliver, J. (2021). Greece sells first 30-year bond since 2008 financial crisis. *Financial Times*. https://www.ft.com/content/c31bac51-d065-421f-a600-943c7356c2e2

Baker, A., & Murphy, R. (2020). Modern Monetary Theory and the changing role of tax in society. *Social Policy and Society, 19*(3), 454–469. https://doi.org/10.1017/S1474746420000056

British Broadcasting Corporation. (2020). UK quarterly borrowing hits record high. *BBC News*. https://www.bbc.co.uk/news/business-53482895

Brown, W. (2015). *Undoing the demos: Neoliberalism's stealth revolution*. MIT Press.

Cenzatti, M. (2008). Heterotopias of difference. In M. Dehaene & L. De Cauter (Eds.), *Heterotopia and the city—Urban theory and the transformations of public space*. Blackwell.

Chen, C. (2022). Naming the ghost of capitalism in sport management. *European Sport Management Quarterly*, 1–22. https://doi.org/10.1080/16184742.2022.2046123

De Bosscher, V., Shibil, S., Westerbeek, H., & van Bottenburg, M. (2015). *Successful elite sport policies: An international comparison of the SportsPolicy factors Leading to International Sporting Success (SPLISS 2.0) in 15 nations*. Meyer & Meyer Verlag.

Dean, M. (2010). *Governmentality: Power and rule in modern society* (2nd ed.). Sage.

Flyvbjerg, B., Budzier, A., & Lunn, D. (2021). Regression to the tail: Why the Olympics blow up. *Environment and Planning A, 53*(2), 233–260. https://doi.org/10.1177/0308518X20958724

Giardina, M. D., & Cole, C. (2012). Race, class, and politics in post-Katrina America. In D. L. Andrews & M. L. Silk (Eds.), *Sport and neoliberalism* (pp. 57–74). Temple University Press. http://www.jstor.org/stable/j.ctt14bt86n.6

Green, M., & Houlihan, B. (2006). Governmentality, modernization, and the "disciplining" of national sporting organizations: Athletics in Australia and the United Kingdom. *Sociology of Sport Journal, 23*(1), 47–71. http://ezproxy.lib.monash.edu.au/login?url=http://search.ebscohost.com/login.aspx?direct=true&db=s3h&AN=21368895&site=ehost-live&scope=site

Hammond, A. M. (2020). Financing sport post-COVID-19: Using Modern Monetary Theory (MMT) to help make a case for economic recovery through spending on sport and recreation. *Managing Sport and Leisure*. https://doi.org/10.1080/23750472.2020.1850326

Hammond, A. M., Jeanes, R., Penney, D., & Leahy, D. (2019). 'I feel we are inclusive enough': Examining swimming coaches' understandings of inclusion and disability. *Sociology of Sport Journal, 36*(4), 311–321. https://doi.org/10.1123/ssj.2018-0164

Hammond, A. M., Penney, D., & Jeanes, R. (2020). Sport coaches as policy actors: An investigation of the interpretation and enactment of disability and

inclusion policy in swimming in Victoria Australia. *Sport, Education and Society, 25*(5), 570–585. https://doi.org/10.1080/13573322.2019.1628013
Hawzen, M. G., McLeod, C. M., Holden, J. T., & Newman, J. I. (2018). Cruel optimism in sport management: Fans, affective labor, and the political economy of internships in the sport industry. *Journal of Sport and Social Issues, 42*(3), 184–204. https://doi.org/10.1177/0193723518758457
Houlihan, B. (2014). Achieving compliance in international anti-doping policy: An analysis of the 2009 World Anti-Doping Code. *Sport Management Review, 17*(3), 265–276.
Jedwab, J. (2017). Vive le québec libre @ 50: The rise and decline of québec's independence movement, 1967–2017. *Canadian Issues*, 36–40.
Kalman-Lamb, N. (2019). Athletic labor and social reproduction. *Journal of Sport and Social Issues, 43*(6), 515–530. https://doi.org/10.1177/0193723519850879
Kelton, S. (2011). Limitations of the government budget constraint: Users vs. issuers of the currency. *Panoeconomicus, 1*, 57–66. https://doi.org/10.2298/PAN1101057K
Kelton, S. (2015). 2. The failure of austerity: Rethinking fiscal policy. *Political Quarterly, 86*, 28–46. https://doi.org/10.1111/1467-923X.12231
Kelton, S. (2020). *The deficit Myth*. John Murray.
Keynes, J. M. (2007). *The general theory of employment, interest and money*. Palgrave Macmillan for the Royal Economic Society. https://search.ebscohost.com/login.aspx?direct=true&db=cat08605a&AN=uelc.b1662516&site=eds-live&authtype=sso&custid=s9814295
Kidd, B. (1992). The culture wars of the Montreal Olympics. *International Review for the Sociology of Sport, 27*(2), 151–162. https://doi.org/10.1177/101269029202700205
Macintosh, D., & Bedecki, T. (1988). *Sport and politics in Canada: Federal govenrment involvement since 1961*. Mcgill-Queen's Press.
Mankiw, N. G. (2019). *Macroeconomics* (10th ed.). Macmillan.
Meren, D. (2012). *With friends like these: Entangled nationalisms and the Canada-Quebec-France triangle, 1944–1970*. UBC Press.
Miller, T. (2012). A distorted playing field. In D. L. Andrews & M. L. Silk (Eds.), *Sport and neoliberalism* (pp. 23–37). Temple University Press. http://www.jstor.org/stable/j.ctt14bt86n.4
Mitchell, W., Wray, L. R., & Watts, M. (2016). *Modern monetary theory and practice: An introductory text*. Centre for full employment, University of Newcastle.

Murphy, R. (2019). Tax and modern monetary theory. *Real-World Economics Review, 89*(1), 138–147. https://rwer.wordpress.com/comments-on-rwer-issue-no-89/

Nauright, J., & Schimmel, K. S. (2005). *The political economy of sport*. Palgrave Macmillan.

Newman, J. I. (2014). Sport without management. *Journal of Sport Management, 28*(6), 603–615. https://doi.org/10.1123/jsm.2012-0159

Newman, J. I., & Bunds, K. S. (2016). Special issue foreword: On the political economy of amateur athletics. *Journal of Amateur Sport, 2*(1), 1–§§. https://doi.org/10.17161/jas.v2i1.5696

Newman, J. I., & Giardina, M. D. (2010). Neoliberalism's last lap? NASCAR Nation and the cultural politics of sport. *American Behavioral Scientist, 53*(10), 1511–1529. https://doi.org/10.1177/0002764210368082

OECD. (2021). *OECD Economic Outlook, Interim Report March 2021, Strengthening the recovery: The need for speed* (OECD Economic Outlook). OECD. https://doi.org/10.1787/34BFD999-EN

Papadopoulos, K. (2021). Greece records highest government debt to GDP ratio at more than 200%. *Greek City Times*. https://greekcitytimes.com/2021/08/02/greece-records-highest-government-debt-to-gdp-ratio-at-more-than-200/

Parnell, D., May, A., Widdop, P., Cope, E., & Bailey, R. (2018). Management strategies of non-profit community sport facilities in an era of austerity. *European Sport Management Quarterly, 19*(3), 312–330. https://doi.org/10.1080/16184742.2018.1523944

Rowe, D. (2004). *Sport, culture and the media: The unruly trinity*. McGraw-Hill Education.

Rowe, D. (2020). Subjecting pandemic sport to a sociological procedure. *Journal of Sociology*. https://doi.org/10.1177/1440783320941284

Sharma, D., Bouchaud, J.-P., Gualdi, S., Tarzia, M., & Zamponi, F. (2021). V–, U–, L– or W–shaped economic recovery after Covid-19: Insights from an Agent Based Model. *PLOS ONE, 16*(3), e0247823. https://doi.org/10.1371/JOURNAL.PONE.0247823

Sharpe, T. P., & Watts, M. (2013). Unconventional monetary policy in the UK: A modern money critique. *Economic Issues, 18*(2), 41–64.

Silk, M., & Andrews, D. L. (2012). Sport and the neoliberal conjuncture: Complicating the consensus. In D. L. Andrews & M. Silk (Eds.), *Sport and neoliberalism: Politics, consumption, and culture* (pp. 1–19). Temple University Press.

Silk, M., Francombe, J., & Andrews, D. L. (2014). Slowing the social sciences of sport: On the possibilities of physical culture. *Sport in Society, 17*(10), 1266–1289. https://doi.org/10.1080/17430437.2014.849649

Smith, R. (1999). Visible and invisible cultures of parliamentary ethics: The "sports rorts" affair revisited. *Australian Journal of Political Science, 34*(1), 47–62. https://doi.org/10.1080/10361149950452

Smyth, J. (2020). Covid blamed for Australia's largest budget deficit since the war. *Financial Times*. https://www.ft.com/content/73ccc06d-18f0-4d1e-95a0-79736f05556a

Stenling, C. (2013). The introduction of drive-in sport in community sport organizations as an example of organizational non-change. *Journal of Sport Management, 27*(6), 497–509. https://doi.org/10.1123/jsm.27.6.497

Stewart, B., Nicholson, M., Smith, A., & Westerbeek, H. (2004). *Australian sport: Better by design? The evolution of Australian sport policy*. Routledge.

Thatcher, M. (1983). *Speech to Conservative Party Conference*. https://www.margaretthatcher.org/document/105454

Thibault, L., & Harvey, J. T. (2013). The evolution of federal sport policy from 1960 to today. In L. Thibault & J. T. Harvey (Eds.), *Sport policy in Canada* (pp. 11–35). University of Ottawa Press.

Toomey, J. (2012). *Change You Can Really Believe In: The Obama Legacy of Broken Promises and Failed Policies*. AuthorHouse.

Wheelock, D. (2020). Comparing the COVID-19 recession with the great depression. *Economic Synopses, 39*. https://doi.org/10.20955/es.2020.39

Whitson, D., & Horne, J. (2006). Underestimated costs and overestimated benefits? Comparing the outcomes of sports mega-events in Canada and Japan. *Sociological Review, 54*(2_Suppl), 73–89. https://doi.org/10.1111/j.1467-954x.2006.00654.x

Widdop, P., King, N., Parnell, D., Cutts, D., & Millward, P. (2017). Austerity, policy and sport participation in England. *International Journal of Sport Policy and Politics, 10*(1), 7–24. https://doi.org/10.1080/19406940.2017.1348964

Yoon, L. (2019). *Mount Gariwang: An Olympic casualty—UBC Library Open Collections* [University of British Columbia]. https://open.library.ubc.ca/cIRcle/collections/ubctheses/24/items/1.0378394

Yoon, L. (2020). Understanding local residents' responses to the development of Mount Gariwang for the 2018 PyeongChang Winter Olympic and Paralympic Games. *Leisure Studies, 00*(00), 1–15. https://doi.org/10.1080/02614367.2020.1743741

Yoon, L., & Wilson, B. (2019). Journalism, environmental issues, and sport mega-events: A study of South Korean media coverage of the Mount Gariwang development for the 2018 PyeongChang Winter Olympic and Paralympic Games. *Communication and Sport, 7*(6), 699–728. https://doi.org/10.1177/2167479518811381

21

Furlough, Food Banks and Vaccine Hesitancy: Sport in Britain During the COVID-19 Pandemic

Jon Dart

Introduction

This chapter discusses sport in the UK during the first two years of the COVID-19 pandemic, focusing on the activities of sports fans, athletes, clubs, national governing bodies and the UK government. I explore the response of football fans to the announcement by some elite clubs that they would apply to the UK government's 'furlough' scheme and continue to pay the million-pound salaries of their star players while making their lowest paid staff redundant. I then consider the response of football fans to proposed Pay-Per-View (PPV) arrangements during the second national lockdown. The role of athletes in expressing their support for, or opposition to, the vaccination programme is also discussed. As in other workplaces the 'no jab, no job' scenario has made explicit the employee/employer relationship within professional sport and raises important questions on employment rights, individual human rights, and collective

J. Dart (✉)
Leeds Beckett University, Leeds, UK
e-mail: J.J.Dart@leedsbeckett.ac.uk

D. L. Andrews et al. (eds.), *Sport and Physical Culture in Global Pandemic Times*, Global Culture and Sport Series, https://doi.org/10.1007/978-3-031-14387-8_21

responsibility. Much of the discussion draws upon football (soccer) because the sport is omnipresent in British popular culture, often to the all-but-total exclusion of other sports and leisure activities. Soccer is the UK's richest and most popular sport with the global audience of the English Premier League (EPL) making it the UK's most recognised and popular global brand / icon (British Council, 2018).

In the first 18 months of the COVID-19 pandemic, the UK experienced very high death rates as well as high vaccination rates. The chapter adopts a materialist approach in which the economic conditions are seen as foundational to forming the social conditions. Employing a political economy focus, I discuss how responses to the pandemic show that capitalism will always seek to profit from a crisis. History is the organised actions of people and the social conditions, and while people are actively involved in creating their social environment, they enter existing arrangements of production. For Marx, historical developments and social processes emerge from concrete realities (realism), which necessitates using a materialist approach, which is used here to understand how social relationships are reflections of deeper economic mechanisms. Whilst not necessarily identifying themselves as Marxists, Beamish (1982), Boykoff (2013), Carrington and McDonald (2009), Collins (2013), Marqusee (1994), and Zirin (2005, 2008, 2010, 2013), have all shown how political economy and class relations are essential to an understanding of modern sport. More explicit Marxist critiques, in which competitive sport has few to no redeeming features, have been offered by Brohm (1978), Gruneau (1983), Hargreaves (1986), Hoch (1972), Lavalette (2013) and Pearlman (2012), the latter arguing that capitalism uses sport to flatten everything its path and who compares sport to a plague.

The Context

In the UK, at the beginning of March 2020, a full programme of football matches took place, as did five horse race meetings and a Six Nations Rugby match between England and Wales. In the days immediately prior to the UK's first national lockdown, two sporting events took place that were quickly described as 'super-spreader' events. Generating millions of pounds of revenue, the UEFA Champions League tie between Liverpool FC and Atlético Madrid (March 11th), drew a crowd of 52,000 people to Anfield, including 3000 fans who travelled from Madrid—despite that city being the epicentre of the COVID-19 outbreak in Spain, which had closed its schools two days earlier (Chadwick, 2015; Conn, 2020).

In the same week as the Liverpool-Atlético game, the four-day Cheltenham (horse racing) Festival took place (March 10th and 13th) with the 250,000 race-goers generating over £100m for the regional economy (University of Gloucester, 2016). Amid criticism at staging this event, the race organisers cited UK Prime Minster Johnson's contemporaneous attendance at an international rugby match as a reason *not* to cancel the event. Simultaneously, England's Chief Scientific Officer, Sir Patrick Vallance, said he was opposed to further restrictions and that 'our aim is to… build up some kind of herd immunity'; the UK government quickly changed their approach once they became aware of how many people would die before they reached 'herd immunity' (Stewart & Busby, 2020).

In an attempt to keep the economy 'alive' the government provided 'income' to workers (quickly termed 'furlough'). However, because this was only 80% of their wages, many workers could not afford to stay home if they had COVID-19; as a consequence, many were forced to continue working and thus spread the virus. One option available to national governments, as noted by Dave Zirin (2020), was to provide full wages, funded by a 'wealth tax' on those whose fortunes had increased during the pandemic. During the pandemic, the wealth of the world's richest 1% (including Jeff Bezos, Amazon; Elon Musk, Tesla; and Mark Zuckerberg, Meta), rose by trillions of dollars (i.e., ten to the twelfth power); at the same time the poorest in society grew poorer and more insecure. Despite attempts by central governments, the pandemic triggered high levels of layoffs, and whilst sections of the job market did begin to recover, along with a rise in global stock markets and house prices, the economic outlook has improved for the wealthiest, whilst worsening for the poorest and most precarious, nationally and globally (Rushe, 2021).

While statistical modelling might prove or disprove the wisdom in allowing these sporting events to take place, they show how the UK government were often 'behind the curve' and unwilling to take measures that would impact upon the economy (such as halting these two events, their slowness in 'locking down' and their eagerness to lift lockdowns). The decision to allow thousands of people from across the UK, and from abroad, to mingle, cheer and sing, is an example of the UK government's approach in the early stages of the pandemic. Before continuing, it might be useful to note the author's positionality in respect of the COVID-19 pandemic and vaccine. No-one has been untouched by this virus and as someone with immediate family members working on the frontline in the education system and NHS, I am fully supportive of the vaccination programme (and have been 'double-jabbed'); I did subsequently catch the virus, but fortunately, I was not significantly unwell.

Like many governments across the world, the UK's Conservative government were wholly unprepared for the pandemic. However, in 2016 senior health officials, having 'role-played' a large-scale outbreak, found the UK was unprepared in terms of PPE, a functioning contact tracing system and the ability to screen foreign travellers, and lacked guidelines on the prioritisation of specialist treatments (for example, oxygenation); the report also recommended setting up 'sleeping contracts' that would facilitate the rapid development of vaccine (Booth, 2021). Despite the mantras they were 'following the advice of the scientists' and they would 'stay home, protect the NHS', there were repeated breaches by politicians and advisors of their own guidelines (Allegretti, 2021; BBC News, 2020a; BBC News, 2020b). Repeated high-profile breaches constantly undermined what were intended to be clear messages on the importance of maintaining isolation rules, wearing masks, and adhering to guidelines on social distancing. Government ministers delayed implementing safety measures and instead prioritised the economy and profits before people's health. The wish to keep as many people as possible in work was seen in the government's decision to close schools too late and reopen them too soon; the motive was to keep parents in their workplaces and keep company profits flowing. In October 2020, Prime Minister Johnson was reported as saying he would prefer to 'let the bodies pile high in their thousands' rather than impose another lockdown' (Elgot & Booth, 2021). Public confidence was weakened by the government's tendency to make an announcement one day, only to reverse their decision twenty-four later. Aside from generating one of Europe's highest death tolls from the virus, public confidence was damaged by the failure of the Prime Minster to deliver a 'world beating test and trace system'. The government allocated £37 billion to the system, which was subsequently found to have made very little progress in minimising the impact of the pandemic. As the pandemic developed, more and more examples were reported of (self-) serving politicians lobbying on behalf of companies hoping to benefit from the pandemic. Contracts worth millions of pounds were found to have been 'awarded' to friends and supporters of the Conservative government. Throughout the pandemic, the British public were subjected to a government whose actions were incoherent and insincere.

The following timeline summarises key events since the COVID-19 virus was first identified at the end of 2019. The timeline presents some facts in an emerging world of alternative realities and post-truths. Timelines have become even more important given the emergence of those who seek to avoid debates based on objective facts (truths) and instead appeal to individual emotions and personal beliefs. Arguing for 'different interpretations', their intention is to draw attention away from key events (ranging from the purchase of faulty PPE, see Dyer, 2021, to the hosting of 'Christmas parties that were not parties' see Cowper, 2021). Naomi Klein (2007) has shown how capitalists will exploit crisis for personal enrichment and push through neo-liberal legislation with little scrutiny (see also Griffin, 2021; Miller, 2020). Mainstream media, with their rolling 24-hour news schedules, are complicit with their fetishization of 'breaking news' whilst silencing those events that are less obvious. This timeline helps in 'connecting the dots' and understanding when events took place and how they are related. This is necessary to call out those who advance alternative histories; we knew at the time what was happening and why.

Timeline

- 8th December 2019: First patient develops symptoms of Wuhan coronavirus.
- 31st December: China alerts the World Health Organisation about several pneumonia cases.
- 1st January 2020: Wuhan wholesale seafood market shuts down.

- 7th January: Identification of new virus, named COVID-19.
- 11th January: First death in China recorded.
- 13th January: First case outside China was reported in Thailand.
- 31st January: First two cases of COVID-19 are confirmed in the UK.
- 5th March: First UK death from COVID-19 confirmed.
- 10th March: start of four-day Cheltenham Festival (crowd 250,000+).
- 11th March: COVID-19 declared a pandemic by WHO. UEFA Champions League game between Liverpool and Atlético Madrid takes place in Liverpool (crowd c.52,000).
- 13th March: All football leagues in the UK suspended.
- 17th March: UEFA announces postponement of Euro 2020 (due to take place in the summer 2020) to summer 2021.
- 23rd March: All UK schools close.
- 24th March: IOC and Tokyo Organizing Committee of the Olympic and Paralympic Games (TOCOG) announce the 2020 Summer Olympics and Paralympics would be rescheduled.
- 26th March: Start of the first national lockdown in the UK.
- 1st April: Wimbledon cancelled (due to take place between 29 June and 12 July 2020.
- 4th April: The cancelled Grand National horse race was replaced by a virtual race.
- 5th May: UK surpasses Italy to become the country with the highest declared death toll in Europe with more than 32,000 deaths.
- 13th May: Lockdown relaxed to allow outdoor exercise with one other person from another household.
- 28th September: Global death toll exceeds 1 million.
- 5th November: Start of second lockdown in England.
- 2nd December: Second lockdown ends.
- 8th December: Margaret Keenan becomes first British person to receive a COVID-19 vaccine outside a clinical trial.
- December: UK vaccination programme begins.
- 6th January 2021: Start of third lockdown.
- 13th January: UK death toll exceeds 100,000 people (deaths within 28 days of a positive COVID-19 test).
- 11th June–11th July: the UEFA European Football Championship (Euro 2020) takes place in 11 cities across Europe.

- 21st June: All restrictions of social contact removed.
- July: Australia and New Zealand withdraw from Rugby League World Cup (set to be held in the UK in October), citing coronavirus concerns.
- November 2021: UK COVID-19 death toll:142,553.

Furlough

Responding to surging infection rates, on March 13th football's governing body, FIFA, advised that international matches should be postponed indefinitely. In a statement FIFA stated,

> To avoid any unnecessary health risks and also situations of potential sporting unfairness, we therefore recommend that all international matches previously scheduled to take place in March and April should now be postponed until such time that they can take place in a safe and secure environment, both for players and for the general public. The final decision on this issue rests with the respective competition organisers or relevant member association in case of friendlies. (FIFA, 2020)

On the same day, football authorities, including the FA and EPL began to suspend football activity across the country. Prioritising the health and welfare of players, staff and supporters, the English Premier League, the English Football League, the Women's Super League, and football in Wales was suspended until April. In Scotland all professional and grassroots football was suspended until further notice. Two weeks later the country entered its first national lockdown. Sport like other sectors in the economy, when the gates/ doors were closed, saw little to no revenue generation.

Those countries who could afford to, set up furlough payment schemes which were designed to avoid thousands of workers becoming unemployed and collapse national economies. In the UK, the 'Coronavirus Job Retention Scheme' (often shortened to 'furlough pay / scheme'), would pay the wages of workers who were unable to work due to coronavirus. The UK government began paying up to 80 per cent of the wages of those who could not work, or whose employers could no longer afford to pay them. Football fans reacted to the decision by some English Premier League (EPL) clubs to lay-off some of their staff, then to accept the UK government's 'furlough' payments, while continuing to pay the million-pound salaries of their star players. When it was launched, football clubs from all levels in the football pyramid began to apply to access the government's furlough scheme. While it was understandable that clubs outside the English Premier League (EPL) would seek to access the scheme, it was less clear why some of the world's richest sports clubs also applied. Premier League sides Tottenham Hotspur FC, Newcastle United FC, AFC Bournemouth and Norwich City FC were amongst the first to apply to access government funds (Guardian Sport, 2020). These clubs were seen as being able to afford to pay its staff from their own reserves and were subsequently accused of seeking to profit from the crisis.

Liverpool FC also announced they would apply to the furlough scheme to cover 80 per cent of their staff's wages whilst they would pay the remaining 20 per cent. Liverpool FC had intended to put around 200 non-playing staff on furlough, and that they would *consider* reimbursing any funding received at a later date (Hunter, 2020a; Liverpool Football Club, 2020). The club posted a pre-tax profit of £42m on an increased turnover of £533m for 2018–2019. In 2019, they paid £43.8m in agents' fees and had a £310m wage bill; by putting their staff on the furlough scheme, they stood to save up to £1.5m (Hunter, 2020b; Ingle, 2019). The decision by the owners of the seventh-richest football club in the world, Fenway Sports Group, to apply to the furlough scheme was met with disapproval by supporters, writers and fans of rival clubs. Many argued that in seeking to access state funds to pay their staff, the club was betraying its values, with some claiming this decision was damaging the club's reputation, values and weakening its claimed socialist ethos (This Is Anfield, 2020; Steinberg, 2020). When Tottenham Hotspur FC also sought to access the furlough scheme, its Supporters' Trust (THST) appealed to them to follow Liverpool's lead, and posted '*we have been saying consistently—pause and rethink. We are now saying it clearly and in public—do not further damage the Club's reputation, listen to your fans*' (in a tweet posted by THST, April 6, 2020). The negative publicity surrounding these events led to both clubs reversing their initial decisions and apologise to their supporters.

Some clubs who began to furlough some of their non-playing staff did not, initially, consider reducing their players' wages. In an attempt to deflect attention away from the UK government's mismanagement of the pandemic, its poorly-performing Health Secretary, Matt Hancock MP, questioned the clubs decision to accept furlough payments, and going further, invited football players to take a pay cut in the fight against coronavirus. The EPL's Chief Executive, Richard Masters, was asked by government minsters to 'take action' on player wages, with those clubs who were furloughing non-playing staff, but not imposing cuts on player wages, threatened by the introduction of a 'windfall tax' if they did not change their approach (BBC Sport, 2020a).

In response to calls for players to have their wages reduced, the Professional Footballers' Association (PFA), misjudging the public mood, stated that 'instances where clubs have the resources to pay all staff, the benefit of players paying non-playing staff salaries will only serve the business of the club's shareholders' (PFA, 2020). Away from the elite level, Roan (BBC Sport, 2020a) suggested that the PFA shift its focus to the dire situation in the lower leagues. While the chairmen of the wealthy EPL clubs did not anticipate how their fans would react to their decision to apply to the government's furlough scheme, a more long-standing issue is that most of the richest EPL clubs paid their workers 'minimum wage' before and throughout the pandemic. One waits to see if football fans are willing to organise around the issue of clubs paying their workers a living wage, especially those working at those clubs in London where the cost of living is much higher (BBC Sport, 2020b; Goldblatt, 2020; Hodges, 2015).

Pay-per-view Football and Food Banks

One of the most visible instances of fan disapproval was in response to proposed Pay-Per-View (PPV) arrangements for English Premier League (EPL) matches during the second national lockdown. During the first national lockdown the EPL's official broadcasters (Sky Sport, BT Sport and Amazon Prime) agreed to make all matches accessible to supporters when it restarted in June 2020; more than a third of EPL games were broadcast free-to-air on the BBC. Although recognising the positive public relations aspect of this arrangement, the EPL were frustrated at the 'free offering' of their valuable product.

During the second lockdown (5th November to 2nd December 2020) there were calls for the reintroduction of the free-to-air broadcast model that operated at the end of the first lockdown. However, the financial implications of the COVID-19 pandemic, and the fact that the EPL clubs were unable to allow fans to return to their stadia, both the clubs and broadcasters hoped to recoup some of the lost revenue by introducing a new PPV scheme that charged £14.95 ($20 US; €17.50) for each additional match. However, these 'extra' live games would not be part of customers' existing subscription packages. Football fans quickly worked out that the addition of 170 PPV games would cost them c.£3399 to watch all the available games (Marland, 2020). During the planning stage of the new PPV model, only one club, Leicester City FC, voted against the £14.95 charge.

The planned charge proposed by the clubs and broadcasters quickly backfired. The Football Supporters' Association called for the EPL to reconsider the PPV pricing model with fan-sites actively encouraging supporters not to watch the game and instead to find a free (or illegal) stream and/or to listen to the games on the radio (FSA, 2020). With the hashtag #BoycottPPV trending on social media, some activists suggested the £14.95 charge be donated to local food banks and charities (PA Media, 2020; Pope, 2020). As a result hundreds of thousands of pounds was given to food banks and local charities. In response to the fans activity, and recognising the public relations damage being done to the broadcasters (Sky Sports and BT Sport), and EPL brand, those proposing this scheme admitted the fee was too high (ESPN, 2020) and subsequently shelved their plans.

In addition to challenging the EPL's PPV plans, fans (and some clubs) were active in mitigating the effects of the pandemic in their local community by launching food banks, offering free tickets, and allowing club facilities to be used as vaccination sites. All levels of the football pyramid were involved including smaller clubs such as Whitehawk FC, Guernsey FC, Raith Rovers and Dulwich Hamlet, who through local activity raised funds for local food banks and mental health charities (Outside Write, 2020). Other clubs, including Motherwell (playing in the Scottish

Premiership) offered free tickets to NHS staff (Storey, 2020). The work of football fans in their communities was recognised by some Members of the UK Parliament who proposed:

> That this House pays tribute to the invaluable role played by football fans in supporting communities, frontline workers and protecting the most vulnerable people in the COVID-19 crisis; notes that more than 100 tonnes of food have been donated to local foodbanks since the start of lockdown by Fan Supporting Foodbanks groups from many football clubs including Manchester City, Manchester United, Newcastle United, West Ham United, Huddersfield Town, Everton and Liverpool. (EDM, 2021)

The MPs also noted that fans were working in conjunction with clubs to drop off care packages, ring elderly and vulnerable neighbours, and drop off medical prescription. The MPs statement concluded by noting that Scottish football fans had donated more than £1m to their clubs to help them survive during the COVID-19 pandemic.

On 19 November 2020, the UK government announced they would fund a £300m support scheme to some of those sports that were in financial difficulties because of the absence of spectators caused by the pandemic. While both Rugby League and Union clubs, along with the horse racing industry received support, cricket clubs and football clubs playing in the EPL and EFL did not receive any initial support from the government (BBC News, 2020c). Partly in response to the absence of government support, the following month the EPL and EFL launched a £250m support package for clubs in the lower leagues.

Beyond sport, the Covid-19 pandemic caused significant damage to the UK's arts, cultural and entertainment industries in terms of the infrastructure, institutions and workforce. The Coronavirus Job Retention Scheme and the Self-Employment Income Support Scheme acted as important, albeit temporary, lifelines to those unable to work in the creative and entertainment industries. Subsequently, the UK government, through its Department for Culture Media Digital and Sport (DCMS), announced a 'Culture Recovery Fund' which would provide £1.57 billion emergency funding to support the country's cultural, arts and heritage institutions (Hutton & Woodhouse, 2021).

Athletes Supporting the Vaccination Programme

Throughout the pandemic some athletes sought to use their high profile to 'make a difference'. As US sports journalist Dave Zirin (2020) commented they could do this by 'shaming the billionaire class to support their workers through the hardship of covid'. Zirin went on to suggest that athletes could raise awareness of the hardships caused by the pandemic, of the need for a vaccine, and the need to support in less fortunate positions. In the UK the COVID-19 virus was exposing and exacerbating existing inequalities (TUC, 2020). One of the clearest example of an athlete using their 'star power' for social change was the Manchester United F.C. player, Marcus Rashford, who embarrassed the government over the issue of child hunger during the school holidays when free school meals were not available (Richardson, 2020).

During the first few months of the pandemic, some football players offered to take a pay cut (ranging from 10 to 39 per cent), with others participating in a financial support scheme whereby they would donate a percentage of their wages to NHS frontline workers and charities, under the banner of #PlayersTogether (BBC Sport, 2020c). Clubs were active in their communities with ex-football players calling up fans who were isolating, along with supporting other activities in their communities. Notwithstanding the decision by Liverpool FC to apply for furlough wages for its low paid staff, the team manager, Jürgen Klopp, along with senior players that included Jordan Henderson, James Milner, Virgil van Dijk and Georginio Wijnaldum, advised the club's owners, Fenway Sport Group, they would accept a pay cut to ensure no-one at the club would be made redundant.

At the same time as some players and clubs were supporting efforts to mitigate the impact of the COVID-19 pandemic, there were some negative news reports of players (along with politicians and media personalities) who had broken the government's isolation guidelines / rules. There were calls for football clubs to enforce stronger punishments on those players who breached coronavirus protocols; when asked if football players were role models and should be held to a higher standard, Manchester

City FC manager Pep Guardiola disagreed, stating that 'I don't think footballers are more important than doctors, architects or teachers, so they only have the same responsibility as everyone else in the world' (BBC Sport, 2020d, 2021).

In March 2020 some of the country's leading sports stars did lend their support to the government's '*Stay at Home, Protect the NHS and Save Lives*' campaign. Sports stars also supported a government campaign which encouraged more people to volunteer at COVID-19 vaccination sites across the country, some of which were located at local sports grounds. Some individual athletes showed their support for the NHS, with clubs allowing their facilities to be used for medical use and as accommodation for NHS staff, as well as supporting the distribution of food and medicines in their communities. Several football stars (albeit ex-players) took part in a government campaign which promoted the NHS vaccination programme and urged people to 'get a jab' (UK Government, 2021). Prior to the pandemic, the manager of the English Men's national team, Gareth Southgate, was praised when he declared English players have a 'duty' to interact with the public on issues such as equality, inclusiveness and racial justice and that they would continue to 'take a knee' before matches (Parveen, 2021). In July 2021 Southgate joined a campaign to encourage people to have the vaccine. However, he later explained that he was not,

> going to get too involved in this because I was asked to do a video supporting the vaccination programme, which I thought was responsible, and of all the things that I've received abuse for over the summer, of which there's been several, that's probably the one I've received the most abuse over. So I'm probably going to keep out of that argument for the time being. (Quoted in Olley, 2021)

Vaccinated athletes might have been able to act as what health officials call 'trusted messengers' in the promotion of the vaccine (Du-Lieu & Grassi, 2021). Given that elite athletes are recognisable public figures and, as a consequence, are seen by many as role models (Leng & Phua, 2022), the UK government (via sport NGBs) could have encouraged athletes to act as 'influencers' and help ensure its citizens received accurate information and understand the importance of getting vaccinated. Using their celebrity status and social media platforms, they would be more likely to appeal to those demographics who might not engage with mainstream government campaigns on vaccine promotion. Because athletes are seen to be fit and healthy, they have significant leverage in the promotion of the vaccine in that if they were vaccinated, they could share experiences and help promote the societal benefits of everyone being vaccinated. While there was some individual support for the vaccination programme by a few high-profile sports stars, there was not a coordinated campaign that fully exploited the power of sporting stars. There was little in terms of vaccine promotion that could be compared to the activity that was seen around the Black Lives Matter movement, or the campaign led by Manchester United footballer, Marcus Rashford, on the issue of feeding hungry school students.

Vaccine Hesitancy

In this section I discuss the issue of vaccine-hesitancy amongst some athletes and why there was limited support amongst high-profile athletes for a national vaccination programme. While football managers, often older and in a higher risk group, were generally supportive of the vaccine, their players were much less vocal. One of the most vocal supporters of the vaccination was Liverpool's manager Jurgen Klopp who argued there was a social responsibility to be vaccinated, and that unless there was a medical reason, it over-rode any personal decision; he compared having the vaccine with citizens abiding by the speed limit, and not driving whilst under the influence of alcohol. However, many others, when asked about mandatory vaccines, added a caveat to their initial supporting response by stating that the decision to be vaccinated (or not) was a matter of individual choice.

Research by Rumsby (2021) highlighted a perception that many football players were simply too 'lazy' to get themselves vaccinated. Rumsby reported how a Chief Executive from a Championship club had got seven of his football players vaccinated by arranging for them to be immunised at their training ground (rather than relying on the players to arrange their own vaccination). The culture within dressing rooms was highlighted as a possible reason for vaccine-hesitancy (Rumsby, 2021). An argument was advanced that players did not want to cause any tension by going against the views of the more experienced players within a club. As a consequence, younger players were thought to be subjected to peer pressure with views on the vaccine contingent on whether the 'leaders' in the dressing room were pro- or anti- vax (Rushden, 2021). Sports changing/dressing rooms can act as an echo chamber, with the senior professionals often setting the tone and dynamic and influencing whether a club's vaccination rate was closer to 50 per cent or 100 per cent. Recognising the importance of targeting those with the most influence in football's dressing rooms, England's Deputy Chief Medical Officer, Professor Van-Tam, met with the captains of all 20 EPL teams in an attempt to counter the disinformation and the COVID-myths that were circulating, and on the importance of getting vaccinated. However, while the captains of the EPL teams were briefed, those in the second tier, the EFL, were not invited.

Most of the UK population were willing to receive a COVID-19 vaccine, albeit varying by social class, age and ethnicity, with only a small minority having no intention of getting vaccinated. While there has always been misinformation about vaccines since they were first developed by Jenner and Pasteur, anti-vaxxers misinformation did not make a significant impact in the UK. Rather than conspiracy and misinformation, there were some legitimate reasons for vaccine hesitancy within the general population: a lack of transport to vaccination centres, the limited opening hours of vaccination centres (especially for those working shifts, or multiple jobs), the lack of the right information in the right language, a lack of trust within some minority ethnic groups ('cultural memory') towards the medical establishment, and individuals not being registered with a GP (doctor) surgery, which acts as the main point of entry into the NHS. There were concerns over the high number of deaths from COVID-19 in some minority ethnic communities with a range of factors seen to be contributing to the high death rate (Butcher & Massey, 2020). Although specific minority communities are (under)represented in certain sports, it was significant when English cricketer, Moeen Ali, participated in a video promoting the importance of being vaccinated to Britain's South Asian communities (BBC News, 2021a).

In sport there was less public support for the anti-vax movement with very few athletes publicly stating their opposition to the vaccine. Globally, the anti-vaccine movement has sought to exploit the distrust of, and disengagement with, mainstream political structures. However, they were unable to find many athletes who were willing to publicly align themselves against the vaccine; even tennis player Novak Djokovic who did not get vaccinated, stated it was a matter of 'personal choice'. Vaccine hesitancy was more prevalent among the young who thought that being younger and healthier would enable them to manage the virus. Elite athletes have a 'strange' relationship with their bodies and are constantly required to be responsible for what they put into their mouths and arms. It was therefore little surprise that some alighted on the perceived lack of testing and that there were, potentially, unknown side-effects to the vaccine which might affect their performances, in addition to possible long-term effects. It might be noted that while athletes will often trust their medical team on most health-related issues, for unknown reason(s), some were less willing to trust the medical experts on the COVID-19 vaccination.

Some of those opposed to being vaccinated cited misinformation they had gleaned from their social media feeds. Typically, they would claim that the vaccine had not been sufficiently tested, and instead shared myths, including one that claimed that the vaccine would affect an individual's fertility and virility—despite there being no scientific evidence to support these untruths (Willingham, 2021). Although rare, there were some examples of footballers sharing their 'vaccine-hesitancy' and distrust of the government's vaccination programme. In September 2021, it was reported that some players had been sharing misinformation, via WhatsApp, with the head of the Players Football Association (Ziegler & Joyce, 2021). Everton's Fabien Delph republished a quote on his Instagram account that it was now a 'conspiracy theory to believe that the immune system is capable of doing the job it was designed to do'. A lower league player, Leon Legge (Port Vale FC), also shared anti-vaccine (dis) information on his social media platforms. Bristol City FC said they would educate their staff after one of their players, Nahki Wells, shared anti-vaccine information (Draper, 2021).

No Jab = No Job?

One emerging issue has been the clearer delineation of the relationship between clubs and their players, as employers and workers, and whether a club (as the employer) could mandate their athletes (as employees) to be vaccinated. As in other workplaces the prospect of 'no vaccine, no job' has generated a number of questions linked to employment rights, an individual's human rights, and collective responsibility.

All those working within the sports industry have a responsibility to ensure that their workplaces are safe for all staff and customers. Most workplaces needed to consider how to approach staff who were either vaccine-hesitant or out-right refused to be vaccinated. At the time of writing, employees in the health care sector who elected not to be vaccinated were being made redundant (Baynes, 2021). In an attempt to make their workplaces safe employers have used a combination of explanation, incentive, and encouragement to engage their vaccine-hesitant employees. For professional sports clubs and their staff, the prospect of not being able to travel will have motivated some of those who were vaccine-hesitant, with elite clubs needing all their players to be vaccinated in order to travel and compete in international events (and avoid having to quarantine before/after the competition). One of the clearest examples of this was shown in September 2021 during a FIFA World Cup qualifying game between Brazil and Argentina. The game was suspended after seven minutes when Brazilian health officials walked onto the pitch to protest at the presence of three British-based Argentinean players. The three players who had recently arrived from England had failed to follow the Brazilian COVID-19 guidance which required anyone who had recently been in the UK to quarantine upon arrival for a fortnight.

Football's global governing body, FIFA stated that it did not want any player to be prevented from participating in its 2022 World Cup finals tournament because of their (un)vaccinated status; FIFA's starting point was to look at alternatives to being fully vaccinated, including proof of recovery from COVID-19 or negative tests (Palmer, 2021). The influential football players trade union, the Professional Footballers Association, stated its support for the vaccination programme, but at the same time that it supported the right of its members to individually choose whether to be vaccinated; they concluded that they would not support any move to mandate its members to be vaccinated (Naylor, 2021).

The 'no jab, no job' refrain became increasingly common in 2021, but most employers, including professional football clubs, had not (yet) imposed mandatory vaccinations for their players. One option would be to require all staff to be vaccinated on 'health and safety grounds'—arguing that the well-being of a single player would be trumped by the well-being of the whole squad. Towards the end of 2021 several clubs had begun to explore whether they could make vaccination against COVID-19 a condition of employment. UK employment laws do not have any specific regulation that can require a worker to undergo medical treatment to ensure workplace safety; this means that mandatory vaccinations for players is (at the time of writing), 'unworkable' and that 'forcing an employee to get a vaccine takes away their autonomy to make decisions regarding their health and welfare' (Pasricha & Alexiou, 2021). It is recognised that there are some individuals who cannot safely have the vaccine due to a pre-existing health condition. Therefore, any attempt to mandate a vaccine could lead to claims of discrimination on the grounds of disability. Similarly, if the clubs, as employers, sought to make redundant an employee who refused to be vaccinated, they could face legal action on the grounds of unfair dismissal or constructive dismissal' (Pasricha & Alexiou, 2021). Mandatory vaccination is likely to prove the wrong approach; increasing vaccine uptake needs to be done through persuasion, not punishment, and investing the time and resources needed to offer better education to ensure people understand the risks, precautions and benefits.

Conclusion

The most effective advances in public health are often linked to the global vaccination programmes. Vaccines have significantly reduced the deaths from polio, diphtheria, smallpox, measles, mumps, rubella, and tetanus (Orenstein & Ahmed, 2017). The vaccines should not be seen as an affront to civil liberties but instead a routine part of modern life—essential for people to go to school, work, to travel and for the resumption of sport. Some athletes did speak up and promote the '*Stay at Home, Protect the NHS and Save Lives*' message and support the vaccination programme; others were either quiet or questioning. As Leng and Phua (2022) have noted, individual sports men and women will need to reflect on their role and responsibilities to society during the COVID-19 pandemic. More research is needed in understanding how effective they were in promoting positive social change, specifically on promoting vaccine adoption; this question can be extended to sports clubs and governing bodies: 'What did you do during the COVID-19 pandemic'?

The coronavirus pandemic brought into sharp relief the increasing disconnect and distrust between citizens and their governments. Prior to the pandemic there were already significant inequalities based on class, gender, and ethnicity (Jimenez-Martinez, 2021). In the UK, the COVID-19 pandemic arrived on the back of a 10-year government programme of austerity which devastated the health and social services across the UK (Widdop et al., 2018). During the 10 years of austerity, successive governments underfunded the NHS in an attempt to make privatisation seem the only practical option available to 'protect it'. The impact of COVID-19 on working class people became more evident as they lost their jobs and income, found their access to health care reduced, and rent / mortgage defaults leading to more evictions and homelessness. The Marxist adage of 'the rich getting richer' still applies given how the billionaires became trillionaires over the course of the pandemic.

The British government, wanting to keep the economy open, initially tried for 'herd immunity' but quickly abandoned this strategy and went on to make a succession of catastrophic errors. These failings included, but were not limited to, sending elderly hospital patients, known to be infected with the virus, into care homes; locking down too late and opening up too early; purchasing faulty PPE from family and friends (resurrecting claims of parliamentary sleaze, corruption, nepotism and cronyism, see Vidal, 2021). The government spent £37 billion on a 'track and trace' system, branded by Prime Minster Johnson as 'world beating and operated by NHS', but was neither; it was subsequently described by a Parliament spending watchdog as having 'no effect' in combatting COVID-19 infection levels (Tiggle, 2021). The government hoped that its vaccination programme would restore public confidence in those whose were responsible for causing the deaths of over 140,000 of its citizens.

This chapter has explored vaccine-hesitancy amongst professional athletes, but there is a more important discussion to be had about who is able to access the vaccine. The deep inequality surrounding the distribution of vaccines reflects a hierarchy of wealth and power. The wealthy western nations have controlled and restricted access to the vaccines, with the G7 countries offering boosters while many people in the Global South continue to wait for their first. Vaccines are produced for profit by 'big pharma' (Pfizer, BioNTech, Moderna), who have made billions of dollars of profits during the pandemic; these profits are justified on the basis that they are a necessary incentive to develop new drugs. Many countries in the Global South are reliant on the 'COVID-19 Strategic Preparedness and Response Program' (World Bank, 2021). Recognising that there is no such thing as 'herd immunity' in one country and that 'no-one is safe until everyone is safe', one immediate advance would be to remove the patents on the vaccines so that poorer countries could manufacture their own supplies.

Prior to the pandemic's arrival in the UK, and throughout the pandemic, people took to the streets to protest. They were driven by an array of often contradictory grievances, including calls to protect and expand the NHS, support for BLM and against racial injustice, opposition to restrictions on personal freedoms (and the compulsory use of masks in public), opposition to mandatory vaccination, and opposition to immigration. Towards the end of 2021, much of the public's attention had shifted to the climate crisis with protestors engaging in direct-action tactics, most notably Extinction Rebellion activists (BBC News, 2021b). At the time of writing there was no end in sight to the pandemic; it is too early to make a full assessment of the British government's mis-handling of the pandemic, and too early to rule out another surge in cases, particularly if a new strain/s develop that evade the current vaccines. We do not know to what extent COVID-19 will change sport, but we can expect the profit motive will be central to understanding what form the 'new normal' and 'building back better' will take.

References

Allegretti, A. (2021). Anger as Boris Johnson does not isolate after Staffer's positive covid test. *The Guardian*. https://www.theguardian.com/politics/2021/aug/06/boris-johnson-will-not-isolate-after-staffer-tests-positive-for-covid

Baynes, M. (2021). Thousands of care home staff to lose their jobs as mandatory COVID-19 vaccine deadline passes. *Sky News*. https://news.sky.com/story/thousands-of-care-home-staff-to-lose-their-jobs-as-mandatory-covid-19-vaccine-deadline-passes-12465668

BBC News. (2020a). Dominic Cummings: Did he break lockdown rules? *BBC News*. https://www.bbc.co.uk/news/uk-politics-52784290

BBC News. (2020b). Coronavirus: Prof Neil Ferguson quits government role after 'undermining' lockdown. *BBC News*. https://www.bbc.co.uk/news/uk-politics-52553229

BBC News. (2020c). Coronavirus-hit sports to benefit from £300m emergency funding rescue package. https://www.bbc.co.uk/sport/54998979

BBC News. (2021a). British Asian celebrities unite for video to dispel Covid vaccine. *BBC News*. https://www.bbc.co.uk/news/entertainment-arts-55809355

BBC News. (2021b). What is extinction rebellion and what does it want? *BBC News*. https://www.bbc.co.uk/news/uk-48607989

BBC Sport. (2020a). Coronavirus: Premier League players should take a pay cut—Matt Hancock. *BBC Sport*. https://www.bbc.co.uk/sport/football/52142267

BBC Sport. (2020b). Manchester clubs urged to pay staff 'real living wage'. *BBC Sport*. https://www.bbc.co.uk/news/uk-england-manchester-54847859

BBC Sport. (2020c). Leeds United staff volunteer for wage deferral because of coronavirus outbreak. *BBC Sport*. https://www.bbc.co.uk/sport/football/52048216

BBC Sport. (2020d). NHS: Premier League players' initiative to generate & distribute funds. https://www.bbc.co.uk/sport/football/52219771

BBC Sport. (2021). COVID-19 breaches: Football clubs 'need to be tougher'. *BBC Sport*. https://www.bbc.co.uk/sport/football/55523891

Beamish, R. (1982). The political economy of professional sport. In J. Harvey & H. Cantelon (Eds.), *Not just a game: Essays in Canadian sport* (pp. 141–158). University of Ottawa Press.

Booth, R. (2021). Coronavirus report warned of impact on UK four years before pandemic. *The Guardian*. https://www.theguardian.com/politics/2021/oct/07/coronavirus-report-warned-of-impact-on-uk-four-years-before-pandemic

Boykoff, J. (2013). *Celebration capitalism and the Olympic Games*. Routledge.

British Council. (2018). The Premier League of British icons. https://www.britishcouncil.org/research-policy-insight/insight-articles/premier-british-icons
Brohm, J.-M. (1978). *Sport a prison of measured time*. Ink Links.
Butcher, B., & Massey, J. (2020). Why are more people from BAME backgrounds dying from coronavirus? *BBC Reality Check*. https://www.bbc.co.uk/news/uk-52219070
Carrington, B., & McDonald, I. (Eds.). (2009). *Marxism, cultural studies and sport*. Routledge.
Chadwick, S. (2015). Hard Evidence: How much is the Champions League worth? *The Conversation*. https://theconversation.com/hard-evidence-how-much-is-the-champions-league-worth-42376
Collins, T. (2013). *Sport in capitalist society*. Routledge.
Conn, D. (2020). It was wrong to play against Atlético, says Liverpool's public health director. *The Guardian*. https://www.theguardian.com/football/2020/apr/02/wrong-to-play-liverpool-v-atletico-says-citys-public-health-director-matthew-ashton
Cowper, A. (2021). When is a Christmas party not a Christmas party? When it's in Downing Street. *BMJ, 375*, bn3056.
Draper, R. (2021). Premier League players will NOT be forced to have a Covid-19 jab amid fears an outbreak could lead to the season unravelling. *Daily Mail Online*. https://www.dailymail.co.uk/sport/football/article-9872655/Vaccine-refusal-ruin-footballs-return-majority-players-not-jabbed.html
Du-Lieu, L., & Grassi, A. (2021). COVID vaccine: Celebrity endorsements work—Even if people don't like it. *The Conversation*. https://theconversation.com/covid-vaccine-celebrity-endorsements-work-even-if-people-dont-like-it-151130
Dyer, C. (2021). Covid-19: Government wasted millions on poor quality ppe, spending watchdog finds. *BMJ, 372*, bn399.
EDM. (2021). Support of football fans for communities during the Covid-19 outbreak. *EDM* (Early Day Motion) 714: Tabled on 13 July 2020. https://edm.parliament.uk/early-day-motion/57241/support-of-football-fans-for-communities-during-the-covid19-outbreak
Elgot, J., & Booth, R. (2021). Pressure mounts on Johnson over alleged 'let the bodies pile high' remarks. *The Guardian*. https://www.theguardian.com/politics/2021/apr/26/pressure-mounts-on-boris-johnson-over-alleged-let-the-bodies-pile-high-remarks

ESPN. (2020). Premier League backing off pay-per-view plans, says CEO Masters. *ESPN*. https://www.espn.co.uk/football/english-premier-league/story/4231733/premier-league-backing-off-pay-per-view-planssays-ceo-masters

FIFA. (2020). FIFA statement. https://www.fifa.com/about-fifa/organisation/media-releases/fifa-statement-x8681

FSA. (2020). Top-flight fans message to Premier League: "Let us watch our teams!" https://thefsa.org.uk/news/top-flight-fans-message-to-premier-league-let-us-watch-our-teams/

Goldblatt, D. (2020). Football clubs must pay staff the living wage. *The Guardian*. https://www.theguardian.com/football/2020/feb/11/football-clubs-must-pay-staff-the-living-wage

Griffin, J. (2021). UK introducing three laws that threaten human rights, says UN expert. *The Guardian*. https://www.theguardian.com/law/2021/jun/24/uk-introducing-three-laws-that-threaten-human-rights-says-un-expert

Gruneau, R. (1983). *Class, sports and social development*. University of Massachusetts Press.

Guardian Sport. (2020). Pay cuts, furlough or deferrals: What are the Premier League clubs doing? *The Guardian*. https://www.theguardian.com/football/2020/apr/02/pay-cuts-furlough-or-deferrals-what-are-the-premier-league-clubs-doing

Hargreaves, J. (1986). *Sport, culture and ideology*. Polity.

Hoch, P. (1972). *Rip off the big game*. Doubleday.

Hodges, C. (2015). Jeremy Corbyn with football fans protesting for workers to earn the living wage. *The Mirror*. https://www.mirror.co.uk/sport/gallery/jeremy-corbyn-football-fans-protesting-6793328

Hunter, A. (2020a). Liverpool under fire for furloughs while PFA points to pay-cut tax trap. *The Guardian*. https://www.theguardian.com/football/2020/apr/04/liverpool-become-latest-premier-league-club-to-furlough-non-playing-staff

Hunter, A. (2020b). Liverpool announce £42m pre-tax profit despite record £223m spend on players. *The Guardian*. https://www.theguardian.com/football/2020/feb/27/liverpool-42m-pre-tax-profit-record-223m-spend-on-players-financial-year-2018-19

Hutton, G., & Woodhouse, J. (2021). *Covid-19 and the arts and culture sectors Research Briefing*. House of Commons Library. https://commonslibrary.parliament.uk/research-briefings/cbp-9018/

Ingle, S. (2019). Liverpool paid agents £43.8m in last year—£17m more than next rival. *The Guardian*. https://www.theguardian.com/football/2019/apr/04/liverpool-paid-43m-agents-spurs-113m-profit-record

Jimenez-Martinez, J. (2021). The public as a problem: Protest, public diplomacy and the pandemic. *Place Branding and Public Diplomacy*. https://doi.org/10.1057/s41254-021-00235-1; https://www.thenation.com/article/society/coronavirus-athletes/

Klein, N. (2007). *The shock doctrine: The rise of disaster capitalism*. Penguin.

Lavalette, M. (2013). *Capitalism and sport: Politics, protest, people and play*. Bookmarks.

Leng, H. K., & Phua, Y. X. P. (2022). Athletes as role models during the COVID-19 pandemic. *Managing Sport and Leisure, 27*(1-2), 163-167. https://doi.org/10.1080/23750472.2020.1762330

Liverpool Football Club. (2020). A letter from Peter Moore to Liverpool supporters. https://www.liverpoolfc.com/news/announcements/392368-a-letter-from-peter-moore-to-liverpool-supporters

Marland, D. (2020). Premier League are under pressure to cancel pay-per-view football during second England lockdown. *Sport Bible*. https://www.sportbible.com/football/football-news-premier-league-are-under-pressure-to-cancel-pay-per-view-football-20201102

Marqusee, M. (1994). *Anyone but England: Cricket and the national malaise*. Verso.

Miller, G. (2020). Boris Johnson is using the Covid crisis as a pretext for a power grab. *The Guardian*. https://www.theguardian.com/commentisfree/2020/oct/07/boris-johnson-covid-power-grab

Naylor, A. (2021). Explained: The Premier League and compulsory Covid-19 vaccinations. *The Athletic*. https://theathletic.com/2722921/2021/07/23/explained-the-premier-league-and-compulsory-covid-19-vaccinations/

Olley, J. (2021). England Boss Gareth Southgate reveals abuse over Covid-19 Vaccine Push. *ESPN*. https://www.espn.co.uk/football/england-eng/story/4462548/england-boss-gareth-southgate-reveals-abuse-over-covid-19-vaccine-push

Orenstein, W., & Ahmed, R. (2017). Simply put: Vaccination saves lives. *Proceedings of the National Academy of Sciences of the United States of America, 114*(16), 4031–4033. https://doi.org/10.1073/pnas.1704507114

Outside Write. (2020). Progressive football: Whitehawk FC. *Outside Write*. https://outsidewrite.co.uk/progressive-football-whitehawk-fc/

PA Media. (2020). Newcastle fans boycott pay-per-view and donate fees to local food bank. *The Guardian*. https://www.theguardian.com/football/2020/oct/19/newcastle-fans-boycott-pay-per-view-and-donate-fees-to-local-food-bank

Palmer, D. (2021). Qatar could ban players who are not fully vaccinated from 2022 FIFA World Cup. *Inside the Games*. https://www.insidethegames.biz/articles/1113261/qatar-fifa-world-cup-2022-vacciantions

Parveen, N. (2021). 'Southgate's team represents real England': Three Lions unite country. *The Guardian*. https://www.theguardian.com/world/2021/jul/09/southgates-team-represents-real-england-three-lions-unites-country

Pasricha, M., & Alexiou, J. (2021). COVID-19 vaccinations—What can clubs offer or enforce—Navigating through the minefield? *Mackrell Solicitors*. https://www.mackrell.com/press-releases/covid-19-vaccinations-what-can-clubs-offer-or-enforce-navigating-through-the-minefield/

Pearlman, M. (2012). *Barbaric sport: A global plague*. Verso.

PFA. (2020). @PFA Twitter. 2 April 2020. https://twitter.com/pfa/status/1245784987246497795

Pope, C. (2020). Premier League fans raise hundreds of thousands of pounds for food banks in pay-per-view boycott–here's what every club is doing. *FourFourTwo*. https://www.fourfourtwo.com/features/premier-league-fans-pay-per-view-boycott-charity-food-bank-fundraising

Richardson, H. (2020). Marcus Rashford welcomes school holiday support climbdown. *BBC News*. https://www.bbc.co.uk/news/education-54841316

Rumsby, B. (2021). Why are some footballers not getting vaccinated against Covid? *Telegraph Sport*. https://www.telegraph.co.uk/football/2021/09/02/footballers-not-getting-vaccinated-against-covid/

Rushden, M. (2021). Unvaccinated footballers are putting lives at risk. Is it time to stop picking them? *The Guardian*. https://www.theguardian.com/sport/blog/2021/oct/07/unvaccinated-footballers-putting-lives-at-risk-maybe-its-time-to-stop-picking-them-covid

Rushe, D. (2021). The richest Americans became 40% richer during the pandemic. *The Guardian*. https://www.theguardian.com/media/2021/oct/05/richest-americans-became-richer-during-pandemic

Steinberg, J. (2020). Liverpool challenged by Spirit of Shankly fan group over staff furlough. *The Guardian*. https://www.theguardian.com/football/2020/apr/05/liverpool-challenged-by-spirit-of-shankly-fan-group-over-staff-furloughs

Stewart, H., & Busby, M. (2020). Coronavirus: Science chief defends UK plan from criticism. *The Guardian*. https://www.theguardian.com/world/2020/mar/13/coronavirus-science-chief-defends-uk-measures-criticism-herd-immunity

Storey, D. (2020). Motherwell and their free season tickets: A community club like no other. https://inews.co.uk/sport/football/motherwell-free-season-tickets-scottish-football-1157169

T.U.C. (2020). The new class divide—How Covid-19 exposed and exacerbated workplace inequality in the UK. https://www.tuc.org.uk/blogs/new-class-divide-how-covid-19-exposed-and-exacerbated-workplace-inequality-uk

This Is Anfield. (2020). Liverpool reverse decision to furlough staff. https://www.thisisanfield.com/2020/04/liverpool-reverse-decision-to-furlough-staff/

THST. (April 6, 2020). Tottenham Hotspur Supporters' Trust. https://twitter.com/THSTOfficial/status/1247238005997346821

Tiggle, N. (2021). Covid-19: NHS test and trace 'no clear impact' despite £37bn budget. *BBC News*. https://www.bbc.co.uk/news/health-56340831

UK Government. (2021). *Football stars hail Covid-19 vaccine as the 'best defence' of 2021*. GOV.UK. https://www.gov.uk/government/news/football-stars-hail-covid-19-vaccine-as-the-best-defence-of-2021

University of Gloucester. (2016). The festival—Worth over £100m to the Gloucestershire economy. https://www.glos.ac.uk/content/festival-worth-over-100m/

Vidal, J. (2021). 'If You Wanted to Design a Virus Dispersion Hub, You Could Do Worse': The Cheltenham festival, one year on. *The Guardian*. https://www.theguardian.com/world/2021/feb/20/virus-dispersion-hub-packed-racecourse-cheltenham-festival

Widdop, P., King, N., Parnell, D., Cutts, D., & Millward, P. (2018). Austerity, policy and sport participation in England. *International Journal of Sport Policy and Politics, 10*(1), 7–24. https://doi.org/10.1080/19406940.2017.1348964

Willingham, E. (2021). COVID-19 vaccines show no signs of harming fertility or sexual function. *Scientific American*. https://www.scientificamerican.com/article/covid-vaccines-show-no-signs-of-harming-fertility-or-sexual-function/

World Bank. (2021). World Bank group's operational response to COVID-19 (coronavirus)—Projects list. https://www.worldbank.org/en/about/what-we-do/brief/world-bank-group-operational-response-covid-19-coronavirus-projects-list

Ziegler, M., & Joyce, P. (2021). Premier League players told to ignore anti-vaccination 'myths and lies' by PFA chief executive Maheta Molango. *The Times*. https://www.thetimes.co.uk/article/premier-league-players-told-to-ignore-anti-vaccination-myths-and-lies-by-pfa-chief-executive-maheta-molango-gmcxnzr0c

Zirin, D. (2005). *What's my name, fool? Sports and resistance in the United States*. Haymarket.

Zirin, D. (2008). *People's history of sports in the United States; 250 years of politics, protest, people, and play*. New Press.

Zirin, D. (2010). *Bad sports: How owners are ruining the games we love*. Scribner.

Zirin, D. (2013). *Game over: How politics has turned the sports world upside down*. The New Press.

Zirin, D. (2020). Athlete activists respond to the coronavirus pandemic. *The Nation*. https://www.thenation.com/article/society/coronavirus-athletes/

22

COVID-19, the Anthropocene, and the Need for Post-Sport

Samuel M. Clevenger, Oliver J. C. Rick, and Jacob J. Bustad

The COVID-19 pandemic, in all its needless horrors and historical significance, has provided further evidence that global society is embroiled in a calamitous moment marked by the deleterious consequences of unrestrained, capital-seeking, biosphere-degrading human and corporate activities. The origins of COVID-19 and other "emerging diseases with pandemic potential," according to scholar Li Zhang, lay in the "complex entanglements of state-making, science and technology, and global capitalism" (2021, p. 3), particularly the "specific political ecologies of capitalist agribusiness" that have increased the risk of viral transmission between humans and wildlife in the name of development and capital accumulation (p. 5). Diseases with "pandemic potential" existed and circulated well before what the British historian Eric Hobsbawm once called "the age of

S. M. Clevenger (✉) • J. J. Bustad
Towson University, Towson, MD, USA
e-mail: sclevenger@towson.edu

O. J. C. Rick
Springfield College, Springfield, MA, USA

D. L. Andrews et al. (eds.), *Sport and Physical Culture in Global Pandemic Times*, Global Culture and Sport Series, https://doi.org/10.1007/978-3-031-14387-8_22

capital" (1996), but the continued and accelerating anthropogenic destruction of the environment and wildlife habitats is increasing the frequency of potential pandemics and creating what researchers are calling "novel opportunities" for more widespread, dangerous viral transmission between species (Carlson et al., 2022; Wallace et al., 2020). Deadly pathogens arise from conditions shaped by a multitude of factors, processes, and biological-cultural entanglements. However, the changing and degrading of land and sea habitats due to global capitalist activity is accelerating the evolution and dispersal of deadly pathogens, creating new pathways of transmission and fueling more infectious, more dangerous variants (Wallace, 2016, p. 12). As the scholar Mike Davis noted, the global circulation of capital, tourism, agribusiness, and urban development are "[h]uman-induced environmental shocks" that are facilitating the degradation of planetary ecosystems and the growth in range and quantity of dangerous, highly mutable pathogens like COVID-19 (2005, p. 8).

Despite its dramatic and horrific demonstration of the deleterious consequences of anthropogenic, globalized economic activity, the pandemic has not ushered in a rethinking of the various interdependent industries of the capitalist world-system, including the global sport industry. Scholars and researchers continue to underscore that the anthropogenic aspects of the global sport industry and the ways it is actively contributing to the degradation of the planet, the disruption and displacement of wildlife, and the circulation of pathogens (Cardazzi et al., 2020; Gibson, 2020; McCullough & Kellison, 2018; Wilson & Millington, 2020). Though there was a brief, fleeting suspension of live sporting events and an open questioning of whether sports would return in their pre-pandemic forms during the early months of the pandemic (Leitch, 2020), we are now witness to a renewed, hyper-capitalist sport industry dictated by the endless pursuit of economic growth, market expansion, and profit maximization. Despite disruptions due to the pandemic and the suspension of live events, the global sport industry remains dominated by and dependent on highly corporatized, commercialized, consumer-, media-, and celebrity-driven, carbon-emitting professional and elite sporting spectacles (Andrews, 2019). When all levels of sporting organizations adjusted and continued their business activities during the initial waves of the pandemic, the adjustments were business-oriented, rationalized strategies to re-align events and operations to the pandemic-shaping conditions without disrupting their focus on the generation of revenue and the consumption of sporting commodities. The International Olympic Committee (IOC) promoted the 2020 Games in Tokyo as an opportunity to showcase the role of sport in building sustainable societies (International Olympic Committee, 2021), even as the hyper-commercial, growth-oriented spectacle enflamed environmental, social, epidemiological, and political crises within Japan (Boykoff & Gaffney, 2020). When the National Basketball Association (NBA) and Ultimate Fighting Championship (UFC) decided to relocate their regular-season games and contests to self-contained, bio-secure "bubbles" in 2020, this constituted an attempt to maintain their pre-pandemic business commitments and relationships with corporate sponsors and media partners through a circumventing of travel restrictions and strict testing and quarantine protocols (Beer, 2020; Reuters, 2020). Meanwhile, the National Football League (NFL) and National Collegiate Athletic Association (NCAA) recklessly decided to continue with their fall 2020 football schedules despite the onslaught of the pandemic, transparently demonstrating the organizations' prioritizing of capital over human welfare (Kalman-Lamb et al., 2020; Seifert, 2020).

It is a problem that the dominant, neoliberal capitalist forms of organized sport have been reinforced and re-articulated by corporate and commercial sporting organizations, particularly when we situate industry activities within the anthropogenic crisis that urgently requires a drastic reduction of human activity and a careful consideration of human and more-than-human entanglements,. If human society is to envision and build alternative physical cultural forms and practices capable of promoting more sustainable relations between humans, more-than-humans, and environments—including relations that require a restriction or reduction in human physical activities—perhaps this compels scholars and researchers to engage in some healthy skepticism of the sustainability of the sport industry as we know it. In addition to critically examining, analyzing, and critique sporting contexts, perhaps we need to engage in the thought experiment of asking what is "*after* sport" and what an "after sport" might, and should, entail. Questioning the future of sport can complement contemporary "new materialist" scholarship on the ways in which the material, environmental, and more-than-human are never simply subjugated and objectified by human activity but are always enmeshed in complex interactions and networks with the cultural and the physical (Newman et al., 2020). It also can complement approaching sports as contested, dynamic cultural phenomena, revealing how sporting iterations such as popular and emerging "lifestyle" sports, presenting alternative practices, experiences, and identities, can potentially challenge "traditional ways of 'seeing', 'doing' and understanding sport" (Wheaton, 2013, p. 1). The pressing, multivariate, and calamitous pressures of global environmental change demand that we both continue to challenge and complicate what is occurring within sporting contexts *and* expand our imaginative horizons for the possibility of new, ecological, democratic, pleasurably limiting physical cultures.

As part of an initial attempt to engage in such a thought experiment, the goal of the present chapter is twofold. First, we suggest that the re-permutation of the sport industry following the initial suspension of live sporting events in 2020 highlights the glaring contradiction between the growth- and achievement-driven dictates of the dominant athletic, capitalist sports models and the necessary limitations to human activity required to live sustainability in the epoch of the Anthropocene (Bonneuil & Fressoz, 2016). If we "already live in the Anthropocene" and must "get used to this ugly word and the reality it names" (p. 8), we must also be critical of what is going on within sport in the Anthropocene *and* come to terms with its limitations as a way of conceptualizing physical-material-cultural practices. We must ponder the possibility of life after sport, if only to become more aware of the necessary limits of our sporting present and expand our imaginative horizons of the physical cultural. Second, the chapter engages with the late scholar Brian Pronger's (1998) concept of "post-sport," exploring its utility as a conceptual tool for identifying and valorizing embodied practices that, to borrow Pronger's words, potentially counterpose modern sport's "aggressive socio-cultural resourcing of the body" (p. 291). By revisiting Pronger's work on post-sport and the work of scholars and researchers who have also engaged with post-sport physical cultures, the chapter contends that the concept of post-sport emphasizes the transgressive and liberatory elements of physical culture and energizes its relevance for our current, pressing concerns.

Post-sport offers not only a conceptual pathway to re-envisaging sports as sites of "joyful energy" (Newman, 2014), but a way of contemplating the possibility that our physical cultural futures in the Anthropocene may need to include embracing the pleasurable limits of non-sporting and "idle" practices.

Sport and the Anthropocene

We did not need COVID-19 to expose the ways in which human-centered activities and actions are causing widespread planetary disruptions and degrading its finite resources. As early as 1700s C.E., scientists and thinkers were already contemplating the possibility that human-led historical processes, notably the industrial revolution, had transformed human society into a geological force (Lewis & Maslin, 2015). In the 1820s, the French philosopher Henri de Saint-Simon pointed to industrialization as the catalyst of a new historical epoch defined by the anthropogenic destruction of the planet. Saint-Simon warned that the "object" of the industrial revolution and its self-interested entrepreneurs was "the exploitation of the globe … the appropriation of its products for the needs of man; and by accomplishing this task, it modifies the globe and transforms it" (quoted in Bonneuil & Fressoz, 2016, p. 8). According to Marxist scholar John Bellamy Foster, Karl Marx observed in the mid-nineteenth century that the growth of both "large-scale industry and large-scale agriculture under capitalism" was contributing to a "rift" in what he called the "metabolic interaction between man [sic] and the earth" and "robbing" the soil of the elements necessary to restore itself (2000, p. 156). A few years prior to the arrival of COVID-19, the philosopher and critical theorist McKenzie Wark (2015) wrote that global society had arrived at the "the end of pre-history," meaning the end of a theologically-informed worldview that posits we live amidst a global ecology that is "self-correcting, self-balancing and self-healing" (p. 9). The pandemic merely added further emphasis to the realization, already established by an untold number of philosophers, researchers, writers, and observers, that there are not enough resources on Earth to sustain the activities of all nations and corporations (Latour, 2018). The limitations of the planet, Wark writes, are "really coming to bear on the ever-expanding universe of the commodification of everything" (2015, p. 9).

In 1992, the Russian geologist Aleksei Pavlov was reportedly the first to specifically use the neologism "Anthropocene" to classify a new geological epoch of anthropogenic change (Lewis & Maslin, 2015, p. 173). The atmospheric chemist Paul Crutzen and the biologist Eugene Stoermer are credited with using the term to designate the end of the Holocene, a geological epoch of 11,700 years, and the beginning of an "Anthropocene" in which "mankind[sic] had become a force of telluric amplitude" (Bonneuil & Fressoz, 2016, p. 13; Demos, 2017, p. 7). The warming of the Earth due to the enrichment of the atmosphere with carbon dioxide, nitrous oxide, methane, and other "greenhouse gases," the acidification of the oceans, the breaking down of the planet's biosphere and the biodiversity of its habitats and ecosystems, and the disruption of the global water and nitrogen cycles can be linked to the human-centered historical processes of industrialization and urbanization, including the extraction and burning of fossil fuels and the "unprecedented upsurge in energy mobilization" since industrialization (Bonneuil & Fressoz, 2016, p. 18). While the degree to which humans have impacted the planet has been the subject of ongoing research in various fields of study, there is an increasingly accepted general notion across fields that the practices and movements of human beings has a primarily deleterious effect on the environment. Following Heyd (2021), "we are increasingly finding that activities that at first seem innocuous, such as heating our homes, travelling to our places of work and leisure, industrially exploiting resources to supply ourselves with useful products … cumulatively are having global and long-lasting effects" (p. 23), resulting in the present existential crisis for human and more-than-human wellbeing (Chakrabarty, 2021). Scientists and researchers continue to debate the originating event(s) that ushered in an epoch of human dominance, noting both the advent of the industrial revolution, with its ties to greenhouse gas emissions, urbanization, and the modern capitalist world-system, and the arrival of Europeans in the Americas in 1492 C.E., a key moment in the advent of Western colonialism, the genocide, enslavement, and imperial conquest of non-Western peoples, and the "massive rearrangement of life on [E]arth" that resulted (Demos, 2017, p. 8), as possible starting points for the Anthropocene epoch. If we view the arrival of COVID-19 from the standpoint of the Anthropocene, the pandemic is less a singular biological and cultural phenomenon than characteristic of a contemporaneous historical and geological epoch defined by the disruption of wildlife habitats, ecosystems, and the consequent transformation of interactions between human and non-human species, including the transmission of infectious diseases (O'Callaghan-Gordo & Antó, 2020).

As a term for describing our present condition, the Anthropocene is contested and by no means universally accepted. Numerous scholars and writers point to its problematic "reinforcement of anthropocentric actionable worldview that generated 'the Anthropocene'—with all its looming emergencies—in the first place" (Crist, 2016, p. 1). Eileen Crist contends that the discourse on the Anthropocene too often results in a kind of "Promethean self-portrait" that presents homo sapiens as "an ingenious if unruly species, distinguishing itself from the background of merely-living life, rising so as to earn itself a separate name … and whose unstoppable and in many ways glorious history … has yielded an 'I' on a par with Nature's own tremendous forces" (p. 4). The term, in effect, serves to naturalize the dominance of human society over the Earth and its multitude of inhabitants, bestowing the species with god-like powers to direct the course of geological time. The only recourse to avoid catastrophe "lies in humanity embracing a managerial mindset and active stewardship of earth's natural systems" (p. 2). Historian Jason W. Moore (2017) argues that the dominant rendition of the Anthropocene represents a "comforting story with uncomfortable facts," in that the story rests on a "Nature/Society" dualism that presupposes human society as first separate from, and now impacting, "Nature" (p. 2). Thus, the Anthropocene recapitulates what Moore (2016) calls "capitalism's either/or organization of reality" (p. xv), limiting its ability to offer to conceptual pathways out of the logical frameworks of capitalist development. Moore offers an alternative: the Capitalocene, which, according to scholar T.J. Demos, "foregrounds how capitalism evolved within and against nature's web of life, as well as brought ecological transformations to it" (2017, p. 86). As an alternative to the Anthropocene, Moore's Capitalocene places responsibility for the disruption of the planet's ecological systems and cycles on the modern capitalist world-system, its corresponding and unsustainable processes of expansive commodification, resource extraction, labor exploitation, and unquenchable consumption, and its profiting from imperialist conquest, colonization, and military conflict. Philosopher Donna Haraway (2016) also critiques Anthropocene discourse, writing that it is "not simply wrong-headed and wrong-hearted in itself; it saps our capacity for imagining and caring for other worlds, both those that precariously exist now … as well as those we need to bring into being in alliance with other critters, for still possible recuperating pasts, presents, and futures" (p. 50). Haraway offers a third term that extends from the Capitalocene: Chthulucene, a multi-species emphasis on the "stories and practices of becoming-with in times that remain at stake, in precarious times, in which the world is not finished and the sky has not fallen—yet" (p. 57). The compelling critiques offered by the Capitalocene and Chthulucene underscore that the Anthropocene has raised important questions as to the future of human activities that contribute to the disruption and degradation of the planet.

This discussion of the Anthropocene, Capitalocene, and Chthulucene unsettles and necessarily complicates preexisting historical narratives on the origins of modern sporting forms. First, by engaging with the idea that the origins of anthropogenic environmental change are tied up in the processes of a capitalist world-system that is within, not separate from, nature's web of life, we can see (perhaps unintentionally) an anthropocentric framing in the historical contention that modern sports were "initially a product of the British industrial revolution" (Cronin, 2014, p. 30; Collins, 2013). Such narratives, by their very design, tend to present the modernization and rationalization of sporting forms as an outgrowth of historical developments endemic to human-centered activity (the advent and codification of rules, the commodification and rationalization of preexisting games and contests)—and, as a result, rely on a similar "Nature/Society" dualism noted previously with Anthropocene discourses. Thus, historical accounts of the links between modern sports and notions of human desires for "control" of "mastery"—for example, historian Tony Collins contends that games "developed from humanity's efforts to master nature and sustain life" (2013, p. 1)—can be re-read as an anthropocentric understanding of organized physical culture that reifies capitalism's dualist logic and need to valorize human mastery over a nonhuman nature. The crisis of the Anthropocene and the dangers it poses to all forms of planetary life means that it is perhaps no longer enough to link the history of modern sporting forms to modes of capitalist production and their socially-sanctioned boundaries. If historical narratives on modern sport are to serve as resources for imagining post-capitalist sporting cultures, this may require that we, to misquote Moore (2015), understand how "the mosaic of relations that we call capitalism [and sport] work *through* nature; and how nature works *through* that more limited zone, capitalism [and sport]" (p. 11).

Contemporaneously, the Anthropocene exposes the unsustainable orientation and drive for economic growth within capitalist sporting organizations. This problem extends from the ideological operations of the global sport industry as what Andrews (2019) terms "a multi-faceted agent of macro-political reproduction" (p. 4). The ongoing marketization, corporate structuring, and commercialization of sport stems from an industry logic based on relentlessly pursuing the accumulation of capital and the multiplication of consumer opportunities and revenue streams through the commodification of virtually all forms of sport and athletic contests (Newman, 2014). When we situate and view the global sport industry through the lens of the Anthropocene, we are compelled to consider the environmental and more-than-human aspects of economic growth in the industry. There are, for example, immense extractive, polluting, and carbon-emitting dimensions to recent economic estimates that the global sport industry will grow from US$388.3 billion in 2020 to US$826 billion in 2030 due to consumer growth in the esports market, "emerging economies," and the increase in viewership on personal digital devices (Research and Markets, 2021). The sports merchandise market, estimated to grow at a yearly rate of 3.4% this decade, from US$22.3 billion in 2020 to US$27.2 billion in 2026 (Research and Markets, 2022), is part of the global fashion and apparel industries, which comprise 10% of all yearly greenhouse gas emissions (McFall-Johnsen, 2020). Just in terms of the waste-creating activities of their fans, the major professional sports organizations in North America generate tens of thousands of tons of carbon dioxide every year (Henczel, n.d.). This also does not include international mega-events like the Olympic Games and the World Cup, which generate millions of tons of CO_2 per event (White & Rathi, 2022; Berners-Lee, 2010). Thus, researchers are already warning that international sporting mega-events like the Olympics will need to drastically reduce their size and carbon footprint to become sustainable (Müller et al., 2021).

The sport industry's ongoing contributions to anthropogenic climate change is compounded by a seeming inability to imagine alternatives to contemporary, prevailing sporting forms. For example, the field of sport management, as arguably "*the* overarching instructional and institutional frame for sport-related inquiry, pedagogy, and practice" in U.S. higher education (Newman, 2014, p. 603), serves as the conceptual framework through which undergraduate and graduate students in the U.S. learn about the economic, political, and sociocultural contexts of sport. The growth of the discipline, typically to the detriment of (sub)fields such as physical education, sport history, sport philosophy, and sport sociology, can be linked to market-based pressures to supply the industry with trained managers and administrators (p. 606). As scholar Chen Chen (2022) recently notes, sport management academics and practitioners rarely question or even acknowledge the role of capitalism as "the predominant mode of economic organizing that structures and conditions the 'management' of sport activities" (p. 3). The prevailing values and ideals of capitalism, Chen argues, "materially undergirds the sport 'industry' and conditions the various issues, topics, and identities that are of interest to, and examined by sport management scholars" (p. 8). Beyond its dictates of capital accumulation and growth and its demands for entry-level managerial workers, the logics of the capitalist sport industry constricts the horizons of the possible by presenting sport in terms of industry performance and growth. The result is a kind of pervasive sporting "capitalist realism" in which the permanence and adaptability of the sport industry in its dominant, capitalist form is assumed (Fisher, 2009).

The problem is that the anthropogenic processes driving climate change—namely, the pursuit of endless growth, productivity, and accumulation—target both the material *and* the psychopolitical conditions of life on earth. Contemporary capitalism exploits not just the material resources of the planet but also the psychic resources of its human inhabitants, resulting in what the Swiss-German philosopher Byung-Chul Han terms a compulsive, destructive "death drive" for growth in economic, material, as well as non-material psychological terms (Han, 2021, p. 11). The neoliberal dictates of efficiency and productivity are not only exploiting and degrading our biosphere in the name of capital accumulation but exploiting our psyches in the name of optimal performance in work and life (Han, 2017). Thus, it is not surprising that Han terms twenty-first century society an achievement-obsessed "burnout society" replete with pervasive and systemic "neuronal violence" (2015, p. 7), as the "imperative to achieve" and be productive under neoliberal capitalism leads to widespread mental health maladies such as depression, anxiety, fatigue, and hyperactivity (p. 10). We are exploiting and exhausting ourselves as we exploit and exhaust the planet. This means that questions concerning the sustainability of the sport industry need to consider not just what some sport management researchers term the "bidirectional" relationship between the sport industry and natural environments (McCullough et al., 2020), but the relations between our physical cultures and the unsustainable "imperative to achieve" under capitalism. This line of thinking has led us to consider Pronger's notion of post-sport as a possible generative avenue for imagining more ecologically- and psychopolitically-sustainable ways of being physically active.

Post-Sport Physical Cultures

Our engagement with post-sport is informed in large part by the work of Brian Pronger, notably a chapter of his titled "Post-Sport: Transgressing Boundaries in Physical Culture" in Genevieve Rail's 1998 edited volume *Sport and Postmodern Times*. In his chapter, Pronger argued that modern sports are what he called projects of "socio-cultural boundary maintenance" (1998, p. 177): highly rationalized sporting practices and spaces that play a key role in the reproduction and reinforcement of boundaries, from the establishment of "order" out of "chaos" through codified rules, to the re-presentation of gender, racial, ethnic, class, and ableist hierarchies, to cultural definitions of what constitutes a "healthy" or "sick" body (p. 281). Pronger does not include this boundary formation in his original chapter, but we would also include the valorization of activity, and, in turn, the denigration of inactivity or "idleness," as another important socio-culturally defined boundary maintained and re-presented by modern sports. In Pronger's view, modern sports have been integral to and have furthered the historical processes of modernization by serving as ideological vehicles and instruments for the rationalization of the active body: by facilitating the inscription of bodies with cultural discourses (p. 279), sports do the important cultural work of hegemonizing the dictates and ideologies of modern, capitalist life. Further, modern sports are agents in the exploitation of the human body by targeting bodies as "cultural resources" for reproducing socio-cultural discourses (p. 289). In the critical study of sport, Pronger's conception of modern sports as projects of socio-cultural boundary maintenance gels with existing scholarship on the links between sport and modernity (Gruneau, 2017), the reproduction of capitalist processes and values (Andrews & Silk, 2012), colonialist and Eurocentric epistemologies and hierarchies (Carrington, 2015), racial, gender, and sexual divisions (Hawkins, 2010; Cahn, 1994; Pieper, 2016), nationalist identities and international relations (Sotomayor, 2016), and the wide array of other important social relations.

Pronger argued that the task of helping make the "realities of cultured bodies a little freer" requires not only recognizing the ways in which active bodies transgress and help destroy the socio-cultural boundary formations within modern sports (p. 277), but also aiding in the imagining and constructing of what he called "new 'postmodern' physical activities" (p. 291). Pronger was a scholar who was influenced by the works of postmodern thinkers like Donna Haraway (1985) and the postmodern contention that there is pleasure and value to be gained by confusing and transgressing socio-cultural boundaries. Thus, scholar Lucen Liu (2021) contends that in his elucidation of the concept, Pronger used "post-sport" and "postmodern sport" interchangeably to describe physical cultural expressions that unsettle "the dichotomous boundary projects" of modern sports and the ways in which they reproduce and maintain socio-cultural discourses linked to the modernization process.

Post-sport was arguably Pronger's key conceptual contribution to the task of imagining new and highlighting existing postmodern, boundary-transgressing physical cultures. Calling on researchers, specifically schools of physical education, to engage in the "postmodernization of the modern body" (p. 293), Pronger presented post-sport as forms of physical cultures that seem to slip within the grips of sport's socio-cultural discourses and demarcations. As a conceptual lens for viewing physical cultural realities, post-sport both enlivens our attention to physical cultural pursuits that transgress or play with the rules and boundaries of modernized sporting practices (Pronger, 1998, p. 291), as well as points to the need for such forms of postmodern physical culture. Further, post-sport recasts the meaning of pleasure and its emanation from the embodied experience. Though he acknowledged that modern sporting activities can be pleasurable and produce a sense of ecstasy—for example, the joy that can arise from successfully finishing a difficult race or climbing a mountain—pleasure can also be experienced through what Pronger called the "the irony of resisting the limits of discourse, in the wild eroticism that moves passionately through discourse, through boundary projects" (p. 292). Throughout the chapter, Pronger seems to hint at a definition of what constitutes a post-sport without defining it beyond the notion of postmodernizing sport. This, perhaps, may have been the author's intention, for not only is the nature of "post-sport" difficult to pin down, but, considering the boundary-making nature of a published volume of scholarly knowledge, perhaps he also found pleasure knowing he was not fully abiding by some of the socio-culturally sanctioned rules of academic discourse.

A few researchers and scholars of sport and physical culture have engaged with post-sport in their research on alternative physical cultures, providing further elucidation of the concept and its utility. For example, scholar Belinda Wheaton notes in her study of "lifestyle" sports— alternative, participatory physical cultural expressions such as surfing, parkour, skateboarding, and climbing—that the practices often "retain characteristics that are different to the traditional rule-bound, competitive, institutionalised, Western 'achievement' sport cultures" (2013, p. 29). As part of Wheaton's study of the cultural, economic, and political dimensions of lifestyle sports, she engaged with Pronger's post-sport concept to explore how lifestyle sports appear to resemble mainstream sports, in terms of their relations to capitalist processes and the consumption of commodities, and yet exhibit "nonmainstream" characteristics. For Wheaton, post-sports "help to clarify and extend our understanding of the boundaries of contemporary lifestyle sports, reminding us that our understanding of what lifestyle sports are (and might become), their boundaries and their needs to be continually reviewed in the light of emerging research" (p. 28).

Perhaps the most developed example of post-sport scholarship within sport-related disciplines is scholar Michael Atkinson's exploration of yoga and fell running, a physically strenuous, difficult practice involving "cross-country, trail, mountain and, at times, wilderness running" in rugged highland areas, as constituting post-sport physical cultures (2010a, p. 1255). Atkinson situates post-sport fell running within the conditions of late modern, neoliberal society, "a world over-saturated by global commodities and cultural flows" that leads one to "question whether stable, enduring, inter-subjective styles of life with definitive boundaries are possible" (p. 1250). The late modern context of ubiquitous commodity circulation and destabilized cultural forms, Atkinson writes, "may indeed allow for a mass destabilization of many mainstream sport forms" and a "fertile social environment" for "a variety of non-traditional, boundary-crossing physical cultural practices that might loosely be called 'post-sport athletics'" (p. 1250). Fell running, for Atkinson, is a "non-mainstream" physical cultural form that does not "perfectly emulate or replicate hyper-competitive, hierarchical and patriarchal modernist sports" (2010b, p. 112). Through participation in the practice, he noticed and experienced firsthand a sense of community bonding that is energized by the rugged outdoor spaces; a sense of "communion," of "co-producing and experiencing desires and spirituality with others" through the running (p. 118); a physical and emotional suffering that is seen by running participants as a "vehicle for self-exploration and transcendence" and escaping from some of the more coercive effects of modern existence (p. 188). Fell running does not suggest a post-sport physical culture because it is totally detached from the rationalizing, competitive, masculine, consumerist impulses of modernist sports, but because the practice also harbors "existential, democratic and community-building" possibilities that have been not extinguished and can be energized and embraced by participants (p. 129).

Lucen Liu's (2021) recent ethnographic exploration of the Māori practice of waka ama (outrigger canoe) paddling extends the study of post-sport physical cultures by relating the concept to the issue of Indigenous understandings of physical activity, as well as human interactions with the environmental and the more-than-human through physical culture. For Liu, post-sport became a useful conceptual tool for studying waka ama because the practice seemed difficult to define using just traditional, Western-centered conceptions of sport: both "the competitiveness of sport and Māori cultural practices" seemed to coexist in and through waka ama (p. 139). Using post-sport to help form her critical analytical lens, Liu argues that Māori waka ama practices transgress modernist sporting boundaries in multiple ways. For one, she wrote that waka ama paddlers "often invite the uncontrollable and sometimes unpredictable natural forces of bluespaces into their physical activity," embracing "non-human forces and agencies of wind, air, frost, land, and ocean" and inviting those forces and agencies "to enable and ensure the smooth process of the human activity" (p. 146). This acknowledgement and embracing of more-than-human actants complicates modernist dualisms distinguishing human "culture" from "nature". The Māori waka ama participants, Liu writes, seemed to "act like post-sport athletes," with the boundaries separating their identities as athlete and Indigenous Māori blurred in and through their interactions with and respect for the agentic force of the ocean (p. 149). As part of her research framework, post-sport helped Liu highlight how waka ama participants complicate traditional, Western-centered notions of more-than-human "nature" as a static backdrop to human cultural expressions or an obstacle to conquer through masculine activity.

At the same time, Liu's study also highlights an important limitation to post-sport that is particularly relevant to the question of sport's future in the Anthropocene. In the conclusion of her study, Liu contends that post-sport "has limited ability in examining the nonhuman world or the mutual transgression between human and nonhuman worlds" (p. 155). She specifically pointed to what seems like an anthropocentric framing within Pronger and Atkinson's conceptions of post-sport:

> In Pronger's conceptualization of post-sport, the human actors take the initiatives, deploying various disruptive strategies to shake the modern boundaries, such as bringing the pleasure of chaos back to physical education or bringing the profaned and primordial bodies back to sport,

> whereas the nonhuman factors are weak in influencing or participating in the boundary transgression. The human-centered conceptualization is also reflected in Atkinson's discussion of what a post-sport athlete may look like. Without the integration of Māori indigenous cultural concepts, which do not separate human and natural worlds, the concept of post-sport alone will be insufficient to illustrate the natural actors crossing the boundary and moving toward the human actors in the bluespaces. (p. 155)

Liu's critique is notable on at least two fronts. First, she points to the need to rethink the concept through a recognition of the inherent entanglements between the human and more-than-human within physical culture, a necessary development if post-sport is to be useful in imagining post-anthropocentric, ecologically-attuned physical cultures in the Anthropocene. Second, her critique underscores the subtle ways postmodern deconstructions of modernist boundaries and categories can still reproduce Western-centered knowledge forms through their frameworks of analysis (Mignolo & Walsh, 2018). In the case of post-sport, its human-centered approach to transgressing modern sport, assuming that human actors will take the lead in "deploying various disruptive strategies to shake the modern boundaries" (Liu, 2021, p. 155), obscures Indigenous, non-Western, and other alternative perspectives that may complicate and challenge the notion of sport as a priori and inherently anthropocentric.

If we question the future of sport in the Anthropocene, however, there is additional layer of complexity to post-sport that, to date, has not been addressed in existing scholarship. Similar to the broader study of sport and physical culture in its myriad forms and expressions, the post-sport scholarship discussed above assumes that the post-sport will take the form of some kind of physical activity or active body practice, from Pronger's (1998) contention that "physical activity needs to play with the pleasure of chaos" (p. 293), to Atkinson's exploration of the extremely physical active and strenuous practice of fell running (2010a, 2010b), to Liu's study of waka ama paddling in oceanic bluespaces (2021). A notable exception is Atkinson's study of Ashtanga yoga (2010a), but even in that study Atkinson approaches yoga as a "potential post-sport athletic practice" and an "intense practice designed to cultivate and shape one's body, to calm the mind and discover universal energy" (p. 1256). Iterations of active human physicality are the assumed sites for empirical, theoretical, and philosophical inquiry.

This tendency to absolutize physical activity in the study of both sport and post-sport leaves uncontested and maintained an important boundary in Western, modern, and late modern capitalist social relations: the separation of "activity" and "inactivity" and the denigration of forms of inactivity as immoral, unproductive "idleness". The Irish philosopher Brian O'Connor (2018) argues that idleness can be a form of human freedom and pleasurable, playful activity, but only if idleness is wrestled from its denigration under capitalism as unproductive laziness and redefined as an experienced and embodied activity that is without a "guiding purpose" and characterized by a general "feeling of noncompulsion and drift" (p. 5). According to O'Connor, this definition of an idle experience, entailing some kind of autonomy from coercive notions of economic productivity or "disciplined self-monitoring," offers a "bolder image of freedom" because it suggests a way of living that offers human beings a "liberating possession of ourselves, free of pressure, and evidently content" (p. 7), particularly in terms of the stress-inducing compulsions of "busyness, self-making, usefulness, and productivity" that typify late modern capitalist society (p. 3). To the best of our knowledge, the notion of idleness as a form of physical culture does not appear in the existing published scholarship on sport, post-sport, and the academic and political project of Physical Cultural Studies (PCS) (Silk et al., 2017). Pronger's presentation and elucidation of post-sport, however, seems amenable to questions concerning the idle and the inactive. After all, Pronger (1998) evocatively asserted that "the academic focus on sport rather than alternative forms of physical activity" reinforces the "privileged status of sport as a socio-cultural practice" and excludes other physical cultures that exist at or transgress the boundaries of sport in its modernist iterations (p. 288). The privileging of sport in its modern, rationalized forms does the work of "hegemonizing" a particularly Western-centered, capital-driven iteration of sport and restricts the horizon of imagination concerning human physical culture (p. 287). The importance of post-sport physical cultures, following Pronger, is that they "introduce into the world of modern sport the very things modern sport has tried to keep out: chaos, inefficiency, irrationality, sex, and other illicit pleasures" (p. 288). Today, in a moment shaped by the deterioration of the biosphere, we should increasingly look towards radical embodiments and expressions of idleness, particularly those that can and already do manifest in decidedly anti-capitalist, pleasurably limited, democratic, and anti-productivist forms, as not just expressions of physical culture but practices potentially offering ecologically, communally, socially mindful "illicit pleasures" (Odell, 2019; O'Connor, 2018).

Parting Vision: Towards Idleness as Post-Sport Physical Culture

The limitations of this chapter prevent us from doing more than suggest that idleness is a possible generative post-sport physical culture in terms of its ontological relation to living in conditions demanding restrictions on human activity and its potential expressions as a physical cultural and illicit pleasure. Idleness can potentially be approached as a post-sport physical culture because idle practices can cross the rational, modernist boundary supposedly separating activity and inactivity. As Amelia DeFalco (2016) notes, "there is some slippage between the terms" idleness and activity (p. 93), especially when idleness is recast in terms of its health-giving, ecological, and humanistic qualities (Russell, 2004). Idleness can be imagined as a kind of post-sport practice of "joyful energy" that necessarily slips within modern and postmodern sport's compulsions for consumer and commercial growth (Newman, 2014). There is even more value and potential in post-sport as an analytical concept than perhaps Pronger imagined if we use it to envisage forms of human physical culture that are decidedly oppositional to sport in its prevailing capitalist forms and capable of promoting practices with reduced ecological footprints. Any exploration of idleness as post-sport physical culture should not take the place of new materialist and other researches seeking to "flatten" the entanglements and interactions between humans, animals, more-than-human agents, and environment. Rather, the study of radical forms of idleness can and should productively complement such researches, while devoting scholarly energies to practices that potentially deliberately and pleasurably limit human impacts on the more-than-human universe.

The relevance of idleness in this age of the Anthropocene/Capitalocene/Chthulucene stems from the possibility of valorizing idle physical cultural practices in terms of the pleasures of limited, non-compulsive, non-growth-driven human activities. This has only become more relevant to us as we witnessed a momentary glimpse of the benefits of limited human activity in the first year of the pandemic. During the initial lockdown measures instituted by various governments in response to the novel coronavirus—which, as we remember, occurred in conjunction with the widespread suspension of live sporting events—there was what researchers have termed a "considerable global slowing of modern human activities" (Rutz et al., 2020): a brief "anthropause", an interruption of contemporary patterns of human action and interaction as a result of the mobility and travel restrictions of lockdown measures. Media outlets reported animals reclaiming environments, returning to habitats where they had been previously displaced due to human development and tourism, or encroaching within urban spaces (British Broadcasting Corporation, 2020). For an all-too-brief moment, the anthropause provided visual, and perhaps overly celebratory evidence of some possible positive effects on ecosystems and more-than-human livelihoods due to a reduced human footprint.

The pandemic, however, has also demonstrated the firmly non-idle nature of contemporary capitalist life. First, the Economic Policy Institute asserted that COVID-19 has "highlighted and exacerbated underlying disparities in the health and economic wellbeing of people across the country" (Gould & Kandra, 2021, para. 1), finding that African American and Hispanic workers were less likely to be able to work from home during the first year of the pandemic. In other words, the notion of being able to partake in idleness is importantly marked by divisions according to race, class, gender, ableism, and other intersecting social factors. Second, the brief anthropause was superseded by a resurgence and acceleration of consumer growth and carbon-emitting human activity, particularly outdoor recreation participation rates and sales. During a year of lockdowns, suspensions, rising COVID-related death rates, and social strife, the outdoor recreation industry generated $688 billion in revenues, with "record sales and unprecedented growth" in sports such as hunting and fishing, as well as biking, boating, camping, and RVing (RV Industry Association, 2021). In short, the pandemic experience has underscored for us that the collective task of constructing and embracing more sustainable, equitable, and pleasurable physical cultural practices requires thinking about the pleasures of limited, local, non-anthropocentric, and non-consumer-driven practices. Perhaps the study of idle physical cultures could help supply clues and resources for such an urgent task.

References

Andrews, D. L. (2019). *Making sport great again: The Uber-sport assemblage, neoliberalism, and the Trump conjuncture*. Palgrave Macmillan.

Andrews, D. L., & Silk, M. L. (Eds.). (2012). *Sport and neoliberalism: Politics, consumption, and culture*. Temple University Press.

Atkinson, M. (2010a). Entering scapeland: Yoga, fell and post-sport physical cultures. *Sport in Society, 13*(7–8), 1249–1267.

Atkinson, M. (2010b). Fell running in post-sport territories. *Qualitative Research in Sport and Exercise, 2*(2), 109–132.

Beer, T. (2020, October 20). Report: NBA's bubble prevented $1.5 billion in losses. *Forbes*. https://www.forbes.com/sites/tommybeer/2020/10/20/report-nbas-bubble-prevented-15-billion-in-losses/

Berners-Lee, M. (2010, June 10). What's the carbon footprint of … the World Cup? *The Guardian*. https://www.theguardian.com/environment/green-living-blog/2010/jun/10/carbon-footprint-world-cup

Bonneuil, C., & Fressoz, J.-B. (2016). *The shock of the Anthropocene: The Earth, history and us*. Verso.

Boykoff, J., & Gaffney, C. (2020). The Tokyo 2020 Games and the end of Olympic history. *Capitalism Nature Socialism, 31*(2), 1–19.

British Broadcasting Corporation. (2020, April 29). Coronavirus: Wild animals enjoy freedom of a quieter world. Retrieved from https://www.bbc.com/news/world-52459487

Cahn, S. K. (1994). *Coming on strong: Gender and sexuality in twentieth-century women's sport*. Harvard University Press.

Cardazzi, A., Humphreys, B., Ruseski, J. E., Soebbing, B. P., & Watanabe, N. (2020). Professional sporting events increase seasonal influenza mortality in US cities. *Economics Faculty Working Papers Series, 49*. https://researchrepository.wvu.edu/econ_working-papers/49

Carlson, C. J., Albery, G. F., Merow, C., Trisos, C. H., Zipfel, C. M., Eskew, E. A., Olival, K. J., Ross, N., & Bansal, S. (2022). Climate change increases cross-species viral transmission risk. *Nature*. https://doi.org/10.1038/s41586-022-04788-w

Carrington, B. (2015). Post/colonial theory and sport. In R. Giulianotti (Ed.), *Routledge handbook of the sociology of sport* (pp. 105–115). Routledge.

Chakrabarty, D. (2021). *The climate of history in a planetary age*. The University of Chicago Press.

Chen, C. (2022). Naming the ghost of capitalism in sport management. *European Sport Management Quarterly*. https://doi.org/10.1080/16184742.2022.2046123

Collins, T. (2013). *Sport in capitalist society: A short history*. Routledge.

Crist, E. (2016). On the poverty of our nomenclature. In J. W. Moore (Ed.), *Anthropocene or capitalocene? Nature, history, and the crisis of capitalism* (pp. 1–24). PM Press.

Cronin, M. (2014). *Sport: A very short introduction*. Oxford University Press.

Davis, M. (2005). *The monster at our door: The global threat of avian flu*. The New Press.

DeFalco, A. (2016). In praise of idleness: Aging and the morality of inactivity. *Cultural Critique, 92*, 84–113.

Demos, T. J. (2017). *Against the Anthropocene: Visual culture and environment today*. Sternberg Press.

Fisher, M. (2009). *Capitalist realism: Is there no alternative?* Zero Books.

Foster, J. B. (2000). *Marx's ecology: Materialism and nature*. Monthly Review Press.

Gibson, K. (2020). Animals, sport, and the environment. In B. Wilson & B. Millington (Eds.), *Sport and the environment* (pp. 103–121). Emerald Publishing Limited.

Gould, E., & Kandra, J. (2021, June 2). *Only one in five workers are working from home due to COVID*. Economic Policy Institute. https://www.epi.org/blog/only-one-in-five-workers-are-working-from-home-due-to-covid-black-and-hispanic-workers-are-less-likely-to-be-able-to-telework/

Gruneau, R. (2017). *Sport and modernity*. Polity Press.

Han, B.-C. (2015). *The burnout society* (E. Butler, Trans.). Stanford University Press.

Han, B.-C. (2017). *Psychopolitics: Neoliberalism and new technologies of power* (E. Butler, Trans.). Verso.

Han, B.-C. (2021). *Capitalism and the death drive* (D. Steuer, Trans.). Polity Press.
Haraway, D. (1985). A manifesto for cyborgs: Science, technology, and socialist feminism in the 1980s. *Socialist Review, 80*, 65–108.
Haraway, D. J. (2016). Staying with the trouble: Anthropocene, capitalocene, chthulucene. In J. W. Moore (Ed.), *Anthropocene or capitalocene? Nature, history, and the crisis of capitalism* (pp. 26–80). PM Press.
Hawkins, B. (2010). *The new plantation: Black athletes, college sports, predominantly white NCAA institutions*. Palgrave Macmillan.
Henczel, T. (n.d.). The environmental impact of professional sports. *The Environmentor*. https://blog.tentree.com/the-environmental-impact-of-professional-sports/
Heyd, T. (2021). COVID-19 and climate change in the times of the Anthropocene. *The Anthropocene Review, 8*(1), 21–36.
Hobsbawm, E. (1996). *The age of capital, 1848–1875*. Penguin Random House.
International Olympic Committee. (2021, December 22). Tokyo 2020 goes beyond carbon neutrality and helps create a more "sustainable society". https://olympics.com/ioc/news/tokyo-2020-goes-beyond-carbon-neutrality-and-helps-create-a-more-sustainable-society
Kalman-Lamb, N., Silva, D., & Mellis, J. (2020, October 22). College football feels all too normal during the pandemic. *TIME*. https://time.com/5901657/college-football-covid-19/
Latour, B. (2018). *Down to Earth: Politics in the new climatic regime*. Polity.
Leitch, W. (2020, March 15). How will sports recover from this hiatus? *The New York Times*. https://www.nytimes.com/2020/03/15/opinion/sports-coronavirus.html
Lewis, S. L., & Maslin, M. A. (2015). Defining the Anthropocene. *Nature, 519*(7542), 171–180.
Liu, L. (2021). Paddling through bluespaces: Understanding waka ama as a post-sport through Indigenous Māori perspectives. *Journal of Sport & Social Issues, 45*(2), 138–160.
McCullough, B. P., & Kellison, T. B. (Eds.). (2018). *Routledge handbook of sport and the environment*. Routledge.
McCullough, B. P., Orr, M., & Kellison, T. (2020). Sport ecology: Conceptualizing an emerging subdiscipline within sport management. *Journal of Sport Management, 34*(6), 509–520.
McFall-Johnsen, M. (2020, January 31). *These facts show how unsustainable the fashion industry is*. World Economic Forum. https://www.weforum.org/agenda/2020/01/fashion-industry-carbon-unsustainable-environment-pollution/

Mignolo, W. D., & Walsh, C. E. (2018). *On decoloniality: Concepts, analytics, praxis*. Duke University Press.
Moore, J. W. (2015). *Capitalism in the web of life: Ecology and the accumulation of capital.* Verso.
Moore, J. W. (2016). *Anthropocene or capitalocene? Nature, history, and the crisis of capitalism.* In J. W. Moore (Ed.), *Anthropocene or capitalocene? Nature, history, and the crisis of capitalism* (pp. xiii–xxvi). PM Press.
Moore, J. W. (2017). The Capitalocene, part I: On the nature and origins of our ecological crisis. *The Journal of Peasant Studies, 44*(3), 594–630.
Müller, M., Wolfe, S. D., Gaffney, C., Gogishvili, D., Hug, M., & Leick, A. (2021). An evaluation of the sustainability of the Olympic Games. *Nature Sustainability, 4*, 340–348.
Newman, J. I. (2014). Sport without management. *Journal of Sport Management, 28*(6), 603–615.
Newman, J. I., Thorpe, H., & Andrews, D. L. (Eds.). (2020). *Sport, physical culture, and the moving body: Materialisms, technologies, ecologies.* Rutgers University Press.
O'Connor, B. (2018). *Idleness: A philosophical essay*. Princeton University Press.
O'Callaghan-Gordo, C., & Antó, J. M. (2020). COVID-19: The disease of the Anthropocene. *Environmental Research, 187*, 109683. https://doi.org/10.1016/j.envres.2020.109683
Odell, J. (2019). *How to do nothing: Resisting the attention economy.* Melville House.
Pieper, L. P. (2016). *Sex Testing: Gender policing in women's sport.* University of Illinois Press.
Pronger, B. (1998). Post-sport: Transgressing boundaries in physical culture. In G. Rail (Ed.), *Sport and postmodern times* (pp. 277–298). State University of New York Press.
Research and Markets. (2021, July 22). Global sports market opportunities and strategies report 2021: Sports market forecast to reach $599.9 billion by 2025 as COVID-19 lockdowns ease. Yahoo! https://www.yahoo.com/now/global-sports-market-opportunities-strategies-080800261.html
Research and Markets. (2022, January 14). Global licensed sports merchandise market report 2022: U.S. market is estimated at $5.4 Billion in 2021, while China is forecast to reach $4.1 billion by 2026. PR Newswire. https://www.prnewswire.com/news-releases/global-licensed-sports-merchandise-market-report-2022-us-market-is-estimated-at-5-4-billion-in-2021%2D%2Dwhile-china-is-forecast-to-reach-4-1-billion-by-2026%2D%2D301461234.html

Reuters. (2020, June 9). Mixed martial arts: White says Abu Dhabi 'Fight Island' to host UFC 251. https://www.reuters.com/article/us-health-coronavirus-mma-ufc/mixed-martial-arts-white-says-abu-dhabi-fight-island-to-host-ufc-251-idUSKBN23G2SP

Russell, B. (2004). *In praise of idleness and other essays*. Routledge. (Original work published 1932).

Rutz, C., Loretto, M.-C., Bates, A. E., Davidson, S. C., Durate, C. M., Jetz, W., et al. (2020). COVID-19 lockdown allows researchers to quantify the effects of human activity on wildlife. *Nature Ecology and Evolution, 4*, 1156–1159.

RV Industry Association. (2021, November 9). New economic report showcases outdoor recreation economy's strength & resiliency during difficult year. https://www.rvia.org/news-insights/new-economic-report-showcases-outdoor-recreation-economys-strength-resiliency-during-difficult-year

Seifert, K. (2020, July 10). The plan to start the 2020 NFL season: What we know and what we don't know. *ESPN*. https://www.espn.com/nfl/story/_/id/29440970/the-plan-start-2020-nfl-season-know-know

Silk, M. L., Thorpe, H., & Andrews, D. L. (Eds.). (2017). *Routledge handbook of physical cultural studies*. Routledge.

Sotomayor, A. (2016). *The sovereign colony: Olympic sport, national identity, and international politics in Puerto Rico*. University of Nebraska Press.

Wallace, R. (2016). *Big farms make big flu: Dispatches on infectious disease, agribusiness, and the nature of science*. NYU Press.

Wallace, R., Liebman, A., Chaves, L. F., & Wallace, R. (2020, May 1). COVID-19 and circuits of capital. *Monthly Review*. https://monthlyreview.org/2020/05/01/covid-19-and-circuits-of-capital/

Wark, M. (2015). *Molecular red: Theory for the anthropocene*. Verso.

Wheaton, B. (2013). *The cultural politics of lifestyle sports*. Routledge.

White, N., & Rathi, A. (2022, February 16). China says the winter Olympics are carbon neutral. They aren't. Bloomberg. https://www.bloomberg.com/news/articles/2022-02-16/beijing-olympics-carbon-neutral-claim-is-based-on-junk-offsets

Wilson, B., & Millington, B. (Eds.). (2020). *Sport and the environment: Politics and preferred futures*. Emerald Publishing Limited.

Zhang, L. (2021). *The origins of COVID-19: China and global capitalism*. Stanford University Press.

23

A Syndemics Approach to NCAA Collegiate Sport Participation During COVID-19

Caitlin Vitosky Clarke, Kaitlin Pericak, Brynn C. Adamson, and Kassidy Mahoney

Introduction

This chapter focuses on a syndemics (Singer, 1994, 1996) approach to college athlete health, specifically football, in the United States (U.S.) collegiate sport system as a new framework for understanding sport participation during an infectious disease outbreak, epidemic, or pandemic. We have two main objectives: describe the syndemics framework and key scholarly contributions of biological social factors (Bio-Social) and provide a preliminary application to the U.S. collegiate sport system during

C. V. Clarke (✉) • K. Mahoney
University of Illinois at Urbana-Champaign, Champaign, IL, USA
e-mail: vitosky@illinois.edu

K. Pericak
North Carolina Wesleyan University, Rocky Mount, NC, USA

B. C. Adamson
University of Colorado Colorado Springs, Colorado Springs, CO, USA

D. L. Andrews et al. (eds.), *Sport and Physical Culture in Global Pandemic Times*, Global Culture and Sport Series, https://doi.org/10.1007/978-3-031-14387-8_23

the COVID-19 pandemic. Since the pandemic is ongoing, we draw from examples during the U.S. Fall 2020 college sport season.

Here, we propose a syndemics approach to sport participation by offering a case study of the NCAA's neoliberal model of U.S. collegiate sport, with a particular interest in decision-making during the COVID-19 pandemic. The syndemics framework focuses on disease *concentrations*, and disease *interactions* or comorbidities which are exacerbated (or sometimes caused) by large-scale social conditions. We focus on the disease concentrations in college athletes and the interactions of SARS-CoV-2 (COVID-19) with chronic health conditions (e.g., pulmonary disease, obesity, diabetes, psychiatric disorder, etc.), myocarditis and head trauma, exacerbated by the social condition: the neoliberal U.S. collegiate sport model and the decision to play during the pandemic. While the pandemic landscape continues to change rapidly, we are entering the third-year mark. Furthermore, the frequency of emerging infectious diseases with pandemic potential will increase due to climate change (Jain et al., 2018). Therefore, the syndemics framework provides a useful lens for future consideration of other infectious disease epidemics and sport participation. To lay the groundwork for this conceptualization, we first provide the social context of collegiate sport during the COVID-19 pandemic. Then we move to discuss the specifics of the syndemics framework, including previously demonstrated syndemic interactions. Finally, we discuss the ethical implications of continued sport participation during infectious disease epidemics.

The Social Context of U.S. College Sport and the COVID-19 Pandemic

The U.S. collegiate sport system is unique in that sports generate immense revenue, but the athletes are unpaid college students (Leroy, 2021). Building on Goffman's (1961) concept, Hatteberg (2018) argues that the U.S. collegiate sport system is a total institution. The National Collegiate Athletic Association (NCAA) is part of the U.S. collegiate sport system and oversees collegiate championships, provides safety and health recommendations, and athletic scholarships. Within the NCAA are the "Power 5" conferences which are the five largest and most financially profitable conferences in the Football Bowl Subdivision (FBS). The Power 5 conferences include the Big 12, Pac-12, ACC, SEC, and the Big Ten.

In the U.S., college football starts in early September. During July and August 2020, decisions were made not to play in the regular fall season by 54 of 130 teams in the FBS, (Division I-A: the most competitive level), to prevent the spread of COVID-19. However, by September 16th, the majority of the 130 teams had decided to play. While the NCAA moved the fall championships for 5 other collegiate sports to the spring, football and basketball carried on despite the pandemic's spikes in cases. In the U.S., a peak in positive COVID-19 cases occurred in late November 2020 through March 2021 during this season. Despite football being designated as a high-contact risk, and the continued rise of COVID-19 morbidity throughout the season, some cast playing as an 'opportunity' because they were willing to assume and mitigate the risk (Zucker, 2020; Blinder et al., 2020). However, the risk here was not framed as long-term.

American football requires large groups of athletes to interact regularly and directly. Close-quarters interactions also occur in other collegiate athlete-specific spaces. Through these spaces, numerous daily sport-specific interactions occurred and complicated maintaining a "COVID-19 bubble," in which a person intentionally limits their interactions to a select group of people and keeps that bubble as small as possible to reduce the likelihood of disease transmission. Former President Trump refused to mandate COVID prevention measures at the federal level (Victor et al., 2020), leaving each state to govern mandates if they so choose (and many chose to do nothing). Consequently, decisions about mandated or suggested preventive measures varied widely across the U.S. college landscape (IHE Staff, 2020; Thomason & O'Leary, 2021). Attempts to mitigate risk through COVID bubbles were fraught everywhere in the U.S. because of inconsistent definitions of what it meant to "bubble" in any given state (Gutman, 2020). Furthermore, such bubbles only worked to the extent that athletes and related staff maintained the bubble, leaving athletes effectively incarcerated to perform their athletic labor for the public who, athletic organizations worldwide claimed, desperately needed sport to continue amid the pandemic (Pavlidis & Rowe, 2021). As well, full games with travel eventually occurred and expanded the "bubble". This was quite different from the varied U.S. state-level mandates for households. For example, in Illinois citizens were directed by Governor Pritzker to limit interactions between different households, to keep gatherings outdoors, and limited to less than 10 people (Restore Illinois, 2020).

Even though most U.S. collegiate athletics programs eventually implemented testing protocols and additional preventive measures for their collegiate athletes at the conference level, the wide range of approaches to COVID-19 protocols for the general student population and wider university community may have contributed to possible exposures on campus. The variations in preventive measures and testing protocols were/are compounded by public pressure to continue competitive sport seasons during the COVID-19 pandemic in the Fall 2020 semester and beyond. Indeed, the pressure was so great that the Big Ten Conference member school presidents held meetings on the Big Ten Network private VPN network to avoid being subjected to the Freedom of Information Act open meeting laws (Giambalvo & Maese, 2021). Like the Australian Football League (Pavlidis & Rowe, 2021), there was obvious financial pressure and political pressure to allow college and professional sport to continue such that former U.S. President Trump pressured the Big 10 conference to return to competitive play in August of 2020 (Giambalvo & Maese, 2021). Such pressure resulted in several national sporting events including the NCAA Division I college football season, the National Football League competitive season, the National Basketball Association (NBA), and later, in 2021, the NCAA Division I March Madness National Basketball Tournament. However, college athletic programs and public COVID bubbles were drastically different from the NBA or NCAA March Madness bubbles, in which players, coaches, training staff, and even sports news reporters were required to remain in one space during their entire competitive season (e.g., NBA), (Golliver, 2020) or the entire Tournament (Maese et al., 2021).

In the lead-up to the U.S. Fall 2020 college sport season, although the news media often framed COVID-19 as a greater risk for aging populations, by August 5th of 2020 at least 800 college football players had tested positive for COVID-19 including many with moderate to severe symptoms (Dellenger, 2020). Hundreds of players in the Power 5 conferences were vocal on social media about their expectations and demands for appropriate conditions needed to protect their safety in the event of a regular season otherwise they would boycott the season (Nadkarni, 2020). Additionally, over 1000 players in the Big Ten, proposed the Unity Proposal—lambasting the NCAA for their lack of preparation for a safe season and proposing 26 actions to ensure player safety amidst an in-person season during the pandemic (#BigTenUnited, 2020). These actions included third-party testing, social distancing requirements, mandatory mask-wearing by all parties interacting with athletes, quarantine guidelines, whistleblower protections, banning the use of COVID-19 liability waivers, and coverage COVID related medical expenses. On the other hand, athletes at The Ohio State University responded by stating these demands did not represent their experiences and rejected the narrative of being exploited as collegiate athletes, affirming their decision to assume risks and play. By the end of November 2020, The Ohio State University went from essentially zero COVID-19 cases to pausing all football operations in a period of 48 hours (the head coach tested positive at the same time) because of increased cases. Over the 2020 football season, 139 games were canceled due to the increased spread of COVID-19.

The decision to play puts the health of college athletes at risk. Over 6600 positive COVID-19 cases were publicly reported among college athletes in the U.S. during the 2020–2021 academic year, however, U.S. reporters noted a lack of transparency in total positive case counts (Blinder & Witz, 2020). The lack of transparency, combined with a wide variety of contexts and outcomes across individual college campuses, makes it difficult to assess the complete impact of the decision to play. On one campus, outbreaks among college athletes were a driving factor in campus outbreaks (Hertel et al., 2021). At another, there was a demonstrated lack of spread among college athletes above the regular campus rates (Dixon et al., 2021). However, social gatherings among unvaccinated students are associated with increased spread, including specific cases related to U.S. college sport events such as the 2020 NCAA March Madness Tournament (O'Donoghue, 2021). Furthermore, colleges, regardless of sport participation, were and continue to be a major source of COVID-19 spread, given that by mid-December 2020, The New York

Times reported over 397,000 positive cases across 1800 colleges (NYT, 2020). Yet, even the popular sports magazine, Entertainment and Sports Programming Network (ESPN) reported on the difficulty in accessing positive case data for athletes in the Power 5, stating that a total of 30 out of 65 schools declined to share their athletics program COVID-19 data (Lavigne & Schlabach, 2020).

The NCAA provided some guidance and universal policies aimed at protecting athlete health. Importantly, the decision was made in August 2020 to extend all college athlete eligibility by an additional year and to allow all college athletes to elect not to compete during the 2020–2021 year without penalty. While the choice to not play was made by individual athletes (circumscribed by a neoliberal sporting context of "risk it for the biscuit"), it became complicated as they navigated power dynamics and social pressures from teammates, coaches, family, and even fans to continue to compete rather than sit out that year. Additionally, football athletes could already "redshirt," meaning they can play up to four games and still maintain an extra year of eligibility to compete as an NCAA athlete. In the NCAA, athletes have five years to complete four years of eligibility. However, since the NCAA granted an *additional* year of eligibility, the athletes impacted by COVID could have six years to complete five years of eligibility.

Decisions to play were exceptionally fraught despite attempts to mitigate risk and protect those who opted not to play. Therefore, we now turn to interrogate risk in the context of U.S. collegiate sport and COVID-19. Specifically, we consider historical conceptions of racialized bodies in physical culture. James Short's, 1984 presidential address at the American Sociological Association (ASA) meeting and subsequent publication of "The Social Fabric at Risk" (Frey, 1991; Short, 1984) spurred James Frey's acknowledgment of the rise of risk research in the sociology of sport. Nixon II (1993) extended this discussion by addressing the dominant "culture of risk" in sport through a content analysis of *Sports Illustrated* articles, in which he found that athletes are socialized to adopt a specific set of beliefs about risk and pain (Nixon II, 1993). However, much of the work on risk to date has focused on sport-related physical injury rather than on infectious disease. This is where the syndemic framework is useful.

Syndemics as a Theoretical Framework

A syndemic is "the aggregation of two or more diseases or other health conditions in a population in which there is some level of deleterious biological or behavioural interface that exacerbates the negative health effects of any or all of the diseases involved" (Singer et al., 2017, p. 941). The framework, originally conceived by Merrill Singer (1994), related to substance abuse, violence, and AIDS (SAVA). Its purpose was to refocus attention "on the multifaceted interactions that occur among the health of a community, political and economic structures, and the encompassing physical and social environment" (Singer, 2009, p. xiii). Rather than investigating one specific health disparity, syndemics scholars attempt to consider "the full array of the health and social problems suffered by an individual or a community and assess the nature of the interconnections among the parts, including the intricate ways in which they promote and reinforce each other and thereby create a complex and burdensome web of entwined health and social problems" (Singer, 2009, p. xiv).

Singer explains the development of the framework was driven by an understanding that epidemic entities and social problems are in fact inseparable, often driven or exacerbated by social factors. At times, this Bio-Social interaction can even lead to the development of additional diseases but at the very least leads to increased avoidable suffering. One example demonstrates a syndemic within Latinx populations in Chicago involving interactions between exposure to community violence, depression, and the onset of type II diabetes (Mendenhall, 2013). That specific syndemic suggests diabetes prevention programs failed to address two major underlying contributing factors, namely, grief and declines in mental health-related to the loss of loved ones to gun violence.

Syndemics is distinct from Bronfenbrenner's (1979) social-ecological model, which involves consideration of multiple levels of influence from micro (e.g., individual factors) through the macro-level (e.g., the five major social institutions). Syndemics scholars are concerned with the *clustering* of diseases in relation to social factors and how the social factor either drives those diseases or exacerbates them. Bronfenbrenner's model does not account for Bio-Bio interactions or Bio-Social interactions that lead to a new disease or preventable increased suffering. A "true" syndemic demonstrates both the Bio-Bio and the Bio-Social pathways of interaction in addition to explaining the contribution of the social or structural factor to negative health outcomes within a specific social context (Singer et al., 2020). A syndemic cannot be addressed by only considering one part or diseases as separate entities that simply co-occur or perhaps interact but in isolation from the social context.

Methodology

Establishing a "true" syndemic involves statistical modeling with robust epidemiological data (Mendenhall & Singer, 2020). Considering that data are still being compiled and analyzed related to short and long-term health outcomes associated with COVID-19, the purpose of this chapter is *not* to provide that type of analysis for establishing a true syndemic interaction. Indeed, as noted above, the NCAA did not track COVID-19 cases and individual schools often concealed their positive case numbers among athletics programs from the public. Yet, Singer (2009) already demonstrated an existing syndemic between severe acute respiratory syndrome (SARS), the first major coronavirus outbreak in 2003, and chronic diseases including diabetes mellitus, hypertension, coronary heart disease, and chronic obstructive pulmonary disease (COPD). Considering previous related syndemic interactions such as this and despite limited available data regarding positive SARS Cov-2 (COVID-19) cases among college athletes, we suggest that the syndemics framework, as a theoretical lens, is an important contribution to sociological analyses of sport participation and theorizing health risk, particularly during infectious disease epidemics and pandemics. We propose the driving social factor is the neoliberal model of college sport, discussed below.

In the context of unknown risk and decision-making regarding the health of vulnerable populations, we believe that demonstrating the preliminary evidence for syndemic interactions is warranted to influence future sport participation. Recently, Gravlee's (2020) proposed syndemic involving systemic racism, chronic disease, and COVID-19 share many of our concerns. However, Gravlee does not consider sport, let alone the neoliberal college sports model in the U.S. as a driving social and structural factor. Therefore, we outline a preliminary application of the syndemics framework via demonstrated and potential Bio-Bio and Bio-Social pathways in a U.S. collegiate sport context.

To this end, we offer a case study approach utilizing data sources from news outlets, the Centers for Disease Control (CDC), peer-reviewed literature (where available), University websites, publicly available NCAA documents/press releases, etc. to provide preliminary evidence of the existence of syndemic interactions between COVID-19 and other chronic and acute health conditions which are exacerbated by the decision to proceed with a fall 2020 football season. We discuss Bio-Bio interactions between COVID-19 and several health conditions including psychiatric disorders (especially depression), pulmonary disease (especially asthma), myocarditis, long-term COVID-19 symptoms, and hypertension among others; Bio-Social interactions between health, socioeconomic status, race, grief and trauma from COVID-19-related loss, grief and trauma from exposure to racist violence, and stress from exposure to racism; as well as the structural and social factors which amplify, exacerbate and contribute to the clustering of COVID-19 and other chronic conditions. We discuss the need to address known health inequities in the Black community including higher rates of hypertension, diabetes, and chronic lung diseases (Williams & Sternthal, 2010) that are risk factors for severe COVID-19 symptoms (CDC, 2020). We intentionally use the term health inequities defined as "systematic differences in health that could be avoided by reasonable means" (Arcaya et al., 2015). Meanwhile, the risk of playing football in the U.S. collegiate sport system during COVID-19 is under investigation given limited data on the long-term effects of COVID-19.

Incorporating the syndemics paradigm into the sociology of sport enables our understanding of the effects of COVID-19 and may extend to international sporting contexts which also align with neoliberal values and exploitative processes. Specifically, we theorize the potential for creating a syndemic through pressures to return to in-person collegiate play, which is a conflation of a "return to normal American life" using NCAA football to signify normalcy during a pandemic (Kalman-Lamb et al., 2020). We argue that amidst COVID-19, the continuation of collegiate football is a public health concern and a potential social factor driving the emergence of new disease interactions and increased preventable suffering. Utilizing the syndemic paradigm demonstrates that the perceived social "need" for sport *performance* led to the implementation of *policies* aimed at returning to competitive seasons. Thus, the syndemic *paradigm* explains the connection between *policies* and *performance* amid a public health crisis. We now outline the Syndemics Framework and its application to the NCAA decision surrounding continued play throughout the COVID-19 pandemic.

Syndemics in Action: NCAA U.S. Collegiate Sport Continuation and COVID-19

To build the case for this syndemic interaction, the following sections will use data both within and outside the U.S. collegiate sporting context. Bio-Bio interactions are established mainly outside of the sporting context, Bio-Social interactions are established both within and outside the sporting context, but the structural/social context *is* the sporting context. Therefore, the following sections will start with a wide lens and will narrow to the decision to play in the pandemic as the ultimate focus.

Bio-Bio Interactions

Starting with the wide lens of general population health risks during the pandemic, we consider biological interactions between comorbid or multimorbid diseases including COVID-19. These do not specifically address athletes but are common health problems in the U.S., thus likely to impact athletes. Bio-Bio interactions between COVID-19 and chronic diseases follow the already demonstrated syndemic interactions between SARS (the 2003 coronavirus outbreak) and the same chronic diseases (see Singer, 2009, pp. 60–65). Currently, there are significant associations between cardiovascular disease, diabetes, anxiety disorder, and severe COVID-19 symptoms leading to higher rates of hospitalization and death (Kompaniyets et al., 2021). Similar associations between pulmonary disease (such as asthma, Chronic Obstructive Pulmonary Disease (COPD), interstitial lung disease, cystic fibrosis, and pulmonary hypertension) and COVID-19 have also been demonstrated (CDC, 2021a). Lastly, since the publication of the first round of results from the Big Ten COVID-19 Cardiac Registry, there has been some concern regarding the potential increased risk for athletes to develop myocarditis after testing positive for COVID-19 (Daniels et al., 2021).

There is also a concern for chronic respiratory diseases and interactions with COVID-19. For example, there is demonstrated overlap between asthma and COPD among women as they age (T et al., 2018). This overlap increases the risk of developing COPD with exacerbations related to asthma (Park et al., 2018). For women, these are also associated with an increased risk of developing rheumatoid arthritis (Ford et al., 2020). Given the demonstrated interactions between SARS CoV-2 and COPD leading to an increased risk of severe COVID-19 symptoms (Lippi & Henry, 2020), athletes with asthma have reason to be concerned about potential health outcomes should they test positive for COVID-19.

Gravlee's (2020) proposed syndemic, discussed above, is most concerned with Black and Latinx populations in the U.S. that are disproportionately affected by COVID-19. It highlights connections between the impact of racism on cardiometabolic disease outcomes, seen in work on *weathering* (Geronimus et al., 2006), and structural factors such as overcrowded housing, poor air and water quality, food insecurity, essential worker jobs, and health care access/quality that led to greater exposure to and worsened outcomes of COVID-19. Weathering occurs through disproportionate increases in allostatic load, which is the cumulative physical wear and tear on the body because of stress and "as a consequence of the cumulative impact of repeated experience with social or economic adversity and political marginalization," which is demonstrated via disparities in two biomarker categories (Geronimus et al., 2006, p. 826).

Gravlee (2020), despite being focused on the general population, provides important analysis related to interactions between diabetes, hypertension, and COVID-19. Possible pathways include the renin-angiotensin system, inflammatory dysregulation, and the endothelium, which relate to both hypertension and diabetes in such a way that may be the consequence of increased disease severity for those who contract COVID-19

(Gravlee, 2020, p. 3). Gravlee also acknowledges the potential pleiotropic effects of SARS-CoV-2 on glucose metabolism that may complicate diabetes or lead to new onset, creating a bidirectional relationship between COVID-19 and diabetes (Rubino et al., 2020). Furthermore, coronaviruses, including SARS-CoV-2, are known to result in long-term cardiovascular problems including changes in lipid metabolism (Wu et al., 2017) and increased risk of hypertension and heart diseases. Although such information may be less relevant to most actively competing athletes, retired football athletes and those who gain weight are at risk for cardiometabolic disease such as diabetes (Trexler et al., 2018) and for developing cardiovascular disease and hypertension (Kim et al., 2019).

One disease interaction of particular concern for contact sport athletes is the development of encephalitis and encephalopathy. A study by scholars involving 232 COVID-19 patients with neurological symptoms found that "encephalopathy and encephalitis are among the complications most frequently reported in the registry" such that "more than one-third of patients presented mild or moderate confusional syndrome" (Abenza Abildúa et al., 2021). While the development of increased cerebrospinal fluid (CSF) and encephalitis or encephalopathy is rare compared to more common COVID-19 symptoms (e.g., fever and cough), there is concern regarding an increase of neurological complications in part because of observations of SARS Cov-2 patients developing encephalitis with atypical parkinsonism and "distinctive brain metabolic alterations" (Morassi et al., 2021, p. 1).

COVID-19-related neurological concerns related overlap with mental health concerns related to COVID-19 *and* head trauma, the long-term results of which are still being investigated. Early work indicates an interaction between anxiety disorder and COVID-19 (Kompaniyets et al., 2021) as well as a bidirectional relationship between COVID-19 and psychiatric disorder (Taquet et al., 2021). Athletes face unique risks for depression and have more recently reported higher rates of depression (Gill et al., 2020) with injured athletes at the highest risk (Appaneal et al., 2009). Studies consistently indicate a positive relationship between a history of concussions and/or Traumatic Brain Injuries (TBI) and depression (Hutchison et al., 2018). This nexus alone—COVID-19, head trauma, neurological disorders, and psychiatric disorders—introduces substantial ethical dilemmas for college athletic programs and their athletes moving forward, which we discuss below.

Bio-Social Interactions: Sport Participation as the Social and Structural Factor

Here we turn to Harry Edwards' work on the exploitation of the Black athlete (Edwards, 1969). Edwards's work predates syndemics but informs our proposed syndemic, which is largely driven by the neoliberal model of college sport and exploitation of the Black athlete related to the continuation of collegiate sport during COVID-19. We argue that football is the best example for understanding the concerns about exploitative practices because, in the U.S. context, it is one of the most profitable revenue-generating college sports. This racialized neoliberal model can be seen in the way the NCAA and universities profit from the labor of collegiate athletes, many of whom are Black. For example, in 2019 the NCAA reported that of men's DI football athletes, 49% were Black, 37% were White, and 15% were "other". In 2020, 40% of 183,755 Division I college athletes self-identified as Black, Hispanic, Asian, or Multi-Racial (NCAA Demographics Database, 2021), meaning 73,502 college athletes were at higher risk for being exposed to COVID-19 as well as the above-described diseases and chronic conditions.

Connecting to syndemics and the COVID-19 pandemic, COVID-19 positive case rates, especially hospitalizations and mortality rates, were highest among low socioeconomic status groups and communities of color (Liao & de Maio, 2021). While some of the diseases outlined in the Bio-Bio section may not currently affect collegiate athletes at disproportionate rates, those who come from low-SES communities and/or communities of color are already at disproportionate risk of developing these health conditions later in life and continue to be disproportionately affected by COVID-19 (Mahajan & Larkins-Pettigrew, 2020). These health inequities are related to lower quality housing (Ahmad et al., 2020) and environmental living conditions, which make necessary preventive measures more difficult, whether in terms of size of household, type of housing, the physical condition of housing, type of work and/or in/

ability to work remotely, health insurance status, access to quality healthcare, healthy literacy, water equity (Zhang et al., 2022) and many other related factors. The mortality burden of COVID-19 on communities of color persists even when analyses controlled for SES but were especially high for those living with racialized economic inequity (Feldman & Bassett, 2021).

Multiple variants caused additional surges in cases even among fully vaccinated individuals and increased severe symptomatic cases and hospitalizations among the unvaccinated. One major concern regarding in-person instruction and sport participation on college campuses has been and continues to be the unpredictable nature and emergence of new variants. Consequently, an important future consideration will be the efficacy of the existing vaccines that received FDA Emergency Use Authorization (e.g., Pfizer and Moderna) (Bernal et al., 2021) and any variant's ability to infect and spread (Brown, 2021). With the Delta variant, such factors led the CDC on July 27, 2021, to reinstate mask recommendations for all individuals in indoor public spaces regardless of vaccination status (CDC, 2021b). Such recommendations have continued during the emergence of the Omicron variant.

For this reason, we suggest analyzing collegiate sport participation from a syndemic framework allows consideration beyond individual-level concerns and incorporates interpersonal, community-level, and structural contributions to Bio-Bio interactions and health inequities. Most importantly, we argue that this framework requires us to consider U.S. collegiate sport participation from a holistic perspective and to broaden college athletics programs' attention to athlete health beyond the limits of four years of NCAA competitive eligibility.

Neoliberal U.S. Collegiate Sport as a Syndemic Social Factor

Having outlined the Bio-Bio and Bio-Social interactions above, we now discuss how the neoliberal U.S. collegiate sport model as a social phenomenon during COVID-19 may exacerbate the existing Bio-Bio interactions or lead to new disease development. When we consider the above-outlined interactions between the biological and social factors, the importance of attending to these interactions as more than just comorbidities or structural violence clarifies the utility of this syndemics framework.

We argue that the primary social factor in this proposed syndemic is the neoliberal model of NCAA college sports, which places intense pressure on collegiate athletes to accept no obstacles, play through pain, and win at all costs (Coakley, 2015; Nixon II, 1993). While neoliberal sport models are not unique to the U.S., scholars argue the neoliberal sport model "has its ideological and figurative core in the U.S." (Andrews & Silk, 2012, p. 1). A large component of this ideology focuses on capital-labor relations, in which popular perceptions of success hinge on the bootstrap mentality (e.g., those who experience financial success do so through their own individual hard work and fiscal responsibility rather than through any amount of social privilege or structural inequalities). Conversely, those who do not achieve this 'American Dream' are believed to have personally failed to work hard enough or to be fiscally responsible, thereby absolving the success of any role in the life struggles experienced by marginalized groups with low socioeconomic status. This, in turn, bolstered justifications for reframing social problems as individual problems and the promotion of deregulated free markets (Andrews & Silk, 2012). Sport, particularly in the U.S., has been a central tool in the diffusion of this ideology. What makes this social factor uniquely localized to the U.S. is the NCAA Division I sports teams' network. In addition, the broader business model for colleges and universities in the U.S. is centered around a tuition and fee system designed to fund a substantial component of the annual budget per institution, placing the burden of accessing a college degree on the individual who can afford tuition or can 'earn' a scholarship either via academic merit or athletics. Thus, unpaid college athlete's labor has been theorized as a form of social reproductive labor (Kalman-Lamb, 2019).

The neoliberal model of the university (Giroux, 2002) and the associated racism integral to that model have been theorized at length (Hamer & Lang, 2015). In the interest of social mobility via scholarships and the elusive allure of professional league contracts after college, many BIPOC collegiate athletes are encouraged to accept recruitment offers to the extent that Hawkins (2010) has termed these institutions "the New Plantation". As a result, collegiate athletes, especially BIPOC collegiate football athletes, were expected to participate in a grand COVID-19 college sport experiment, in which some conference commissioners explained that positive COVID-19 cases were "a given" (Scarborough, 2020). Where other professional and college sports competitive seasons were canceled, delayed, or substantially modified due to COVID-19, significantly different decisions were made for college football, which as discussed above appeared to be based on decisions related to revenue. Such decisions would be less ethically questionable had a clearer risk assessment of all sports been made available.

Ethical Implications for Future Sport Participation from a Syndemics Framework Perspective

Through defining this collegiate sport-specific syndemic, we argue the syndemics framework is an important tool for considering the ethical implications of expecting, even encouraging, collegiate athletes to continue playing their competitive season throughout the COVID-19 pandemic.

There is a long history of unethical treatment of athletes (Byers & Hammer, 1995), and specifically Black athletes (Hawkins, 2010). Knowing that many collegiate athletes rely on their athletic scholarship to fund their undergraduate academic degree, which is dependent upon their commitment to competitive U.S. collegiate sport participation, colleges and conferences that chose to remain open for the 2020–2021 Academic Year competitive season constrained athletes' ability to avoid potential Bio-Bio and Bio-Social interactions described above. The consequences are still unfolding. However, like the other known long-term health effects of repeated head trauma from contact sports such as football, we should expect that these problems do not cease once an individual collegiate athlete's season or career ends.

We now discuss the ethical implications of the syndemics framework on future sport participation during COVID-19 and other infectious disease epidemics or pandemics:

1. Concussion epidemic compounded by COVID-19.
2. Informed consent and athletic labor exploitation.
3. Ethics of care.

Concussion Epidemic

Prior to the COVID-19 pandemic, the concussion crisis dominated health-related scholarly discussions on sport (Malcolm, 2018). This issue remains a looming problem that appears to be confounded by potential interactions with SARS CoV-2 in relation to the impact of COVID-19 on collegiate athletes. For example, while long-term symptoms of COVID-19 include memory loss, confusion, headache, it is currently unknown how concussions and COVID-19 interact, let alone how this may impact the development of Chronic Traumatic Encephalopathy (CTE).

Informed Consent and Athletic Labor Exploitation

Those who do test positive for COVID-19 and develop long COVID symptoms may risk losing their ability to advance to professional leagues because of lingering physical impairments. For example, Clemson University's Justin Foster was expected to return to play after the required 14-day quarantine period when he tested positive for COVID-19 but instead ended up with long-haul COVID symptoms that ended his NFL career aspirations (Quinn, 2021). This makes the decision to play more complicated. Failure to adequately educate college athletes regarding the risks posed to them via their choice to participate in in-person training or competitive season activities would be a failure to achieve informed consent. We argue that conversations about athlete health must extend the conversation about risk beyond that of physical injury or the immediate competitive season. Such conversations must include a holistic approach to the athlete's health and wellbeing and must include discussion of potential future risks as they age in relation to testing positive for COVID-19 (and any other diseases, disorders, or injuries that they may incur either during or post-competitive play).

Programs that decided to continue to play assumed there would be positive cases. However, the inequality in those health disparities was assumed to be a result of personal choice (e.g., personal choice to play, personal choice to ignore preventive measures) rather than the policy-level decisions made. Furthermore, it is unclear the extent to which changing risk information was provided to college athletes as evidence was amassed. Without appropriate informed consent of the risks involved with sport participation during an infectious novel disease pandemic, U.S. college athletics programs only perpetuate the disproportionate power dynamic between the universities and the college athletes. The U.S. collegiate sport system has already been accused of exploiting athletic labor. That exploitation, when combined with incomplete information regarding participation risks in pandemic circumstances, is potentially exacerbated by health inequities among marginalized populations.

Ethics of Care

The NCAA (2020) is self-described as a "member-led organization dedicated to the well-being and lifelong success of college athletes" ((NCAA), 2020). The neoliberal model of the NCAA is evidenced in the organization's 16 principles for the conduct of intercollegiate athletics which have been adopted into bylaws, which are internal rules for how the organization operates and sanctions members ((NCAA), 2021c). One of these, "Student-Athlete Well-Being," states, "intercollegiate athletics programs shall be conducted in a manner designed to protect and enhance the physical and educational well-being of student-athletes" ((NCAA), 2021b). Within the bylaw, "Health and Safety," the NCAA claims, "it is the responsibility of each member institution to protect the health of, and provide a safe environment for, each of its participating student-athletes" ((NCAA), 2021a). In these bylaws, the NCAA puts the responsibility onto each individual institution that houses NCAA-level athletics. Moreover, the NCAA dictates what the goals should be (e.g., student-athlete well-being) but each individual school has the autonomy to make decisions for how to carry out this goal. Consequently, the application of the bylaws is highly varied by school.

We argue that this neoliberal "hands-off" model fails to adequately protect college athletes from COVID-19. Instead, the neoliberal model of sport implemented by the NCAA is a way to absolve themselves of responsibility. Indeed, analysis of the effect of preventive measures (e.g., masks, social distancing, etc.) for the general U.S. population implemented between March 15th, 2020, through May 3rd, 2020, found that the U.S. could have prevented 601,667 positive COVID-19 cases and 32,335 COVID-19 deaths if "observed control measures [had] been adopted 1 week earlier [to the first week of March 2020]"(Pei et al., 2020). This is the most important aspect of the syndemic framework, that a large-scale social factor, such as a failure to implement observed control measures and/or the choice to encourage college athletes to continue to play, leads to exacerbated interactions between disease entities and/or leads to new interactions thereby causing suffering that would have not otherwise occurred.

Wren and Waller (Wrenn & Waller, 2017) argue that an ethic of care is pathological in neoliberalism. This is opposed to an ethic of care being normal or natural, to which the Universities contribute and, therefore, should be responsible for helping care for athletes. Further, the approach suggested by the NCAA regarding medical care among collegiate athletes is an "athlete-centered care," approach (NCAA, 2021a). Athlete-centered care is similar to "patient-centered care" which is a practice that seeks to focus medical attention on the specific patient's needs and concerns, as opposed to the doctor's (Bardes 2012). Even though the NCAA states that their focus is on the athletes and the athletes' care, responsibility of care is given to each individual institution. Therefore, it is difficult for the NCAA to understand if athlete health is at the forefront for each institution. This highlights the need to look at athlete health holistically which can be better achieved by looking at athlete health during the pandemic through the lens of a syndemic framework that accounts for the Bio-Bio *and* the Bio-Social.

Conclusion

The use of a syndemic framework provides insight into the consequences of collegiate athletes of color being exploited in a racial neoliberal society during an infectious disease pandemic. Specifically, this framework illuminates the interactions between biological and social entities. We have outlined previously demonstrated syndemics and the biological interactions of concern for this specific U.S. collegiate sporting context—NCAA Division I athletics programs in the U.S., namely COVID-19, diabetes, hypertension, myocarditis, and depression. We have, furthermore, outlined the social and structural factors that are specific to college sports in the U.S., namely the exploitation of athletic labor within neoliberal collegiate sport and the high percentages of athletes of color in revenue-generating sports such as football. Thus, from this syndemic framework, we argue that future sport participation must better address these interactions as an inextricable *whole* rather than addressing only parts of this syndemic, or indeed what may be symptoms of these collective interactions.

References

Abenza Abildúa, M., Atienza, S., Carvalho Monteiro, G., Erro Aguirre, M., Imaz Aguayo, L., Freire Álvarez, E., García-Azorín, D., Gil-Olarte Montesinos, I., Lara Lezama, L., Navarro Pérez, M., Pérez Sánchez, J., Romero Delgado, F., Serrano Serrano, B., Villarreal Vitorica, E., & Ezpeleta Echávarri, D. (2021). Encephalopathy and encephalitis during acute SARS-CoV-2 infection. Spanish Society of Neurology COVID-19 registry. *Neurologia (Barcelona, Spain), 36*(2), 127–134. https://doi.org/10.1016/J.NRL.2020.11.013

Ahmad, K., Erqou, S., Shah, N., Nazir, U., Morrison, A. R., Choudhary, G., & Wu, W. C. (2020). Association of poor housing conditions with COVID-19 incidence and mortality across US counties. *PLoS One, 15*(11). https://doi.org/10.1371/JOURNAL.PONE.0241327

Andrews, D. L., & Silk, M. L. (Eds.). (2012). *Sport and neoliberalism: Politics, consumption, and culture*. Temple University Press.

Appaneal, R. N., Levine, B. R., Perna, F. M., & Roh, J. L. (2009). Measuring postinjury depression among male and female competitive athletes. *Journal of Sport & Exercise Psychology, 31*, 60–76. https://doi.org/10.1123/jsep.31.1.60

Arcaya, M. C., Arcaya, A. L., Subramanian, S., & v. (2015). Inequalities in health: Definitions, concepts, and theories. *Global Health Action, 8*(1). https://doi.org/10.3402/gha.v8.27106

#BigTenUnited. (2020, August 5). The players' tribune. https://www.theplayerstribune.com/articles/big-ten-covid-19-football-season

Bardes, C. (2012). Defining "Patient-Centered Medicine". New England Journal of Medicine, 366, 782–783. https://doi.org/10.1056/NEJMp1200070

Bernal, J. L., Andrews, N., Gower, C., Gallagher, E., Simmons, R., Thelwall, S., Stowe, J., Tessier, E., Groves, N., Dabrera, G., Myers, R., Campbell, C. N. J., Amirthalingam, G., Edmunds, M., Zambon, M., Brown, K. E., Hopkins, S., Chand, M., & Ramsay, M. (2021). Effectiveness of Covid-19 vaccines against the B.1.617.2 (delta) variant. https://doi.org/10.1056/NEJMoa2108891, NEJMoa2108891.

Blinder, A., Higgins, L., & Guggenheim, B. (2020, December 11). *College sports has reported at least 6,629 virus cases—The new york times.* https://www.nytimes.com/2020/12/11/sports/coronavirus-college-sports-football.html

Blinder, A., & Witz, B. (2020, August 10). In push to play, college football stars show sudden unity—The New York times. *The New York Times.* https://www.nytimes.com/2020/08/10/sports/ncaafootball/coronavirus-college-football-players.html

Bronfenbrenner, U. (1979). *The ecology of human development : experiments by nature and design.* Harvard University Press. https://www.hup.harvard.edu/catalog.php?isbn=9780674224575

Brown, C. M. (2021, July). Outbreak of SARS-CoV-2 infections, including COVID-19 vaccine breakthrough infections, associated with large public gatherings—Barnstable county, Massachusetts. In *MMWR. Morbidity and Mortality Weekly Report* (vol. 70 (31)). https://doi.org/10.15585/MMWR.MM7031E2.

Byers, W., & Hammer, C. (1995). *Unsportsmanlike conduct: Exploiting college athletes.* University of Michigan Press.

(CDC), C. for D. C. and P. (2020). *COVID-19 hospitalization and death by race/ethnicity.*

Centers for Disease Control. (2021a). *Certain medical conditions and risk for severe COVID-19 illness.* https://www.cdc.gov/coronavirus/2019-ncov/need-extra-precautions/people-with-medical-conditions.html

Centers for Disease Control. (2021b). *Interim public health recommendations for fully vaccinated people*. CDC.
Coakley, J. (2015). Assessing the sociology of sport: On cultural sensibilities and the great sport myth. *International Review for the Sociology of Sport, 50*(4–5), 402–406. https://doi.org/10.1177/1012690214538864
Daniels, C. J., Rajpal, S., Greenshields, J. T., Rosenthal, G. L., Chung, E. H., Terrin, M., Jeudy, J., Mattson, S. E., Law, I. H., Borchers, J., Kovacs, R., Kovan, J., Rifat, S. F., Albrecht, J., Bento, A. I., Albers, L., Bernhardt, D., Day, C., Hecht, S., et al. (2021). Prevalence of clinical and subclinical myocarditis in competitive athletes with recent SARS-CoV-2 infection. *JAMA Cardiology*, 1–10. https://doi.org/10.1001/jamacardio.2021.2065
Dellenger, R. (2020, August 5). College football players speak out on coronavirus symptoms—Sports Illustrated. *Sports Illustrated*. https://www.si.com/college/2020/08/05/college-football-coronavirus-covid-cases-opt-outs
Dixon, B. C., Fischer, R. S. B., Zhao, H., O'Neal, C. S., Clugston, J. R., & Gibbs, S. G. (2021). Contact and SARS-CoV-2 infections among college football athletes in the Southeastern conference during the COVID-19 pandemic. *JAMA Network Open, 4*(10), e2135566–e2135566. https://doi.org/10.1001/JAMANETWORKOPEN.2021.35566
Edwards, H. (1969). *The revolt of the black athlete*. The Free Press.
Feldman, J. M., & Bassett, M. T. (2021). Variation in COVID-19 mortality in the US by race and ethnicity and educational attainment. *JAMA Network Open, 4*(11), e2135967–e2135967. https://doi.org/10.1001/JAMANETWORKOPEN.2021.35967
Ford, J., Liu, X., Chu, S., Lu, B., Cho, M., & EK, S., KH, C., CA, C., & JA, S. (2020). Asthma, chronic obstructive pulmonary disease, and subsequent risk for incident rheumatoid arthritis among women: A prospective cohort study. *Arthritis & Rheumatology (Hoboken, N.J.), 72*(5), 704–713. https://doi.org/10.1002/ART.41194
Frey, J. (1991). Social risk and the meaning of sport. *Sociology of Sport Journal, 8*, 136–145.
Geronimus, A. T., Hicken, M., Keene, D., & Bound, J. (2006). "Weathering" and age patterns of allostatic load scores among blacks and whites in the United States. *American Journal of Public Health, 96*(5), 826–833. https://doi.org/10.2105/AJPH.2004.060749
Giambalvo, E., & Maese, R. (2021, March 5). Big Ten presidents kept return-to-school football communications out of public eye. *The Washington Post*.

Gill, E. L., Wasielewski, E., & Parker, K. L. (2020). *2020 power five conference behavioral/mental health providers race & gender report card.*
Giroux, H. (2002). Neoliberalism, corporate culture, and the promise of higher education: The university as a democratic public sphere. *Harvard Educational Review, 72*(4), 425–464.
Golliver, B. (2020, July 18). What's it like in the NBA's Disney bubble? For me, hotel room workouts and lots of time to think. *The Washington Post.*
Gravlee, C. C. (2020). Systemic racism, chronic health inequities, and COVID-19: A syndemic in the making? *American Journal of Human Biology, 32*(5), 1–8. https://doi.org/10.1002/ajhb.23482
Gutman, R. (2020, November). Are COVID-19 bubbles a good idea? *The Atlantic.*
Hamer, J. F., & Lang, C. (2015). Race, structural violence, and the neoliberal university: The challenges of inhabitation. *Critical Sociology, 41*(6), 897–912. https://doi.org/10.1177/0896920515594765
Hatteberg, S. J. (2018). Under surveillance: Collegiate athletics as a total institution. *Sociology of Sport Journal, 35*(2), 149–158. https://doi.org/10.1123/ssj.2017-0096
Hawkins, B. (2010). *The new plantation: Black athletes, college sports, and predominantly white NCAA institutions.* Palgrave Macmillan.
Hertel, A. T., Heeter, M. M., Wirfel, O. M., Bestram, M. J., & Mauro, S. A. (2021). Athletes drive distinctive trends of covid-19 infection in a college campus environment. *International Journal of Environmental Research and Public Health, 18*(14). https://doi.org/10.3390/ijerph18147689
Hutchison, M. G., Di Battista, A. P., McCoskey, J., & Watling, S. E. (2018). Systematic review of mental health measures associated with concussive and subconcussive head trauma in former athletes. *International Journal of Psychophysiology, 132,* 55–61. https://doi.org/10.1016/j.ijpsycho.2017.11.006
IHE Staff. (2020, October 29). *Live updates archive: Aug. 2020—Oct. 2021 COVID-19 and higher education.* Inside Higher Ed. https://www.insidehighered.com/news/2021/10/29/live-updates-archive-aug-2020-oct-2021-covid-19-and-higher-education
Jain, V., Duse, A., & Bausch, D. G. (2018). Planning for large epidemics and pandemics: Challenges from a policy perspective. *Current Opinion in Infectious Diseases, 31*(4), 316–324. https://doi.org/10.1097/QCO.0000000000000462

Kalman-Lamb, N. (2019). Athletic Labor and Social Reproduction. *Journal of Sport and Social Issues, 43*(6), 515–530. https://doi-org.proxy2.library.illinois.edu/10.1177/0193723519850879

Kalman-Lamb, N., Silva, D., & Mellis, J. (2020). College Football Feels All Too Normal During the Pandemic. *Time.*

Kim, J. H., Hollowed, C., Liu, C., Al-Badri, A., Alkhoder, A., Dommisse, M., Gowani, Z., Miller, A., Nguyen, P., Prabakaran, G., Sidoti, A., Wehbe, M., Galante, A., Gilson, C. L., Clark, C., Ko, Y. A., Quyyumi, A. A., & Baggish, A. L. (2019). Weight gain, hypertension, and the emergence of a maladaptive cardiovascular phenotype among US football players. *JAMA Cardiology, 4*(12), 1221–1229. https://doi.org/10.1001/jamacardio.2019.3909

Kompaniyets, L., Pennington, A. F., Goodman, A. B., Rosenblum, H. G., Belay, B., Ko, J. Y., Chevinsky, J. R., Schieber, L. Z., Summers, A. D., Lavery, A. M., Preston, L. E., Danielson, M. L., Cui, Z., Namulanda, G., Yusuf, H., & Gundlapalli, A. V. (2021). Underlying medical conditions and severe illness among 540,667 adults hospitalized with COVID-19, march 2020-march 2021. *Preventing Chronic Disease: Public Health Research, Practice, and Policy, 18*(E66), 1–13.

Lavigne, P., & Schlabach, M. (2020, September 3). Nearly half of Power 5 won't disclose COVID-19 test data. *ESPN.* https://www.espn.com/college-sports/story/_/id/29745712/nearly-half-power-5-disclose-covid-19-test-data

Leroy, M. H. (2021). Harassment, abuse, and mistreatment in college sports: Protecting players through employment Laws. *Berkeley Journal of Employment & Labor Law, 42*(1), 117. https://doi.org/10.15779/Z385H7BV2X

Liao, T. F., & de Maio, F. (2021). Association of Social and Economic Inequality with coronavirus disease 2019 incidence and mortality across US counties. *JAMA Network Open, 4*(1), 1–10. https://doi.org/10.1001/jamanetworkopen.2020.34578

Lippi, G., & Henry, B. (2020). Chronic obstructive pulmonary disease is associated with severe coronavirus disease 2019 (COVID-19). *Respiratory Medicine, 167.* https://doi.org/10.1016/J.RMED.2020.105941

Maese, R., Giambalvo, E., & Galocha, A. (2021, March 16). How the NCAA tournament built its 'bubble' in Indianapolis—Washington Post. *The Washington Post.* https://www.washingtonpost.com/sports/interactive/2021/ncaa-tournament-bubble-covid-indianapolis/

Mahajan, U. V., & Larkins-Pettigrew, M. (2020). Racial demographics and COVID-19 confirmed cases and deaths: A correlational analysis of 2886 US counties. *Journal of Public Health, 42*(3), 445–447. https://doi.org/10.1093/PUBMED/FDAA070

Malcolm, D. (2018). Concussion in sport: Public, professional and critical sociologies. *Sociology of Sport Journal, 35*(2), 141–148. https://doi.org/10.1123/SSJ.2017-0113

Mendenhall, E. (2013). *Syndemic suffering: Social distress, depression, and diabetes among Mexican immigrant women.* Routledge.

Mendenhall, E., & Singer, M. (2020). What constitutes a syndemic? Methods, contexts, and framing from 2019. *Current Opinion in HIV and AIDS, 15*(4), 213–217. https://doi.org/10.1097/COH.0000000000000628

Morassi, M., Palmerini, F., Nici, S., Magni, E., Savelli, G., Guerra, U., Chieregato, M., Morbelli, S., & Vogrig, A. (2021). SARS-CoV-2-related encephalitis with prominent parkinsonism: Clinical and FDG-PET correlates in two patients. *Journal of Neurology.* https://doi.org/10.1007/S00415-021-10560-3

Nadkarni, R. (2020, August 10). *Inside college football players fight to save the season—Sports Illustrated.* Sports Illustrated. https://www.si.com/college/2020/08/10/ncaa-football-season-we-want-to-play-united

NCAA Demographics Database. (2021).

(NCAA), N. C. A. A. (2020). *What is the NCAA?* https://www.ncaa.org/about/resources/media-center/ncaa-101/what-ncaa

(NCAA), N. C. A. A. (2021a). *Bylaw 2.2.* https://web3.ncaa.org/lsdbi/reports/getReport/90008

(NCAA), N. C. A. A. (2021b). *Bylaw 2.2.3.* https://web3.ncaa.org/lsdbi/bylaw?bylawId=2456&division=1&adopted=0

(NCAA), N. C. A. A. (2021c). *The 16 Principles for Conduct of Intercollegiate Athletics.* https://www.ncaa.org/about/16-principles-conduct-intercollegiate-athletics

Nixon, H. L., II. (1993). Accepting risks of pain and injury in sport: Mediated cultural influences on playing hurt. *Sociology of Sport Journal, 10,* 183–196.

O'Donoghue, A. L. (2021). Association of University Student Gatherings with Community COVID-19 infections before and after the NCAA march madness tournament. *JAMA Network Open, 4*(10), e2130783–e2130783. https://doi.org/10.1001/JAMANETWORKOPEN.2021.30783

Pavlidis, A., & Rowe, D. (2021). The Sporting Bubble as Gilded Cage: Gendered Professional Sport in Pandemic Times and Beyond. *M/C Journal, 24*(1). https://doi.org/10.5204/mcj.2736 (Original work published March 13, 2021).

Park, J., Kim, E., Kim, M., Kim, T., & JH, C., YJ, R., SW, L., YM, O., SJ, Y., WI, C., KH, Y., & JH, L. (2018). Increased risk of exacerbation in asthma predominant asthma-chronic obstructive pulmonary disease overlap syndrome. *Tuberculosis and Respiratory Diseases, 81*(4), 289–298. https://doi.org/10.4046/TRD.2017.0064

Pei, S., Kandula, S., & Shaman, J. (2020). Differential effects of intervention timing on COVID-19 spread in the United States. *Science. Advances, 6*(49). https://doi.org/10.1126/SCIADV.ABD6370/SUPPL_FILE/ABD6370_SM.PDF

Quinn, T. J. (2021, September). *"Is this my life now?": Clemson defensive end Justin Foster's—And my—Struggle with long-haul COVID*. ESPN. https://www.espn.com/college-football/story/_/id/32127148/clemson-defensive-end-justin-foster-my-struggle-long-haul-covid

Restore Illinois. (2020). State of Illinois. https://coronavirus.illinois.gov/restore-illinois.html.

Rubino, F., Amiel, S. A., Zimmet, P., Alberti, G., Bornstein, S., Eckel, R. H., Mingrone, G., Boehm, B., Cooper, M. E., Chai, Z., Prato, S. Del, Ji, L., Hopkins, D., Herman, W. H., Khunti, K., Mbanya, J.-C., & Renard, E. (2020). New-onset diabetes in Covid-19. *383*(8), 789–790. https://doi.org/10.1056/NEJMC2018688.

Scarborough, A. (2020, August 1). *SEC tells football players positive coronavirus tests on all teams are "a given."* ESPN. https://www.espn.com/college-football/story/_/id/29578644/sec-tells-football-players-positive-coronavirus-tests-all-teams-given

Short, J. (1984). The social fabric at risk: Toward the social transformation of risk analysis. *American Sociological Review, 49*(6), 711–725.

Singer, M. (1994). AIDS and the health crisis of the U.S. urban poor: The perspective of critical medical anthropology. *Social Science & Medicine, 39*, 931–948.

Singer, M. (1996). A dose of drugs, a touch of violence, a case of AIDS: Conceptualizing the SAVA syndemic. *Free Inquiry in Creative Sociology, 24*, 99–110.

Singer, M. (2009). *Introduction to syndemics : a critical systems approach to public and community health* (1st ed.). Jossey-Bass.

Singer, M., Bulled, N., & Ostrach, B. (2020). Whither syndemics?: Trends in syndemics research, a review 2015–2019. *Global Public Health, 15*(7), 943–955. https://doi.org/10.1080/17441692.2020.1724317

Singer, M., Bulled, N., Ostrach, B., & Mendenhall, E. (2017). Syndemics and the biosocial conception of health. *The Lancet, 389*(10072), 941–950. https://doi.org/10.1016/S0140-6736(17)30003-X

T, T., J, Z., N, G., LY, F., PJ, V., C, L., A, G., & AB, M. (2018). Asthma and chronic obstructive pulmonary disease overlap in women. Incidence and risk factors. *Annals of the American Thoracic Society, 15*(11), 1304–1310. https://doi.org/10.1513/ANNALSATS.201802-078OC

Taquet, M., Luciano, S., Geddes, J. R., & Harrison, P. J. (2021). Bidirectional associations between COVID-19 and psychiatric disorder: Retrospective cohort studies of 62 354 COVID-19 cases in the USA. *The Lancet Psychiatry, 8*(2), 130–140. https://doi.org/10.1016/S2215-0366(20)30462-4

The New York Times. (2020, December 11). Tracking the coronavirus at U.S. colleges and universities—The New York Times. *The New York Times*. https://www.nytimes.com/interactive/2020/us/covid-college-cases-tracker.html

Thomason, A., & O'Leary, B. (2021, August 2). Live coronavirus updates. *Chronical of Higher Education*. https://www.chronicle.com/blogs/live-coronavirus-updates/heres-a-list-of-colleges-that-will-require-students-to-be-vaccinated-against-covid-19?cid2=gen_login_refresh&cid=gen_sign_in

Trexler, E. T., Smith-Ryan, A. E., Defreese, J. D., Marshall, S. W., Guskiewicz, K. M., & Kerr, Z. Y. (2018). Associations between BMI change and cardiometabolic risk in retired football players. *Medicine and Science in Sports and Exercise, 50*(4), 684–690. https://doi.org/10.1249/MSS.0000000000001492

Victor, D., Serviss, L., & Paybarah, A. (2020, October 2). What Trump has said about wearing masks and Covid-19—The New York Times. *The New York Times*. https://www.nytimes.com/2020/10/02/us/politics/donald-trump-masks.html

Williams, D. R., & Sternthal, M. (2010). Understanding racial-ethnic disparities in health: Sociological contributions. *Journal of Health and Social Behavior, 51*(1), S15–S27. https://doi.org/10.1177/0022146510383838

Wrenn, M. V., & Waller, W. (2017). Care and the neoliberal individual. *Journal of Economic Issues, 51*(2), 495–502. https://doi.org/10.1080/00213624.2017.1321438

Wu, Q., Zhou, L., Sun, X., Yan, Z., Hu, C., Wu, J., Xu, L., Li, X., Liu, H., Yin, P., Li, K., Zhao, J., Li, Y., Wang, X., Li, Y., Zhang, Q., Xu, G., & Chen, H. (2017). Altered lipid metabolism in recovered SARS patients twelve years after infection. *Scientific Reports 2017, 7*(1), 1–12. https://doi.org/10.1038/s41598-017-09536-z

Zhang, X., Warner, M. E., & Grant, M. (2022). Water shutoff moratoria lowered COVID-19 infection and death across U.S. *States. American Journal of Preventive Medicine, 62*(2), 149. https://doi.org/10.1016/J.AMEPRE.2021.07.006

Zucker, J. (2020, August 16). Nebraska football parents push for big ten to play 2020 season in open letter | bleacher report | latest news, videos and highlights. *Bleacher Report*. https://bleacherreport.com/articles/2904964-nebraska-football-parents-push-for-big-ten-to-play-2020-season-in-open-letter

24

On the Politics and Embodiments of Longing: Snapshots from a Digital Photo Diary Study of Australians' Movement Experiences During Lockdown

Marianne Clark

The COVID-19 pandemic, marching determinedly into its third year at time of writing, has disrupted any number of daily routines. Work, care, and leisure practices have been reconfigured to limit the spread of the virus and spaces usually associated with recreation and fitness, such as commercial gyms and community centres, have lurched in and out of lockdown. In some parts of Australia (and other countries around the world) travel limits have been periodically placed on how far people can travel from home.

These new restrictions drastically curtailed opportunities for incidental physical activity and disrupted the exercise routines of avid fitness buffs and recreational movers alike. In response and at the urging of public health advice encouraging people to remain active to protect both

M. Clark (✉)
Acadia University, Wolfville, NS, Canada

University of New South Wales, Sydney, NSW, Australia
e-mail: marianne.clark@acadiau.ca

D. L. Andrews et al. (eds.), *Sport and Physical Culture in Global Pandemic Times*, Global Culture and Sport Series, https://doi.org/10.1007/978-3-031-14387-8_24

physical and mental health (Australian Government, 2020; World Health Organization, 2020), people have had to imagine and create new pandemic fitness practices. This process has involved both embracing and eschewing the influx of online fitness offerings, purchasing new home exercise equipment, and cobbling together makeshift gym set-ups in whatever space is available (Clark & Lupton, 2021; Newbold et al., 2021).

Such creative improvisations have prompted new engagements with indoor and outdoor spaces and yielded a range of affective and embodied experiences (Clark & Lupton, 2021; Thorpe, 2022). In this chapter I explore these experiences through insights gleaned from a digital ethnographic project exploring Australians' improvised pandemic fitness routines. Specifically, I pay attention to a palpable sense of longing that flowed through participants' stories. Conceptualised here as an affective force, longing both emerges and is expressed through people's moving encounters with outdoor spaces. It arises in unexpected ways as bodies respond to the extraordinary conditions wrought by the COVID-19 pandemic and prompts new practices, relations, and sense-making processes.

In what follows I explore longing and consider what longing might do in the context of the COVID-19 crisis. Specifically, I consider the bodily and relational dimensions of longing and how it might contribute to the collective emotional vocabulary required to make sense of these extraordinary times. To do so, I draw on data collected through digital photo diaries that sought to explore how people's pandemic movement practices and their meanings. Attending to the expressions of longing that flowed through people's stories, I highlight the centrality of everyday movement routines in sense making processes and further consider the capacity of longing to prompt new relations and modes of being.

To organise this chapter, I first outline the ways physical activity and engagement with outdoor spaces have been positioned during the COVID-19 pandemic. I then introduce the concept of longing and describe how I understand longing as an embodied affective force. Here I draw upon feminist understandings (Ahmed, 2013; Hemmings, 2005) of affect as deeply corporeal, relational and socio-political. This allows me to consider how longing emerges through human encounters with human and more than human bodies and environments and attend to its visceral and corporeal dimensions. Such perspectives also encourage analyses that account for broader socio-political conditions and the power relations through which they are produced (Thorpe et al., 2020b). Finally, I provide details of the photo digital diary methodology employed and present analysis of the diary content.

Keep Active and Get Outside! (Even During a Pandemic)

During the COVID-19 pandemic public health advice encouraged regular engagement in exercise and physical activity despite the practical constraints posed by social distancing conditions (Black Dog Institute, 2022; World Health Organization, 2020). As the body—that fleshy, breathing, exerting entity—emerged as site of risk and contagion, increased attention was paid to where and when it moved and the other bodies and spaces it encountered. This scrutiny can be conceptualized as what Robert Esposito refers to as the "spatiality of biopoliticized flesh" (2008, p. 160). Inspired by Esposito and other theorists concerned with the ways biopower targets and operates through human bodies, Newman et al. (2015) consider the biomedical discourses that proliferated in response to the increasing community spread of methicillin resistant Staphylococcus aureus (CA-MRSA). The authors trace how the body is conceptualised through popular biopolitical discourse as a "site of transmission, inoculation, and isolation—as a living ecological and pathological vessel" (p. 155).

Similarities can be observed in context of COVID-19, as bodily mobilities, proximities boundaries come to matter in increasingly intensified ways. At the same time, neoliberal logic continues its machinations and individual bodies are urged to 'take care' of themselves by participating in regular exercise, so as long as the body is appropriately contained and moving in and through permissible spaces. Within this public health discourse, the importance of getting outside was particularly highlighted, with the potential of time spent outdoors to preserve and improve both physical and mental health emphasised in popular and medical discourse (Centers for Disease Control and Prevention, 2022; The Victoria Health

Promotion Foundation, 2022). Early in the pandemic, the ritual of the daily walk became a cultural touchstone with newspaper columns and personal essays documenting people's reflections on their regular outdoor forays, describing fleeting moments of joy and (re)invigorated relationships with their neighbourhoods, natural environments, and other humans (Brinson, 2020; Dunn, 2020).

Research supports the idea that engaging in some form of physical activity during the COVID pandemic indeed yields physical and mental health benefits (Maugeri et al., 2020; Young et al., 2022). A survey study in Canada found those who were more physically active during the pandemic reported greater mental health scores (Lesser & Nienhuis, 2020). This same study also found those individuals who performed more of their activity outside exhibited lower levels of anxiety. Similarly, an Austrian-based study reported found time spent outdoors during the pandemic was associated with improved mental health (Haider et al., 2021).

These findings are unsurprising given it has been well established that people are generally more physically active when outside and that time spent in parks, bushland and other green spaces yields physical and mental health benefits (Lee & Maheswaran, 2011; Van den Berg et al., 2010; M. White et al., 2019). Engagement with blue spaces, a term used to refer to watery environments found in in both urban and wilderness settings (e.g., oceans, lakes, rivers, fountains), is similarly believed to promote health and wellbeing (Foley & Kistemann, 2015; Olive & Wheaton, 2021; M. P. White et al., 2013) Physical cultural scholars have illustrated how activities performed in and around coastal and blue spaces (e.g., surfing and swimming) can foster positive emotional, social, and embodied experiences (Britton & Foley, 2021; Wheaton et al., 2017), calling attention to the sensory, immersive, and connected experiences active engagement with such spaces can prompt.

While this research underlines the important role of green and blue spaces in fostering well-being and meaningful fitness and leisure pursuits, access to such spaces is always mediated by myriad social, economic and geo-political conditions (Coen et al., 2021; Evers, 2008; Olive & Wheaton, 2021). In their introduction to a special issue devoted to the relationship between blue spaces, physical activity and wellbeing, Olive and Wheaton (2021) remind us that these spaces are always implicated in the production of health inequities. This is particularly important to remember in the context of Covid-19 during which (health) inequity has played out dramatically; different bodies live the pandemic in drastically different ways (Braidotti, 2020). Although popular and public health discourse espouse the benefits of time spent in outdoor spaces, it is often overlooked that aesthetically pleasant and safe outdoor spaces—and their associated health benefits—are not accessible to everyone. For example, research conducted in the Australian state of Victoria while its residents endured a strict and prolonged lockdown in 2020 found that upwards of 135,000 homes in the city of Melbourne alone had little or no access to parkland within their allowed 5 km radius (Lakhani et al., 2020). Consequently, people in those households and neighbourhoods risk missing out on or having limited access to the health benefits associated with such spaces.

Writing about the social and cultural geographies of physical activity during COVID, Coen et al. (2021) consider the argument there may be more pressing matters than whether people remain active as the virus wreaks its destruction on lives and livelihoods. However, the authors extend this line of thinking to astutely wonder if perhaps the more pressing question is not whether people *should* worry about physical activity but rather who *is able* to? What socio-material conditions enable some people to prioritise physical activity? I keep this question in mind and situate my discussion of pandemic fitness and affective flows of longing within broader discussions around access to and the meaning of outdoor spaces during the pandemic. In what follows below I articulate how I conceptualise longing.

Longing as Affective Force

Qualitative investigations of pandemic physical activity practices suggest people create and engage in these practices as part of their emotional and embodied response to the shifting social, emotional, and material conditions of the COVID crisis (Clark & Lupton, 2021; Jeffrey et al., 2021). For some, the benefits yielded by these practices exceed instrumental framings provided by public health discourse. For example, a survey study of adults aged 50 years and older who participated in online Pilates classes in England suggests people engaged in these classes to maintain a sense of routine and to connect with others (Taylor et al., 2021). In their feminist examination of the experiences of five women yoga practitioners in Aotearoa New Zealand, Jeffrey et al. (2021) describe how physical, mental and ethical dimensions of regular Yoga practice provided deep emotional support to women as they navigated the various challenges of life during COVID. Results from the larger study informing this chapter also reveal how exercise provided Australian adults with a sense of emotional and embodied escape, albeit fleeting, from the weight of pandemic conditions (Clark & Lupton, 2021).

When writing about escape I noted engaging in physical activity (both inside and outside of the home) acted to transform the affective atmosphere daily life, to provide a brief reprieve through the kinaesthetic and sensory dimensions of movement. Closely related to this notion of escape was the visceral sense of longing that flowed through participant accounts; a longing to move, to be outside, to be reunited with loved ones stranded across sealed borders, and quite simply for things to be different. While not all participants named it as such, the restless yearning or desire we might associate with longing was unmistakable.

Philosopher Emmanuel Levinas (1969) describes longing as a 'metaphysical desire' where metaphysical refers to that which exceeds human perception or observation. Levinas is not particularly interested in what people long for nor is longing something that is prompted (or eased) by the lack or presence of a specific person, place, or thing. Rather longing is an embodied frisson, a visceral interruption to subjective experience. It calls attention to conditions and sensations that might otherwise go unnoticed and prompts acknowledgement of one's own subjectivity and vulnerability (Dalton, 2009). Levinas (1969) suggests longing is implicated in the process of becoming a higher or 'true' self as it this disruption of subjectivity that draws attention to possibility.

In his book *Longing for the Other: Levinas and Metaphysical Desire*, philosophy scholar Drew Dalton (2009) paraphrases Levinas for us, explaining "metaphysical desire can be read as awakening a subject from the slumber of ontological actuality into the true life of ethical potentiality" (p.42) Longing reveals the limits of our subjective existence through interruption and disruption. In doing so it can shift our attention and move us towards other, possibly more fulfilling, ways of being.

A small body of research exists within the caring sciences and health psychology that draws on these understandings of longing (Hemberg et al., 2020; Venke Ueland, Dysvik, & Furnes, 2020; V Ueland et al., 2018; V Ueland, Rørtveit, et al., 2020). In this literature, scholars examine the phenomenon of longing from an individual perspective in people living with and surviving cancer as well as those living with obesity. These qualitative studies take a phenomenological approach to consider what people in these circumstances might long for and what longing might do in and for their respective journeys towards health and/or illness. Findings suggest people feel a longing for life prior to illness and for what has been lost, for a return to normality, and even for seemingly mundane things like spending time in natural environments and outdoors spaces. Longing also emerges as a resource called upon for survival as it orients attention and energy towards creating deeper relations and connections in everyday life (Ueland et al., 2018).

The authors suggest such insights can help health providers better understand the experiences and needs of individuals living with chronic health conditions. In turn, this understanding can help care providers support individuals in living their lives more meaningfully. Importantly, longing in this arrangement is not quite a human-centric feeling that resides within an individual, rather it is always deeply situated within and emergent through specific social conditions. What people long for is always socially and materially contingent. As Ueland and colleagues (2020) point out, longing may reflect the desire for an ordinary life, but what constitutes 'ordinary' is always situated, negotiated and contested. Authors further suggest longing for different possibilities of 'normality' can be understood as a performance of resistance to disciplinary social norms.

In this way longing does something. It emerges as a restless yearning but is not characterized by absence or lack. Instead, it prompts new attentional orientations and imaginaries of possibility. It is also, I argue, particularly relevant to discussions within physical cultural, embodiment and health studies for its corporeal and socio-political dimensions. Therefore, in this chapter I borrow from and extend the above understandings and further conceptualise longing as an affective force with transformative capacities. I examine how longing might materialise, emerge, and be expressed through bodily encounters with human and more-than-human others in the context of COVID-19. Drawing from Spinozian (Spinoza, 1994) understandings I understand affect as deeply corporeal and imbued with the potential *to do* something. Elaborating on this understanding I consider the writings of feminist scholars who remind us that affect is also deeply social and political (Ahmed, 2013; Brennan, 2015; Hemmings, 2005). While Brennan (2015) suggests affect can be understood as flows of energy transmitted through relational encounters between bodies, she insists emotional and affective experiences cannot be disentangled from social context. Similarly, Ahmed and Hemmings suggest affect cannot be understood "as something prepersonal that flows between bodies in a generic sense. Rather, some bodies generate different affective responses in a particular context than others"(Åhäll, 2018, p. 40). These differences are produced through power relations and always implicated in the ways we encounter and form relations with human and non-human others.

Conceptualising longing as an affective—but always politicised—force encourages analyses that consider the relational dimensions of longing and the ways it materialises and is expressed through deeply situated bodily encounters. I argue it further prompts consideration of what longing might 'do' and the social, material, and geo-political conditions through which it emerges. Given these possibilities I use it to guide my analysis of the digital photo diaries created and shared by participants. In so doing I turn my attention to the relational encounters been bodies, movement and indoor and outdoor spaces while considering the socio, geo-political and material context in which these practices occur. I now outline the methodological approach taken to achieve this.

Methodological Details

In this chapter I draw from empirical material collected between July and September 2020 as part of a broader study examining pandemic fitness practices, space, and digital technologies (Clark & Lupton, 2021). The purpose of this project was to explore how, where, and why Australians engaged in fitness during COVID, the kinds of technologies and equipment they used, and the meanings these practices held for them. Participants were recruited via social media and the study was open to all adults 18–64 years of age currently living in Australia and currently engaging in any form of physical activity for at least 20 minutes a day, two times or more per week. A total of 16 people participated, aged 30–56 years.

Data collection involved online interviews and virtual tours of the activity space (see Clark & Lupton, 2021) as well as digital photo diaries. In this chapter I focus specifically on material collected through the digital photo diaries. This methodological approach takes inspiration from diary-based research methods used by qualitative health and psychology researchers to examine insights into health behaviours and practices across time and space (Day & Thatcher, 2009; Herron et al., 2019; Milligan et al., 2005). Diary methods lend insight into aspects of daily life that might be overlooked or considered less important in an interview setting and offer participants the opportunity to actively guide the research process by deciding when, where and to what extent certain moments or events will be explored (Markham & Couldry, 2007). In my study, digital photo diaries were employed to explore the materialities and spatialities of people's pandemic fitness and the feelings and sensations that emerged. While these diaries provided some practical solutions to conducting field work during the pandemic, they also offered unique strengths and capacities for eliciting rich insights across time and space and for capturing the more-than-human forces that shaped pandemic fitness and the emotional responses they evoked.

This method also draws from visual social research methods that have the potential to deepen and extend our understanding of our social worlds (Phoenix, 2010; Pink, 2013). Visual approaches to knowledge creation both accommodate alternative ways of knowing that exceed logo-centric approaches reliant on language to construct and communicate knowledge (Knowles & Sweetman, 2004). Phoenix (2010) advocating for the use of visual methods within physical cultural studies, suggests "images are powerful in that they can *do* things. Images can evoke a particular kind of response" (p. 94). It was my intent to access thoughts and feelings that may be just out of reach of words, particularly as it felt at times as though we were all grasping at the right words to make sense of the world around us. I also wanted to see where else people were moving. The virtual tours were fascinating and disrupted the sedentariness of the interview but were confined to the spatialities and temporalities of the online interview. Here diaries are used to capture and convey relationships between bodies and social and material worlds and in attempt to access deeply felt responses to kinaesthetic sensations of physical movement and affective encounters with various outdoor spaces.

Procedures

Eight of the 16 participants from the larger project took part in the digital photo diary exercise. Six women, two men, four from Melbourne and four from Sydney. After informed consent was obtained participants received an email every day for 7–12 days until at least five entries were collected. The email contained a link to an online form that invited participants to upload a photo related to their physical activity practice. Participants were then asked to provide information about when and where the photo was taken, what the photo depicts, a caption, and brief description about how they felt when the photo was taken and/or what the photo means to them. Participants could choose how to take their photos (e.g., by smartphone or digital camera) so long as the photos could be uploaded to the online platform used. The daily form provided unlimited space for diary entries, however most participants provided two-to-three paragraphs.

Analysis considered both the visual and text-based material (Pink, 2004) and was informed by the guiding concepts such as affect, movement and relationality. A relational approach meant analysis also recognised and actively sought to attend to the distributed agentic capacities of the human, more than human, social and environmental forces implicated in people's pandemic fitness improvisations. This means it was not only *what* appeared in the photos that became the object of analysis, but rather how the various elements identified in both photos and text became intertwined in the production and performance of pandemic fitness and its multiple meanings.

Analysis

Sarah Pink (2013) suggests "the purpose of analysis is not to translate 'visual evidence' into verbal knowledge, but to explore the relationship between visual and other knowledge" (p. 96). Inspired by Pink but also drawing pragmatically on Harrison (2004) and Phoenix (2010) who suggest some form of verbalisation is often necessary to communicate the meanings of an image I engage both the visual elements and the text provided in my analysis. In doing so I seek to gain insight into the various relations unfolding in the image and understand how they might be produced through and productive of embodied pandemic fitness experiences and their meanings. This method also seeks to help invoke those senses and feelings not captured easily through image or text but that nevertheless contribute to the production of knowledge and experience (e.g., sound, smell, touch).

While this digital method was designed in part to accommodate the constraints to field work posed by pandemic conditions, Hine (2020) reminds us that the digital is always embodied. I was particularly interested in how the physical performance of movement during the pandemic and the embodied encounters with various spaces shaped people's sense making processes. This digital method therefore allowed me to tune into the materiality of space, bodily sensations and relationalities that emerged in people's stories. The text and images work in tandem to produce evocative insights and narratives about not only pandemic fitness practices and the spaces they occurred but also how people lived and experienced the pandemic through the moving body. I now present insights gleaned from the photo diaries, paying particular attention the sense of longing that emerged.

Findings

In what follows I share my analysis of the expressions of longing that emerged in the digital photo diaries; a longing to move, to be outdoors, to be reunited with loved ones, for things to be otherwise. This sense of longing was deeply bodily and visceral. It was expressed through improvised movement practices and often entangled with the spaces in which and through which people moved. Analysis focuses the relationships these practices created, and the ways longing was felt and articulated. I further consider what longing might *do* in these stories and in the context of the COVID-19 pandemic. I share a total of three diaries entries, two from Evie (pseudonym) an employed 39-year-old mother of two living in Sydney with her husband and children and one from Jane, an employed 29-year-old from Melbourne who shares a flat with a friend.

Longing for the Sea, 'wildness', and Catharsis

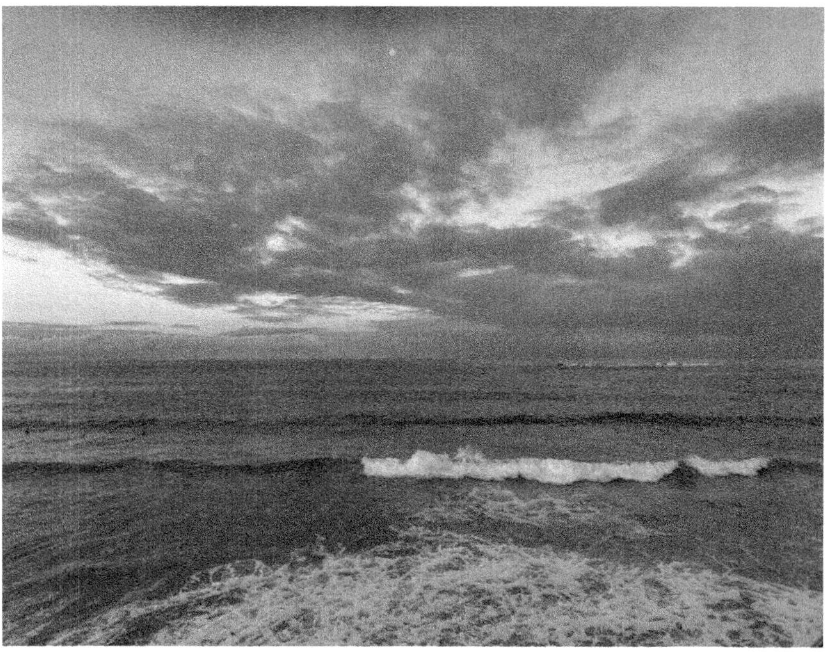

Diary Entry: Evie

Please describe the photo and share why is it meaningful to you: This picture is from my walk today. Sometimes I run but today I walked my usual route along the coast. The ocean was choppy and wild and it was very windy. In this picture I try to capture the energy, but it doesn't do it justice. You can't feel the wind or hear or smell the ocean. But it's all part of this picture. I love it when it's wild like this. It's like the ocean is restless and it's cathartic just to be close to it. You can't see this in the photo, but it was part of the moment and inspired me to take this photo.

I was feeling restless today and tired and worried. With everything going on it's hard to focus on work and I'm exhausted from home schooling and worry. But by the end of the day my legs are just longing to move, I long to get out of the house and to be by the ocean. By the end of the day I long to get out of the house and to get up to the coast. Walking or running here is cathartic and I love being in this wide-open space. The world feels so heavy but the energy of the wind and the wildness of ocean carries some of that weight away for me. I like sunny days but I like these darker days too. I think they capture something we're all feeling but can't really express. I need these moments of release. After my walk I can go home and get dinner on the table and feel like I can get through one more day.

When was this photo taken:? 4:40pm

What appears in the photo (e.g., people, place, objects)?: Wavy ocean, sky appear in the photo.

How were you feeling when you took the photo?: restless, energized, soothed

Evie's photo image shows a vista of the ocean on the east coast of Sydney on an early spring day. The accompanying text describes what elements appears in the picture (e.g., textured ocean, sky), how she was feeling, and situates the encounter that prompted this entry specifically in the context of the pandemic. Evie acknowledges the heavy affective atmosphere and sense of exhaustion that characterise life during the pandemic (Clark & Lupton, 2021; Jeffrey et al., 2021), and the resulting emotional responses (e.g., tired, worried). There also lives a sense of longing in this entry, manifesting viscerally in aching legs and a palpable sense of restlessness.

This sense of longing in turn prompts an embodied doing that involves changing geographic location and seeking out specific outdoor spaces (in this case, coastal spaces). Moving through these spaces transforms Evie's embodied and emotional experience which is largely shaped by the conditions of the pandemic. She describes feeling exhausted with worry and acknowledges the additional labour of home schooling presented by the public health measures introduced to limit the spread of the virus. This sense of exhaustion was also present in Jeffrey and colleagues' examination of yoga practitioners' experiences during the pandemic and speaks to the deeply corporeal ways this exhaustion manifests. In Evie's story, these sensations prompted a longing to move and to be elsewhere. In turn, her physical practice (walking by the ocean) provides release and catharsis. This sensation emerges not only through physical movement, but through the relational encounters and responses to more than human forces such as wind and oceanic currents. Evie describes being moved by this intangible, but deeply affective 'wild' energy and her interactions with these elemental forces prompt a sense of catharsis or release. They also become implicated in—and transformative of—her capacities to make sense of and cope with everyday life during the pandemic.

Evie's reflections align with previous research on experiences of longing in the frail elderly, who described longing to be outdoors in nature as it provided them with a sense of wellbeing and vitality (Hemberg et al., 2020). Her experience also resonates with existing research done with people who engage in coastal activities like swimming or surfing and describe similarly emotional and sensory experiences (Britton & Foley, 2020; Foley, 2017; Throsby, 2013). While Evie does not describe immersive experiences like swimming, the ocean plays a central role in her stories. It appears in her diary visually and is a lively presence and force, along with weather-related elements like wind and sunshine, that shape and shift her pandemic movement practices and capacities to make sense of and cope with the pandemic.

Importantly, Evie was able to access the beach easily from her home and felt safe and comfortable being in and engaging in this space. As mentioned previously, access to such spaces is often contingent upon overlapping social, cultural, geographical, and political factors. As Sydney locked down some of its beaches for weeks at a time in 2020, only those bodies able and interested in performing what might be recognised as legitimate forms of exercise were allowed on the beach. I have previously articulated how these closures shifted the affective atmospheres of coastal communities and contributed to constraining and ableist notions of what 'counts' as physical activity (Clark, 2021). They are also implicated in the (re)production of beaches and blue spaces as deeply exclusionary spaces. During COVID, Evie's access to and engagement with these spaces shaped her capacities to care for herself and others and enabled practices that facilitated experiences of wellbeing. While this is important to emphasise, it also draws attention to and raises questions around who *might not* have access to these spaces and therefore who does not have access to the associated benefits. These questions are not only relevant in the context of Australia, or more specifically Sydney, where Evie lives, but can be asked in the broader, global context. Who has access to environments that are safe, physically pristine or viable, to temperatures that allow exposure. How are these experiences implicated in broader balances of power, resources, and economics?

Longing for Others and for Things to Be Otherwise

Diary Entry: Kate

Please describe the photo and explain why it is meaningful to you: My diary entry is two pictures today. The first is a picture of the sky that I took on my walk. I spend a lot more time walking outside these days and notice things like the sky and how pretty the light is at certain parts of the day. The second picture is of my phone and my running shoes because these two objects are important to my pandemic walks. I wear these runners everyday and I always take my phone. Sometimes I listen to music but today I talked to my Mum. I don't know when I'll see her next because she lives in WA [Western Australia] and I really miss her. Whenever she visits we always walk together and that's the last thing we did together, on this path. Now we've both started walking a lot during COVID. Sometimes we'll talk or send photos to each other of things we see on our walk. One day she sent a photo of the moon rising and said 'We're looking at the same moon'. It made me cry. But it also made me feel connected to her so sometimes I look at the sky and think 'we're looking at the same sky.'

When was this photo taken?: 12 noon and 4pm and

What appears in the photo?: photo 1. Clouds and blue sky photo 2 Running shoes and black iPhone

How did you feel when you took this photo?: missing, sad, hopeful

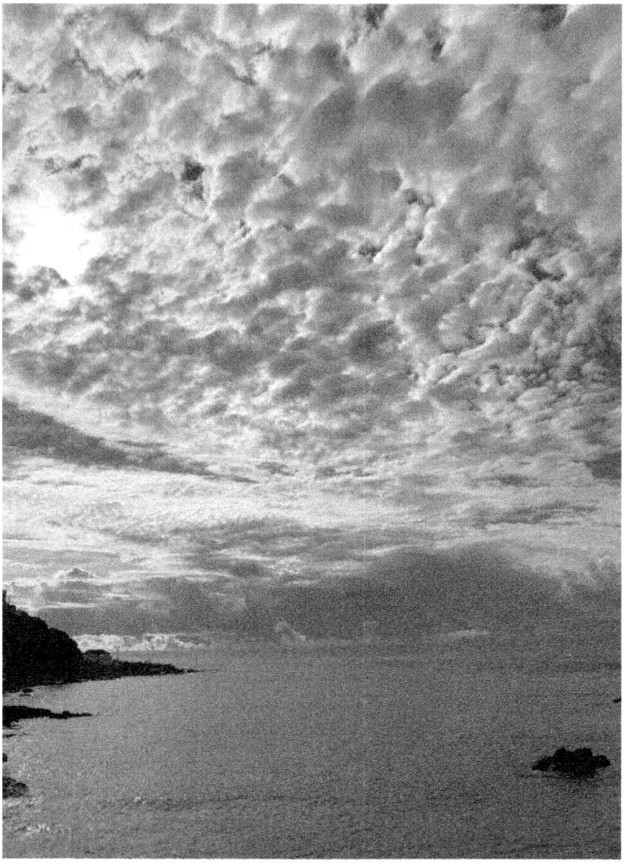

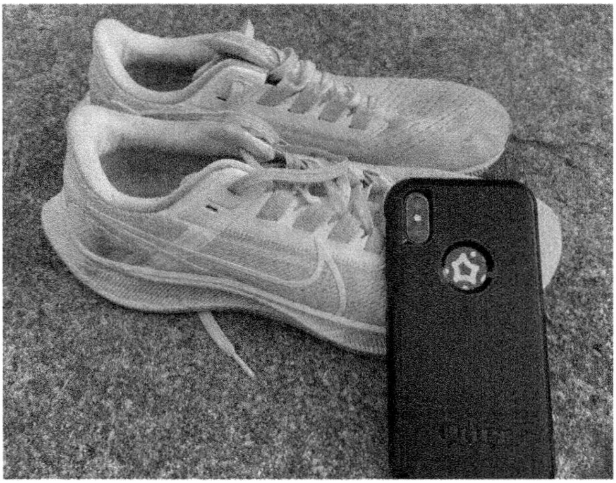

During the pandemic borders and mobilities came to matter in new ways. Australia not only sealed its international borders for almost two years but domestic borders were closed for months, in some cases years, separating families and loved ones and wreaking havoc on personal, professional and economic lives (Boscaini, 2021; Jeffries, 2022). These policies illustrate how the COVID-19 public health response was, in many cases, shaped by forces of nationalism and immigration and migration policies (Boucher et al., 2021). In Kate's diary entry, these forces materialise in her expressions of longing for her mother who lives in Western Australia, a state that imposed hard border closures, including to its own residents, for stretches of time during the pandemic.

Kate's entry is tinged with grief and longing. Like participants in the studies cited earlier by Ueland et al. (2018, 2020). Kate longs for something lost—the ability to see her mother, to travel freely across domestic borders—and a previous way of life. Longing emerges and is expressed through movement as Kate's walking routines both call attention to and are taken up in response to the absence of her mother. It is also implicated in the sense of connection created through the recollection of shared, past experiences. Through participating in asynchronous walking routines and exchanging digital photos taken on their walks via text message, Kate and her mother responded to the desire to see each other performed embodied, digitally mediated act of sharing and connecting. While state borders separated them, seeing, and living under 'the same moon' and the 'same sky' allowed for some sense of connection.

These improvised acts of sharing and connection emerged in part from the flows of longing experienced by Kate. In alignment with Dalton's reading of Levinas (Dalton, 2009), longing 'interrupts' Kate and orients her to a different set of practices. In this way, I argue, longing *does* something. It both prompts and transforms, giving way to Kate's movement practices, outdoor engagements and sharing of digital photos that in turn yield new forms of connection.

While longing in Kate's example can be associated with absence (of her mother) and lack (the inability to move freely across domestic borders) it is also related to the creation of connection, possibility, and hope. It flows and shifts with Kate's moving, relational encounters with other human, celestial, and technological bodies and gives way to more hopeful orientations and glimmers of possibility. However, and importantly, these hopeful gleanings are in part enabled by her access to safe and pleasant outdoor spaces. Like Evie, Kate can easily get to a walking path safely and 'legally' under Melbourne's 5km radius restrictions. However, as mentioned previously, a substantial number of households in Melbourne have no access to green spaces in this radius (Lakhani et al., 2020).

Consequently, both Kate's and Evie's embodiments and expressions of longing must be situated within a broader politics of privilege that acknowledges the multiple geo-political, historical, social and material conditions through which these expressions emerge. Australia was one of many countries that imposed strict lockdown rules that dictated when, where and for how long people could leave their homes. But, unlike many countries, the island nation of Australia enjoys moderate temperatures all year around and is surrounded by ocean, meaning coastal landscapes, and the associated benefits, are available to at least part of the population. At the same time, the privilege of being able to live in and access these spaces is entangled with fraught geo-politics, violent colonial-settler histories and legacies of white privilege (Bonds & Inwood, 2015; Peake & Ray, 2001). Therefore, while Evie and Kate may long for a sense of normalcy, and find shards of hope in their leisure practices and outdoor encounters, these capacities for hope are always contingent upon overlapping socio-material, geographical, historical and political forces (Clark & Southerton, 2021) and the pandemic renders visible the stark inequalities and inequities both inherent to and produced by our most powerful social systems and structures. Consequently, it is imperative to resist romanticising, universalising, or depoliticising discussions about the benefits of physical activity and/or engagement with outdoor, blue, and green spaces during the pandemic. Doing so risks exacerbating and naturalising the processes through which exclusion and privilege are produced and materialise through embodied experiences of enabled or constrained wellbeing.

Conclusion

In this chapter I share two digital photo diary entries shared by participants of my broader examination of Australian's pandemic fitness practices and trace the affective flows of longing. I draw on the concept of longing articulated by Levinas (1969) and later Dalton (2009) who suggest longing holds the capacity to interrupts us and put something new in motion. My analysis reveals how longing, as part of the affective response to the pandemic, indeed interrupted and moved participants, prompting new (physical) practices, encounters, and forms of connection. Importantly, longing here was not merely the desire for something or someone missing or absent. Nor could its contours be definitively traced. Rather, longing emerged, shifted, and was expressed through entangled temporalities, moving bodies, elemental forces, and more-than-human objects and technologies.

Blue and green spaces, in the form of coastal trails and parkland, as well as elemental and celestial forces (e.g., wind, currents, the sun and sky) were central to participants' diary entries. These forces were not always visible (e.g., wind) or even articulable (vaguely referred to by Evie as 'energies'), but important, nonetheless. They evoked, transformed, and at times eased the sense of longing and contributed to the production of embodied experience. I argue attending to these more-than-human forces can offer start to elaborate how and why encounters with blue and green spaces can contribute to wellbeing in deeply embodied, situated and sometimes intangible ways (Finlay et al., 2015; Foley, 2017; Olive & Wheaton, 2021). I also attempt to articulate how the associated benefits of physical activity and outdoor engagement during the pandemic are contingent on the same socio-material, political and economic systems and processes implicated in the production of health inequities (Coen et al., 2021).

Keeping this mind, I have sought not to romanticise or universalise the positive experiences reported by participants, but instead provide analysis that attends to specificity and acknowledges the human and more-than-human forces at work in the production of people's pandemic fitness practices and the embodied experiences of longing. I further suggest that in addition to considering how blue and green spaces are implicated in the production of *human* health inequities it is imperative we consider seriously the wellbeing of our planet. So often green and blue spaces are mined for their capacities to enhance our health, but it is growing increasingly clear we need to do more to care for them (Evers, 2019; Neimanis, 2019; Olive & Wheaton, 2021; Thorpe et al., 2020a). At the time of wrapping up this chapter, southeast Australia was experiencing a significant rain event causing devastating flooding along the New South Wales and Queensland coasts that claimed multiple lives and destroyed the property and livelihoods of many. Touted by some politicians as a '1 in 1000-year event' (Morton & Readfearn, 2022), this flooding occurred not even three years after the devastating bush fires of 2019/2020 fires scorched Australia, blanketing large swathes of the country in toxic smoke, filling oceans with plumes of ash that clung to surfing and swimming bodies, and causing extraordinary harm to human physical health that continues to unfold (Borchers Arriagada et al., 2020). As these climate-related events bookend the COVID-19 pandemic, which can also be understood as a consequence of human-driven processes related to climate change (Rodó et al., 2021), it becomes increasingly and alarmingly clear human-planetary relations cannot continue as they are. The forces and processes of modernity, intensified capitalism, and globalisation must be disrupted, unsettled, and somehow augmented or replaced.

In thinking about the stories of longing shared above, they cannot be disentangled from or meaningfully made sense of without also considering these broader geo-socio-political conditions. What people long for and how that longing is expressed or materialised is always socially and materially contingent and implicated in the politics of privilege. However, in efforts to think again, what longing might *do*, I hope, and wonder if perhaps longing might prompt radical practices of care. If longing is, as demonstrated above, imbued with the potential to transforms, perhaps it can alter us, dis/orient us, unsettle us. As movement, in and of itself, perhaps longing can urge us to create space for something new.

References

Åhäll, L. (2018). Affect as methodology: Feminism and the politics of emotion. *International Political Sociology, 12*(1), 36–52. https://doi.org/10.1093/ips/olx024

Ahmed, S. (2013). *The cultural politics of emotion*. Routledge.

Australian Government, D. o. H. (2020). Exercising and staying active during coronavirus (COVID-19) restrictions | Australian Government Department of Health. https://www.health.gov.au/news/health-alerts/novel-coronavirus-2019-ncov-health-alert/ongoing-support-during-coronavirus-covid-19/exercising-and-staying-active-during-coronavirus-covid-19-restrictions

Black Dog Institute. (2022). During COVID-19, you can exercise your way to better mental health – Black Dog Institute. https://www.blackdoginstitute.org.au/news/during-covid-19-you-can-exercise-your-way-to-better-mental-health/

Bonds, A., & Inwood, J. (2015). Beyond white privilege: Geographies of white supremacy and settler colonialism. *Progress in Human Geography, 40*(6), 715–733. https://doi.org/10.1177/0309132515613166

Borchers Arriagada, N., Palmer, A. J., Bowman, D. M., Morgan, G. G., Jalaludin, B. B., & Johnston, F. H. (2020). Unprecedented smoke-related health burden associated with the 2019–20 bushfires in eastern Australia. *Medical Journal of Australia, 213*(6), 282–283.

Boscaini, J. (2021, August 12). 'It has changed my perception of Australia': What migrants think of pandemic border closures. https://www.abc.net.au/news/2021-12-09/australian-visa-holders-considered-leaving-country-covid-border/100653474

Boucher, A., Hooijer, G., King, D., Napier, I., & Stears, M. (2021). COVID-19: A crisis of borders. *PS. Political Science & Politics, 54*(4), 617–622. https://doi.org/10.1017/S1049096521000603

Braidotti, R. (2020). "We" are in this together, but we are not one and the same. *Journal of Bioethical Inquiry, 17*(4), 465–469. https://doi.org/10.1007/s11673-020-10017-8

Brennan, T. (2015). *The transmission of affect*. Cornell University Press.
Brinson, K. (2020, June 5). One foot in front of the other: How a daily walk helps us Cope (Published 2020). *The New York Times*. https://www.nytimes.com/2020/05/06/us/coronavirus-stress-daily-walk.html
Britton, E., & Foley, R. (2020). Sensing water: Uncovering health and well-being in the sea and surf. *Journal of Sport and Social Issues, 45*(1), 60–87. https://doi.org/10.1177/0193723520928597
Britton, E., & Foley, R. (2021). Sensing water: Uncovering health and well-being in the sea and surf. *Journal of Sport and Social Issues, 45*(1), 60–87.
Centers for Disease Control and Prevention. (2022, 2022-02-01T07,46:22Z). Coping with Stress. https://www.cdc.gov/mentalhealth/stress-coping/cope-with-stress/index.html
Clark, M. (2021). Signs, beaches and bodies in pandemic times. *Media International Australia, 178*(1), 8–15. https://doi.org/10.1177/1329878x20949980
Clark, M., & Lupton, D. (2021). Pandemic fitness assemblages: The sociomaterialities and affective dimensions of exercising at home during the COVID-19 crisis. *Convergence, 27*(5), 1222–1237. https://doi.org/10.1177/13548565211042460
Clark, M., & Southerton, C. (2021). *Lingering in the 'bad feelings' for good reason: What might bad feelings do?* Paper presented at the The Australian Sociological Association Symposium: Hope and Empathy in Uncertain Times Australia.
Coen, S. E., Cook, S., & Hayes, S. J. (2021). Pandemic geographies of physical activity. In G. J. Andrews, V. A. Crooks, J. R. Pearce, & J. P. Messina (Eds.), *COVID-19 and similar futures: Pandemic geographies* (pp. 165–172). Springer International Publishing.
Dalton, D. M. (2009). *Longing for the other: Levinas and metaphysical desire*.
Day, M., & Thatcher, J. (2009). "I'm really embarrassed that you're going to read this…": Reflections on using diaries in qualitative research. *Qualitative Research in Psychology, 6*(4), 249–259.
Dunn, A. (2020, August 9). In Melbourne's interminable lockdown, my daily walks have gone from a chore to a delight | Amanda Dunn. *The Guardian Australia*. Retrieved from http://www.theguardian.com/commentisfree/2020/sep/08/in-melbournes-interminable-lockdown-my-daily-walks-have-gone-from-a-chore-to-a-delight
Esposito, R. (2008). Bios: Biopolitics and philosophy. Minneapolis, MIN: University of Minnesota Press.

Evers, C. (2008). The Cronulla Race Riots: Safety maps on an Australian Beach. *South Atlantic Quarterly, 107*(2), 411–429. https://doi.org/10.1215/00382876-2007-074

Evers, C. (2019). Polluted leisure and blue spaces: More-than-human concerns in Fukushima. *Journal of Sport and Social Issues, 45*(2), 179–195. https://doi.org/10.1177/0193723519884854

Finlay, J., Franke, T., McKay, H., & Sims-Gould, J. (2015). Therapeutic landscapes and wellbeing in later life: Impacts of blue and green spaces for older adults. *Health & Place, 34*, 97–106. https://doi.org/10.1016/j.healthplace.2015.05.001

Foley, R. (2017). Swimming as an accretive practice in healthy blue space. *Emotion, Space and Society, 22*, 43–51. https://doi.org/10.1016/j.emospa.2016.12.001

Foley, R., & Kistemann, T. (2015). Blue space geographies: Enabling health in place. *Health & Place, 35*, 157–165.

Haider, S., Smith, L., Markovic, L., Schuch, F. B., Sadarangani, K. P., Lopez Sanchez, G. F., ... & Grabovac, I. (2021). Associations between physical activity, sitting time, and time spent outdoors with mental health during the first COVID-19 lock down in Austria. *International Journal of Environmental Research and Public Health, 18*(17), 9168.

Harrison, B. (2004). Photographic visions and narrative inquiry. *Considering Counter-Narratives: Narrating, Resisting, Making Sense, 4*, 111–136.

Hemberg, J., Nyqvist, F., Ueland, V., & Näsman, M. (2020). Experiences of longing in daily life and associations to well-being among frail older adults receiving home care: A qualitative study. *The International Journal of Qualitative Studies on Health and Well-being, 15*(1), 1857950. https://doi.org/10.1080/17482631.2020.1857950

Hemmings, C. (2005). Invoking affect: Cultural theory and the ontological turn. *Cultural Studies, 19*(5), 548–567.

Herron, R., Dansereau, L., Wrathall, M., Funk, L., & Spencer, D. (2019). Using a flexible diary method rigorously and sensitively with family carers. *Qualitative Health Research, 29*(7), 1004–1015.

Hine, C. (2020). *Ethnography for the internet: Embedded, embodied and everyday*. Routledge.

Jeffrey, A., Thorpe, H., & Ahmad, N. (2021). Women Yoga practitioners' experiences in the pandemic: From collective exhaustion to affirmative ethics. *Sociology of Sport Journal, 1–10*. https://doi.org/10.1123/ssj.2020-0207

Jeffries, R. (2022). *Border closures should not be Australia's default response*. Retrieved from The Lowy Institute: https://www.lowyinstitute.org/the-interpreter/border-closures-should-not-be-australia-s-default-response

Knowles, C., & Sweetman, P. (2004). *Picturing the social landscape*. Routledge.

Lakhani, A., Wollersheim, D., Kendall, E., & Korah, P. (2020, August 11). 340,000 Melburnians have little or no parkland within 5k of their home. The Conversation https://theconversation.com/340-000-elburnians-have-little-orno-parkland-within-5km-of-their-home-144069

Lee, A. C., & Maheswaran, R. (2011). The health benefits of urban green spaces: A review of the evidence. *Journal of Public Health, 33*(2), 212–222.

Lesser, I. A., & Nienhuis, C. P. (2020). The impact of COVID-19 on physical activity behavior and well-being of Canadians. *International Journal of Environmental Research and Public Health, 17*(11), 3899. https://www.mdpi.com/1660-4601/17/11/3899

Levinas, E. (1969). *Totality and Infinity: An Essay on Exteriority, Alphonso Lingis* (trans.), Pittsburgh: Duquesne University Press.

Markham, T., & Couldry, N. (2007). Tracking the reflexivity of the (dis) engaged citizen: Some methodological reflections. *Qualitative Inquiry, 13*(5), 675–695.

Maugeri, G., Castrogiovanni, P., Battaglia, G., Pippi, R., D'Agata, V., Palma, A., et al. (2020). The impact of physical activity on psychological health during Covid-19 pandemic in Italy. *Heliyon, 6*(6), e04315. https://doi.org/10.1016/j.heliyon.2020.e04315

Milligan, C., Bingley, A., & Gatrell, A. (2005). Digging deep: Using diary techniques to explore the place of health and well-being amongst older people. *Social Science & Medicine, 61*(9), 1882–1892.

Morton, A., & Readfearn, G. (2022). *The Guardian*. https://www.theguardian.com/australia-news/2022/mar/04/are-eastern-australias-catastrophic-floods-really-a-one-in-1000-year-event

Neimanis, A. (2019). *Bodies of water: Posthuman feminist phenomenology*. Bloomsbury Publishing.

Newbold, J. W., Rudnicka, A., & Cox, A. (2021). Staying active while staying home: The use of physical activity technologies during life disruptions. *Frontiers in Digital Health, 3*. https://doi.org/10.3389/fdgth.2021.753115

Newman, J. I., Shields, R., & McLeod, C. M. (2015). The MRSA epidemic and/as fluid biopolitics. *Body & Society, 22*(4), 155–184. https://doi.org/10.1177/1357034X14551844

Olive, R., & Wheaton, B. (2021). Understanding blue spaces: Sport, bodies, wellbeing, and the sea. *Journal of Sport and Social Issues, 45*(1), 3–19. https://doi.org/10.1177/0193723520950549

Peake, L. M., & Ray, B. K. (2001). Racializing the Canadian landscape: Whiteness, uneven geographies and social justice1. *Canadian Geographer, 45*, 180–186.

Phoenix, C. (2010). Seeing the world of physical culture: The potential of visual methods for qualitative research in sport and exercise. *Qualitative Research in Sport and Exercise, 2*(2), 93–108. https://doi.org/10.1080/19398441.2010.488017

Pink, S. (2004). Visual methods. *Qualitative research practice*, 391–406.

Pink, S. (2013). *Doing visual ethnography*. Sage.

Rodó, X., San-José, A., Kirchgatter, K., & López, L. (2021). Changing climate and the COVID-19 pandemic: More than just heads or tails. *Nature Medicine, 27*(4), 576–579. https://doi.org/10.1038/s41591-021-01303-y

Spinoza, B. d. (1994). *A Spinoza reader: The Ethics and other works*. Princeton University Press.

Taylor, L., Raisborough, J., Harrison, K., & Dulson, S. (2021). 'It's like Going to the Regular Class but without Being there': A Qualitative Analysis of Older people's Experiences of Exercise in the Home during Covid-19 Lockdown in England. *International Journal of the Sociology of Leisure, 4*(3), 177–192.

The Victoria Health Promotion Foundation. (2022). What is nature bathing and how does it benefit our health? http://www.vichealth.vic.gov.au/be-healthy/what-is-nature-bathing

Thorpe, H. (2022). The challenges and benefits of outdoor recreation during NZ's coronavirus lockdown. *The Conversation*. http://theconversation.com/the-challenges-and-benefits-of-outdoor-recreation-during-nzs-coronavirus-lockdown-134892

Thorpe, H., Brice, J., & Clark, M. (2020a). Feminist ethics, the environment, and vital respondings. *Feminist New Materialisms, Sport and Fitness*, 177–207.

Thorpe, H., Brice, J., & Clark, M. (2020b). *Feminist new materialisms, sport and fitness: A lively entanglement*. Palgrave Macmillan.

Throsby, K. (2013). 'If I go in like a Cranky Sea Lion, I Come out like a Smiling Dolphin': Marathon Swimming and the Unexpected Pleasures of Being a Body in Water. *Feminist Review, 103*(1), 5–22. https://doi.org/10.1057/fr.2012.23

Ueland, V., Dysvik, E., & Furnes, B. (2020). Living with obesity: Expressions of longing. *SAGE Open Nursing, 6*, 2377960819901193.

Ueland, V., Nåden, D., & Lindström, U. (2018). Longing – A dynamic power in the becoming of health when suffering from cancer. *The Scandinavian Journal of Caring Sciences, 32*(2), 924–932. https://doi.org/10.1111/scs.12527

Ueland, V., Rørtveit, K., Dysvik, E., & Furnes, B. (2020). Life after cancer treatment – Existential experiences of longing. *The International Journal of Qualitative Studies on Health and Well-being, 15*(1), 1838041. https://doi.org/10.1080/17482631.2020.1838041

Van den Berg, A. E., Maas, J., Verheij, R. A., & Groenewegen, P. P. (2010). Green space as a buffer between stressful life events and health. *Social Science & Medicine, 70*(8), 1203–1210.

Wheaton, B., Roy, G., & Olive, R. (2017). Exploring critical alternatives for youth development through lifestyle sport: Surfing and community development in Aotearoa/New Zealand. *Sustainability, 9*(12), 2298.

White, M., Alcock, I., Grellier, J., Wheeler, B., Hartig, T., Warber, S., et al. (2019). Spending at least 120 minutes a week in nature is associated with good health and wellbeing. *Scientific Reports, 9*, 7730. https://doi.org/10.1038/s41598-019-44097-3

White, M. P., Alcock, I., Wheeler, B. W., & Depledge, M. H. (2013). Coastal proximity, health and well-being: Results from a longitudinal panel survey. *Health & Place, 23*, 97–103.

World Health Organization. (2020). #HealthyAtHome. https://www.who.int/campaigns/connecting-the-world-to-combat-coronavirus/healthyathome

Young, D. R., Hong, B. D., Lo, T., Inzhakova, G., Cohen, D. A., & Sidell, M. A. (2022). The longitudinal associations of physical activity, time spent outdoors in nature and symptoms of depression and anxiety during COVID-19 quarantine and social distancing in the United States. *Preventive Medicine, 154*, 106863. https://doi.org/10.1016/j.ypmed.2021.106863

25

Playing Through a Pandemic: Football Bodies, Racialized Violence, and Institutionalized Care

Tracie Canada

As an alumna of Duke University and the University of Virginia, a former researcher at the University of North Carolina, and a current faculty member at the University of Notre Dame, I openly claim an investment in the athletic teams of the Atlantic Coast Conference (ACC) institutions. At this point, it would be difficult to deny. Specifically, though, I pay close attention to the football teams at these universities.

I followed along with the entire 2020 football season by watching as many games as possible. While I prefer to attend games in person, I watched on television and this decision afforded me an opportunity not provided to those who physically attended: I got to see the commercials. And during this particular football season, each ACC match up featured a specific one.

"We at the ACC know that change needs to occur," the first voice begins. Others continue: "Despite our rivalries, this is the time to unite.

T. Canada (✉)
Duke University, Durham, NC, USA
e-mail: tracie.canada@duke.edu

D. L. Andrews et al. (eds.), *Sport and Physical Culture in Global Pandemic Times*,
Global Culture and Sport Series, https://doi.org/10.1007/978-3-031-14387-8_25

We need to come together to conquer biases, as well as oppression. We are committed to seeing each other as equals, and treating each other with respect and dignity at all times. We must hold ourselves and those around us to a higher standard because racism and bigotry will not be tolerated. We must fight for racial and social justice." The 30 second spot ends poignantly: "We at the ACC will fight for unity."

The voices in this commercial belong to the 15 head football coaches in the ACC in 2020, with each offering a line or two of this script. Each man, as they are all male, would flash on the screen, with his name and team affiliation, as he read off his part. Words and phrases like 'unite,' 'conquer biases,' 'oppression,' and 'racism and bigotry' were meant to be highlighted, as they were captioned across the bottom of the screen as they were spoken by the respective coach. Finally, the conference's new branding image flashed on the screen before it faded to black: "Unite," in all uppercase letters, crosscut by "ACC," with the logos of each university careful spaced underneath.

This commercial was particularly interesting because of the underlying tensions and disconnects that even allowed for it to occur. First, it was only shown once during every game and it only played during halftime. Save for the annual Super Bowl, halftime is not an ideal time to show content that might attract interaction and engagement; this commercial was shown during the time that fans would most likely take a break from the television screen since play was paused.

Second, the reason I did not attend any games in person during the 2020 season and was able to watch these commercials was because, of course, this was the "pandemic season," one marked and defined by the ongoing coronavirus pandemic. By the time play resumed in early-November 2020 for all 65 teams at Power Five universities, data show that more than 200,000 people had died, with Black, Indigenous, and Latinx people disproportionately affected. Power Five universities, of course, are the biggest, most popular, and most profitable football schools in the country, all belonging to the Division I Football Bowl Subdivision (FBS). Despite the pandemic, young men, disproportionately young Black men (Harper, 2018), ran onto college gridirons almost every Saturday in fall 2020 to participate in a high-contact sport that cannot be played without the consistent coming together of bodies. According to the annual report from The Institute for Diversity and Ethics in Sport, Black men accounted for 48.5% of Division I FBS football athletes during the 2020 season (Lapchick, 2021, p. 13). At stake with this decision, in addition to the health and well-being of the players, was capital for all of the institutional parties invested in the football system. Data published by *USA Today* state that at least $4.1 billion in fiscal-year revenue was at risk for athletic programs had the Power Five football season been canceled and those players not taken the field (Berkowitz, 2020).

But it is important to note that this commercial was not about the pandemic. It was pointing to a third tension, another issue that had reached international news and made its way onto the gridiron. The summer of supposed racial reckoning required that college football programs respond, in some way, to the police murder of George Floyd in May 2020. These programs, after all, statistically rely on laboring young Black men in order to subsist. George Floyd's murder was particularly relevant to the lived reality of the athletes on their teams, as it was such a blatant display of fatal anti-Blackness and state-sanctioned violence. The visuals of the commercial further support the paradox of the message: the majority of the coaches represented in the commercial are white, specifically 13 of the 15. Syracuse University and University of Miami are the only institutions with a head coach of color. In fact, during this 2020 season, only 16.2% of all head coaches in Division I FBS football were of color (Lapchick, 2021, p. 13).

These bio-physical, economic, and racial issues were braided together and on full display in a spectacular way during the pandemic season, as were the administrative responses to these sensational violent and threatening events. However, motivated by anthropologist Laurence Ralph's provocation to "fixate on those more ordinary forms of violence as a way to reimagine our social worlds" (Humanities Unbounded, 2020), I ask: how do these issues play out and how are they responded to on every other non-pandemic football Saturday? How do football institutions' pandemic responses to spectacular violence and harm mirror their responses to ordinary forms of violence that always impact the sport? Triangulating Black Studies and sports studies literatures with ethnographic observations helps to answer these questions.

Everyday Violence and Institutionalized Care in College Football

As an anthropologist who specializes in the intersections of race and sport, the pandemic football season of 2020 was both a fascinating and deeply problematic object of inquiry. I have spent almost ten years learning about the ways that Black college football players navigate their lives both on and off the gridiron, given the ways that time on the field inevitably bleeds into and affects time off it. Unfortunately, what I witnessed during the pandemic season—from afar and from the luxury and safety of my own home—was familiar because it reinforced the normalized responses to the mundane injury and violence that have come to define the sport. As sport scholars Chris McLeod and colleagues argue, football is defined by violent and dangerous "practices which we understand as normal within this space but outside of which constitute an aberration" (2014, p. 229). American football has normalized violence in a way that treats what should be exceptional as incredibly mundane. Thus, the administrative and institutional responses to violence and injury in football did not begin with the pandemic.

There were tangible similarities that connect the pandemic season to what I witnessed while conducting sustained ethnographic research a few years ago during the 2017–18 football season. Together, these point to the ways that care is performed by football programs and institutions to convince players that they are invested in their well-being. Conversely, I argue that these parties are interested only in profiting off these players' labor and are thus acting with this sole mission in mind.

* * *

I ended up with a broken arm in January 2018. This was unfortunate for various reasons, but most relevant here, the accident occurred about halfway through fieldwork for my dissertation research. I spent the fall 2017 playing season with Black college football players at Mellon University,[1]

[1] Pseudonyms for institutions and people are used throughout.

a Division I institution in the southeastern United States, learning how they navigated their everyday lives. In the new year, I wondered how my injury, combined with the end of the football season and the beginning of the spring semester, would shape the later months of my research.

As I walked to the Football Center on my first day back on campus after my injury, I struggled to maneuver my awkward cast and bulky sling. Amidst my fidgeting and slow movement forward, I saw Isaiah from afar. As we approached one another and he noticed my arm, he chuckled after finding out I was okay. "You'll fit right in with us," he explained. "A lot of guys are in slings right now because of their surgeries. Carter is one of them. You should find him."

I soon learned that Carter had undergone shoulder surgery in late-January for an injury he sustained in mid-September. When I asked why he waited so long to go through with it, Carter downplayed the seriousness of the injury.

"I tore the labrum in my shoulder, so it was just a minor injury," he claimed, listing at least five other teammates who had the same injury to highlight how common it was.

I made sure to tell him that perhaps the injury seemed ordinary because of who he was surrounded by, but outside of football, that was not common. He laughed, acknowledging the truth of my statement. "Even so," he continued, "plenty of guys play with it torn and that's what I did. If I could, I wanted to play through the season."

The team's athletic trainers informed Carter that as long as he was careful, he could finish the season and have the surgery afterward. So, rather than sit out during his redshirt junior year, he opted to postpone the surgery. And he was taken care of: Carter was carefully monitored to ensure the injury did not get worse as he continued to play, and the football program covered the surgery and rehab expenses. But learning of his situation, and being more aware of others on the team, I realized there was strategy involved in this decision. This, and other decisions like it, are exploitative because the program sought to guarantee its ability to extract as much labor as possible from Carter's football-playing body during the season. Not only are coaches' careers "built (or broken) by athletes' labor in the stadium" (Hatton, 2020, p. 71), the team's and university's reputation were also on the line. By surveiling Carter's condition and encouraging a later surgery date, Mellon increased its chance of winning more games because it successfully kept him playing.

Isaiah's quip about my ability to blend in with other recovering players—as so many were marked by braces and slings because of their post-season surgeries—and Carter's explanation of the timing of his surgery point to ways that football programs carefully strategize when and how they patch players up so they're able to produce on the field. As mentioned, it is not that care for them is not exhibited, but it is a kind of care that is based upon a capitalist sensibility because the aim is to win games, garner revenue, and secure prestige. Also, as college athletes "are often seen as creators of capital," it is a care that depends upon disciplining and surveilling the injured players, which follows that "the primary goal of their subjugation is *exploitation*" (Hatton, 2020, p. 128). Carter's predicament, I came to realize, epitomizes a concern for maximizing the potential of each sporting body for the benefit of the coaches, the team, and the university.

While I was conducting fieldwork in 2017–18, there was no way to predict the reality of the current moment that led to such remarkable shifts in our daily social lives. Beginning in March 2020, various changes were made to the landscape of higher education in an attempt to keep students, staff, and educators safe in the face of an unpredictable and unknown virus. Most pressing, in the spirit of social distancing, shifts were made to accommodate and encourage physical isolation from one another, as sharing space presented an unprecedented risk. But this precaution did not apply to those students who also played football for Power Five universities.

In the world of college football, the pandemic season felt disturbingly similar to the pre-pandemic world because 2020 gridiron play relied on the same principles and ideals that structured play at any other time. College athletes' status as 'amateurs' is central because it points to the social position that these players maintain for the system to persist. The hallmark of intercollegiate sport in the United States is the notion of amateurism, which distinguishes these athletes from those at the professional level through its supposed focus on the playful, non-serious, and uncompensated aspects of sport (Camp, 1901; Roosevelt, 1900). However, intercollegiate athletics have developed into big-time college sports that are now highly visible and commercialized, and ruled by high stakes competition, huge budgets and revenue, highly compensated coaches, and inflated media contracts and coverage (Clotfelter, 2011). Rather than reform, administrations and bureaucracies have doubled down on the reliance upon this foundational principle of amateurism. Thus, in its current iteration, amateurism is rooted in exploitation, as players themselves have gained little to no more rights and privileges within this scaled up and immensely popular system.

Take, for instance, the school song controversy at University of Texas-Austin to consider this exploitative disconnect. Following the police murder of George Floyd, Black athletes at the university in June 2020 demanded that a number of issues be addressed in order to "make Texas more comfortable and inclusive for the black athletes and the black community that has so fervently supported this [athletics] program" (Cramer & Diaz, 2020). Included in the request was that the institution's alma mater, "The Eyes of Texas," be replaced because of its racist and anti-Black foundations. Anthropologist Gabby Yearwood has analyzed the song as exhibiting "embodied surveillance in the lyrics" while being "used to control the bodies of Black student-athletes" (2018, p. 679). The playing of this song, which has roots in minstrelsy and dates back to the Confederacy, was a postgame tradition that Black athletes were no longer supporting.

There was much debate about the song during the 2020 football season, with athletes and band members openly protesting it during games, and administrators disagreeing about its role in athletic fanfare. Donors and alumni also became involved and hundreds of their angry emails to the university president were released. The messages showed that they threatened to pull their financial contributions in all different forms, complaining that the president "was not forcefully defending the song and school traditions enough" (McGee, 2021), even though the president had announced the song would remain in place. The only change made was that he initiated a university committee that would research the song's origins.

This controversy, and the song itself, are prime examples of what occurs when "racist anti-Black sentiment becomes normalised as heritage or tradition" (Yearwood, 2018, p. 680). Black athletes were rightfully defending themselves against an act they deemed harmful, but the university's administration did not support them in any way that led to structural change. Instead, they secured future donations by placating alumni and donors who had a vested interest in a particular history and memory of UT-Austin that current Black students were actively speaking out against. To further exaggerate the point that money is more important than the well-being of athletes, it is of note that the university still brought in $98.2 million in football revenue during the 2020–21 athletic year (Davis, 2022).

The exploitation at the heart of the amateur system is clearly on display. The ridiculous amount of capital involved in this calculus, whether through donations or ticket sales or media rights, all benefited the university and the athletics program at the expense of the players whose labor powers the enterprise. Black athletes are already particularly vulnerable in the college athletics system, but in this situation at UT-Austin, they were not protected or supported by their university because of administrative practices meant to ensure capitalist gains. Thus, this poignant example on one college campus during the pandemic season points to ways that power is exercised and wielded at all times to protect the bottom line, no matter the cost, because of the way these big-time programs operate.

The creation of and dependence on the term "student-athlete" only furthers this capitalist manipulation. Universities and the NCAA traffic in the utility of the dually indexed "student-athlete" identity to perform their care for one's success in both the classroom and on the playing field. While in practice this is far from the truth—as many have argued that much more time, energy, attention, and resources are devoted to the 'athlete' rather than the 'student'—the term is just as problematic in theory because of its origins. In September 1955, Ray Dennison, a right guard for the Fort Lewis A&M Aggies, died from a head injury sustained during a game against Trinidad Junior College. Dennison was a scholarship athlete and upon his death, his widow sued the university for worker's compensation benefits. Rather than grant the requests made in the lawsuit, the Colorado Supreme Court ruled that Dennison was not eligible for benefits because the school was "not in the football business." To further prove this point and highlight college players' roles as not-employees, the idea of the "student-athlete" was born. Walter Byers, the first Executive

Director of the NCAA, led the charge for this term to enter the public lexicon and encouraged the organization's transition to the moneymaking machine it is today (Branch, 2011; Given, 2017; Slothower, 2014; The Daily Tar Heel Staff, 2020).

Realistically, the notion of the "student-athlete" is a fallacy that relies on the feigned interest in one's student identity before their athlete identity; regardless, it was and is still driven by a capitalist impulse. The terminology is rooted in maintaining these players' status as amateurs who can be exploited, disciplined, and controlled in ways that would not be possible if they were considered employees or professionals. Further, amateurism allows for status coercion to occur, a practice that sociologist Erin Hatton argues defines the labor relations that exist in college athletics, as coaches have the power to "discharge them from a particular status [...] and thereby deprive them of the rights, privileges, and future opportunities that such status confers" (2020, p. 13). This is an argument that prioritizes how labor and work are manipulated for the benefit of those in power, which "helps *create* the vulnerable and compliant workers on whom neoliberal precarity relies" (Hatton, 2020, p. 20). It is because of this vulnerability and precarity that football players feel the need to put themselves at risk on the gridiron.

The lack of security in players' status and role on the team encourages risky behaviors that can lead to individual injury; there is pressure to compete to maintain their status as football players, their playing time, and the potential opportunities that can come from it all. Athletes, after all, "understand their coaches as having control over their education and future employment, as well as the much-sought-after chance to play their sport at the elite collegiate level" (Hatton, 2020, pp. 72–73). But the prospect of potential future opportunities, particularly participation in professional sport, is a lenient way of framing this. The most recently released NCAA data noted that the probability of a Division I football player being drafted to the National Football League (NFL) is 1.5% (NCAA, 2020). This is quite the slim possibility of 'making it,' but the risks are seen as worth the potential pay off.

The pandemic only exacerbated existing issues in this already precarious situation. Even though football play became riskier because of the uncertainty of an airborne virus, players were mandated by their universities to sign liability waivers before returning to campus for workouts, only to protect the institutions against potential litigation if players contracted the coronavirus (Dellenger, 2020). Given how the "student-athlete" moniker developed, this is a familiar approach for college football institutions. In response to this absolution of responsibility and disregard for players' health, several individual players opted out of play while Power Five teams were announcing their decisions to participate in the 2020 season. By September 2020, at least 150 FBS players chose to opt-out (Prewitt, 2021). A group of these players were featured in a *Sports Illustrated* issue in April 2021. They were not applauded for avoiding further risk and sitting out the season, but were instead highlighted because opting out of the season might have impacted their potential NFL status, as the decision had been framed as letting down their college teams. Together, these waivers and the bashing of those players who opted out squarely placed the responsibility and blame on individual athletes who noted the risks of pandemic play, thereby demonstrating a practical application of status coercion.

Layered with this understanding of their deliberate identification as "student-athletes" is the fact that risk of injury and harm are foundational to the sport. In his investigation of the interconnectedness of fandom, injury, spectacle, and business in hockey, sociologist Nathan Kalman-Lamb writes that "injury is a structural feature of team spectator sport. It validates a spectator's investment by demonstrating how much is at stake through the very fact that violence, pain, and injury are literally enacted upon the bodies that participate" (2018, p. 12). The same can be said of American football. Whether an injury attained during play that physically ails a player or the contraction of a virus with unpredictable consequences on future health, these risks have been treated the same by football institutions, as care is performed for players in the immediate moment to ensure they're able to take the field. Michael Bennett, former NFL player, takes this argument even further. Bennett states that because of the lack of Black administrators, coaches, managers, and staff, at all levels of football, and subsequent abundance of Black players, football is not an integrated sport. This means that the pain and violence witnessed by fans is most often enacted upon Black bodies, people who are divorced of their humanity and only valued for their entertainment purposes (Bennett & Zirin, 2019).

Therefore, player exploitation is multi-fold. Not only are these young men participating in an inherently violent sport that has the potential to cause irreparable harm to their physical bodies, they are also navigating various sporting institutions, at different levels, that are taking advantage of their desire to participate in the game in hopes of progressing to the next level of play. Very few real protections are in place. In the current pandemic landscape, this is even more obvious. Journalist and former professional basketball player Etan Thomas (2021) poignantly illuminates this fact in his conversation about college basketball players:

> The harsh reality is that the school is not concerned with their health long-term. That's evident by the borderline-reckless COVID-19 protocol that the NCAA has enacted. Rather than having a universal COVID protocol that every university must follow, they are leaving it up to the individual schools and conferences to come up with their own health-and-safety protocols, which is absolutely insane.

The lack of standardized protocols across universities, despite the bureaucratic power held by the NCAA, makes clear the true focus of the rush to return to the football field.

This continued insistence on one's value to the team and university through his labor and bodily production on the gridiron is a kind of violence. Hatton argues that this rhetoric of care from football programs actually contributes to athletes' experiences of dehumanization and commodification (2020, p. 134). McLeod and colleagues would expand this analysis to describe this dehumanization as "the rational, logical production of the body, requiring specialization, expertise, and specific *types* of bodies" (2014, p. 233) in order to produce on the field. Therefore, despite institutions' performances of care for players—through public virtue signaling, financial support for surgeries, resources to help balance classwork with field work—this all points to the inherent violence of the system.

Media scholar Jennifer McClearen closes her book-length account of female UFC fighters with a rumination on the violence leveled against these women, not because of what happens in the cage, but because of how the bureaucracy of the sport violently exploits them. She writes, "I contend that neoliberal business practices that place organizational growth and accumulation of wealth above human interests are inherently violent" (McClearen, 2020, pp. 164–165). This tension applies to college football. The systems and spaces that rely on the athletic bodies of these young Black men are concerned with their labor on the field, but not their lived experiences off it. No matter how these institutions and bureaucracies claim to be committed to their players' well-being, there is overwhelming evidence to the contrary to show the limits of that care.

Racialized Violence On and Off the Gridiron

When the Power Five decisions to play during the pandemic were announced and I actually saw players take the field on Saturdays during fall 2020, I was immediately reminded of Carter and his surgery because the response to dealing with the virus mirrors the continued response to treating injury. Given the risk of contracting the coronavirus and myocarditis (Cunningham, 2020; Rajpal et al., 2021), and the unknown effects of what we now call long-haul COVID (Quinn, 2021), football programs went on the offensive to make sure their players could play through an entire season. For instance, they tried to ensure that the season could continue by doing regular testing, as evident in the higher rates at which athletes were tested when compared with other students on campus (Babb, 2020; Kelderman, 2020). This only further speaks to the tension of the term "student-athlete," given the exaggerated ways this disconnect was blatantly put on display in the differing treatments of students and athletes on campuses around the country. It also points to just one demonstration of how administrators rationalize players' "spectacular and exceptional violence, injury, [and] dehumanization" (McLeod et al., 2014, p. 233), to thereby normalize the harmful treatment they receive.

Let's consider the Sugar Bowl game, played January 1, 2021, to think about the overlapping interests that presented themselves during a high profile college football game, with 'amateur' athletes, during a pandemic.

This game was played between Ohio State University, the 4th ranked team, and Clemson University, the 3rd ranked team. Ohio State quarterback Justin Fields suffered a tremendous tackle and nasty hit to the ribs during the second quarter that clearly left him in pain. He struggled to walk straight and throw the ball effectively. When asked at halftime about Fields' condition, Ohio State head coach Ryan Day told ESPN's Maria Taylor, "He's got the heart of a lion and he's gotta play for 30 more minutes. This is a good start, but this is a championship team we're playing. So we know that no matter what happens at half time, we're going to have to play another 30 minutes" (Gulick, 2021). It was reported that Fields did not receive an x-ray or a diagnosis during halftime (Lyons, 2021), but did receive multiple shots in the tent to help him finish the game (Schrotenboer, 2021). Ohio State won and Fields finished with six touchdowns and 385 passing yards. It was later determined that he suffered a hip pointer injury. After some rehabbing, Fields and Ohio State played in the championship game 10 days later and lost to University of Alabama.

Fields, a Black college quarterback on one of highest ranked teams in the nation, was expected to (and perhaps made to) play through a traumatic injury. Further, he was doubly at risk, given the persistent threat of contracting COVID around other unmasked individuals and the chance of suffering a worse injury during play. His participation in these two games could have had very real implications for his potential to play professional football, had he been more severely injured. Thankfully, his past performances on the gridiron and the fact that he healed from the injury helped to ensure that he remained a highly-sought after quarterback in the league; he was selected #11 in the 2021 NFL Draft by the Chicago Bears.

Fields' selection in the draft meant that all of his hard work would finally and literally pay off; because of his status as an "amateur student-athlete," he was not compensated for his actual physical labor during either college playoff game. However, his coaches, the television networks, and his university definitely made money. At the end of the calendar year, *Forbes* reported that the head coaches from Alabama, Clemson, Ohio State, and Notre Dame—the final four teams vying for the national championship—collectively made almost $26 million during 2020

(Andrzejewski, 2020). Further, according to a new study conducted by the National College Players Association, "between 2017–2020, approximately $10 billion in generational wealth will have been transferred from college football and men's basketball players, the majority of whom are athletes of color, to coaches, athletics administrators, and college administrators who are predominantly White or to institutions and programs that serve majority White constituencies" (Huma et al., 2020, p. 3). These statistics speak to a particular kind of extraction and exploitation, as the bodies of young Black men are fueling the present financial success of individual white men and institutions, all while their own future families suffer. Not only do football players experience physical harm while participating in an inherently violent sport, but the value they produce from their bodily labor is transferred away, to coaches, institutions, and administrators who claim to care about their well-being. Because of the financial benefits they reap, it comes as no surprise that the NCAA maintains that college athletes should not be allowed to unionize to advocate for their own economic rights (NCAA, 2021).

This blatant disconnect between who gets paid for athletic labor explains just one of the reasons for *NCAA* v *Alston*, the Supreme Court case which questions whether the lack of compensation for collegiate athletes violates antitrust laws. The second page of the brief succinctly outlines these issues, stating:

> The NCAA and its member conferences and schools receive billions of dollars every year through the hard work, sweat, and sometimes broken bodies of student-athletes. Coaches, assistant coaches, and athletic directors take millions in salaries. Yet the schools have agreed among themselves to limit what student-athletes may receive for their work in generating these extraordinary revenues. (*National Collegiate Athletic Association v Alston*, et al., 2020, p. 2)

This case deals with one of the most pressing issues in college sport right now: the ability for athletes to gain compensation for their own labor on the field of play. While this seemed to be placated with the passing of name, image, likeness (NIL) laws in July 2021, advocates of college athletic labor compensation argue this is far from enough. As sociologists

Nathan Kalman-Lamb and Derek Silva describe, with NIL, college athletes "earn revenue related to non-sports things. They have to hustle and go on their own [...] in separate work, work unrelated to their athletic endeavors. And at the end of the day they're still not compensated in any real way for the actual labor, which is violent labor that leads to injury and harm" (2021). These scholars point to the limits of NIL and the changes that still need to occur to even feign actual payment for athletic labor. Therefore, the decision in this Supreme Court case is fundamental to the ways the college sport system progresses.

Together, responses to suffering from mundane injury, attempts to nullify the impacts of contracting COVID, and dealing with calls for racial justice embody the institutionalized form of care that football teams, coaches, administrators, and institutions of higher education show for these athletes. It is the way that football invests in and cares for its players, not for their individual well-being, but to secure financial gain from their free labor on the field. Whether that manifests as postponed surgeries or mid-game shots, daily team COVID tests or public displays of solidarity, there is a clear concern for the ability and desire of the player to actually take the field. In short, while it can be classified as care, it is a rubric of care that sees and uses athletic bodies as commodities and invests in these bodies to keep them healthy and interested enough to play. This care is intended to have long-term benefits for the team and the university, with wins as the desired outcome, no matter how individual players are harmed in the process.

With that, it is important to reconsider the racial dynamics of this situation alongside scholar Billy Hawkins' metaphor of the new plantation. In his foundational book, Hawkins argues that predominantly white institutions are the new plantations for Black athletes because of the capitalist exploitations they experience within the colonial system perpetuated on campuses of higher education. These historically white institutions "function like plantation systems that internally colonize and exploit the athletic resources of Black athletes, [to such an extent that] they return to their communities injured (physically or psychologically) or poorly educated; despite the athletic expenditures they have given to these institutions" (Hawkins, 2010, p. 19). Through this argument, it is clear that white coaches, administrators, and institutions extract value from Black athletes' labor in a way that limits their opportunities for success once they are no longer recognized as college football players.

Comparisons to and metaphors of the plantation logics of American football, at both the college and professional levels, are not new. In 1995, Walter Byers wrote in his memoir: "Today, the NCAA President's Commission is […] firmly committed to the neoplantation belief that the enormous proceeds from college games belong to the overseers (the administrators) and supervisors (coaches). The plantation workers performing in the arena may receive only those benefits authorized by the overseers" (Byers & Hammer, 1995, pp. 2–3). This scathing critique of the bureaucracy that governs college sport has been kept in circulation. Complementary to Hawkins' theorization of college athletes, journalist William Rhoden provocatively describes professional Black male athletes as forty million dollar slaves. With the historically rooted power dynamic that has allowed for white executives and administrators to make millions from Black athletes' labor, even in an "era of multimillion-dollar salaries, slavery remains the model for the power relationship between athletes and their owners," (2007, p. 237). Civil Rights historian Taylor Branch analyzes the NCAA, specifically, as a "classic cartel" and denounces the college sport system for having "an unmistakable whiff of the plantation" that can most appropriately be compared to colonialism (2011). In his co-written memoir that details his experiences with various football institutions, Super Bowl champion Michael Bennett compares the NFL combine to "slave auctions" and explains that his brother Martellus, also a pro player, nicknamed the league 'Niggas For Lease' because of how it underpays and discards its players (Bennett & Zirin, 2019, p. 70).

I have argued elsewhere that if we extend the metaphor of the plantation logics to its limits, then the injuries that Black athletes sustain, along with their side effects, can be classified as the afterlives of slavery, in the words of Saidiya Hartman (Canada & Carter, 2021). According to Hartman, "Black lives are still imperiled and devalued by a racial calculus and a political arithmetic that were entrenched centuries ago. This is the afterlife of slavery—skewed life chances, limited access to health and education, premature death, incarceration, and impoverishment" (2007, p. 6). This is a theorization that disrupts the concept of linear chronological time, implying that those events of the not-so-distant past continue to have tangible effects in the not-so-different present. In this case, the years that a player spends on the gridiron very directly affect his physical outcomes off it. The injuries that he sustains from either breaks, tears, bruises, sprains, concussions, or viruses will have a lasting impact and will influence the way that he must navigate his everyday life as he lives through injury (Ralph, 2014).

It is important to highlight that the conditions created by the pandemic are not novel in the way of anti-Black racism in the United States; this is not a new phenomenon. The sports we watch, the medical institutions we visit, the media we engage, the history we learn, and Black folks' everyday lived realities have consistently been implicated by interactions with white supremacist systems. This is so pervasive that scholar Christina Sharpe (2016) describes this as a holistic environment, known as "the weather," which presents an atmospheric anti-Blackness that Black folks must navigate. Therefore, the theorization of the plantation logics of American football only adds to the notion that Black athletes' lives are fundamentally shaped and changed by their experiences with college football. These injuries and bodily harm are just one way that the anti-Black racism that circulates in these sporting spaces and institutions will continue to impact athletes long after they graduate and are no longer affiliated with their teams. Thus, the anti-Black framework of the college football system cannot be substantially addressed with pitiful performances of care that come on behalf of football institutions and administrators. It is not enough to play a commercial during halftime or excessively test for a deadly virus or increase attention paid to the physical bodies of athletes.

The 2020 season plainly laid bare all that football programs have attempted to hide behind the masquerade of egalitarianism, meritocracy, fair play, and rationality, all elements that are claimed to be representative of modern sport (Guttmann, 1978). No matter how convincing the system's attempt at caring for players is, it is now difficult to deny that staple tenets of football are promoted through a spectacle which actualizes social hierarchies and inequalities, anti-Blackness, labor exploitation, and structural violence.

Conclusion

I write this conclusion at the beginning of the 2021 college football season. A few ACC match ups have already occurred, and yet, the commercial from the 2020 season, the one played each halftime, has not been shown. What this absence signals to me is that the conference and the NCAA feel that even the bare minimum performance of this kind of care for their Black athletes is no longer relevant. They have shifted their attention away from issues of racism and anti-Blackness, both in and out sport, perhaps in hopes of signaling to the public that they no longer exist.

When I reflect on my immersive fieldwork from several years ago alongside the season(s) of pandemic play, it is interesting to note how little seems to have changed in institutional responses to player-specific issues that impact experiences both on and off the gridiron. Despite a global pandemic, national civil and racial unrest, calls to reform the entire collegiate athletic model, and ever-increasing evidence of the dangers of gridiron play, the capitalist machine that drives college football continues to forge forward at full speed. As long as those in the system with power perform a certain kind of care, they seem to argue, there will always be players willing to sacrifice their bodies and expend their labor on the playing field. What happens, I wonder, if and when those players are no longer willing.

**Portions of this work were previously published online in *SAPIENS* and *Black Perspectives*.

References

Andrzejewski, A. (2020, December 30). Head football coaches at Alabama, Clemson, Ohio State & Notre Dame collectively made $25.9 million. *Forbes*. https://www.forbes.com/sites/adamandrzejewski/2021/12/30/top-four-football-coaches-in-ncaa-national-playoff-collectively-made-259-million/?sh=61125bb131d8

Babb, K. (2020, December 3). *As thousands of athletes get coronavirus tests, nurses wonder: What about us?* The Washington Post. https://www.washingtonpost.com/sports/2020/11/27/nurses-athletes-sports-coronavirus-tests/

Bennett, M., & Zirin, D. (2019). *Things that make white people uncomfortable*. Haymarket Books.

Berkowitz, S. (2020, April 15). Major public college football programs could lose billions in revenue if no season is played. *USA Today*. https://www.usatoday.com/story/sports/ncaaf/2020/04/14/college-football-major-programs-could-see-billions-revenue-go-away/2989466001/

Branch, T. (2011, October). The shame of college sports. *The Atlantic*. https://www.theatlantic.com/magazine/archive/2011/10/the-shame-of-college-sports/308643/

Byers, W., & Hammer, C. (1995). *Unsportsmanlike conduct: Exploiting college athletes*. University of Michigan Press.

Camp, W. (1901). *Walter Camp's book of college sports*. The Century Co.

Canada, T., & Carter, C. R. (2021). The NFL's racist 'race norming' is an afterlife of slavery. *Scientific American*. https://www.scientificamerican.com/article/the-nfls-racist-race-norming-is-an-afterlife-of-slavery/

Clotfelter, C. T. (2011). *Big-time sports in American universities*. Cambridge University Press.

Cramer, M., & Diaz, J. (2020, June 13). Texas football players call on university to drop a song steeped in racist history. *The New York Times*. https://www.nytimes.com/2020/06/13/us/eyes-texas-racist-longhorn-football.html

Cunningham, A. (2020, September 11). College athletes show signs of possible heart injury after COVID-19. *Science News*. https://www.sciencenews.org/article/covid19-coronavirus-heart-injury-college-athletes-sports

Davis, B. (2022, January 25). COVID hit Texas football, other sports with financial shortfall. *Hook Em*. https://www.hookem.com/story/sports/football/2022/01/25/accounting-data-shows-how-much-pandemic-squeezed-texas-athletics/9218078002/

Dellenger, R. (2020, June 17). Coronavirus liability waivers raise questions as college athletes return to campus. *Sports Illustrated*. https://www.si.com/college/2020/06/17/college-athletes-coronavirus-waivers-ohio-state-smu

Given, K. (2017, October 13). *Walter Byers: The man who built the NCAA, then tried to tear it down*. WBUR. https://www.wbur.org/onlyagame/2017/10/13/walter-byers-ncaa

Gulick, B. (2021, January 1). Ryan Day's halftime comments to ESPN. *Sports Illustrated*. https://www.si.com/college/ohiostate/football/ohio-state-football-ryan-day-halftime-interview-sugar-bowl-vs-clemson

Guttmann, A. (1978). *From ritual to record: The nature of modern sports*. Columbia University Press.

Harper, S. R. (2018). *Black male student-athletes and racial inequality in NCAA Division I college sports*. USC Race and Equity Center. https://abfe.issuelab.org/resources/29858/29858.pdf

Hartman, S. (2007). *Lose your mother: A journey along the Atlantic slave trade*. Farrar, Straus and Giroux.

Hatton, E. (2020). *Coerced: Work under threat of punishment*. University of California Press.

Hawkins, B. (2010). *The new plantation: Black athletes, college sports, and predominantly white NCAA institutions*. Palgrave Macmillan.

Huma, R., Staurowsky, E. J., & Montgomery, L. (2020, July 31). *How the NCAA's empire robs predominantly Black athletes of billions in generational wealth*. National College Players Association. https://drive.google.com/file/d/1z97vhcjErrHIvuO3Nu2wUWbG90bFKnm_/view

Humanities Unbounded. (2020, September 23). *Whiplash: Anthropology in/of Disaster* [Video.] Youtube. https://www.youtube.com/watch?v=kSy-Cqt-430

Kalman-Lamb, N. (2018). *Game misconduct: Injury, fandom, and the business of sport*. Fernwood Publishing.

Kalman-Lamb, N., & Silva, D. (Hosts). (2021, July 9). Episode 72: College Sport 'Apocalypse' (No. 72). [Audio podcast episode]. In *End of Sport Podcast*. https://www.theendofsport.com/episodes/episode-72-college-sport-apocalypse

Kelderman, E. (2020, September 17). 'A scene out of gladiator': Big Ten football players get daily coronavirus tests, but other students don't. *The Chronicle of Higher Education*. https://www.chronicle.com/article/a-scene-out-of-gladiator-big-ten-football-players-get-daily-coronavirus-tests-but-other-students-dont

Lapchick, R. E. (2021). *The 2020 DI FBS leadership college racial and gender report card: The lack of diversity within collegiate athletic leadership continues*. Institute for Diversity and Ethics in Sport. https://43530132-36e9-4f52-811a-182c7a91933b.filesusr.com/ugd/138a69_a7d5807e08804005960a584bb2fb261d.pdf

Lyons, D. (2021, January 1). *Justin Fields reportedly did not get an x-ray at halftime*. The Sun by Sports Illustrated. https://thespun.com/big-ten/ohio-state-buckeyes/justin-fields-injury-ribs-james-skalski-hit-x-ray-ryan-day-ohio-state-clemson

McClearen, J. (2020). *Fighting visibility: Sports media and female athletes in UFC*. University of Illinois Press.

McGee, K. (2021, March 1). 'UT needs rich donors': Emails show wealthy alumni supporting 'Eyes of Texas' threatened to pull donations. *Texas Tribune*. https://www.texastribune.org/2021/03/01/ut-eyes-of-texas-donors-emails/

McLeod, C., Lovich, J., Newman, J. I., & Shields, R. (2014). The training camp: American football and/as spectacle of exception. *Journal of Sport and Social Issues, 38*(3), 222–244.

National Collegiate Athletic Association v Alston, et al., 20-512 U.S. 2. (2020). https://www.supremecourt.gov/DocketPDF/20/20-512/160131/20201109144114249_Brief%20in%20Opp_pdfA.pdf

NCAA (2020, April 20). *Football: Probability of competing beyond high school.* https://www.ncaa.org/about/resources/research/football

NCAA (2021, May 27). *NCAA statement on Murphy-Sanders bill.* https://www.ncaa.org/about/resources/media-center/news/ncaa-statement-murphy-sanders-bill

Prewitt, A. (2021, April 7). What happens now to the NFL prospects who opted out of their final college season? *Sports Illustrated.* https://www.si.com/nfl/2021/04/07/daily-cover-nfl-draft-opt-out-covid

Quinn, T.J. (2021, September 3). 'Is this my life now?': Clemson defensive end Justin Foster's – And my – Struggle with long-haul COVID. *ESPN.* https://www.espn.com/college-football/story/_/id/32127148/clemson-defensive-end-justin-foster-my-struggle-long-haul-covid

Rajpal, S., Tong, M. S., Borchers, J., Zareba, K. M., Obarski, T. P., Simonetti, O. P., & Daniels, C. J. (2021). Cardiovascular magnetic resonance findings in competitive athletes recovering from COVID-19 infection. *JAMA Cardiology, 6*(1), 116–118. https://doi.org/10.1001/jamacardio.2020.4916

Ralph, L. (2014). *Renegade dreams: Living through injury in gangland Chicago.* University of Chicago Press.

Rhoden, W. C. (2007). *Forty million dollar slaves: The rise, fall, and redemption of the black athlete.* Penguin Random House.

Roosevelt, T. (1900, May). What we can expect from the American man. *St. Nicholas.*

Schrotenboer, B. (2021, January 2). Ohio State quarterback Justin Fields says 'whole right torso messed up' after record Sugar Bowl performance. *USA Today.* https://www.usatoday.com/story/sports/ncaaf/2021/01/02/ohio-state-justin-fields-college-football-title-game-alabama/4110769001/

Sharpe, C. (2016). *In the wake: On blackness and being.* Duke University Press.

Slothower, C. (2014, September 24). Fort Lewis' first 'student-athlete.' *The Durango Herald.* https://www.durangoherald.com/articles/fort-lewis-first-student-athlete/

The Daily Tar Heel Staff. (2020, August 9). *The Daily Tar Heel will no longer use the term 'student athlete.'* The Daily Tar Heel. https://www.dailytarheel.com/article/2020/08/student-athlete-term-editorial

Thomas, E. (2021, February 17). More NCAA players should look out for themselves like Duke's Jalen Johnson. *BasketballNews.com*. https://www.basketballnews.com/stories/ncaa-duke-university-blue-devils-college-basketball-jalen-johnson-coach-k-mike-krzyzewski-syracuse-jim-boeheim-bourama-sidibe-etan-thomas-nba-covid-2021-nba-draft

Yearwood, G. M. H. (2018). Heritage as hate: Racism and sporting traditions. *Leisure Studies, 37*(6), 677–669. https://doi.org/10.1080/02614367.2018.1497683

26

Mapping the Geographies of Combat Sport during COVID-19: Dana White, Trumpism, and the Landscapes of the UFC

Ted Butryn, Matthew A. Masucci, and jay a. johnson

Introduction

Early into the pandemic, as businesses were being shuttered, public services halted, and states were urging their citizens to stay home in a collective bid to ward off the rising COVID-19 infection numbers in the United States, President Donald Trump started proclaiming the importance of resuming live sporting events. For Trump and his supporters, the push represented a (misguided) conceptualization of the meaning of successfully emerging from the ongoing quagmire of the pandemic for America and Americans. One of the first ambassadors Trump named to his newly created Sports Advisory Committee (Lutz, 2020) was Dana

T. Butryn (✉) • M. A. Masucci
San José State University, San Jose, CA, USA
e-mail: theodore.butryn@sjsu.edu

j. a. johnson
University of Manitoba, Winnipeg, MB, Canada

D. L. Andrews et al. (eds.), *Sport and Physical Culture in Global Pandemic Times*, Global Culture and Sport Series, https://doi.org/10.1007/978-3-031-14387-8_26

White, former co-owner and current President of the Ultimate Fighting Championship (UFC). Rarely do the heads of major sporting organizations run towards political controversy, when the politics may threaten to alienate a percentage of your audience and put the health and welfare of athletes at risk (Zirin, 2020). However, Dana White did just that, careening towards media battles regarding COVID-19 with the underpinnings and outward rhetoric of Trumpism virtually tattooed on his kingpinesque persona.

While most professional sporting organizations quickly postponed their seasons in compliance with public health guidelines related to COVID-19, the UFC approach to the crisis mirrored the spectacle of Donald Trump's daily pandemic news briefings, particularly given the cavalier manner in which Dana White openly dismissed the grave impact of the coronavirus. Further, White's friendship with Trump arguably influenced Florida Governor and (then) fellow Trump supporter, Ron DeSantis to declare the World Wrestling Entertainment (WWE) an "essential service," (i.e., a public service that is necessary for the functioning of a community), and allowed them to continue taping live events. The UFC were beneficiaries of this decision as well, as they were able to promote several events in Florida at the time, which is perhaps not surprising given the close relationship that White and Trump have shared over the years (Proffitt et al., 2021).

Moreover, this decision provides an opportunity to closely examine how Trumpism's influence on a sport organization impacted the policies, performances, and physicalities involved in the establishment of two hubs where the events have taken place to accommodate both North American and International fighters. Most have occurred in a venue constructed and owned by the UFC called UFC APEX in Las Vegas and the second site was what was dubbed "Fight Island" in Abu Dhabi, UAE. While everyone's future is yet unwritten under the cloud of COVID-19, they vowed to continue to adapt and to find a way for the show to go on.

While Trumpism was always and already present in segments of the UFC and its fanbase, in this chapter we will show how the geographical challenges during COVID-19 accentuated and perhaps extended its presence.

The purpose of this chapter is to unpack the operational decisions and attendant rhetoric that occurred within the UFC organization during the time-frame of the pandemic. By interrogating the unrelenting pursuit of promoting live events, made possible by the utilization of highly controlled event spaces, we articulate the deployment of decidedly Trumpian tactics of media manipulation and a political strategy Gaber and Fisher (2022) call "strategic lying" (p. 461), that ultimately served to exacerbate the (long-standing) exploitation of fighters. Indeed, while other pro sports at least pretended to wrestle with the best ways to resume play while ensuring athlete and spectator health, the UFC's aggressive efforts led to multiple positive COVID-19 tests, in spite of near-constant corporate rhetoric that continually and publicly minimized the severity of the Coronavirus as nothing more than a cold or the flu. Lastly, throughout this chapter, we will speak to the interlaced political, rhetorical, and promotional relationship of Trumpism, Dana White and the UFC in moving forward an unquestioned and acritical message of "bringing sport back" in a march towards normalcy. In doing so, we hope to highlight the important relationship between sport and politics, broadly, but also the multifaceted consequences of Trumpism's tendrils extending into a sporting space like the UFC. In a sense, it is not possible to understand Dana White's rhetoric during the pandemic without considering the ways that his demeanor and overall sensibility overlapped with that of Trump.

Theoretically, we draw from Bale (1994) and Eichberg's (1998) writings on space and bodies as well as Newman et al. (2020) and Andrews' (2019) work to illustrate how the UFC's newly constructed fight venues are central to the "vast and complex web of science, human action and rationality, culture, capital, and spectacle" (Newman et al., 2020, p. 25) that shaped the meanings of various bodies during COVID-19. Finally, following Kalman-Lamb (2018) and others, we discuss how, in his efforts to continue business-as-usual, White's (mediated) words reveal a Trumpian attitude towards athletes-as-laborers that privilege the corporate bottom-line over individual health and agency.

With respect to the crux of the chapter, examining the creation of spaces within which to hold live, nearly spectatorless events during the pandemic, we lean on the work of sport geographer John Bale (1994, 2003) and draw from Henning Eichberg's concept of the sporting trialectic (1998). Bale's work, in particular, is informative in interpreting the meanings of Fight Island and UFC APEX. Indeed, he was one of the first sport studies scholars who championed work that examined sporting environments and that sought "to understand its meaning for people and to 'read' it as a kind of a text'" (Bale, 1994, p. 3). As Bale (2003) noted, the concepts of space and place are fundamental to the understanding of geography, in general, and the geographical environments in which sports take place, specifically. Further, geographical spaces in sport, in this case Fight island and the UFC APEX Center, can never be totally removed from the politics of the places themselves, whether it be controversies over the use of massive plots of public land for municipal golf courses, or the removal of local populace for the benefit of a more "fan friendly" and consumer-ready Olympic games. As media accounts clearly showed, these newly constructed environments in Las Vegas and Abu Dhabi were born of politics, and positioned at the center of larger discourses over the politicization of COVID-19 from the moment they became sites for the UFC's events in July of 2020.

Covid Geographies: Constructing Pandemic Combat Landscapes

UFC APEX, opened for production in June of 2019 (pre-pandemic) on a site in close proximity to UFC headquarters and the UFC Performance Institute. Among other events, Apex was designed to host the new UFC broadcast production called *Dana White's Contender Series*, where unsigned mixed martial arts fighters vie for a UFC contract through combat. According to their website:

> UFC APEX has built-in, advanced production capabilities with an arena space that can be configured to accommodate a variety of live events, including other sports competitions, concerts, stage shows, esports tournaments, and more. The arena can also be converted into a sound stage for use as a rehearsal space for entertainment acts booked throughout Las Vegas. (www.ufc.com/news/ufc-apex-officially-opens-las-vegas)

UFC APEX is a much smaller venue with limited seats for spectators and a smaller octagon size (the space that the 2 fighters perform in) of 25 feet across compared to the usual 30 ft, which according to preliminary data, creates a competition area that facilitates nearly 20% more strikes and more finishes via knockouts, submissions and technical knockouts (MMAmania, May 25, 2020). The availability of this facility, although not intended, was one of the pivotal reasons that the UFC was able to return to production during the pandemic, particularly in the early, more restrictive phase of the Covid-19 response when travel was significantly curtailed or discouraged. It also provided a physical space to manage, control and exploit fighter's bodies and the flow of media messaging, something we address throughout this chapter. Another layer of access and jurisdiction over the system and those in it, was the announcement that the UFC has also purchased additional acreage in the same vicinity of the other structures with the intention of building a hotel to house the fighters in. While travel restrictions and other COVID-19-related regulations, which vary by State, have opened with time, the UFC has not yet reverted back to their pre-pandemic business practice of taking events to cities across the globe, which comes with greater expense. On the reports of a record setting fiscal year, the UFC was lauded (Weprin, 2021) for most likely saving its parent company Endeavor after they struggled financially; missing earnings targets in the wake of going public in April, 2021. Owing, in part, to the profitability of this vertical production model, the UFC most likely pivoted more permanently to adopt this "new way of doing things" given that UFC APEX was already equipped for television broadcast and essentially owned a sporting venue and sophisticated production studio all in one (Dachman, 2020). Consequently, their in-house production capabilities, the high price that they command for exclusive seating, and control over all aspects of production (and safety measures in a post-COVID-19 environment) helped to accelerate utilization of UFC APEX for event programming.

At the beginning of the pandemic when the UFC hosted its first few spectatorless events, there were marked differences and points of impact with the new regulations and COVID-19 restrictions. One of the limiting factors for fights to resume Internationally, both for fighters located outside of the US and for hosting events outside of the US, were restrictive travel bans in and out of the United States and other countries. What this meant for UFC fighters–who, to clarify, are not employees but are classified as independent contractors–is that those located outside of the United States during that period of time, were unable to take part in any of the UFC events. The UFC boasts a roster of close to 600 male and female athletes, living in training in many different countries around the world. To circumvent the limiting landscape of travel opportunity for international fighters that existed at the time, Dana White tweeted that a UFC octagon cage was being constructed on an unknown beach somewhere outside of the US, and that they were building a "Fight Island". Purposively cloaked in intrigue and vague details, White's idea to create an international space for the UFC would allow fighters, particularly those from outside of the US, a place to temporarily resume their fighting careers while further expanding the UFC's business during COVID-19. With an absence of any other professional sports to cover, media reports took to covering the "mystery" of Fight Island and, similar to the so-called "NBA Bubble," began to ask questions about how a space could be created that insured the safety of the athletes (Stonehouse, 2020; Wagenheim, 2020).

When the details of Fight Island were finally revealed, the reality was much more muted than any of the rumours of luxurious spaces which floated around the internet before the final announcement. In short, White and the UFC had brokered a deal with government and private interests in the United Arab Emirates which secured space on Yaz Island in the UAE. The deal apparently bolstered their viewing revenue deal with ESPN and International broadcasters during a period of time when few if any sports were having live events. In addition, the deal involved sponsorship, space, accommodations and travel incentives (all first class), and the entire endeavor from conception through the hosting of the inaugural event was highlighted on the 4 part ESPN documentary titled UFC Fight Island: Declassified. They built this fighting venue on Yaz Island in close proximity to a top-shelf hotel, and everything was integrated in such a way as to seamlessly adhere to the COVID-19 protocols created by the UFC to conform to several governments COVID-19 travel regulations, such as social distancing, masking, and testing protocols (Morgan, 2020).

Finally, the UFC strategically selected journalists, such as John Morgan and Kevin Iole, who have rarely asked critical questions of the UFC, often parroting their scripted and fabricated talking points, to cover the high profile UFC events in Abu Dhabi. Part of their reporting was advertising that they too were being treated to first class amenities, and were lodged in the same hotels, eating in the same spaces and contained under strict UFC COVID-19 protocols, to exist in the newly created and tightly controlled UFC bubble. With the sudden onset of the pandemic and the UFC's pivot to find constructive ways to continue with their business, they were able to fabricate a landscape that completely integrated their desire and ability to control the bodies of all those within the bubble, and to meld and direct the narrative of the UFC to be consumed by a sport starved and unsettled fanbase.

Dana White has a historic propensity to host press conferences before and after events in confined spaces with the reporters that as we indicated previously, he will call out and put on the spot for asking certain questions or writing something unfavorable in an article. Imagine the coercive forces at play within that bubble where there was literally and figuratively no separation between any of the actors within that space, going from the press conference to dinner to any social events as a cohort. In this sense, the UFC's procedures for controlling spaces during the pandemic further tightened and facilitated the control of the messaging from White and the UFC.

This may have come as a surprise to many outside of the Mixed Martial Arts (MMA) community, but upon closer examination, it has been a match forged over several years. Early into the burgeoning sport's existence, Donald Trump, then a high profile property owner, would host UFC events at his Taj Mahal hotel in New Jersey. Later, as he was running for the Republican leadership, he had White speak on his behalf at the Republican National Convention. Throughout his Presidency, he has praised not only Dana White himself, but also several preeminent UFC fighters who have actively supported him and his politics. An example of this was his publicly released call to praise UFC fighter Colby Covington on the heels of his welterweight championship. In recent years, Covington had infamously shifted his persona to a rabid Trump supporter, donning a MAGA hat and mentioning the President's name every time he was in front of the media, a move which coincided with Trump's rise to political power. This culminated in strategic tours with Covington and other Trump-friendly fighters like Jorge Masvidal, a son of Cuban immigrants and a resident of southern Florida who spoke publicly of the connections he had to the Conservative Miami Cuban community supporting Trump and the Republican agenda, and inviting four UFC champions along with Dana White to high profile rallies where Trump would purposely and visibly aligned himself with them and their organization.

While the road back to hosting live UFC events during the pandemic has been anything but a straightforward path (see Butryn et al., 2020), Dana White in his dual roles of UFC President and National Sports Ambassador under the Trump administration, has been able to cobble together an unbroken string of UFC cards, and positioning the organization as one of the first US sports to return to a relatively normal mode of operation. In fact, the UFC is largely recognized as the organization who literally "wrote the book": a 30 page procedural manuscript on how to navigate the treacherous Coronavirus waters in order to host sporting events that protect athletes, staff and media members alike, and a text which they have apparently shared with many other professional sport organizations.

The Trumpian Bubble: Dana White and the Politics of the Venues

In her book, *Donald Trump and the Kayfabe Presidency* (2020), Shannon Bow O'Brien argues that Trump, unlike any of his predecessors in the White house, used his intimate knowledge of professional wrestling to drive home a populist message that resonated with sections of the American public. Indeed, given Trump's thirty-year history with professional wrestling, (Moon, 2020; O'Brien, 2020) his utilization of the tools and techniques of that unique form of sporting entertainment are clearly evident in his messaging, demeanor and rhetoric. These techniques, she argues, helped to shape, through the deft use of social media, a narrative that is highly antagonistic and devoid of fact yet appealing to a particular segment of society, particularly white, non-college educated men.

Moreover, and important for this chapter, is Trump's reliance on the *kayfabe* performance whereby the wrestler/performer (Trump in this case) maintains that "whatever is happening around them is absolutely real" (O'Brien, p. 3) though the audience clearly understands the "performance" to be part of the show. According to Moon:

> In a now lost world in which wrestling competitions were meant to be 'shoot' fights (real contests), kayfabe was the noble lie that excluded outsiders from the industry secret that the 'sport' was, in fact, a 'work' (predetermined). It was also the basis upon which 'bookers' (the promoters who 'book' matches) could generate 'heat' (hype and investment in a wrestler, whether positive or negative) with audiences by pushing 'worked angles' (scripted events which all wrestlers would know and act out), which built financially successful 'programs' between wrestlers. Wrestlers took on 'gimmicks' (characters), playing either 'heels' (bad guys) or 'baby aces' (good guys). "In this world, wrestlers lived their gimmicks inside and outside the ring to avoid 'breaking kayfabe' by letting the public know that the fights were predetermined and the conflicts constructed". (Moon, 2020, p. 51)

In this sense, while at the end of the day the audience is aware that the performance is not reflective of reality, the performer is steadfast in their role to maintain the illusion. It is in this way that Trump, and as we will see, Dana While, are able to unapologetically craft a narrative that, while obviously and objectively untrue, are told (and sold) in such a convincing way to a complicit audience (Moon, 2020), as to serve the broader goal of reshaping the discourse in a way that is impervious to critique or, at least, that the skeptics themselves are seen as villains to be vanquished. Accordingly, this careful and methodical story-shaping follows the techniques that are well known in the wrestling world and have been cunningly deployed by Trump and White to go "all-in" on blatantly false narratives (about COVID-19, fighter rights, and the media for example) in order to deflect legitimate criticism of policy and practice. Indeed, both Trump and White utilize a specific yet critical tool of the kayfabe performance—to identify an individual foil—to further their agendas. Whether it is Trump belittling a political rival or White calling out a journalist that has written an unflattering piece about the UFC, the end goal is to create an ecosystem where truth is what you make it. Of course, as O'Brien points out, this rhetorical style would not be effective if the fans didn't understand and appreciate the kayfabe dichotomy (p. 4). According to her, the complicity of fans "gives the wrestlers tacit approval to behave appallingly while allowing their fans to understand it is all part of the show where stereotypes and truths can be aired without repercussions" (p. 4). Using a page out of the Trumpian kayfabe playbook, Dana White doggedly cast suspicion on COVID-19 and the rules surrounding live events in the wake of ever-restrictive public health mandates in the early days of the pandemic.

As we have explored elsewhere (Butryn et al., 2020), following Trump and other COVID-19-skeptical politicians, White's non-stop bombast helped shape the narrative surrounding the intent to return to sport; casting the argument in terms of individual liberty, pseudoscience, capitalist and entrepreneurial interests and impugning individuals—politicians and journalists alike—who challenged the tenets of his "truth." Within this post-truth framework, the idea to move forward and host a large-scale sporting event began to emerge, as we mentioned above, after attempts to stage a UFC event were thwarted by increasingly strict public health guidelines.

Of course, much like Trump, Dana White's hyperbole relied on a continuous barrage of attacks on mainstream sport media sources, and a reliance on a few chosen media outlets, selected to carry his message to the public. Singleton and Green (2021) explore how the media messages surrounding moving ahead with live events in spite of the pandemic, exemplify a version of this one-dimensional promotional strategy. Their examination revealed that "the most dominant theme was that the show simply must go on and will be justified in their marketing by any means necessary" (p. 16). Moreover, and echoing a Trumpian disdain for any critical examination of messaging that runs counter to advancing the bottom line, Singleton and Green (2021) and Butryn et al. (2020) argue that the consequence of eschewing the very real dangers of the pandemic is born by the fighters themselves who are at the mercy of a precarious and exploitative labor arrangement. More specifically, White and the UFC have utilized the media, in both slickly produced quazi-infomercials (ESPN+ UFC Fight Island: Declassified, 2020) and in the MMA and mainstream press to strategically deploy a kind of "self described" apolitical rhetoric (Singleton & Green, 2021) that is, of course, clearly aligned with a neoliberal framework of individual choice and profit motivation that is the cornerstone of Trumpism. In addition, by calling out MMA journalists by name and dismissing their well-informed critiques questioning the prudence of hosting combat sport events during a pandemic, White and the UFC use a version of the increasingly effective (at least for many of the UFC's core fans) refrain of "fake news" to diffuse legitimate journalistic questions. Moreover, by taking a combative and controversial stance, as we have explored elsewhere (Butryn et al., 2020) and will expand on below, moving forward with events at Fight Island and UFC APEX are politicized in a way to promote an ideological stance and not just a sporting event.

In their media analysis of several videos that the UFC launched in June 2020 to promote their upcoming fights, even as all other sports had ceased operation, Singleton and Green (2021) note that both Trump (who recorded a voiceover introduction to the event) and White seemed to use Fight Island as a symbol of the single-minded "return to normalcy without an explanation of why and how this is to be accomplished under new health and safety protocols" (p. 8). As opposed to the various mainstream outlets that collectively questioned the wisdom and public safety of running these shows, the production of the initial Fight Island and UFC APEX shows in the initial months of the pandemic in 2020 were clearly designed to frame the events as a means of geographically and structurally defying COVID-19, and publicly highlight the efforts of Trump and White to run live events, ostensibly for the fans.

Of Space and COVID-19: Theorizing the UFC's Sporting Landscapes

In the preceding sections, we have established how Fight Island and the UFC APEX came into being, and how White's Trumpian rhetoric and savvy use of media aided his ability to frame these spaces as the sporting equivalent to "making America great again." In this section, we lean on the work of British sports geographer, John Bale (1994, 2003), German scholar Henning Eichberg (1998) and others to examine the meanings of sporting landscapes, and further elucidate the ways that the UFC APEX venue and Fight Island, in particular, became tightly wound up in the politicization of the pandemic and the UFC's intersection with Trumpism.

As Andrews (2019) noted, Trump's attacks on the NFL for becoming "too soft," and his mantra of "making America great again," speak to "a condition of contemporary crisis in need of resolution" (p. 121). Similarly, White's constant rallying against politicians and media critics who would prevent hosting UFC shows, and his verbose attacks on a US populace who have, in his thinking, retreated in fear from the COVID-19, were also framed as (geographical) solutions to a crisis. Not only has White used similar language regarding Americans "hiding" in their homes due to COVID-19, UFC APEX and Fight Island became part of the larger discursive attempt to parrot Trump's rhetoric related to the presumed emasculation of American society, something that speaks directly to how he frames the fighters who are willing to fight in these spaces.

Through his rhetoric and ongoing efforts to frame the UFC as a sort of neoliberal, anti-pandemic role model, White successfully framed these two venues as resolutions to American crises of sporting character and identity. The existence and employment of UFC APEX and Fight island, then, are not merely venues to house UFC bouts, but the geographical manifestations of White's echoing of Trumpian rhetoric.

Newman, Thorpe, & Andrews suggest that, "The material body exists—we can touch it, feel it, cut it, and so on—*and* it has the capacity to produce (representations, material outcomes, social relations, affect). The representational body also exists—we can perceive it, locate its locutions, point to its discursive politics—and it can point back at us" (pp. 11–12). However, what has received less attention from sport studies scholars is the (material) space within which these bodies exist and produce. Andrews (2019) also positions what he calls the "uber-sport integrated spectacle" as a central part of how contemporary sport operates, complete with an intersection array of several sub-spectacles, one of which is "spacial spectacle." (p. 42.) Thus, we argue that the spaces of Fight Island and the UFC APEX—spaces designed to *protect* (from COVID-19), *preserve* (content and profit), and *produce* (violent combat sport and politicized meanings of "opening up the country")—allow these venues to be simultaneously safe and risk-laden; at once unexposed to COVID-19, and exposed to brutal pain and injury.

In Bale's (1994) key text, *Landscapes of Modern Sport*, he highlights ten views of the sports landscape. We focus here on a few that are directly relevant to the ways in which the creation of venues that became politicized means of striving to provide UFC content to fans at a time when most sports throughout the world had ceased production, also became imbued with meanings that relate to Andrews' (2019) notion of the ubersport assemblage and the Trump conjuncture.

One way Bale interprets sporting landscapes relates to the ways that sporting spaces "can be viewed as a reflection of various ideologies" (p. 12). While some stadiums and arenas are ideological in the technocentric sense–meant to show that the internet-ready, plugged-in capable spaces are a step forward from the passive ways in which sport fans watched events in the past, on aluminum benches with hotseats that would never match the cruel frigidity of colder winter climates–other sporting spaces are associated with a more explicit political ideology, the most glaring example being the stadium at the 1936 Berlin Olympics. To an extent, UFC APEX, and most certainly Fight Island are inherently ideological in their conceptualization, structure, and location. They are built not only to provide paying fans an opportunity to watch the events on the newly configured ESPN+ platform, but as a means of publicly chastising the political Left, doubters of White's vision for resuscitating sport during COVID-19, and all other assorted 'sportive snowflakes.'

Indeed, as Bale suggests, sport landscapes do not just appear out of nowhere, absent of the larger sociocultural context and the underlying political machinations of the time. In addition, power, in the form of the control of players or fans, can certainly be reflected in the ways that sporting spaces are constructed, overseen, policed, and framed by sporting organizations. While Bale wrote about various instances in which groups have been excluded from sport spaces based on socioeconomic status, cultural differences, and a myriad of other reasons, in the case of the UFC, the power to exclude the MMA and general sporting press was clearly designed to control the flow of information, and allow the organization to direct the desired narrative. Specifically, White seemed to intentionally select journalists to attend his news conferences during which he railed against those that would get in the way of "bringing sport back," who the UFC felt would frame their efforts in a benevolent, nationalistic light.

Importantly for this chapter, Bale also was one of the first scholars to examine sporting landscapes like the UFC APEX and Fight Island as spectacles, and the notion that sporting spectacles are not merely run of the mill contests, but rather dramatic events that go "beyond the more modest expectations of day to day sport" (Bale, 1994, p. 130). Following the work of John MacAloon (1981), Bale noted that the athletes who inhabit the landscapes of sporting spectacle can come to represent something much larger than athletic excellence. Rather, they may eventually stand in as a kind of "cross-cultural voyeurism" for fans who can observe from a distance the exotic other. In the two UFC venues, the athletes represent a different kind of exotic other, defined less by race or ethnicity than by their very presence as athletes in a world almost devoid of other televised professional sport. Indeed, this was part of Dana White's desire to have the UFC become the first professional sports league to return to live competitions during the pandemic. It was not just about providing sport to the people or any sense of a supposed return to normalcy, as a return to sport was often framed following the terrorist attacks of September 11th, 2001.

This is where the spectacle of the fighters and the landscapes intersect, and contribute to a rare occasion when fans have access to sensory information that they would not have otherwise. UFC APEX Center and Fight Island were, either by design in the case of the latter or ultimately in the case of the former, meant to house a live audience. However, by removing the fans from the venues, a different form of audiovisual spectacle was born, and thus these landscapes served as a literal and figurative *amplification* of a pedagogy of brutality for fans watching at home. While UFC fights often feature blood, clearly broken limbs, and nearly disfigured faces, the experience of seeing and *hearing* this without a live crowd cheering in these spaces made the images more visceral. Moreover, owing to these uniquely deployed fan-less sporting spaces (UFC APEX), the outcomes themselves may have been altered as athletes became attuned to sensory information that is typically not available in the arena full of spectators. For example, fighters could better focus on their coaches' instructions during rounds and even the commentators' feedback, and then alter their strategy and technique accordingly, which heretofore was not possible in a venue filled to capacity with a boisterous crowd.

Viewing the carnage also felt more intimate via auditory stimuli that were seldom heard because of the lack of spectators. The roar of the crowd adds to the collective emotion of viewing the fights, but it also importantly masks the brutality, the almost visceral sound of flesh being rearranged, bones broken and joints dislodged. In this sense, the fans viewing at home, removed from the geographical space yet for the first time witness to particular sensory forms of violence, are forced to experience the consequences of hearing the pounded flesh, of viewing fighters hearing their flesh pounded, and of their bodies "cared for" by a raging kingpin touting his ability to open up sport again safely for the good of the country. In the end, these Covid combative landscapes still house fighters who, win or lose, are ultimately the disposable, bipedal equivalents of Covid test nasal swabs. A negative test means the opportunity to step into the cage with the promise of damage and sometimes not much else, while a positive test means no financial gain and excommunication from the now tainted spaces occupied by the virus.

These landscapes, then, are made safe *from* COVID-19 and made safe *for* violent combat sport, the fights to be consumed not live but solely as mediated spectacle. Meanwhile, the senses, some numbed from COVID-19 (e.g., taste), others amplified due to the lack of crowd noise. From a viewer's perspective, it was like watching a play, not a sporting event, the violence almost out of place without cheers of the spectators. All of this begs the question of who were these fighters sacrificing their bodies for, and whose country were they opening back up?

Eichberg and COVID-19 Sporting Spaces

Another interesting aspect of the social, political, and geographical meanings of Fight Island and UFC APEX involves the question of the implications of their creation to our collective sporting ontological compass. German scholar Henning Eichberg (1998) argued that it was not the need to enhance our timing capabilities that led to the creation of the stopwatch. Rather, it was the creation of this technological device that led to our preoccupation and eventual obsession with time increments that, in everyday life, have far less if any meaning. Similarly, we argue that it was not the pandemic that prompted the creation of the UFC APEX in particular. Rather, the creation of the UFC APEX center prompted Dana White and the UFC to assure themselves that they could put on events in their imperfect bubbled spaces, thus paving the way for the eventual creation and launch of Fight Island.

In his original (1998) notion of the body cultural trialectic, Eichberg noted the relationship between three types of sporting and exercise spaces. The recreational/hygienic space was meant for fitness and recreation, and thus necessitated the creation of newly constructed sporting facilities. The experiential space related to spaces where the running or jumping or moving corporeal self could engage in non-competitive play, by one's self or with others, which occurred in open public areas, whether in the streets (parkour) or parks (games of tag, etc.). Finally, the achievement space was directly tied to performance standards and improvement of existing records or standards, something that necessitated high-tech stadiums that facilitated these efforts and yielded the desired output. The COVID-19 pandemic brought about, for the UFC and other sports, a new space that intersected with the achievement space, which not only related to high-performance sport but also supposedly safe, COVID-19-free spaces within which to, in the case of the UFC, conduct violent contests removed from the larger harmful environment of the "contaminated" exterior setting. Within the trialectic, "elements of play and sensuousness may creep into serious sport; likewise, serious sport may be incorporated into hygienist or welfare body culture (as in physical education) (Bale, 1994, p. 5). However while the work of Eichberg and Bale often centers on the ways that sporting spaces are constructed to discipline its inhabitants, in the case of Fight Island and UFC APEX, the purpose was less to discipline than to liberate athletes from "oppressive" COVID-19 restrictions (thus allowing them to compete), and to protect them from the (often publicly dismissed) dangers of contracting COVID-19 by taking over tight control of event safety protocols (under the auspices of protecting them).

So the question here is that during the pandemic, what sorts of body cultures were born of the pandemic, what bodies do these cultures spawn, and what landscapes follow? As Bale (1994) notes, sporting bodies are not the result of some naturally occurring desire to compete or discipline the body. Rather, "the landscape upon which such body culture takes place is thereby generally regarded as part of the cultural landscape…" (p. 9). In other words, the cultural moment of a global pandemic, for the UFC, prompted a full-on mission to "bring sport back" under Trump's directive, and this yielded, and in fact necessitated, the creation of new spaces after existing venues were no longer an option, whether due to political pressure or other reasons. In this way, the creation of Fight Island was not only born of the pandemic, but of a desire by the UFC and its Trump associate Dana White to create a brick and mortar manifestation of White's infamous 2020 statement, "I don't give a shit about coronavirus," by doubling-down on his stance to single handedly take on the Coronavirus and all of its mutations. Indeed, White stated in the South China Morning Post that, "[We are] through what I'm hoping was the worst of the worst, we cruised right through it," giving himself a pat on the back for guiding the UFC through the earlier phases of the pandemic. "I'm not worried about any of that stuff. I could care less [about the Omicron variant]" (Taylor, 2021, p. 1).

These sporting spaces, then, also produce meaning; meaning politically and economically, meaning of the narrative of opportunity that obscures that risk and arguably exploitative nature of the UFC and perhaps more broadly MMA. The spaces produce pride in not only White, but Trump and a segment of the populace that saw Dr. Anthony Fauci as the enemy and masks as the mark of compliance and blind obedience.

Conclusions

In this chapter, we highlighted the ways that the UFC, and specifically Dana White, took a play out of former US President and ally Donald Trump's playbook in an effort to become the first major sports league to hold live events during the COVID-19 pandemic. We showed the similarities between Trump and White, including their use of harsh and dismissive rhetoric regarding the pandemic, their combative relationship with many media sources, and their attempts to frame their versions of reality in a variety of ways. We also examined, drawing from the work of Bale (1994, 2003) and Eichberg (1998), as well as Andrews (2019), how the creation of the two Venues, UFC APEX and Fight Island, were not simply sporting spaces within which to hold events devoid of fans and, hypothetically, the virus itself.

As Newman et al. (2020) note, "A materialist approach to the analysis of physical culture thus looks to the explicit articulations of the physical (material, physics) and the cultural (political, systems of meaning) within and from active embodiment" (p. 5). In this case the multidimensional relationships between fighter bodies and combat spaces, and the cultural and political forces that imbued both with meaning, conflict, infection and indoctrination, tell a story of Trumpism's impact on uber-sport and the discourses surrounding it (Andrews, 2019).

Spaces built to host events filled with bodies that themselves at times became host to COVID-19, a biological calculus made by fighters seeking to move up the rankings, some stepping in to fight in the UFC for the first time as fighter after fighter had to withdraw due to a positive COVID-19 test or coming into contact with someone (such as their coaches or corner support), who had. Stepping in at a moment's notice became a litmus test for White, and like Trump loyalty was rewarded superficially, and often temporarily. Similarly, Dana White's rhetoric and bombastic persona throughout his tenure as the president of the UFC, and especially during the beginning of the pandemic, are also indivisible from the politicized symbolism of Trumpism that Fight Island the APEX came to represent. While the explicitly racialized elements of Trumpism were most often left to fighters-as-surrogates like Trump supporter Colby Covington and others, White's Trump-infused messages related to the "bringing sport back" rhetoric are ultimately and intimately connected with the ability of these two sporting landscapes to house events that were not merely sporting spectacles, but representations of Trumpism fit for UFC fan consumption.

Andrews (2019) further notes that uber-sport's "generative entanglements with Trumpism" (p. 140) also have ties to the (at the time) proposed return of World Wrestling Entertainment chairman, Vince McMahon's XFL football league that was to, on some level, characterized by Trump's sport-related political rhetoric. While the league did not materialize, we argue that in some key ways the UFC and Dana White became not just a "sporting excrescence of his [Trump's] authoritarian populism," (p. 140) but an even more refined, audacious version of it. Indeed, in late December of 2021, in the same timeframe that the former president was being booed at a speaking event in Texas for admitting that he had received a vaccine booster shot (Paybarah & McCarthy, 2021), White seemed to actually not just take on the Trumpian mantle, but amplify its magnitude. Combined with his ongoing public rhetoric surrounding the controversial topic of UFC fighter pay, and his consultation with UFC announcer and highly influential podcaster Joe Rogan following his own bout with COVID-19, which included promoting and distributing information about nonapproved treatment regimens for bodies that have contracted the virus, further work will be needed to examine how the the UFC's Trumpian mode of operation intersects with the larger geography of MMA, and the bodies that perform within it.

In the end, Fight Island and UFC APEX facilities-which ultimately became less bubble than incubator-also illustrate White's efforts to use his political clout and near-unilateral organizational control to circumvent policies and procedures meant to keep the virus from spreading among fighters and other stakeholders. Control the modes of production, policies, performance, the bodies, the mediated narratives, and thus "truth" itself. All of this is set against the backdrop of Trumpism's totalitarian tendencies.

In the UFC, the meaning of bodies fighting in these newly created COVID-19-era spaces was always and already fraught with political conflict, and the desire to show White as a Trumpian *bro* willing to put on the show that seemingly had to go on, data be damned. But just as these spaces were meant to keep out the almost immediately politicized virus, Fight Island and UFC APEX signified and made readily apparent the very political struggles over the bodies involved in the spectacle. The COVID-19-tested combatants, the controlling and regulating of bodies, and the consuming spectators that were witnesses to the (admittedly successful) petri dish that were UFC PPV events during the pandemic. The two sporting spaces were ultimately part of the larger-scale pandemic rage, angry debates, and violent conflict that eventually played out in a different landscape, as the influence of Trumpism on the UFC made its way back from the Octagon to the US Capital.

References

Andrews, D. L. (2019). *Making sport great again: The uber-sport assemblage, neoliberalism, and the Trump conjuncture*. Cham, Switzerland: Palgrave Macmillan.

Bale, J. (1994). *Landscapes of modern sport*. Leicester University Press.

Bale, J. (2003). *Sports geography*. Routledge.

Butryn, T. M., Masucci, M. A., & johnson, j. (2020). The show must go on: The strategy and spectacle of Dana White's efforts to promote UFC 249 during the coronavirus pandemic. *International Journal of Sport Communication, 13*(3), 381–390.

Dachman, J. (2020, November 13). UFC's IP-based, state-of-the-art broadcast-ops center goes live at UFC APEX despite pandemic. *Sports Video Group News*. https://www.sportsvideo.org/2020/11/13/ufcs-ip-based-state-of-the-art-broadcast-ops-center-goes-live-at-ufc-apex-despite-pandemic/

Eichberg, H. (1998). Body culture as paradigm: The Danish sociology of sport. In J. Bale & C. Philo (Eds.), *Body cultures: Essays on sport, space and identity* (pp. 111–127). Routledge.

Gaber, I., & Fisher, C. (2022). "Strategic lying": The case of Brexit and the 2019 U.K. election. *The International Journal of Press/Politics, 27*(2), 460–477.

Kalman-Lamb, N. (2018). *Game misconduct: Injury, fandom, and the business of sport*. Fernwood Publishing.

Lutz, T. (2020, April 15). "We have to get our sports back": Trump says he is sick of watching baseball repeats. *The Guardian*. https://www.theguardian.com/sport/2020/apr/15/donald-trump-sports-reopen-coronavirus-shutdown

MacAloon, J. (1981). *This great symbol: Pierre de Cubertin and the origins of the modern Olympic Games*. University of Chicago Press: Chicago.

Moon, D. S. (2020). Kayfabe, smartdom and marking out: Can pro-wrestling help us understand Donald Trump? *Political Studies Review*. https://doi.org/10.1177/1478929920963827

Morgan, J. (2020, October 19). *A review of "UFC Fight Island: Declassified" from behind the scenes*. mmmjunkie.usatoday.com. https://mmajunkie.usatoday.com/lists/ufc-fight-island-declassified-documentary-reviewespn

Newman, J. I., Thorpe, H., & Andrews, D. L. (2020). Introduction: Sport, physical culture, and new materialisms. In J. I. Newman, H. Thorpe, & D. L. Andrews (Eds.), *Sport, physical culture, and the moving body: Materialisms, technologies, ecologies* (pp. 1–46). Rutgers University Press.

O'Brien, S. B. (2020). *Donald Trump and the Kayfabe presidency: Professional wrestling rhetoric in the White House*. Palgrave Macmillan.
Paybarah, A., & McCarthy, L. (2021, December 20). Donald Trump said he got a booster shot and his supporters booed. https://www.nytimes.com/2021/12/20/world/trump-supporters-booster-shots.html
Proffitt, J. M., Salazar, N. E., Cortese, J., & Merle, P. F. (2021). The rush to return to live sports events: A political-economic analysis of sports entertainment in the time of COVID-19. *The Political Economy of Communication, 9*(1), 22–40.
Singleton, T., & Green, K. (2021). A lot of people did not want this to happen. *Journal of Emerging Sport Studies, 5,* 1–38.
Stonehouse, G. (2020, June 6). UA-GLEE UFC chief Dana White plans to stay on 'Fight Island' for a month as Abu Dhabi is touted as mystery venue. *The Sun, UK.* https://www.thesun.co.uk/sport/11800775/ufc-fight-island-abu-dhabi/
Taylor, T. (2021, December 19). UFC: Dana White 'could care less' about Omicron variant—'I'm not worried about any of that stuff. *South China Morning Post.* https://www.scmp.com/sport/martial-arts/mixed-martial-arts/article/3160302/ufc-dana-white-could-care-less-about-omicron
Wagenheim, J. (2020, June 11). UFC 251—What we know and don't know about 'Fight Island'. ESPN. https://www.espn.com/mma/story/_/id/29294243/ufc-251-know-know-fight-island
Weprin, A. (2021, June 2). Endeavor swings to slim profit thanks to UFC in first earnings report since IPO. *The Hollywood Reporter.* https://www.hollywoodreporter.com/business/business-news/endeavor-earnings-ufc-q1-2021-1234961779/
Zirin, D. (2020, April 17). Trump's sports advisers represent the worst of the sports world. *The Nation.* https://www.thenation.com/article/society/trump-sports-advisory-coronavirus/

27

Corona Games: The Tokyo 2020 Olympics, Celebration Capitalism, and COVID-19

Jules Boykoff

Introduction

When the Tokyo 2020 Olympic bid team stood before voting members of the International Olympic Committee (IOC) in 2013, it faced a formidable hurdle: the triple-whammy catastrophe in Fukushima—an earthquake, tsunami, and nuclear meltdown that occurred in March 2011—was generating skepticism that Japan would be able to host the Games. The meltdown of three reactors at the Fukushima Daiichi nuclear plant released radioactive cesium and iodine-131 isotopes into the atmosphere, some 80 percent of it landing in the nearby Pacific Ocean, with the rest of it causing havoc and death on land (Christoudias & Lelieveld, 2013). To assuage the anxieties of voting IOC members, Japanese Prime Minister Shinzo Abe directly addressed the situation in his pitch: "Some may have concerns about Fukushima," he said. "Let me assure you, the

J. Boykoff (✉)
Pacific University, Forest Grove, OR, USA
e-mail: boykoff@pacificu.edu

D. L. Andrews et al. (eds.), *Sport and Physical Culture in Global Pandemic Times*, Global Culture and Sport Series, https://doi.org/10.1007/978-3-031-14387-8_27

situation is under control. It has never done and will never do any damage to Tokyo." The Tokyo Games would be dubbed the "Recovery Olympics," a nod to using the mega-event to quicken the rhythms of relief for the affected prefectures (Whiteside, 2013).

Back in Japan, people with direct knowledge of the Fukushima environmental disaster lacked Abe's optimism. Marine ecologists and local residents in the Fukushima region unequivocally contradicted the prime minister's claim that radioactive water gushing out of the nuclear plant and into the ocean was being contained (Hobson & Dewit, 2013; Yogeshwar, 2014). A few years later, former Japanese premier Junichiro Koizumi bluntly stated, "Mr. Abe's 'under control' remark was a lie" (Sieg & Lim, 2016).

Even though the Japanese government did not have the Fukushima situation "under control" in 2013, the IOC selected Tokyo over Istanbul and Madrid. IOC President Jacques Rogge—a Belgian yachtsman, orthopedic surgeon, and the eighth leader of the IOC—exalted Tokyo as "a safe pair of hands" (Whiteside, 2013). And yet, despite their "safe pair of hands" billing, Tokyo 2020 Olympic organizers repeatedly fumbled the torch during their preparations for the Games. Organizers vaulted four times over their initial budget, scrapped expensive stadium blueprints from celebrity architect Zaha Hadid, and became embroiled in a plagiarism scandal over its logo design (Martin, 2021). Then, after all that, the coronavirus forced the IOC and local Olympic organizers to postpone the Tokyo 2020 Olympics by a year.

The Covid-induced delay ramified, impacting the preparation, cost, delivery, and, eventually, even the spectator experience of the Tokyo Games. Olympic organizers were forced to scramble in order to secure Games venues for another year. The Olympic Village, where athletes stay during the Games, was to be converted into private housing in the wake of the Olympics; the delay meant sorting out complications with tenants who planned on moving in after the Paralympics. Due to maintenance costs for Olympic facilities and the extension of labor costs, the additional price tag for postponement hovered around $3 billion (Lies, 2021). Countermeasures to address coronavirus—from rapid testing and masks to cleaning supplies and services—ramped up costs. Expected revenues also dried up. When Olympic organizers chose to forbid Olympic visitors from abroad—aside from journalists, the IOC, and its associates—the tourist and hospitalities industries took a hit. Ticket sales—projected to produce $800 million for Tokyo organizers—essentially dwindled to nil. The decision to also ban local spectators meant cavernous Olympic venues for sporting events, casting a cloud of quietude over what is typically a rambunctious, animated atmosphere.

In this chapter, I situate the Tokyo 2020 Olympics in the wider context of critical, academic scholarship on the politics and economics of the Olympic Games in the twenty-first century. To make sense of why the Tokyo 2020 Games transpired amid a global pandemic, I place this first-ever five-ring postponement in the wider frame of modern Olympic history and its predominant funding model rooted in broadcaster cash, corporate sponsorships, and taxpayer money from the host city and country. I dissect the politics of the postponed 2020 Olympics, grounding this analysis in the theory of celebration capitalism. In a way, the Covid-19 virus was tantamount to a massive injection of dye—as used in an imaging exam—into the Olympics in that it revealed in glaring contrast the imperfections not only in the Tokyo 2020 Olympics, but within the Olympic body more generally. I also trace the upsurge in athlete voice that put pressure on Olympic organizers to delay the Games. By scrutinizing a seemingly anomalous Olympics occurring under extraordinary conditions, one can see with sharper clarity the ingrained problems that plague the Games.

Celebration Capitalism

"Today's hypercapitalism transforms all human existence into a network of commercial relations," writes theorist Byung-Chul Han (2021, p. 21). "There is no area of life that can escape commercialization." The Olympics, of course, are no exception. The Games arrive with a power-slate of corporate partners like Alibaba, Coca-Cola, and Visa that pay millions to benefit from the Olympic halo effect. Each Olympic host gathers a gaggle of domestic sponsors as well, with Tokyo 2020 breaking the all-time record, raking in more than $3 billion (Lau, 2021). Other capitalist firms lace deals with individual athletes and national Olympic committees. The

Tokyo 2020 Olympics laid bare the corporate-capitalist pulse that thumps beneath the shimmering scrim of Olympism. With 73% of its revenues derived from television broadcaster fees and another 18% arriving from its corporate partners (IOC, 2020c, p. 6), the IOC was perfectly willing to hold a made-for-TV event, with Tokyo relegated to an expensive sound stage for the group's profitmaking.

Capitalism is a shapeshifter, and the Olympics provide a window into its divergent formations. Capitalism takes different form depending on political context, geography, and tradition. Political economist Geoff Mann (2013) notes, "In reality, there is a range of actually existing capitalisms" playing out simultaneously (p. 6). At times, economic relations take shape along neoliberal lines, yet at other times, they fail to conform to the norms of privatization, deregulation, financialization, and 'letting the market decide.' The Olympics, as a political-economic phenomenon, are less about neoliberalism and more about the machinations of capitalism in general. The host government, drawing on taxpayer funds, plays a lopsided role in paying for and policing the five-ring spectacle, rather than outsourcing these responsibilities to private entities (Boykoff, 2013).

To fully grasp celebration capitalism, one must first comprehend "disaster capitalism." In *The Shock Doctrine: The Rise of Disaster Capitalism* Naomi Klein (2007) elucidates how neoliberal capitalists capitalize on catastrophe. With "the disaster capitalism complex," Klein argues the goal is to exploit social trauma. Disasters—like wars, hurricanes, military *coups d'état*, terrorist violence, and severe economic downturns—spark collective states of shock that can convince residents to give up what they might otherwise ardently defend during normal political times. In the aftermath of disaster, while the general population is reeling, powerful corporations combine with their collaborators in government to orchestrate the institution of neoliberal policies rooted in privatization and deregulation. Klein argues that disaster capitalists manipulate "the disorientation of rapid political change combined with the collective fear generated by an economic meltdown." This leaves the population vulnerable to "the promise of a quick and magical cure—however illusory" (Klein, 2007, p. 181). Free-market proponents opportunistically convert social instability into a political cudgel that they use to weaken the state and install neoliberal policies and principles where they previously did not exist. While Klein notes that privatization can often "be paid for with public money," her primary contention is that "the ultimate goal" of the corporations at the center of disaster capitalism is to normalize the privatization of the public sphere, to convert government responsibilities into corporate functions (Klein, 2007, pp. 14, 15).

Both disaster capitalism and celebration capitalism occur during states of exception: catastrophe and exuberance respectively. And both modes of capitalism allow politicians to circumvent normal democratic processes and advance unprecedented policies. Sport sociologists have long argued the Olympics are an elite-driven affair with scant opportunity for meaningful public participation. Hayes and Horne (2011) assert that civil society has "rarely been factored into the definition of the Games or Games projects. The role of civic organizations and publics is one of implementation and support, not one of definition and decision." (p. 759). A democracy deficit is endemic to both disaster capitalism and celebration capitalism. It also afflicts the Olympics.

In the context of the Olympic Games, celebration capitalism exhibits six essential elements. First, it occurs during a state of celebratory exception where the normal rules of politics can be temporarily suspended. Second, the IOC and mass media combine as a discursive linchpin that creates and trumpets the political-economic spectacle, fomenting the feel-good factor. A third dimension is festive commoditization that rallies public backing for the Games. Fourth, celebration capitalism depends on public-private partnerships that are lopsided in favor of private entities in terms of input and risk: costs are socialized and benefits are privatized. Fifth, celebration capitalism is buoyed by the feel-good claims of environmental and social sustainability, even though accountability and oversight is often weak. Finally, celebration capitalism uplifts the security industry and state policing units responsible for preventing terrorism, corralling political dissent, and safeguarding the festive spectacle. Celebration capitalism exhibits these six central features, but takes distinctive form depending on the political and historical context. These tenets coalesce into a celebratory socio-political space where social critics and athlete activists are unwelcome (Boykoff, 2013).

Anthropologist Anna Lowenhaupt Tsing (2000) has illuminated "the heterogeneity of capitalism at every moment in time." (p. 143). Such simultaneous heterogeneity applies to disaster capitalism and celebration capitalism. Together, these forms of 'actually existing capitalism' can be dialectically productive, harmonizing into a potent combination, with celebration capitalism clearing a path for disaster capitalism, and vice versa. In short, they can make for a powerful one-two punch. With the evisceration of public services that disaster capitalism wreaks, the population becomes vulnerable to promises of massive social celebration that will ostensibly bring joy to all. With the Tokyo 2020 Summer Olympics, an unprecedented synergy existed between disaster capitalism and celebration capitalism, whereby nationalism, hyper-consumerism, and disaster recovery were fused and refashioned into a powerful political-economic spectacle fueled by feel-good Olympic ideology amid a volatile historical conjuncture (Boykoff & Gaffney, 2020).

Olympic-Sized Problems and the Tokyo 2020 Games

Academic research has illuminated four negative externalities consistently associated with hosting the Olympics: (1) overspending, (2) militarization of the public sphere, (3) forced eviction and gentrification, and (4) greenwashing. These intertwined externalities emerge from the machinations of celebration capitalism, which simultaneously grants Olympic organizers happy-faced, socio-political cover. On one hand, the Tokyo Olympics appear to be a one-off event: the first-ever postponed Olympics that transpired during a massive global-health pandemic. On the other hand, Tokyo 2020 is a case study in celebration capitalism, replete with previously identified, socially deleterious patterns. What follows is an explication of how these patterns entwine in the Tokyo context.

The Tokyo Olympics were originally slated to cost \$7.3 billion, but the official price tag more than doubled to \$15.4 billion. According to a government audit in Japan, however, the actual cost was more like \$26 billion, with all but \$6.7 billion furnished by taxpayers. Postponement added billions more, bringing the total to around \$30 billion (Demsas, 2021). These jaw-dropping cost overruns—well over 200%—not only exceed the historical average for Olympic overspending, but make Tokyo 2020 the most expensive Summer Games to date (Wade, 2020). The "safe pair of hands" ended up being extraordinarily expensive hands, too.

Tokyo 2020 created space for local developers to leverage the Olympic state of exception to relax longtime height restrictions on building in the neighborhood around the National Stadium. In 1970 city officials in Tokyo instituted a 15-meter height limit, in part in so as not to build higher than Meiji-era imperial structures. However, in 2013, to accommodate the new National Stadium design, the height restriction was erased and replaced with an 80-meter limit in the stadium's vicinity (Inagaki, 2019). This regulation, made possible by the Olympics, pried open urban terrain for well-positioned developers. Celebration capitalism trumped imperial tradition.

Tokyo 2020s enormous price tag is symbolized by the organizers' decision to hire celebrity architect Zaha Hadid to design a sleek stadium with costs that escalated to around $2 billion. As public pressure mounted, Hadid downgraded her design's complexity. When negotiations with a domestic construction partner stalled, Japanese architect Kengo Kuma swooped in with blueprints that cost less than half of Hadid's (Rogers, 2016). Meanwhile, the US-based NGO Rainforest Action Network detailed how Korindo, a Tokyo 2020 wood supplier, engaged in unsustainable practices and illegal behavior stoking forest destruction in Indonesia. Wood used to build numerous Olympic venues was unethically sourced (RAN, 2019). In March 2020, eight environmental NGOs spanning the globe issued a joint statement slamming Tokyo 2020 organizers for "fake sustainability." They asserted, "Tokyo 2020s use of large quantities of tropical plywood linked to rainforest destruction for construction of the Olympic venues was a clear violation of its commitment to sustainability" (RAN, 2020).

These damning proclamations link to greenwashing: the public display of concern for the environment and the propensity to claim credit for providing solutions while in actuality doing the bare minimum, if anything, to make material ecological improvements. Beginning in the 1990s, Olympic leaders in Lausanne, Switzerland enfolded environmental rhetoric into their language and plans. Paying rhetorical attention to ecological concerns emerged as a way to both embrace the global zeitgeist of environmentalism and to anesthetize the public to the deleterious impacts of the Olympics (Boykoff & Gaffney, 2020).

One longitudinal assessment of Olympic sustainability at sixteen installations of the Summer and Winter Olympic Games spanning 1992 through 2020 found follow-through wanting (Müller et al., 2021). Researchers broadened the discussion of sustainability to include three axes: ecological, social, and economic. Overall, they found that the Olympic Games achieve "medium" sustainability marks, earning 48 out of 100 points on the nine-indicator scale they construct. More specifically, the ecological dimension averages 44 points while the mean for social and economic sustainability are 51 and 47 respectively. The researchers found that the 2002 Salt Lake City Winter Games were the most sustainable during the time period under study. On the other hand, the least sustainable Olympics were quite recent—the 2014 Sochi Winter Olympics and the 2016 Summer Games in Rio de Janeiro—with the Tokyo 2020 Games ranked third lowest, pointing up the reality that the Olympics have not improved their sustainability performance over time.

This brings us back to Fukushima. While Olympic boosters hoisted the "Recovery Olympics" mantra into the mediasphere, the situation in Fukushima remained grim. In July 2019, I traveled with a group of academics, journalists, and activists to Fukushima. We were accompanied by scientist and professor Fujita Yasumoto who carried a hand-held dosimeter, a device that measures external ionizing radiation levels. As we navigated through Fukushima Prefecture, the dosimeter readings elevated, eventually reaching an apex at the TEPCO decommissioning archive center and museum where radiation levels were eighteen times higher than the recommended standard.

As we traveled through the affected region, we passed roads barricaded by gates and guarded by police. These were the "difficult to return zones" where radioactivity was so high that the federal government has prevented residents' return. Even the fact that the Abe government had raised the allowable standard for exposure to radioactivity from the international benchmark of 1 milisilvert (mSv) annually to 20 mSv did not qualify the area as safe for return. People who reside in the area absorb well over the legal limit. *Scientific American* concluded, "Abe's determination to put the Daiichi accident behind the nation is jeopardizing public health, especially among children, who are more susceptible" (Little, 2019). The Tokyo Olympics incentivized a rushed process to return residents to Fukushima, regardless of public-health perils for the local population. Satoko Itani, a professor of sport, gender and sexuality studies at Kansai University, called the "Recovery Olympics" tagline ironic since "the money and human resources they are spending in Tokyo could help people who survived the 2011 disaster and make communities more resilient to future catastrophes." Instead, Itani noted, "this Olympics is literally taking the money, workers, and cranes away from the areas where they are needed most" (Boykoff & Zirin, 2019).

Across Fukushima Prefecture, we saw thousands of large plastic bags that were piled into what locals dubbed "black pyramids"—enormous stacks of plastic bags containing radioactive topsoil in various stages of decontamination. Many of the bags were ripped from seedlings sprouting through the plastic. The wind lifted contaminants into the air. When a typhoon struck Japan in October 2019, some of the bags from the black pyramids reportedly washed into nearby rivers (Kotegawa, 2019).

In this context, Fukushima can be viewed as a "sacrifice zone," a term that emerged during the Cold War to denote space made unlivable by nuclear fallout (Holifield & Day, 2017). Fukushima can be read as a modern-day capitalist sacrifice zone, and one that was pressed unwillingly into the service of Olympic spectacle.

While Fukushima residents were being encouraged to return to potentially unsafe spaces, the Olympics also displaced residents in Tokyo from communities they adored. The aforementioned change in zoning laws cleared a political path for the elimination of public housing units. More specifically, residents from the Kasumigaoka apartment complex, which sat in the shadow of the new Olympic Stadium, were forced from their public housing and relocated into different communities across the metropolis. Of the 370 residents who were evicted, 60% were over 65 years old and many were widows in their 80s and 90s. Remarkably, two women and a man who lost their homes in Kasumigaoka were also displaced by the 1964 Tokyo Olympics. Meanwhile, the Japanese Olympic Committee built a glassy tower nearby and developers constructed high-end high-rise apartment buildings, benefiting from the new zoning codes.

The Olympics helped Tokyo's developers, landlords, and gentrifiers, not the city's poor and elderly (Zirin & Boykoff, 2019).

Another beneficiary of the Olympics is the security and surveillance industry. The Tokyo Olympics reportedly brought facial recognition systems to every Olympic venue (although some media reports suggested its use was dialed back after overseas spectators were banned from attending the Games). Various levels of government in Japan have long collaborated with technology companies to develop artificial-intelligence-driven securitization measures through public-private partnerships. The Tokyo Metropolitan Police already used biometric surveillance technologies. However, the Tokyo Olympics promised to be the first-ever application of large-scale security that is firmly rooted in artificial-intelligence technologies. ALSOK, Japan's largest private security firm, prepared a fleet of robots to surveil the Games, to patrol crowds, and to deploy an "emotional visualization system" designed to sniff out "jitters" from Olympics-goers. ALSOK was born out of the 1964 Olympics, but positioned itself to cash in at the 2020 Games. It coordinated its efforts with more than a dozen private-security firms (Friedman, 2019; Synced, 2019).

The Tokyo 2020 Games raised serious civil-liberties concerns, spotlighting the Olympics-induced democracy deficit. In 2017, Japanese legislators rammed anti-terrorism legislation through parliament, justifying the rushed nature of its passage by asserting the need to securitize the Olympics. The legislation added hundreds of new crimes to Japanese law, including specific offenses like sit-ins to oppose the construction of new apartment buildings. The UN special rapporteur on the right to privacy said Japan's government had used fear to push through "defective" legislation (McCurry, 2017). Such legislation and the biometric technologies it enabled nudged Japan down a surveillance-state slippery slope. During the Olympics, protests were heavily policed. For instance, activists who wanted to protest on the sidewalk outside the five-star hotel where IOC members stayed during the Games were forced away from the area by security officials, with coronavirus a convenient justification.

As mentioned above, the mass media function as a key component of celebration capitalism, as they heighten public interest in the sport spectacle and rally the feel-good commoditization that is nestled at the core of the Games' political-economic model. Tokyo 2020 benefited tremendously from Dentsu, the mass-media-connected marketing behemoth that rallied a record amount of local corporate sponsorship funding—including from some Japanese media outlets—in its capacity as the exclusive marketing agency for the Tokyo Games (Wade, 2019a). Many firms even signed non-exclusivity contracts, which means that in some cases they were paying exorbitant sponsorship fees only to share marketing space with a rival firm. In a *Financial Times* article titled "Olympic Sponsorship: Japan Inc Pressed into National Service," it was clear that Dentsu was doing the pressing. After all, the company commands approximately one quarter of Japan's domestic advertising market. Using patriotism as a cudgel, and by insinuating that firms that didn't contribute might not be eligible to receive prized Olympic contracts, Dentsu lined up corporate sponsors at a record clip. One marketing director of an official Tokyo 2020 sponsor said, "It was basically a no-option choice that a company of our stature had to do its duty to Japan. Our biggest rival was probably going to do it as well. There was no way we wanted to be left out" (Lewis et al., 2019).

Dentsu's influence expands far beyond marketing circles. According to Japan-based scholar David McNeill (2020), Dentsu plays an "outsized role in molding not just domestic news and popular culture, but also public perceptions of Japan's ruling party." (p. 2). That ruling party, Shinzo Abe's Liberal Democratic Party, was instrumental in securing the 2020 Games for Tokyo. Six Japanese newspapers were Tokyo 2020 sponsors: *Asahi*, *Hokkaido Shimbun Press*, *Mainichi*, *Nikkei*, *Sankei*, and *Yomiuri*. With all these factors pressing in the same pro-Olympics direction, McNeill (2020) asks, "How much faith can be placed in the media's watchdog role, given that all the major media groups are official Olympic sponsors, as are most of the big companies that advertise in those media?" (p. 3). To be sure, Olympic sponsor *Asahi Shimbun* ran an editorial ahead of the Olympics asserting the Games should not transpire because of Covid-19, but by and large, the media remained compliant, if by focusing on sports and not the wider socio-political or biopolitical contexts. In 2019, Dentsu became embroiled in a case brought by French prosecutors alleging vote-buying linked to Tokyo being named the host for the 2020 Olympics. The firm has firm connections to the major players involved in the alleged scheme. The case is wending its way through the French legal system (Wade, 2019b).

The Tokyo 2020 Olympics are a paradigmatic case of celebration capitalism in action, with an additional sprinkling of rhetorical disaster capitalism—through the "recovery Games" public relations-speak around the Fukushima Daiichi nuclear meltdown—worked in for good measure. Lopsided public-private partnerships abounded, as did intensified securitization, a mass media system proliferating the sporting spectacle, and weak claims of environmental sustainability. The Olympic state of exception became a crowbar for corporate power to pry open access to ever-larger profits on the urban terrain. Although these dynamics unfolded in Tokyo, they flowed from entrenched Olympic problems arise in host city after host city in various measure. The Olympic downsides are systemic, even if they do not play out in systematically identical ways with each Olympic host. Covid-19 wedged open discursive space to discuss these critical issues, even during the actual Games.

Coronavirus: State of Emergency and State of Exception

In March 2020, after first asserting that its Executive Board was not even considering "postponement"—let alone cancellation—of the Tokyo 2020 Olympics, the IOC finally faced up to epidemiological reality and announced it would "take the next step in its scenario-planning." Within hours of pronouncing this wiggle room, the Canadian Olympic and Paralympic Committee issued an official statement that it would not send its athletes to the Tokyo Olympics were they staged in summer 2020. This de facto boycott was bold, and soon afterwards, the Australian Olympic Committee followed their lead, notifying its athletes to prepare for a 12-month postponement. The national Olympic committees from Portugal and Germany also followed suit (Zirin & Boykoff, 2020).

These collective declarations followed a groundswell of dissatisfaction from individual Olympic athletes, coaches, and administrators from around the world. USA Track and Field and USA Swimming both demanded postponement. US Olympic track legends Ashton Eaton and Dick Fosbury advocated for postponement on social media, as did US swimmers Nathan Adrian and Jacob Pebley. They were joined by Kaori Yamaguchi of the Japanese Olympic Committee, Spain Olympic Committee President Alejandro Blanco, Irish Olympian Sonia O'Sullivan, India badminton coach Pullela Gopichand, four-time Olympian and CEO of Sport Ireland John Treacy, Norway's National Olympic & Paralympic Committee, Brazil's Olympic Committee, the Slovenian Olympic Committee, and others (Zirin & Boykoff, 2020).

IOC President Thomas Bach was forced to take notice. Although the IOC initially stated it would take four weeks to study the issue, it ended up taking action less than twenty-four hours later. A joint statement by Bach and Prime Minister Shinzo Abe read, "The Games of the XXXII Olympiad in Tokyo must be rescheduled to a date beyond 2020 but not later than summer 2021, to safeguard the health of the athletes, everybody involved in the Olympic Games and the international community" (IOC, 2020a). It must be emphasized that this would not have happened on the same swift timeline were it not for athletes and sports bodies standing up for global public health and athlete safety. After all, earlier in the month, when Bach was asked why he was not taking decisive action to postpone or cancel the Tokyo Olympics, he replied that he was listening to the likes of US President Donald Trump who was assuring the world that coronavirus was a mere epidemiological blip that would pass off the public-health radar by the end of April 2020 (Dunbar, 2020).

When it came to controlling Olympic athletes, the IOC held a key card in its back pocket: a rule in the Olympic Charter that banned political dissent at the Games. Rule 50 of the Olympic Charter states, "No kind of demonstration or political, religious or racial propaganda is permitted in any Olympic sites, venues or other areas" (IOC, 2020b, p. 90). The rule took its current shape a few years after the 1968 Olympics when John Carlos and Tommie Smith famously fired their fists skyward during the national anthem to stand up for Black pride and human rights while Australian sprinter Peter Norman stood by in solidarity wearing an Olympic Project for Human Rights button.

In July 2021, the IOC released new guidelines that simultaneously opened up possibilities for Olympians to "express their views" while also placing limitations on such expression. The new policy allowed Olympians to express themselves "on the field of play prior to the start of competition" as long as their act was "not disruptive" and did not target specific individuals, countries, organizations or "their dignity." Athletes were still prohibited from free expression while on the medal stand, during the opening and closing ceremonies, in the Olympic Village (where athletes reside during the Games), and on the field of play during competition (IOC, 2021). Many Olympics mavens read this shift as a response to a move made by the US Olympic and Paralympic Committee (USOPC) in December 2020 when it announced that it would not sanction US Olympic athletes who protest "peacefully and respectfully…in support of racial and social justice for all human beings" (USOPC, 2020). Being a major power in the Olympic sphere, the USOPC move put pressure on the IOC to reconsider Rule 50.

After first managing the coronavirus with relative success, Japan eventually experienced a serious uptick in Covid infections. By April 2021, less than one hundred days before the Tokyo 2020 opening ceremony, Covid-19 cases were rising across Japan in roughly equal measure with the public anger that the Games were being staged amid a serious public-health crisis. "Cancelling Olympics" trended on Japanese Twitter. Polls consistently found strong majorities—over 70%—opposing the Games. Some elected officials began opening the door to cancelation, although Tokyo organizers remained steadfast that the Games would go on, even claiming that the Olympics were "a beacon of hope to the world" and "the light at the end of the tunnel" (Zirin & Boykoff, 2021a). Again, the Olympics adopted an anti-democratic stance, foisting the Games on a largely unwilling population.

Meanwhile, public-health experts sounded the alarm. Japan had some of the lowest vaccination rates in the Global North. One essay that appeared in the academic journal *The BMJ* argued, "Plans to hold the Olympic and Paralympic games this summer must be reconsidered as a matter of urgency. The whole global community recognizes the need to contain the pandemic and save lives. Holding Tokyo 2020 for domestic political and economic purposes—ignoring scientific and moral imperatives—is contradictory to Japan's commitment to global health and human security" (Shimizu et al., 2021). An editorial in the *New England*

Journal of Medicine excoriated Olympic officials for failing to adopt best scientific practices when it came to protecting Olympic participants (Sparrow et al., 2021).

The Japanese national government issued a state of emergency order in early April 2020 to try to corral the crisis. Nevertheless, new infections continued to surge. The government issued a second state of emergency in January 2021 and a third in April 2021. The state of emergency was extended, and was in place during the actual Olympics and beyond. Satoko Itani, the professor from Kansai University in Japan, said, "It is very difficult not to realize that the effort to control the Covid-19 infection in Japan has been severely compromised or sacrificed because of the Olympics. People also realize that there are seemingly endless resources available when it comes to hosting the Olympics, but very few to save people's lives and livelihoods here in Japan" (Zirin & Boykoff, 2021a).

The Olympics brought the nightmare scenario that so many medical professionals both predicted and feared: skyrocketing coronavirus rates and hospitals stretched to the brink. IOC President Thomas Bach made the quizzical assertion that the Olympics posed "zero" risk of spreading coronavirus in Japan (Slodkowski & Park, 2021). However, during the Games, grim records were set regularly for the number of new coronavirus cases. Even inside the so-called 'Olympic bubble', more than 500 infections were detected (Rich, 2021). Including the Paralympics that followed, well over 800 people tested positive for Covid inside the Olympic zone.

In a sense, two dialectically productive dynamics sat beneath the whirling churn out of news from Tokyo: an Olympics-induced state of exception and a coronavirus-driven state of emergency. Democratic practice was battered by the Games. Japan's Prime Minister, Yoshihide Suga, was rendered powerless by a lopsided host-city contract signed with the IOC well before he arrived in office that gave the Lausanne-based body the unilateral power to cancel the Games. Japan's prime minister was reduced to a contractual supplicant, placing a spotlight on the Olympic state of exception. John Coates, the IOC VP who doubled as the head of the Tokyo 2020 coordination commission said the Olympics would transpire even if Tokyo were under a state-of-emergency order and local medical professionals recommended against staging the Games. In the end, he was correct (Boykoff, 2021).

There were moments when the implicit interplay between the state of emergency and state of exception reared its head. Upon arrival in Japan, IOC president Thomas Bach only quarantined for three days (Rowbottom, 2021). Meanwhile, journalists arriving from abroad were forced to quarantine for 14 days. One *National Public Radio* journalist described strictures this way: "We can sign out of the hotel for a maximum of 15 minutes, but longer could mean we are expelled from the country, and an app on our phones is tracking our every move to make sure we don't break quarantine" (Kennedy, 2021). In contrast, after the Games, while the rest of the country was told to only take necessary excursions, the IOC President was spotted strolling through the posh Ginza area of Tokyo, along with a team of bodyguards ("IOC's Bach,", 2021). Olympic athletes who carried out similar sightseeing escapades faced expulsion from the country ("Bach's Walk,", 2021).

Amid the state of emergency, the International Olympic Committee and local organizers maintained that they were "putting athletes first," as the slogan goes. Yet, Olympic historian David Wallechinsky told the *New York Times*, "The athletes, they're not the priority. Television is the priority," in reference to the fact that holding the Tokyo Olympics in the summer months is advantageous to NBC—which, by some estimates, accounts for 40% of all IOC revenue (Branch, 2021). Olympians, too, saw through the IOC public-relations lingo. US Olympic fencer Race Imboden (2021) wrote in the *Guardian* after the Games, "The IOC adhered to their usual gameplan; as long as everything looks fine to the outside world and no one is complaining publicly, then let's just move along."

Imboden also challenged the IOC's Rule 50. When he stepped to the podium to accept his silver medal, a large X scrawled in a black pen adorned his right hand. In addition, Raven Saunders, the US shot putter who won a silver medal in Tokyo, crossed her arms in the form of an X while she stood on the medal stand. This epic gesture of dissent symbolized, she explained, "the intersection of where all people who are oppressed meet." Saunders added, embracing her role-model status as a member of the LGBTQ community, "For me, just being who I always aspired to be, to be able to be me and not apologize for it [and] show the younger generation that no matter what they tell you, no matter how many boxes they try to fit you in, you can be you." Other athletes also flouted Rule 50. Chinese cyclists Bao Shanju and Zhong Tianshi donned pins featuring Chairman Mao while receiving their gold medals. Hong Kong Olympic badminton athlete Angus Ng Ka-long wore a black T-shirt during competition with the words "Hong Kong, China" on it, instead of the official jersey worn by his teammates; black T-shirts are often linked to the pro-democracy movement in China (Zirin & Boykoff, 2021b).

In the immediate wake of the Tokyo Games, the *New York Times* asserted that the Tokyo Olympics "were often claustrophobic, cut off from society, with capacious venues Tokyo repurposed into cloistered safe houses." The Games were "paradoxical, uncanny and hard to wholly comprehend" (Keh, 2021). Yet, through the double-lens of celebration capitalism and disaster capitalism, the Tokyo Olympics make perfect sense. The coronavirus disaster combined with the media-trumpeted Olympic celebration, shunted public funds into private coffers. Corporate profit spigots remained open, even in the face of a grim surge of Covid-19 that engulfed the host city, the wider country, and even, to a certain extent, the 'Olympic bubble.' Even though the Tokyo Games scored low television audience—NBC received the lowest television ratings for NBC since the 1988 Olympics, while in the UK, the BBC's Olympic audience was lower than the three previous Summer Games—the IOC received its broadcaster fees and the Olympic juggernaut rolled on (Dixon, 2021).

The Olympics, and capitalism more generally, produce what Angela Davis (2016, 107) calls "surplus populations" or "disposable populations," which, Davis argues, are comprised largely of "people of color and immigrant populations from the countries of the Global South." These "surplus populations" are routinely gobbled up and spit out by Olympics-induced celebration capitalism, whether through misdirected tax money that goes to Games rather than homes, or through the brass-knuckle processes of displacement and gentrification. "Disposable populations" crop up in the Global North as well, of course, including in Japan where people who stood up in public against the Games were intensely policed with the weapons and special powers that security forces obtained during the extended Tokyo 2020 Olympic moment.

These surplus populations—from London to Rio de Janeiro to Tokyo—are vulnerable to the maneuverings of plenipotentiaries, corporations, and sport bodies pursuing the goal of generating capital and squeezing profits from the populace. Celebration capitalism, through its mobilization of the media, creates a potent social elixir with a brutal side effect: the marginalization and in some cases even the immiseration of the poor and working class in the Olympic city. In other words, the Olympics—through the tenets of celebration capitalism—generate negative externalities that contribute to what Rob Nixon (2011, 2) calls "slow violence," or "a violence that occurs gradually and out of sight, a violence of delayed destruction that is dispersed across time and space, an attritional violence that is typically not viewed as violence at all." Such "slow violence" has galvanized scalding criticism of the Olympics in cities around the world, increasingly bringing the Games' negative externalities into public view. Tokyo 2020, staged under the shadow of the coronavirus, only amplified such criticism of the Olympics.

References

Bach's Walk around Tokyo Symbolizes Olympics' Shameless 'IOC-first' Mentality. (2021, August 13). *The Mainichi*. https://mainichi.jp/english/articles/20210813/p2a/00m/0op/038000c

Boykoff, J. (2013). *Celebration Capitalism and the Olympic Games*. Routledge.

Boykoff, J. (2021, May 27). Tokyo Is Learning that the Only Force Stronger than a Pandemic is the Olympics. *Washington Post*. https://www.washingtonpost.com/outlook/2021/05/27/tokyo-olympics-pandemic-crisis/

Boykoff, J., & Gaffney, C. (2020). Tokyo 2020 and the End of Olympic History. *Capitalism Nature Socialism, 31*(2), 1–19.

Boykoff, J. & Zirin, D. (2019, July 23). Tokyo's 2020 Olympics are Showing the Nightmare Waiting for L.A. in 2028. *Los Angeles Times*. https://www.latimes.com/opinion/story/2019-07-23/anti-olympic-2028-summit-japan-los-angeles

Branch, J. (2021, July 17). Let the Games…Be Gone? *New York Times*. https://www.nytimes.com/2021/07/17/sports/olympics/tokyo-olympics.html

Christoudias, T., & Lelieveld, J. (2013). Modelling the Global Atmospheric Transport and Deposition of Radionuclides from the Fukushima Dai-ichi Nuclear Accident. *Atmospheric Chemistry and Physics, 13*, 1425–1438.

Demsas, J. (2021, August 1). Hosting the Olympics Comes at a Massive Cost. *Vox*. https://www.vox.com/22599732/olympics-tokyo-2020-summer

Dixon, E. (2021, August 11). NBC's Tokyo 2020 Audience Lowest Since 1988 Olympics. *Sports Pro Media*. https://www.sportspromedia.com/news/tokyo-2020-olympics-nbc-bbc-tv-ratings-audience-peacock-streaming

Dunbar, G. (2020, March 25). Bach Invokes Trump in Defense of Olympic Decision. *AP*. https://apnews.com/article/sports-europe-donald-trump-olympic-games-tokyo-sports-general-9b18f727a72990e735dd0b2a4b59da02

Friedman, S. (2019, August 13). The Olympics Are Coming to Tokyo, and So Is the Movement to Kill the Games Forever. *Deadspin*. https://deadspin.com/the-olympics-are-coming-to-tokyo-and-so-is-the-movemen-1837203511

Han, B.-C. (2021). *Capitalism and the Death Drive*. Polity Press.

Hayes, G., & Horne, J. (2011). Sustainable Development, Shock and Awe?: London 2012 and Civil Society. *Sociology, 45*(5), 749–764.

Hobson, C., & Dewit, A. (2013). The Lid Comes Off Fukushima Daiichi, 'Japan's Ground Zero': The Devastating Consequences of Government Inaction. *The Asia-Pacific Journal, 11*(1), 1–15.

Holifield, R., & Day, M. (2017). A Framework for a Critical Physical Geography of 'Sacrifice Zones': Physical Landscapes and Discursive Spaces of Frac Sand Mining in Western Wisconsin. *Geoforum, 85*, 269–279.

Imboden, R. (2021, August 12). The Olympics Proved the IOC Will Do Anything to Save Face. *Guardian*. https://www.theguardian.com/sport/2021/aug/12/race-imboden-tokyo-olympics-ioc-covid

Inagaki, K. (2019, July 25). 聖火は照らす TOKYO2020)第4部:1 神宮外苑、高層化なし崩し (Torch Illuminates Tokyo 2020: Part 4, Jingu Gaien, No Rise in Height). *Asahi Shimbun*. https://www.asahi.com/articles/DA3S14112168.html

International Olympic Committee. (2020a, March 24). Joint Statement from the International Olympic Committee and the Tokyo 2020 Organising Committee. https://olympics.com/ioc/news/joint-statement-from-the-international-olympic-committee-and-the-tokyo-2020-organising-committee

International Olympic Committee. (2020b, July 17). *Olympic Charter*. https://stillmed.olympics.com/media/Document%20Library/OlympicOrg/General/EN-Olympic-Charter.pdf?_ga=2.51458025.1705170707.1625350084-268416468.1620659316

International Olympic Committee. (2020c). *Olympic Marketing Fact File, 2020 Edition*. https://stillmed.olympic.org/media/Document%20Library/OlympicOrg/Documents/IOC-Marketing-and-Broadcasting-General-Files/Olympic-Marketing-Fact-File.pdf

International Olympic Committee. (2021, July 2). IOC Extends Opportunities for Athlete Expression during the Olympic Games Tokyo 2020. https://olympics.com/ioc/news/ioc-extends-opportunities-for-athlete-expression-during-the-olympic-games-tokyo-2020

IOC's Bach to Return to Tokyo for Paralympics Opening Ceremony. (2021, August 18). *Kyodo News*. https://english.kyodonews.net/paralympics/news/2021/08/a273290634f4-iocs-bach-to-return-to-tokyo-for-paralympics-opening-ceremony.html

Keh, A. (2021, August 7). A Memorable Olympics, but for the Right Reasons? *New York Times*. https://www.nytimes.com/2021/08/07/sports/olympics/covid-closing-ceremony-athletes.html

Kennedy, M. (2021, July 20). What It Takes to Get to Tokyo to Cover the Olympics. *National Public Radio.*. https://www.npr.org/sections/tokyo-olympics-live-updates/2021/07/18/1017472761/what-it-takes-to-get-into-tokyo-to-cover-the-olympics

Klein, N. (2007). *The Shock Doctrine: The Rise of Disaster Capitalism*. Metropolitan Books.

Kotegawa, T. (2019, October 14). Bags of Debris from Fukushima Disaster Swept Away in Typhoon. *Asahi Shimbun*. http://www.asahi.com/ajw/articles/AJ201910140036.html

Lau, Y. (2021, July 23). Japanese Sponsors Poured $3 Billion into the Tokyo Olympics. What Will They Get in Return? *Fortune*. https://fortune.com/2021/07/23/tokyo-olympics-sponsor-toyota-skips-opening-ceremony-cancels-ads/

Lewis, L., Harding R., & Inagaki, K. (2019, August 4). Olympic Sponsorship: Japan Inc Pressed into National Service. *Financial Times* https://www.ft.com/content/dfc917ce-bda9-11e9-b350-db00d509634e

Lies, E. (2021, 10 June). Money, Money, Money: The Cost of Tokyo's Pandemic-Delayed Olympics. *Reuters* https://www.reuters.com/business/media-telecom/money-money-money-cost-tokyos-pandemic-delayed-olympics-2021-06-10/

Little, J. B. (2019, January 16). Fukushima Residents Return Despite Radiation. *Scientific American*. https://www.scientificamerican.com/article/fukushima-residents-return-despite-radiation/.

Mann, G. (2013). *Disassembly Required: A Field Guide to Actually Existing Capitalism*. AK Press.

Martin, A.K.T. (2021, July 5). Twists and Turns: Retracing Tokyo's Tumultuous Path to the Olympics. *Japan Times*. https://www.japantimes.co.jp/sports/2021/07/05/olympics/summer-olympics/road-to-tokyo-olympics-covid19/

McCurry, J. (2017, July 15). Japan Passes 'Brutal' Counter-Terror Law Despite Fears Over Civil Liberties. *Guardian*. https://www.theguardian.com/world/2017/jun/15/japan-passes-brutal-new-terror-law-which-opponents-fear-will-quash-freedoms

McNeill, D. (2020). Spinning the Rings: The Media and the 2020 Tokyo Olympics. *The Asia-Pacific Journal, 18*(5), 1–5.

Müller, M., Wolfe, S. D., Gaffney, C., Gogishvili, D., Hug, M., & Leick, A. (2021). An Evaluation of the Sustainability of the Olympic Games. *Nature Sustainability, 4*, 340–348.

Nixon, R. (2011). *Slow Violence and the Environmentalism of the Poor*. Harvard University Press.

Rainforest Action Network. (2019, January 30). NGO Statement of Concern on Tokyo 2020 Olympics' Revised Timber Sourcing Code. https://www.ran.org/press-releases/ngo-statement-of-concern-on-tokyo-2020-olympics-revised-timber-sourcing-code/

Rainforest Action Network. (2020). Joint NGO Statement on Tokyo 2020 Olympics' 'Fake Sustainability'. https://www.ran.org/press-releases/olympics-fake-sustainability/

Rich, M. (2021, August 19). Paralympic Officials in Tokyo Report the First Virus Case in the Olympic Village. *New York Times*. https://www.nytimes.com/2021/08/19/world/asia/paralympics-virus-case.html

Rogers, M. (2016, August 17). Acrimony Surrounding 2020 Games Already Starting. *USA Today*. https://www.usatoday.com/story/sports/columnist/martin-rogers/2016/08/17/acrimony-surrounding-2020-tokyo-games-already-starting/88915890/

Rowbottom, M. (2021, July 8). Bach Set to Quarantine in Hotel for Three Days after Arriving in Tokyo. *Inside the Games*. https://www.insidethegames.biz/articles/1109907/bach-ioc-tokyo-quarantine-un-speech

Shimizu, K., Sridhar, D., Taniguchi, K., & Shibuya, K. (2021). Reconsider this Summer's Olympic and Paralympic Games. *The BMJ*, 373. https://www.bmj.com/content/373/bmj.n962

Sieg, L., & Lim, M. (2016, September 7). Abe's Fukushima 'Under Control' Pledge to Secure Olympics Was a Lie: Former PM. *Reuters*. https://www.reuters.com/article/us-japan-nuclear-idUSKCN11D0UF

Slodkowski, A. & Park, J. (2021, July 15). IOC's Bach Says 'Zero' Risk of COVID Spreading from Participants. *Reuters*. https://www.reuters.com/lifestyle/sports/iocs-bach-says-zero-risk-covid-spreading-participants-2021-07-15/

Sparrow, A.K., Brosseau, L.M., Harrison, R.J., & Osterholm, M.T. (2021). Protecting Olympic Participants from Covid-19—The Urgent Need for a Risk-Management Approach. *New England Journal of Medicine.*. https://www.nejm.org/doi/full/10.1056/NEJMp2108567

Synced. (2019, July 20). One Year Countdown: Readying AI Security for the Tokyo 2020 Olympics. https://syncedreview.com/2019/07/20/one-year-countdown-readying-ai-security-for-the-tokyo-2020-olympics/

Tsing, A. L. (2000). Inside the Economy of Appearances. *Public Culture, 12*, 115–144.

United States Olympic and Paralympic Committee. (2020, December 10). Team USA Council on Racial and Social Justice Releases First Set of Recommendations, Asks for Rule Change Allowing Athletes to Peacefully Protest and Demonstrate without Sanctions During Olympic and ParalympicGames.https://www.teamusa.org/Media/News/USOPC/Team-USA-Council-on-Racial-and-Social-Justice-releases-recommendations-on-demonstrations

Wade, S. (2019a, 21 July). Tokyo 1-Year Out: Scandal, High Costs But Unrivaled Demand. *AP.* https://apnews.com/80972eed8d7f4aec9ceeaebf992c38bd

Wade, S. (2019b, January 23). French Olympic Probe Raises Questions about Japanese Firm. AP. https://apnews.com/2d55d4f512544c99bd3cf306f56aeeab

Wade, S. (2020, September 3). Oxford Study: Tokyo Olympics Are the Most Costly Summer Games. *AP*. https://apnews.com/article/sports-virus-outbreak-sports-asia-2020-tokyo-olympics-olympic-games-cfd618b2fba9109d01103bd9ecae33a3

Whiteside, K. (2013, September 7). Tokyo will Host 2020 Summer Games. *USA Today.* https://www.usatoday.com/story/sports/olympics/2013/09/07/ioc-election-host-city-2020-olympics/2780311/

Yogeshwar, R. (2014, May 11). Fukushima Disaster Site 'Like a Science Fiction Film. *DW*. http://www.dw.de/fukushima-disaster-site-like-a-science-fiction-film/a-18039892

Zirin, D., & Boykoff, J. (2019, July 23). These Women Have Lost Their Homes to the Olympics in Tokyo—Twice. *The Nation*. https://www.thenation.com/article/archive/tokyo-olympics-displacement/

Zirin, D., & Boykoff, J. (2020, March 23). The Olympics Teeter on the Brink. *The Nation*. https://www.thenation.com/article/world/2020-olympics-coronavirus-cancel/

Zirin, D., & Boykoff, J. (2021a, April 21). The Tokyo Olympics Are in Trouble. *The Nation*. https://www.thenation.com/article/society/tokyo-olympics-pandemic/

Zirin, D., & Boykoff, J. (2021b, August 10). Despite the Ban, Protest Emerges at the Olympics. *The Nation*. https://www.thenation.com/article/society/raven-saunders-olympics-protest/

28

"You realise you tick a lot of boxes": Exploring the Impact of COVID-19 on the Rehabilitating Body Through a Bourdieusian Lens

Joanna Blackwell, Hannah Henderson, Adam Evans, and Jacquelyn Allen-Collinson

Introduction

The COVID-19 pandemic has affected the lives of many people, including their embodied practices and physicality. It has also influenced the places where physical activity practices can be conducted. During the pandemic and specifically the first lockdown in England in 2020,

J. Blackwell (✉)
University of Lincoln, Lincoln, UK

University of Copenhagen, Copenhagen, Denmark
e-mail: JBlackwell@lincoln.ac.uk

H. Henderson • J. Allen-Collinson
University of Lincoln, Lincoln, UK

A. Evans
University of Copenhagen, Copenhagen, Denmark

D. L. Andrews et al. (eds.), *Sport and Physical Culture in Global Pandemic Times*, Global Culture and Sport Series, https://doi.org/10.1007/978-3-031-14387-8_28

vulnerable individuals such as those with serious health conditions were advised to 'shield' for an extended period of time (meaning that these people should not leave their homes, and must minimise face to face contact). Additionally, many National Health Service (NHS) services were suspended, with health professionals redeployed from their usual jobs to support alternative efforts deemed 'business critical', such as the COVID response. The purpose of this chapter is to explore some of the complex and varied impacts of the changes brought about by the pandemic on 'afflicted bodies' during attempts to rehabilitate following a serious health event, such as a cardiac event, and the intersections with bodily practices, physicalities and places.

With the redeployment of certain health care staff to other functions deemed more critical, services like cardiac rehabilitation were largely left to flounder for months on end. Although the degree of this disruption varied according to the NHS provider, there was a definite shift in the prioritisation of risk, with communicable disease taking precedence over non-communicable diseases, such as heart disease (Evans et al., 2020). Whilst there was no indication that cardiac events declined during the height of the pandemic, there was, however, a 40 percent reduction in hospital admissions for cardiac conditions in comparison to pre-pandemic levels (Mafham et al., 2020). The impact of this notable reduction remains to be seen both physically and psycho-socially, but could involve more severe bodily effects, and premature deaths. Such outcomes might also be due to the relationship between COVID-19 and cardiovascular disease, as well as the severity of COVID-19 in its own right. Research by Clerkin et al. (2020) found that rates of COVID-19 increased in those with cardiovascular disease. Further, cardiac issues have been identified in COVID-19 patients, both in terms of the exacerbation of existing issues and triggering inflammatory markers (Akhmerov & Marbán, 2020; Naz & Billah, 2021).

The chapter draws on Bourdieusian perspectives and on data from an ethnographic study exploring socio-cultural influences on exercise and health during the cardiac patient journey. The study comprised participant observations, conducted at cardiac rehabilitation programme sites, and at the homes of those not participating in a cardiac rehabilitation programme, and repeat, in-depth, semi-structured interviews with nine cardiac patients and six of their significant others (as identified by the patients). Reflexive journaling was also conducted and continued throughout data collection and analysis. Half-way through the scheduled six-months of fieldwork, the first lockdown occurred in England, which commenced in March 2020, and thus influenced the methods employed as well as the topics of discussion. Switching from in-person observation and interviewing to virtual methods rendered participant observations difficult when video calls were able to take place, and impossible when interviews were via telephone.

There have been several studies conducted concerning cardiac rehabilitation in COVID times (e.g. Epstein et al., 2021; O'Doherty et al., 2021; Pecci & Ajmal, 2021; Schrack et al., 2020). There is, however, a dearth of research examining factors relevant to those individuals who were post cardiac rehabilitation during the COVID-19 pandemic. This is perhaps understandable, given the evolving situation in the global COVID pandemic, and difficulties in recruiting research participants amidst lockdowns, shielding and social distancing. For the research project, however, the pandemic and first lockdown actually provided an opportunity to investigate the impact upon participants' lives.

As this chapter specifically analyses rehabilitation and the rehabilitating body, it is useful first to set the context for rehabilitation, before proceeding to describe the research process and address the use of a Bourdieusian lens. The discussion then moves to examine some of the data collected in respect of two salient themes that were identified in the findings: bodily practices and physicalities, and space and place. The chapter then presents an overview of what the future might hold for people with long-term conditions, and finishes with some concluding thoughts.

What Is Rehabilitation?

The term 'rehabilitation' derives from the Latin prefix *re*, meaning 'again' and *habitare*, meaning 'make fit' and from the Medieval Latin form: *rehabilitationem*, meaning 'restoration' (Online etymology dictionary, 2021). Rehabilitation has been defined as "a set of interventions needed when a person is experiencing or is likely to experience limitations in everyday functioning due to ageing or a health condition, including chronic diseases or disorders, injuries or traumas" (World Health Organisation, 2020). The Chartered Society of Physiotherapy (2019) further defined rehabilitation with a more positively framed explanation: "[rehabilitation includes] enabling and supporting individuals to recover or adjust, to achieve their full potential and to live as full and active lives as possible". Language such as 'recovery' and 'adjustment' in defining rehabilitation, suggests it is designed to rectify or manage an injury or illness that can be aided, alleviated or improved. Cardiac rehabilitation follows this principle in that through the guidance of health care professionals, individuals have the responsibility to adopt behaviours that enable the slowing or reversal of disease progression (British Association for Cardiovascular Prevention & Rehabilitation, 2023).

Prescriptive exercise (with 'exercise' being the term typically used to describe structured physical activity in the context of rehabilitation) often forms a key part of rehabilitation as part of a medicalised approach. Whilst the association between exercise and health is well established (Hupin et al., 2015; Kelly et al., 2014; Lollgen et al., 2009), regarding exercise as a form of medicine has been trenchantly criticised for the production and reproduction of the discourses of restitution, decline and dependency that so often surround ageing and ill-health, and for perpetuating a culture of responsibilisation. These discourses tend to conceptualise exercise as a personal choice, laying the blame squarely with the individual should they fail to live an active lifestyle (Malcolm, 2014; Williams & Gibson, 2018). The concept of exercise as medicine often fails to consider negative aspects, such as risk of injury, and exacerbation of social inequalities, and downplays the potential significance of socio-cultural influences on health, illness and exercise participation.

Having highlighted the importance of socio-cultural influences, the research process that was undertaken is described below and leads on to a discussion regarding the potential of Bourdieusian theory to provide a useful lens through which to investigate rehabilitating bodies in pandemic times.

The Research Process

The research discussed in this chapter forms part of a larger doctoral study exploring the socio-cultural influences on exercise and health along the cardiac patient journey. Both the first and second authors had substantial prior industry experience of this domain, and a continuing interest in developments in this area. A literature review taking a narrative approach revealed several important aspects: firstly, the value of situating cardiac rehabilitation in the context of a journey, considering the individual's life prior to and after the cardiac event itself; secondly, the relevance of the perspectives of patients' significant others; and thirdly, some of the complexities associated with health care decision making. This review gave rise to the main aim and objectives of the doctoral study. Study objectives included: i) an exploration of the aspects of habitus, capital and field in cardiac patients and their significant others, and how these may influence practice along the cardiac patient journey; and ii) to explore the intersectionality of age, gender and social class in relation to the cardiac patient journey.

Recruited with the assistance of NHS cardiology and cardiac rehabilitation services, participants included patients of these services and their significant others, as identified by the patient. These significant others encompassed spouses, partners, daughters and friends. Demographic information about study participants is provided in the table below.

	Male	Female	18-49 years old	50-64 years old	65 years plus
Patients	8	2	2	3	5
Significant others	1	6	2	3	2

Germane to the use of a Bourdieusian perspective, whilst not every participant wished to discuss their social class background, several identified how they considered their upbringing to have been working-class, but due to improved material conditions (through education and employment) they now felt that others would consider them to be more middle class. Several participants described having retired after leading 'comfortable' lives, although relationship breakdown had impacted their lives.

Others who were still working described the challenges illness had created in terms of employment precarity and maintaining income levels.

The study adopted an ethnographic approach, which involved the first author spending time with study participants over a six-month period, attending the cardiac rehabilitation sessions they attended, and/or visiting them at home. During this time participant observations were undertaken, and repeated one to one semi-structured interviews took place. With reflexivity a central part of the approach, a reflexive diary was maintained throughout the fieldwork and until the conclusion of data analysis. This diary was used to record thoughts and feelings, considering the positionality of the researcher herself, the preconceptions she held, and any challenges to assumptions made. As noted above, fieldwork was disrupted by the advent of the first UK lockdown, and after consideration of the situation and after obtaining the required ethical approvals, data collection moved to synchronous virtual means for the remaining three months. Reflexive thematic analysis described by Braun and Clarke (2006, 2019) assisted in the analysing of data and enabled the identification and construction of eight themes in total, 'the impact of the COVID-19 pandemic on the cardiac patient journey' being one of these. There were both inductive and deductive elements to the approach, both working from and towards theory. In this sense, a Bourdieusian theoretical framework was selected as offering a particularly powerful perspective. The core concepts of this approach which shaped the analysis are now outlined.

Bourdieusian Theory and Rehabilitation in Pandemic Times

Pierre Bourdieu was a French philosopher and sociologist whose work was influenced by many other scholars, including phenomenological theorists such as Schütz and Merleau-Ponty (see for example, Robbins, 2019). Aspects of Marxism, together with the work of Bachelard and Durkheim, can also be observed in his approach (Vandenberghe, 1999). Bourdieu himself named Elias, Goffman, Weber and Kant as influential to his work in the preface of one of his most regarded texts, *Distinction* (Bourdieu, 1984). In contemporary times, Bourdieu's work continues to offer a potent theoretical lens, and research continues to challenge and move forward the ideas he developed (see for example, Angus et al., 2018; Taylor-Smith & Dumas, 2019 for studies relating to cardiovascular rehabilitation).

As a means to bridging the structure and agency divide, Bourdieu harnessed the concepts of habitus, capital, and field. Habitus involves a system of durable dispositions (inclinations, tendencies) offering both structure and structuring (Bourdieu, 1977), with structure based on past social conditions, and structuring shaping present and future practices (Maton, 2014). Dispositions guide one's approaches to physical activity, health, and health care; thus, when experiencing ill-health, the habitus will guide an individual's action. Habitus, for Bourdieu, is interlinked with social class, expressed by the different species of capital. Capital involves resources held by people or groups, which have social value that can be deployed, exchanged and transformed within fields (Bourdieu, 2006). The main forms of capital discussed by Bourdieu comprise cultural, social, economic, and symbolic capital. As a subset of cultural capital, physical capital is also pertinent to the current analysis, as it pertains to the body (Bourdieu, 1978). Bourdieu (1994, p.197) described a field as a social space as: "...objective relations between individuals or institutions who are competing for the same stake". Field theory assists in understanding the interconnections between habitus and capital (Watson & Grenfell, 2016), and thus brings the discussion full circle in considering how agency and structure may be bridged in Bourdieu's theoretical framework.

From the interplay between habitus, capital, and field, specific forms of practice emerge, each intertwined with several other concepts: doxa, a notion describing an individual's taken for granted beliefs about the social world; illusio, one's belief in and knowledge of the significance of the 'game'; hexis, the bodily display of the internalised marks left through time, which leads to embodied habitus; and finally, nomos, the rules of the 'game' (Bourdieu, 1977). Bourdieu likens the social world to a 'game' in its organisation, which involves rules and norms. Taste and distinction are central to his conceptual framework, with taste forming from the habitus and being associated with the capital one holds. When deployed, capital assists in situating one within the field, determining one's position in relation to others, and leads to power hierarchies.

Bourdieusian theory is highly relevant to the exploration of rehabilitating bodies in pandemic times. Whilst one's durable system of dispositions, developed as part of the habitus, assist in guiding choices in respect of exercise, health, and health care, alterations to social conditions can result in extended periods in certain fields (family or local neighbourhood, for example), changes to the structures of fields (social distancing, for example), and even the unavailability of some fields (work or leisure facilities, for example). Thus, the nomos can change, stunting the opportunities for deploying, exchanging, and developing capital along the rehabilitation journey, and influencing the body in many ways.

Bourdieu termed the disjuncture between one's habitus and the nomos, laws and practices of fields, hysteresis (Bourdieu, 1977). Whilst hysteresis may be overcome through reflexivity and adaptation to the habitus, although not in every case, and rarely without challenges, the onset of the pandemic and initiation of social restrictions may well have generated further uncertainty. Understanding the impact of a serious health event on an individual's dispositions towards their own health and health care, and how these might be reformed or adjusted, is complex, without the added complications wrought by the pandemic. Some of these complexities are explored in the sections that follow, which are structured into themes, beginning with bodily practices and physicalities, and moving on to space and place.

Bodily Practices and Physicalities

Participants evocatively described how their body felt weakened by the relative inactivity generated by the lockdown, or a reluctance to continue physical activity without professional support. They also portrayed how their recovery from the cardiac event felt stifled by lingering anxiety about current and future imaginings of physical activity and physical cultures. Deeply embodied responses were also evident, for example in despondent postures and facial expressions displaying frustration, as some of the data presented below demonstrate.

The analogy of moving three steps forward and two steps back seems an apt way to describe how many participants experienced the rehabilitation journey during COVID times, which caused both worry and frustration. Having been diagnosed with angina and undergoing a surgical procedure six months prior to the onset of the pandemic, Sandra, a 58-year-old patient-participant described how she felt during the lockdown:

> I was actually starting to, ya know, put it behind me and live with it [coronary heart disease]. Then obviously with this [COVID] and the uncertainty of, ya know, who it affects, and then you look, and you realise you tick a lot of boxes.

Another patient-participant, Tom, aged 43, who had experienced a Myocardial Infarction (heart attack) expressed similar frustration:

> Obviously, the health issues that I've had I've been kinda erm, enough is enough. I just wanted to have a bit of normality and then this [COVID] comes along, and it can be deadly.

The impact of the pandemic was evident, not just in the words spoken by participants, but also in their demeanour. In the following data, patient-participant Tom talked about his recovery journey following a Myocardial Infarction, and the impact of COVID combined with his cardiac event:

> Suddenly you've got this hanging over ya [COVID] so it's not ideal [sighs]. I'm trying to get a bit more positive I'm trying to er... [struggling for words] but it's difficult because of the situation [appears downcast]. You can't have any normality in your life with this going on just now, so it's just an added... [worry]. But hopefully I'm still hoping to get back to normal. I think I just want more, erm a more enjoyable life, ya know. More travel, more doing stuff, more active... I mean just being able to get on my bike and go out for a bike ride whenever and wherever, without... it's not so much the getting out of breath at the time, 'cause you get out of breath

> doing exercise. But it's the time to take to recover afterwards. And that's, ya know, that's the difficult part when it's taking you longer and you're getting the chest pains and the little niggles, 'cause you've got this constant reminder that you've had this [cardiac] incident happen. So now it's like anytime I get the chest pain or you're like 'well why is that?' 'what's causing that?' so you become very conscious of it.

Participant accounts like this indicated that the concerns and worries of those living with coronary heart disease during the pandemic appeared heightened. The unavailability or perceived unavailability of cardiac rehabilitation staff and health professional support generally meant that the search by individuals for support led to greater reliance on other avenues. Participants talked about engaging with social media support groups and undertaking internet research, not only to gain reassurance about their afflicted bodies, but because their bodies were felt to be additionally vulnerable in COVID times. The aim of this 'personal research' was demonstrated in this account from Sandra, a patient-participant who had recently completed cardiac rehabilitation, and felt that staying active was an important part of her continued recovery. She discussed the websites she had looked at, the news stories she had heard, and using the resources (capital) she gained from attending rehabilitation:

> I think it's the uncertainty of not knowing when you can resume [outdoor physical activity]. Or trying to think of a way that's safe to adapt erm, and of course the government [COVID-19] advice seems very contradictory in many ways. So, trying to work out for myself 'ooh what could be safe and what could apply'.

In this instance, participation in cardiac rehabilitation had given legitimacy to physical activity as a health-giving practice. It had reignited dispositions around trying to build activity into everyday life and provided some cultural and physical capital, in the form of knowledge, confidence, and competency. These resources were carried with the participant when she completed cardiac rehabilitation, however, the advent of the pandemic left her wondering how, where and when she could use them.

Despite not having experienced the effects of COVID directly, some participant accounts revealed how the lack of unstructured and incidental physical activity, brought about by government-imposed restrictions, had an important impact on participants' embodiment, perceptions of health, and feelings of confidence:

> Before this virus I would go out shopping and I would walk round nearly, I could walk all day... but now I do find, ya know, a walk with the dogs especially when its warmer I get out of breath a bit quicker than I used to do. (Elizabeth, 70 years old, patient-participant).
>
> I'm trying to do some of the exercises from cardiac rehab, erm I'm not doing ya know [much], just generally I'm not as active as when I was working. I'd be walking to places and from, so I'm not getting the exercise ya know that I did get. That obviously worries me, the impact that that has on me health-wise. (Sandra, 58 years old, patient-participant).

The latter account indicated how the participant sought to introduce some exercise using the cultural and physical capital acquired whilst undertaking rehabilitation. Although in shielding situations (and indeed in all situations) some of these exercises could be undertaken within a home or garden environment, without equipment (sit to stand movements or step ups, for example), and others adapted (bicep curls using tin cans, or shuttle walks instead of walking on a treadmill, for example), there was some reticence to do this. Whilst participants did not express why this was the case, the home environment might have constituted a new field in which to conduct exercise, and a perceived lack of: professional support, confidence, and support of others, could all be feasible considerations demonstrating the uncertainty of using this field in this context.

Unstructured physical activity such as active commuting, occupational activity, and undertaking errands appeared important to the recovering body. This seemed to be the case particularly for those whose habitus meant they were dispositionally disinclined towards structured physical activity, who may or may not have attended rehabilitation, but whose activity would typically occur incidentally in their everyday life. Participant accounts indicated that the restrictions of the pandemic (working from home, and lockdown orders, for example) substantially affected incidental activity and the impacts of this were noted in relation to corporeal indicators, such as becoming breathless more easily. For those who had not attended cardiac rehabilitation and those without an active habitus (where the bodily schema is supported by dispositions relevant to physical activity), structured physical activity may not be considered important, it may be ill-fitting with the habitus, and there may not be the requisite capital resources to act. Perceived capital resources could include physical competence, and access to clothing or equipment.

Recovery journeys post cardiac event were often described by participants in the study in terms of making plans or getting back to things. The lack of opportunity to participate in hobbies and social occasions, such as birdwatching and meeting wider family, created by the conditions of lockdown, had left any previously held social and cultural (including physical) capital floundering without the availability of these fields. Furthermore, there was little opportunity for the accrual or demonstration of symbolic capital, which requires a social space and an opportunity to be seen by those who would view it favourably (Neveu, 2018). For those rehabilitating, the ability to demonstrate their recovery and/or increased fitness, and receive recognition from others for this, would result in symbolic capital in the cardiac rehabilitation field. An instance of how the pandemic had limited the ability to access the social space and opportunity that may have provided such recognition was demonstrated in this account from patient-participant Sandra:

> All those plans, coming out of winter, better weather, so it seemed a great opportunity [to get out more], as obviously I was improving my fitness and health and anxiety [through cardiac rehabilitation] and everything about doing things was ya know [feeling positive]. I had lots of plans and they were incorporated in that, family days out, going off with the grandson and doing things.

Having explored some of the bodily practice and physicality aspects associated with the impact of the COVID-19 pandemic and the rehabilitating body, the second area of discussion concerns space and place.

Space and Place

The association between space and place has great salience during the pandemic and specifically during lockdown periods, when staying at home and within one's local area became a necessity. Where one resides can have great symbolic value, in addition to physical location. Place may serve to bolster capital resources, and linked to one's habitus, can provide a space where one feels able to 'fit in'. Bourdieu and Wacquant (1992, p.127) used the analogy of the weightlessness a "fish in water" may feel, when there is a comfortable relationship between habitus, practice and field.

In cases where shielding was not taking place, daily exercise in the local area was authorised by the UK Government during lockdowns, and provided an opportunity to use outdoor spaces for (unorganised) exercise, such as walking. Those with dispositions more aligned with physical activity may have chosen to take advantage of this. It could be argued that even those less inclined, but with little else to do, might have decided to take the opportunity to go outside. Patient-participant Robert had attended rehabilitation and expressed his desire to stay active thereafter. He had an active occupation and active hobbies which were unfortunately curtailed by lockdown restrictions, yet described feeling largely unhampered, living "in a small village, so I've only got 50 yards to go to get to the nearest bridleway or footpath". His significant other, Sarah, however, indicated that his intentions started well but then his motivation declined as lockdown progressed:

> We started off doing a lot of walking so I suppose I thought that would carry on... He sits round a lot, doesn't do any walking at the minute. He's just into lockdown mode, I think. He needs to get back to work.

Sarah felt that keeping active was something her partner should be doing following his cardiac event, but she was also aware that his occupation was physically demanding and thus returning to this physical labour would likely serve this purpose, as he did not seem interested by other options.

Some participants described enhanced physical activity practices engendered by furlough or hiatus in employment or a reduction in personal commitments. In these circumstances engagement in physical activity was assisted by perceptions of having 'more time' and the social space and place where these practices could be undertaken:

> We're lucky where we are [rural location]. We can get out when we want and there's the local cycle paths and footpaths so we can get out; we're not really that restricted. (Sarah, significant other-participant).

> It [the lockdown] has had a good impact yes, it's been great erm, I'm not rushing round doing jobs. If I do them all today, I'll have nothing left to do tomorrow! (Mark, patient-participant).

Familiarity with one's surroundings during the pandemic may provide some comfort and safety (Schellenberg & Fonberg, 2020). Feelings of being unrestricted, and being able to abide by social distance requirements with ease whilst in outside spaces, were mentioned by several participants, particularly those living in more rural locations:

> I've been out walking with my friend, we've just kept two metres apart from each other… we've been the only people out, everyone else has been sat indoors! [laughs]. (Sarah, significant other-participant, lives in a small village).

The area where the research was conducted was a large mainly rural county in the east of England, and as such the social class of participants was not as relevant in shaping activity practices as was the physical geography or the location. Rather, the symbolic geography and the perceptions associated with undertaking activity appeared more important factors. Relatedly and as discussed above, there were those in the study who described choosing not to utilise their familiar space as a place to undertake activity, exercising at home or in the garden, for example. This could be linked to the value it holds as a place of comfort and/or safety. The perception of risk outside of the home was noted by patient-participant Sandra, who is living with multimorbidity:

> My anxieties are quite high... I was building my confidence and going out for longer walks and things like that prior to lockdown... [now] I need to shield and social distance and be careful, but then in the back of my mind I'm not as active.

Furthermore, given the uncertainty and worry that accompanied the pandemic, individuals could feel a need to protect their space. This included the people in it and the responsibilities they held in that space, which can provide a sense of purpose and control in uncertain times (Helpard & Meagher-Stewart, 1998):

> I'll hold my hands up and admit that all through this virus thing... my granddaughter still comes up every Friday for the weekend... it gives Debbie [daughter] a break. She's very good, she comes with me and walks the dogs and it's company... she's always done it [from being little]. (Elizabeth, patient-participant, self-identified as working class).

What Might the Future Hold for Those with Long-term Health Conditions?

At the time of writing, the pandemic appears to be far from over, and therefore participants could only speculate about what life might involve for them in the future. Some participants had begun to reflect upon how their ability to travel could be limited in the future, and questioned when they would see loved ones again, and whether they would feel able to do the things they enjoy:

> I wonder whether I'll ever get away [on holiday] again. I think more to do with what restrictions they, others put in place, ya know, thinking 'is it really worth it?' but time will tell [whether it could be safe]. I mean ya know, it [the pandemic] makes you more aware of what potential hazards are out there. (Robert, patient-participant).

Schrack et al. (2020) explored some of the health challenges that are likely to be faced as the world emerges from the pandemic, suggesting how physical activity levels, nutrition, and disease burden have all been negatively affected by COVID. The pandemic has though provided a 'kick-start' in the redesign of health services such as cardiac rehabilitation, with digital options being at the forefront of developments (O'Doherty et al., 2021). Indeed, just as digital connections permitted the continuation of research, they also assisted in providing a means to conduct 'personal research', supporting social connections, and provided the leisure sector with an opportunity to develop its role beyond traditional venue-based activities (Son et al., 2021).

There are, however, a number of pervasive issues raised in health care fields organised around the medical model of illness, and notably, the addition of COVID rehabilitation to the list of NHS services now provided (De Biase et al., 2020; Grund et al., 2021) is relevant to that discussion. Firstly, the segregation of people into specialist groups can create an 'othering' effect (e.g. Bangsbo et al., 2019; Evans & Crust, 2015; Tulle, 2008). Thus, grouping and even segregating people as 'unhealthy' or 'ill' can create marginalisation and stigmatisation, both of which may not only be influential to uptake of, and adherence to physical activity, but may also reaffirm the discourses around decline and dependency related to ageing and illness. From a Bourdieusian perspective, the creation of new fields like those created within health care, such as cardiac rehabilitation and now COVID rehabilitation, demands a new set of rules (nomos) to come into existence. A new hierarchical structure is developed distinguishing different members of staff, volunteers, and patients who have already gained cultural and physical capital via engagement, and new patients who have not yet had opportunities to develop their knowledge about managing their health condition, or competency in performing the required exercises. A pertinent example of how capital can be accumulated, and how the nomos can be confirmed within the social space of cardiac rehabilitation, was noted in this excerpt taken from the first author's field notes:

> Robert [patient] seemed very enthusiastic during the exercise session, he said that he had been struggling to get his heart rate into the required zone [mandated by staff] so he wanted to push himself a bit more and was feeling good to do that. He was certainly more buoyant and confident-looking

> in the gym environment than I have seen before. He was able to get into his heart rate zone, which he seemed really pleased about although at one point he was possibly exceeding it and recognised this and eased off a little. There was one occasion when he started the active rest exercise early but was corrected by the assistant, he made a comment saying 'am I getting a telling off?' to which she replied 'yes you are'. He pulled a face, half smiling and looking towards to me [researcher]. That seems to be the way, that it's very much a 'do as you are told to do' environment and it is accepted that those in red [colour of staff t-shirts] give the instructions.

Secondly, as noted previously, the privileging of communicable disease over non-communicable disease, in terms of NHS services, elevates the health needs of one person over another. Prioritising risks in this way again adds to the sense of 'othering'. It may risk challenges to the doxa surrounding health care, when people perceive health care not to be available to them, or feel they are not the priority for the receipt of this health care. As Lewis et al. (2018) posit, one's sense of self is co-produced, with influences coming from a range of sources, including family and friends, and the media. In Bourdieusian terms, this relates to the formation of the habitus. As noted above, online resources have been a prominent source of information during the pandemic. The availability of and reliance on these sources during significant health events such as the pandemic is likely to have been heightened (an example from the Zika virus is shown in Lwin et al., 2018). The longer the pandemic continues, and the uncertainty remains, adjusted practices may become legitimised (Bowness et al., 2021), as repeated engagement by individuals with different practices will through time develop a belief in that practice: or development of illusio in Bourdieusian terms (Palmer et al., 2021).

Lastly, and linked to the previous point, some of the social inequalities that exist between rich and poor, young and old, and white people and those from ethnic minorities, have been laid bare during the pandemic. Thus, groups, including older adults, those who are economically-disadvantaged, and those from ethnic-minority groups, have disproportionately suffered the effects of coronary heart disease over many years (British Heart Foundation, 2019), and more recently of COVID (Burström & Tao, 2020). The political undertone of some of the decisions taken concerning the pandemic contain a level of what Bourdieu (1998) described as 'symbolic violence', manifested in the power differentials within the social hierarchy, such as inferior treatment or denial of resources (Webb et al., 2002). Combined, these actions indicate the important influence of socio-cultural and socio-structural issues, linked in Bourdieusian terms to class via the tastes and lifestyles associated with the habitus and the capital and thus power held.

In Conclusion

This discussion relates primarily to rehabilitating bodies and the impact of the pandemic, yet it is hoped that it also opens a much wider debate around ill bodies generally, as well as ill bodies in a pandemic, how they are conceptualised, particularly in relation to the medical model of illness. Bourdieu's perspectives provide a useful insight into the importance of capital in terms of power at both a micro and macro level. The salience of field, and specifically of place, as constructs, is evident in the importance of familiarity and safety in uncertain times (like a 'fish in water'), as well as a space to conduct physical activity. One may retreat to a comfort zone when crises hit, and the unfamiliarity created by the pandemic and the ongoing uncertainty seem to have created specific opportunities for those with long-term conditions: some positive, and some not so. In particular, the importance of incidental physical activity alongside digital support may provide useful context for the development of health services and in understanding how to assist 'rehabilitation' and recovery more effectively in the future. The medical model of illness largely neglects the personalised nature of recovery. As some of the main proponents of this model, health professionals and health service managers instead attempt to claim personalisation through their own definition of rehabilitation, and the provision of programming aligned to this definition. Importantly, aspects such as incidental physical activity constitute a part of a person's social world, as opposed to anything specifically created for the purpose of 'rehabilitation'. Consequently, if incidental practices were acknowledged as part of the recovery journey, disruption analogous to that caused by the pandemic might have a much more limited impact.

With familiar practices already formed, there may be, for example, no concern about where to source professional guidance when health professionals or health services are unavailable. There may also be a reduced need for 'personal research' about what physical activity to perform, and thus reduced opportunity for confusion and mixed messages. Capital gained from engaging in these practices in familiar spaces and places could create less potential for hysteresis when crisis events occur. It is of course acknowledged that limitation of leisure and work activities will impact this, as would requirements for vulnerable populations to shield from others. The UK Government-prescribed 'daily exercise' in pandemic times might be felt to be legitimate as a health-giving and/or pleasurable practice for everyone, as a means to deploy capital, such as social capital when meeting a friend for a walk, cultural or physical capital when utilising competency to go for a jog.

Uncertainty and fears about vulnerability are difficult to navigate with public health events of the magnitude of COVID-19. The potential for hysteresis in such times appears great, and when occurring in addition to crisis situations like a cardiac event, the disjuncture between one's habitus and the nomos, laws and practices of unfamiliar fields may be experienced as greater. In other cases, an individual may have begun to reconcile their habitus to the contextual nomos, laws and practices of rehabilitation after an inital period of hysteresis following their cardiac event, only to have everything shaken again by the pandemic. Indeed, in times of crisis the habitus can be fundamentally shaken, meaning that dispositions are challenged (Bourdieu, 2000). The delay in the development of strategies in the face of challenges to social positioning Bourdieu termed the 'Don Quixote effect' (Bourdieu, 1979). Periods of reflection and more importantly reflexivity, assist by enabling the consideration of one's position. The result of this consideration may involve a shift in, or conversely, a reaffirming of the habitus. What is not well understood at present is what the impact of the pandemic might be on dispositions, even to the extent of whether the longevity of the impact of the pandemic may create an opportunity for building upon the primary foundations laid in early life (Bourdieu & Passeron, 1977), and the creation of a secondary habitus. Of course, through the new experiences resulting from the pandemic it is not entirely clear yet whether any such evolutions may create lasting change, and whether this change positively or negatively affects both those rehabilitating their body in contemporary times, and those who might experience such rehabilitation in the future.

Although Bourdieu's theory has been criticised for being deterministic and leaving little room for human agency (Yang, 2014), this chapter has sought to demonstrate how his theory can offer a way to explore how individuals navigate crisis events and what may guide the decisions they make about bodily practices in such circumstances. It does so by acknowledging that change can be effected by "practical efficacy" and the capacity for reflection, and not just by the social conditions and nomos within fields (Shilling, 2010, p.481).

References

Akhmerov, A., & Marbán, E. (2020). COVID-19 and the heart. *Circulation Research, 126*(10), 1443–1455.

Angus, J. E., Dale, C. M., Seto Nielsen, L., Kramer-Kile, M., Lapum, J., Pritlove, C., Abramson, B., Price, J. A., Marzolini, S., Oh, P., & Clark, A. (2018). Gender matters in cardiac rehabilitation and diabetes: Using Bourdieu's concepts. *Social Science and Medicine, 200*, 44–51.

Bangsbo, J., Blackwell, J., Boraxbekk C-J., Caserotti, P., Dela, F., Evans, A.B., Jespersen, A.P., Gliemann, L., Kramer, A.F., Lundbye-Jensen, J., Mortensen, E.L., Lassen, A.J., Gow, A.J., Harridge, S.D.R., Hellsten, Y., Kjaer, M., Kujala, U.M., Rhodes, R.E., Pike, E.C.J … Viña, J. (2019). Copenhagen Consensus statement 2019: Physical activity and ageing. *British Journal of Sports Medicine*, 53(14), 856-858

Bourdieu, P. (1977). *Outline of a Theory of Practice*. Cambridge University Press.

Bourdieu, P. (1978). Sport and social class. *Social Science Information, 17*(6), 819–840.

Bourdieu, P. (1979). Les trois etats du capital culturel. *Actes de la Recherche en Sciences, 30*(1), 3–6.

Bourdieu, P. (1984). *Distinction: A Social Critique of the Judgment of Taste*. Routledge, Kegan and Paul.

Bourdieu, P. (1994). *Sociology in question*. Sage Publications Ltd.

Bourdieu, P. (1998). *Practical reason*. Stanford University Press.

Bourdieu, P. (2000). *Pascalian meditations*. Stanford University Press.

Bourdieu, P. (2006). The Forms of Capital. In H. Lauder, P. Brown, J.-A. Dillabough, & A. H. Halsey (Eds.), *Education, Globalisation and Social Change* (pp. 60–107). Oxford University Press.
Bourdieu, P., & Passeron, J.-C. (1977). *Reproduction in Education, Society and Culture*. Sage.
Bourdieu, P., & Wacquant, L. J. D. (1992). *An invitation to Reflexive Sociology*. Polity Press.
Bowness, J., McKendrick, J., & Tulle, E. (2021). From non-runner to parkrunner: Subjective athletic identity and experience of parkrun. *International Review for the Sociology of Sport, 56*(5), 695–718.
Braun, V., & Clarke, V. (2006). Using thematic analysis in psychology. *Qualitative Research in Psychology, 3*(2), 77–101.
Braun, V., & Clarke, V. (2019). Reflecting on reflexive thematic analysis. *Qualitative Research in Sport, Exercise and Health, 11*(4), 589–597.
British Association for Cardiovascular Prevention and Rehabilitation. (2023). *The BACPR Standards and Core Components for Cardiovascular Disease Prevention and Rehabilitation 2023* (4th Edition). http://www.cardiacrehabilitation.org.uk/docs/BACPRStandards-and-Core-Components-2023.pdf
British Heart Foundation. (2019). Quality and outcomes report. https://www.bhf.org.uk/informationsupport/publications/statistics/national-audit-of- cardiac-rehabilitation-quality-and-outcomesreport-2019
Burström, B., & Tao, W. (2020). Social determinants of health and inequalities in COVID-19. *European Journal of Public Health, 30*(4), 617–618.
Clerkin, K. J., Fried, J. A., Raikhelkar, J., Sayer, G., Griffin, J. M., Masoumi, A., et al. (2020). COVID-19 and cardiovascular disease. *Circulation, 141*(20), 1648–1655.
De Biase, S., Cook, L., Skelton, D. A., Witham, M., & Ten Hove, R. (2020). The COVID-19 rehabilitation pandemic. *Age and Ageing, 49*(5), 696–700.
Epstein, E., Patel, N., Maysent, K., & Taub, P. R. (2021). Cardiac Rehab in the COVID Era and Beyond: mHealth and Other Novel Opportunities. *Current Cardiology reports, 23*(5), 1–8.
Evans, A. B., & Crust, L. (2015). 'Some of these people aren't as fit as us …': experiencing the ageing, physically active body in cardiac rehabilitation. *Qualitative Research in Sport, Exercise and Health, 7*(1), 13–36.
Evans, A. B., Blackwell, J., Dolan, P., Fahlén, J., Hoekman, R., Lenneis, V., McNarry, G., Smith, M., & Wilcock, L. (2020). Sport in the face of the COVID-19 pandemic: Towards an agenda for research in the sociology of sport. *European Journal for Sport and Society, 17*(2), 85–95.

Grund, S., Gordon, A. L., Bauer, J. M., Achterberg, W. P., & Schols, J. M. (2021). The COVID rehabilitation paradox: Why we need to protect and develop geriatric rehabilitation services in the face of the pandemic. *Age and Ageing, 50*(3), 605–607.

Helpard, H., & Meagher-Stewart, D. (1998). The "kaleidoscope" experience for elderly women living with coronary artery disease. *Canadian Journal of Cardiovascular Nursing, 9*(3), 11–23.

Hupin, D., Roche, F., Gremeaux, V., Chatard, J-C., Oriol, M., Gaspoz, J-M., Barthélémy, J-C. & Edouard, P. (2015). Even a low-dose of moderate-to-vigorous physical activity reduces mortality by 22% in adults aged 60 years: A systematic review and meta-analysis. *British Journal of Sports Medicine*, 49, 1262-1267

Kelly, P., Kahlmeier, S., Götschi, T., Orsini, N., Richards, J., Roberts, N., Scarborough, P., & Foster, C. (2014). Systematic review and meta-analysis of reduction in all-cause mortality from walking and cycling and shape of dose response relationship. *International Journal of Behavioral Nutrition and Physical Activity, 11*, 132–136.

Lewis, S., Willis, K., & Collyer, F. (2018). Navigating and making choices about healthcare: The role of place. *Health & Place, 52*, 215–220.

Lollgen, H., Bockenhoff, A., & Knapp, G. (2009). Physical activity and all-cause mortality: An updated meta-analysis with different intensity categories. *International Journal of Sports Medicine., 30*, 213–224.

Lwin, M. O., Lu, J., Sheldenkar, A., & Schulz, P. J. (2018). Strategic uses of Facebook in Zika outbreak communication: Implications for the crisis and emergency risk communication model. *International Journal of Environmental Research and Public Health, 15*(9), 1974.

Mafham, M. M., Spata, E., Goldacre, R., Gair, D., Curnow, P., Bray, M., et al. (2020). COVID-19 pandemic and admission rates for and management of acute coronary syndromes in England. *The Lancet, 396*(10248), 381–389.

Malcolm, D. (2014). Sport, health and medicine: A sociological agenda. *Asia Pacific Journal of Sport and Social Science, 3*(1), 51–63.

Maton, K. (2014). Habitus. In M. Grenfell (Ed.), *Pierre Bourdieu: Key concepts* (pp. 60–76). Routledge.

Naz, A., & Billah, M. (2021). COVID-19 and Coronary Heart Disease. *Encyclopedia, 1*(2), 340–349.

Neveu, E. (2018). Bourdieu's Capital(s): Sociologizing an Economic Concept. In T. Medvetz & J. J. Sallaz (Eds.) *The Oxford handbook of Pierre Bourdieu* (pp. 347–374). Oxford University Press.

O'Doherty, A. F., Humphreys, H., Dawkes, S., Cowie, A., Hinton, S., Brubaker, P. H., Butler, T., & Nichols, S. (2021). How has technology been used to deliver cardiac rehabilitation during the COVID-19 pandemic? An international cross-sectional survey of healthcare professionals conducted by the BACPR. *BMJ open, 11*(4), e046051.

Online etymology dictionary. (2021). *Rehabilitation*. https://www.etymonline.com/word/rehabilitation

Palmer, V., Bowness, J., & Tulle, E. (2021). (Re)conceptualising physical activity as a career. *Ageing and Society, 41*(4), 936–954.

Pecci, C., & Ajmal, M. (2021). Cardiac Rehab in the COVID-19 Pandemic. *The American Journal of Medicine, 134*(5), 559–560.

Robbins, D. (2019). *The Bourdieu paradigm: The origins and evolution of an intellectual social project*. Manchester University Press. www.jstor.org/stable/j.ctvnb7qpj

Schellenberg, G., & Fonberg, J. (2020). *Housing characteristics and staying at home during the COVID-19 pandemic*. Statistics Canada. https://epe.lac-bac.gc.ca/

Schrack, J. A., Wanigatunga, A. A., & Juraschek, S. P. (2020). After the COVID-19 pandemic: the next wave of health challenges for older adults. *The Journals of Gerontology: Series A*

Shilling, C. (2010). Physical capital and situated action: A new direction for corporeal sociology. *British Journal of Sociology of Education, 25*(4), 473–487.

Son, J. S., Nimrod, G., West, S. T., Janke, M. C., Liechty, T., & Naar, J. J. (2021). Promoting older adults' physical activity and social well-being during COVID-19. *Leisure Sciences, 43*(1-2), 287–294.

Taylor-Smith, A., & Dumas, A. (2019). Class-based masculinity, cardiovascular health and rehabilitation. *Sociology of Health & Illness, 41*(2), 303–324.

The Chartered Society of Physiotherapy. (2019). *Rehabilitation.*. https://www.csp.org.uk/conditions/rehabilitation

Tulle, E. (2008). *Ageing, the body and social change: Running in later life*. Palgrave Macmillan.

Vandenberghe, F. (1999). "The Real is Relational": An Epistemological Analysis of Pierre Bourdieu's Generative Structuralism. *Sociological Theory, 17*(1), 32–67.

Watson, J., & Grenfell, M. (2016). Working in the methodological 'outfield': The case of Bourdieu and occupational therapy. *International Journal of Research & Method in Education, 39*(2), 151–169.

Webb, J., Schirato, T., & Danaher, G. (2002). *Understanding Bourdieu*. Allen & Unwin.

Williams, O., & Gibson, K. (2018). Exercise as a poisoned elixir: Inactivity, inequality and intervention. *Qualitative Research in Sport, Exercise and Health, 10*(4), 412–428.

World Health Organisation. (2020). *Rehabilitation*. https://www.who.int/news-room/fact-sheets/detail/rehabilitation

Yang, Y. (2014). Bourdieu, practice and change: Beyond the criticism of determinism. *Educational Philosophy and Theory, 46*(14), 1522–1540.

29

Paradoxical Effects of the Health Crisis within the Esports Industry: How French Esports Organizations Illuminate the Perceived Revenue Growth Façade

Nicolas Besombes and Seth E. Jenny

Context

After nearly two years following the first governmental social distancing restrictions on 5 March 2020 aimed at containing the spread of the COVID-19 pandemic, the esports industry continues to repeatedly be presented through media channels as having benefited from this exceptional global health situation. For example, as early as May 2020, economic journalist Stefan Brambilla Hall reported that the COVID-19 pandemic "*is taking esports to the next level*" (Brambilla Hall, 2020), while in July 2020, University of Pennsylvania Wharton School of Business proclaimed that "*esports gets a lift during [the] pandemic... [and that] while*

N. Besombes (✉)
Institut des Sciences du Sport-Santé de Paris, Université Paris Cité, Paris, France

S. E. Jenny
Slippery Rock University of Pennsylvania, Slippery Rock, PA, USA

D. L. Andrews et al. (eds.), *Sport and Physical Culture in Global Pandemic Times*, Global Culture and Sport Series, https://doi.org/10.1007/978-3-031-14387-8_29

other sports temporarily fade into the background, professional gaming thrives" (Baker, 2020). Likewise, in France, the media narrative was similar. For instance, in March 2020, Le Midi Libre headline read "*E-sport, the big winner of this crisis*" (Gounel, 2020), while in July 2020, Europe 1 titled its column La Rétro Sport: "*E-Sport, the lockdown's big winner*" (Europe 1, 2020).

While esports, or organized competitive video gaming (Jenny et al., 2017), has undeniably shown a remarkable capacity to adapt due to its online capability at a time when all other sports and cultural activities were forced to stop, it also had to face the numerous cancellations or postponements of events. For example, the League of Legends European Championship (LEC), which is traditionally held at the game publisher's (Riot Games) offices in Berlin and gathers the 10 teams of the tournament matches every week, was suspended on 13 March 2020 due to many COVID positive cases among the teams and event commentators. However, it took only one week for Riot Games to ensure that all event production staff and players were able to continue the competition from their own homes, and the championship resumed one week later.

As seen in Fig. 29.1, for the first time since 1998, the aggregated number of esports competitions held globally decreased two consecutive years in 2020 and 2021 across the COVID-19 pandemic. These have been linked to travel and gathering bans, closures of public spaces, border crossing restrictions (e.g., within the Schengen area (Direction Générale de la Migration et des Affaires Intérieures, 2020)) and successive lockdowns and curfews. In this respect, esports LAN (local area network) events (i.e., face-to-face competitions) were subject to exactly the same constraints as other spectator-oriented sports and cultural activities. Examples of major events cancelled or postponed include The International DotA 2 Championships (TI10), the Evolution Championship Series (EVO), the Arena of Valor World Cup (AVWC), the Capcom Pro Tour (CPT), the Fortnite World Cup, the Combo Breaker, the ESL One Los Angeles Major, and the League of Legends Mid-Season Invitational (MSI) (Zalamea, 2020). In France, more than 70 in-person esports events were cancelled or postponed in the weeks following the governmental measures instituted in early March 2020.

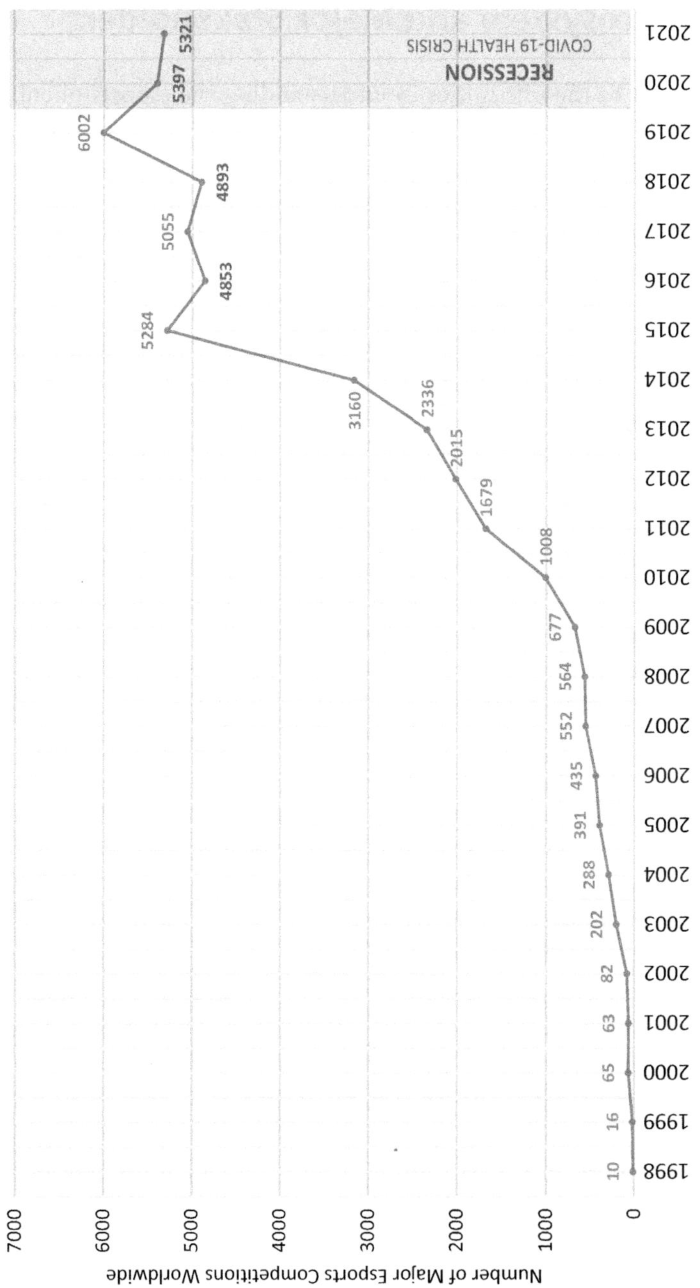

Fig. 29.1 Number of worldwide esports competitions per year between 1998 and 2021 per Esports Earnings (2022)

Esports Ecosystem and Major Stakeholders

However, one of the difficulties in understanding the esports phenomenon lies in the relative complexity of its ecosystem. Indeed, the stakeholders that compose the esports sector's value chain are multiple and form a scattered and fragmented network (Cranmer et al., 2021; Peng et al., 2020; Scholz, 2020). Despite the interdependence of these actors, esports entities operate primarily within a bureaucratic system (Peng et al., 2020) due to the inherently commercial nature of the video games whose intellectual property (IP) belongs to their developers and publishers (Karhulahti, 2017; Lokhman et al., 2018). As shown in Fig. 29.2, the esports ecosystem is composed of a multitude of interrelated stakeholders. We will now provide a brief overview of the esports industry and its stakeholders.

Game Publishers and Video Games. At the center of the esports ecosystem are the game publishers and their video games. Historically, the rights holders were not very involved, or even absent, in the organization and regulation of the esports tournaments and leagues that utilized their games. But, since the 2010s and esports' constant economic and media growth since then, publishers have more recently regained "control" of their IP and are working in concert to varying degrees with the other actors in the value chain (Ahn et al., 2020).

Players, Coaches and Managers. The players are the most visible part of the ecosystem. They are the ambassadors and the stars. Performance-oriented, individually or collectively as a team dependent on the game, they use their physical, cognitive, and social skills to win competitions. They are, with very few exceptions, specialists in a single video game. Their careers are currently relatively short due to both the high amounts of repetitive physical and mental stress they incur, as well as and the general lack of health prevention and promotion within the esports community (Schary et al., 2022). Players generally represent a franchise, team, or club (i.e., esports organization). Professional esports players are paid by these organizations for their competitive activity and also sometimes for complementary activities, such as live-streaming entertainment or sponsor promotion. Upon retirement (some as young as their early 20s), many

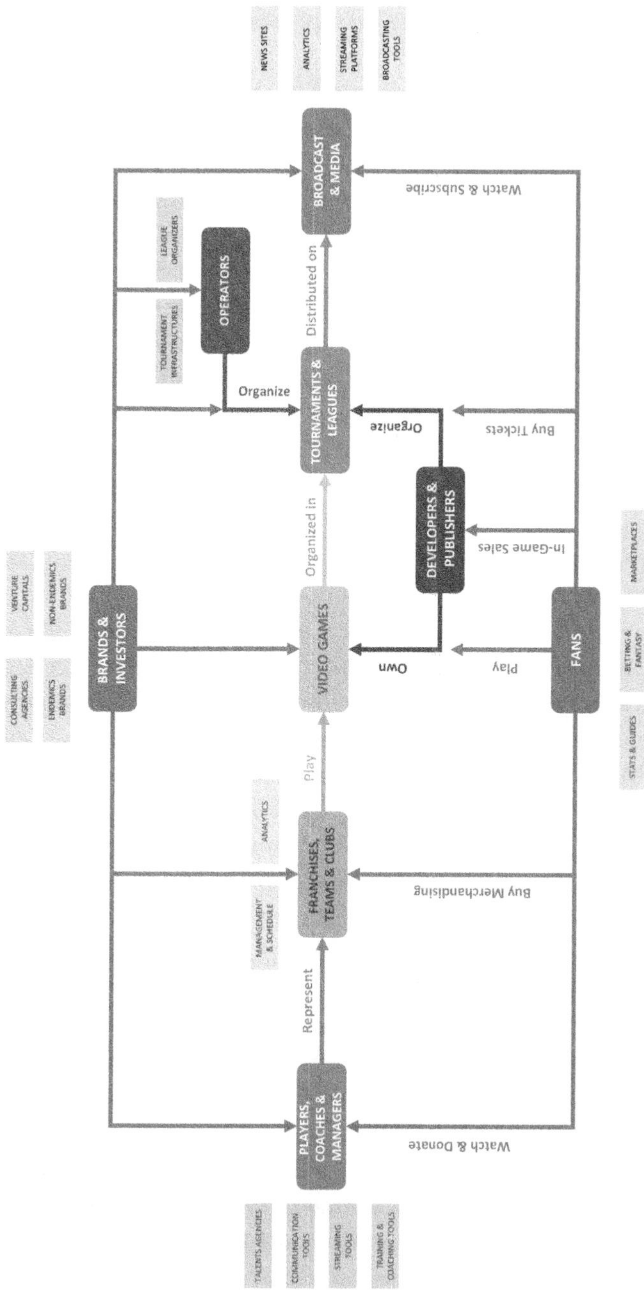

Fig. 29.2 Esports ecosystem at a glance

former professional esports players become coaches, analysts, commentators, or streamers. Talent agencies often act as player agents and support players' careers. Statistical and analytical tool providers can also enable players, coaches, and managers in making informed decisions regarding performance.

Franchises, Teams, and Clubs. Typically, esports franchises and teams refer to for-profit professional esports organizations, while esports clubs are commonly non-profit grassroots entities. In most cases, esports organizations are made up of several players and teams competing across varying video game titles (i.e., "multi-esports" organizations). For example, an esports organization can have a *League of Legends* team, a *Counter-Strike: Global Offensive* team, and a *Rocket League* team, as well as individual players who play the single-player games *FIFA* and *Street Fighter*. Esports teams may also be composed of coaches, managers, and other performance staff (i.e., physical therapist, sport psychologist, etc.), marketing, communication, and social media staff, and human resources and accounting personnel.

Tournaments, Leagues, and Operators. In some cases, the game publisher chooses to delegate the organization of the competitive tournaments and leagues of its video game to third-party organizers, while keeping the regulation of these competitions. Esports event organizers, which can be non-profit or for-profit, are often called operators. The organization of competitions is thus decentralized and the owner of the game IP resides with the game publisher, but is outsourced to operators. Online tournament management platforms may also facilitate the organization of competitions.

Broadcast and Media. Esports competitions are generally broadcasted over the internet through streaming platforms (e.g., Twitch, YouTube). High-speed internet emerged at the end of the 2000s and made esports content widely accessible to many more players and spectators. For many of the biggest global esports tournaments, generally the game publishers and event organizers co-operate the audiovisual production; in the case of national competitions, this is often delegated to local operators and broadcasters who know both the cultural norms and language of the targeted area best. Specialized esports media outlets have surfaced that report on competitions too (e.g., *The Esports Observer*, *Esports Insider*).

Brands and Investors. The esports ecosystem has always been extremely dependent on private funding, from esports dedicated investment funds to brands and advertisers, who are a prime source of revenue for the sector (De Moor et al., 2022). Investment firms often finance various esports-related projects (e.g., building an esports arena, starting an esports league, etc.). However, the nature of partnerships and forms of sponsorship within the esports industry can take very different forms. Historically, the first esports sponsoring brands were "endemic" to esports as they provided products and services directly relating to video gaming (i.e., computer or telecommunications companies). But since the acquisition of Twitch by Amazon in 2014, many progressive investments of "non-endemic" advertisers have entered esports (i.e., companies not directly related to video gaming). Often, their objective is to promote their brand image to Millennials or Generation Z. The sectors from which these brands come from are extremely diverse: the automotive industry, banking, cosmetics, beverages, fast food, aeronautics, insurance, sportswear, betting and gambling, military, etc. Consulting agencies can also act as a link between investors (e.g., Venture Capitals) and the ecosystem.

Fans. Finally, around these key stakeholders are others who have a vital role to play—the fans. This group consumes esports through attending events, spectating online, and purchasing merchandise. Almost all other sectors of the ecosystem target this group.

Gaming and Esports During the Pandemic

Research on recreational video game play prior to and during the pandemic found that players' video game engagement during the pandemic may have assisted with improving player self-perceived vitality (i.e., a measure of wellbeing centered on one's activity and energy levels) and lowering psychological distress (Formosa et al., 2022). Likewise, Nilsson et al. (2022) found that the COVID-19 pandemic resulted in increased video gaming and social media use partly as a function of coping with stress or boredom within Swedish adolescents as they experienced a decline in their self-reported mental health and well-being during lockdown.

Additionally, in an effort to encourage at-home exercise during pandemic lockdown, French game publisher Ubisoft offered free trials of the motion-based video game *Just Dance* while American game developer Niantic updated its mobile games *Pokémon GO* and *Harry Potter: Wizards Unite* (Interactive Software Federation of Europe [ISFE] & European Games Developer Federation [EGDF], 2021). Likewise, some gaming companies attempted to facilitate at-home learning during the pandemic. For instance, the Roblox Corporation included a new teaching remotely resource within their self-titled game while Microsoft Minecraft Marketplace provided new free educational resources (ISFE & EGDF, 2021).

Regarding video gaming attitudes and habits during the pandemic, an online survey study conducted by the Entertainment Software Association (2021) in February 2021 with a representative sample of 4,000 Americans (18 years and older) found the following:

- 55% of video game players reported playing more during the pandemic
- 90% intended to continue to play video games after social distancing regulations were lifted
- 55% reported video games provided stress relief during the pandemic
- 48% reported video games provided a welcome distraction during the pandemic
- 70% of parents reported allowing their child to play more video games during the pandemic

As households around the world were forced to adapt to working, learning, and playing at home, results may have looked similar within European households.

Moreover, during the pandemic, 60% of collegiate esports programs grew and 25% experienced no change in membership numbers, highlighting how the online nature of esports facilitated higher education student engagement in esports across institutions in North America during the pandemic despite more than half never hosting an in-person activity (Postell & Narayan, 2021). However, while participation numbers increased, economic effects of the pandemic resulted in the majority of North American esports collegiate programs experiencing lower annual operating budgets and delayed scheduled renovations or new construction of esports venues on campus (Postell & Narayan, 2021). Similarly, the pandemic caused supply-chain issues of computer and gaming hardware as well as negatively impacted the mass implementation of 5G—the fifth-generation technology standard for broadband cellular networks which can facilitate telecommunication speeds, particularly with mobile esports (NewZoo, 2021).

From a media perspective, esports events have benefited from increased exposure during this period when most other sports and cultural activities were at a standstill. Record online spectatorship was achieved within several major competitive esports circuits. For instance, the League of Legends European Championship Summer Split increased from 177K average viewers and 22M hours watched in 2019 to 301K average viewers and 41M hours watched in 2020 (Esports Charts, 2021). All of these events were held remotely, with each team playing from their own training/performance center, or each player logging into the game from home and coordinating via live voice chat tools like Discord or TeamSpeak.

Moreover, some previously less popular esports game genres emerged for mass public consumption during the pandemic, especially simracing and sports simulation games (Furchgott, 2021). Due to their unprecedented availability, famous international sports athletes competed during some of these sports simulation virtual events, resulting in further promotion of esports amongst the general population (e.g., Charles Leclerc played in the F1 Esports Virtual Grand Prix Series (F1 Esports Series, 2020); Chris Froome played in the Virtual Tour de France (Ballinger, 2020); Andy Murray played in the Mutua Madrid Open Virtual Pro (ESPN, 2020); Denny Hamlin participated in the eNASCAR iRacing Pro Invitational Series (Haislop, 2020)). In some cases—notably eCycling, virtual Formula 1, or eSailing—the federations in charge of these sports (i.e., governing bodies) had already started a shift towards digital versions of their sport years prior, including esports broadcasts. It appeared that some traditional sporting entities discovered during the pandemic that broadcasting the virtual form of sport can be lucrative and help attract new fans, as was the case with the International Basketball Federation (FIBA) and International Olympic Committee (IOC). In many cases, these actors have been assisted and supported by specialized esports stakeholders. For instance, the first Olympic Virtual Series held in

2021 relied on the expertise of DreamHack Sports Games, a Swedish company who organizes major esports events in Scandinavia and throughout the world, to assist in marketing and producing the event (IOC, 2021).

However, these events were not without controversy as some traditional sport athletes who made the transition to esports "behaved badly" during livestreamed events. For example, NASCAR driver Kyle Larson was fired from his racing team after saying a racial slur during a live eNASCAR virtual race broadcast (ESPN News Service, 2020). Also, a series of what appeared to be reckless driving behavior exhibited by professional INDYCAR drivers participating in the INDYCAR iRacing Challenge occurred where drivers seemed to deliberately crash other driver's virtual cars and drive in the virtual environment in ways known to be unsafe in the authentic INDYCAR environment, calling into question the character of some drivers (Witkowski et al., 2021). This only appeared to further increase the media spotlight on these esports events.

Overall, much of the general media reports on gaming and esports during the pandemic glorified surges in player and viewer statistics with little attention to the objective economic impact of COVID-19 lockdown regulations of mid-size and smaller companies within the esports ecosystem.

Literature Gap and Research Questions

While there were some overt negative ramifications, the pandemic and related lockdown requirements appeared by many outsiders to have only positive economic effects on the global and local video game markets due to increased media coverage, viewership, and levels of engagement of online gaming. Internationally, the video gaming market saw a 19.6% growth over 2019 (i.e., pre-pandemic), representing a consolidated revenue of $174.9 billion USD (Wijman, 2020). Similarly, within France, the game publisher trade union reported revenues of 5.3 billion euros for 2020, representing a growth of 11.3% from the previous year (SELL, 2021). Therefore, according to aforementioned esports-hyped media reports (i.e., focusing on increased participation of online gaming and streaming, but not resultant economic impacts), one might assume even higher revenues for the esports industry across the COVID-19 pandemic.

Unfortunately, little past research has investigated the pandemic's economic impact on the esports industry. Past research in this area has been limited to mere audience statistics (e.g., Geyser, 2021) or the entire video gaming industry sales (e.g., Dealessandri, 2021), which has been influenced by increased time spent at home due to social distancing restrictions. Therefore, this study was guided by the following research questions: What were the economic consequences of the pandemic upon the esports market? Did the additional media exposure that esports received during the pandemic period (i.e., March 2020 to February 2021) have a positive effect upon esports market revenue? Has the pandemic had the same or varied impact on the different types of esports stakeholders, based upon their activities, legal status, or size? Answers to these questions, therefore, help in understanding the interweaving of the health, social, and economic issues impacted by the pandemic within the case of esports. Results from this research may allow for the implementation of tools and systems that would help promote the sustainability of the esports industry and its related stakeholders (Nyström et al., 2022).

While these questions may apply globally, this study targeted impacts specifically within the French esports ecosystem. Although esports is a global phenomenon, it is nonetheless crossed by many cultural and geographical specificities. In this respect, the case of France constitutes a fertile ground for esports analysis due to its dynamic domestic esports industry. France holds a unique presence in the global esports ecosystem as numerous stakeholders of the esports value-chain reside there. First, there are several international video game publishers headquartered in France (e.g., Ubisoft, Ankama). Also, there are plethora of French esports organizations (e.g., Vitality, Karmine Corp., LDLC OL), as well as a well-developed non-profit esports ecosystem (e.g., Futurolan, Lyon Esport, 3 Hit Combo) that has resided in France for more than twenty years. More importantly, the biggest global video game publishers and gaming console providers have branch offices in France, such as Riot Games, Electronic Arts, Capcom, Activision Blizzard, Microsoft Xbox, and Sony PlayStation. Moreover, local public authorities and the French government have supported esports legislative, economic, and social development since the 2016 law for a Digital Republic (Vansyngel et al., 2018). As a result, France is now one of the major esports markets of Europe, alongside Great Britain, Germany and Denmark.

Methodology and Data Collection

To evaluate the economic impact of the health crisis on the French esports sector, a targeted online survey was conducted via purposive sampling method, disseminated both by email and social media networks among French esports industry stakeholders (e.g., esports clubs or teams, event organizers, equipment manufacturers, service providers, agencies, and specialized media). Several targeted follow-ups were also performed using snowball-sampling techniques acquired by the first author within the surveyed population.

This 10-question quantitative survey centered on questions relating to estimated losses and gains in revenue of these French esports stakeholders (e.g., *What is your raw estimation of the economic impact of the health crisis on your activity, either in terms of decrease OR increase of revenues for the year?*), the organizational adaptations they have made (e.g., *What business-related measures has your organization taken in response to the pandemic?*), and the French governmental support measures they favored most (e.g., *Among the various support measures put in place by the government, which have been most beneficial?*). In addition to these economic questions, demographic questions were asked about the legal status of the organization, the number of Full-time Equivalent (FTE) positions (described in more detail in the discussion below), and the main esports-related business activities provided. The questionnaire was distributed via Google Form while data analysis (i.e., flat and cross sorting as well as descriptive statistics) were performed using Microsoft Excel.

Data collection was conducted over two time periods, first between 30 March and 5 May 2020. Then, between 19 January and 2 February 2021, respondents were given the opportunity to revise their first responses in order to improve accuracy. Overall, 101 questionnaires were collected (72 in the first period and 29 in the second). Fifteen responses were discarded due to duplication. Thus, 86 total responses were utilized for data analysis.

Main Findings and Discussion of Results

Sample demographics

The majority of respondents represented private esports-related companies (59.3%; n = 51), while 24.4% worked for non-profit esports organizations (i.e., associations) (n = 21), 15.1% were self-employed individuals who work within the French esports industry (n = 13), and one respondent (1.2%) preferred not to answer.

As Fig. 29.3 illustrates, the sample was involved in multiple esports-related business activities, with respondents reporting an average of 2.1 (± 1.0) activities. For example, although the main activity of esports teams is to manage players' performance, many of them diversify their activities by also broadcasting content on streaming platforms, organizing physical or online entertainment events, or assisting advertisers or investors with their esports communication strategies. The majority of the sample disclosed being involved with esports event organization, with other commonly reported esports-related activities being consulting

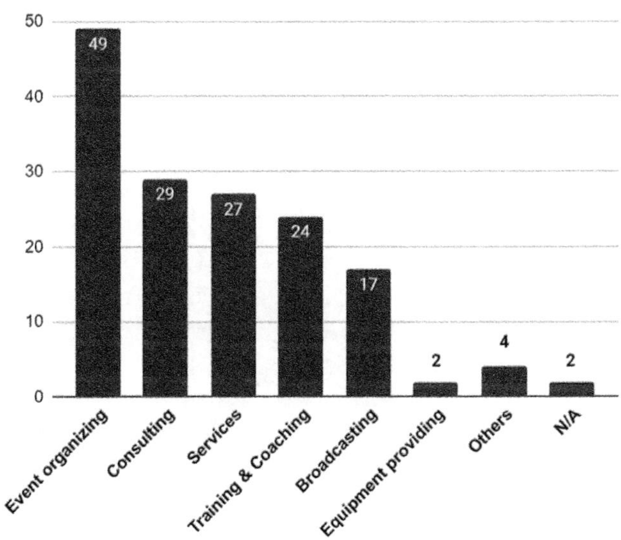

Fig. 29.3 Respondents' main esports activities

(e.g., communication, marketing, career management consulting), esports services (e.g., tool development, online coaching platforms), esports training and coaching, and esports content distribution.

Estimation of the Health Crisis Effects on the French Esports Market

Findings listed in Fig. 29.4 display the respondents reported revenue loss or gain as a result of the COVID-19 pandemic. Results revealed that the vast majority (89.5% and n = 77) of the sample reported that the health crisis had a negative impact on their income. Strikingly, nearly one third of respondents (32.6% and n = 28) estimated their losses to be more than 50% of their typical pre-pandemic revenues. Conversely, only 4.7% of respondents (n = 4) reported that the pandemic positively impacted revenues.

These reported massive losses may be explained by: 1) the multiple cancellations or postponements of (inter)national esports in-person

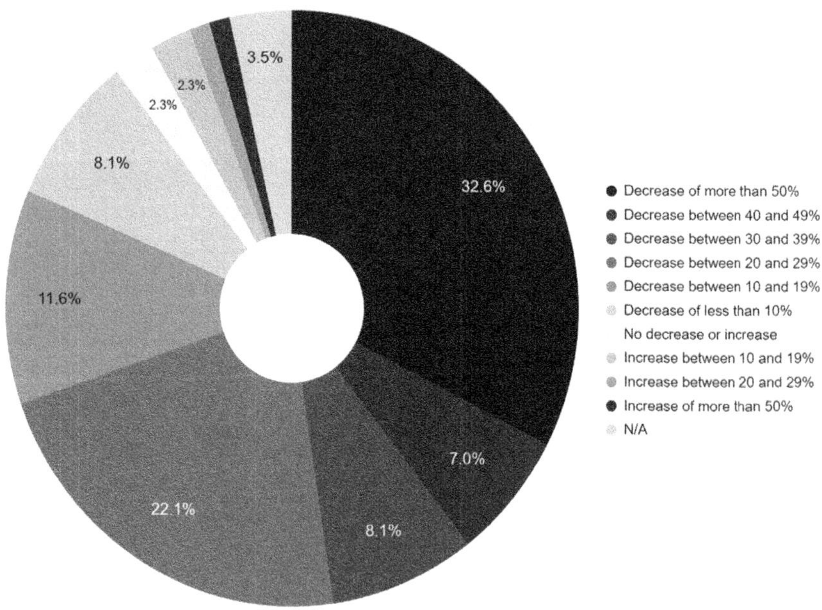

Fig. 29.4 Estimated percentage loss or gain in revenues per respondent

events within France and surrounding regions that could have resulted in a lack of ticketing and other on-site revenues; and, 2) the suspension or postponement of economic partnership agreements with teams or tournament organizers. As Mangeloja (2019) notes, the esports industry is heavily dependent on sponsorships and private investors. It appears that the reduction of non-endemic esports sponsors and investors (i.e., entities whose primary purpose are not esports-related activities) has led to the need for these organizations to make financial compromises (i.e., securing their own employee's salaries) rather than investing in or marketing through esports. In other words, companies outside of esports (e.g., Nike, Renault) may focus on spending money paying their employees rather than providing money to an esports organization or esports event organizer as a sponsor. Beyond the loss of funding which has made many esports stakeholders insecure, the successive shutdowns of public spaces, associated with the lack of awareness concerning possible reopening, have forced some entities to cease all activities, including, for example, the Toulouse Esport Concept in May 2020 and the Esport Stadium in Paris in February 2021—both of which have terminated as businesses.

Moreover, based upon survey responses, Table 29.1 provides a measure of the economic impact of the health crisis on the French esports market. Here, respondents report the amount of lost or gained revenue due to the COVID-19 pandemic. While just shy of one quarter of the respondents (24.4%) estimated that they had lost less than 10,000 euros, nearly a third (29.1%) estimated their loss of earnings at more than 100,000 euros. Across the respondents who reported losses (88.4% and n=76), total losses ranged from 6.95 million to 13.24 million euros. Conversely, the total cumulative gains of the 4.7% of respondents (n = 4) who reported an increase in income over the period only ranged from 110,000 to 240,000 euros. When aggregated, the overall impact of the health crisis on the surveyed sample is between 6.71 million (minimum losses + maximum gains) and 13.13 million euros (maximum losses + minimum gains).

Within a French esports market estimated between 47.5 and 53.3 million euros in 2019 (Cepheïd, 2021)—including professional teams, event organizers, content producers and broadcasters, and multi-activities stakeholders—this represents an estimated loss of 13.4% to 26.3% in revenue. These results parallel other findings observed in Spain where esports

Table 29.1 Estimated amount of lost or gained revenue per respondent

	Number of Respondents	%	Minimum Amount	Maximum Amount
Loss of more than 1M€	2	2.3%	-2 000 000 €	-2 000 000 €
Loss of 500K to 1M€	1	1.2%	- 500 000 €	-1 000 000 €
Loss of 200K to 500K€	14	16.3%	-2 800 000 €	-7 000 000 €
Loss of 100K to 200K€	8	9.3%	- 800 000 €	-1 600 000 €
Loss of 50K to 100K€	7	8.1%	- 350 000 €	- 700 000 €
Loss of 40K to 50K€	4	4.7%	- 160 000 €	- 200 000 €
Loss of 30K to 40K€	6	7.0%	- 180 000 €	- 240 000 €
Loss of 20K to 30K€	3	3.5%	- 60 000 €	- 90 000 €
Loss of 10K to 20K€	10	11.6%	- 100 000 €	- 200 000 €
Loss of less than 10K€	21	24.4%	0 €	- 210 000 €
TOTAL LOSSES	**76**	**88.4%**	**-6 950 000 €**	**-13 240 000 €**
No loss or gain	2	2.3%	0 €	0 €
Gain of less than 10K€	2	2.3%	0 €	20 000 €
Gain of 10K to 20K€	1	1.2%	10 000 €	20 000 €
Gain of 20K to 30K€	0	0.0%	0 €	0 €
Gain of 30K to 40K€	0	0.0%	0 €	0 €
Gain of 40K to 50K€	0	0.0%	0 €	0 €
Gain of 50K to 100K€	0	0.0%	0 €	0 €
Gain of 100K to 200K€	1	1.2%	100 000 €	200 000 €
Gain of 200K to 500K€	0	0.0%	0 €	0 €
Gain from 500K to 1M€	0	0.0%	0 €	0 €
Gain of more than 1M€	0	0.0%	0 €	0 €
TOTAL GAINS	**4**	**4.7%**	**110 000 €**	**240 000 €**
Prefer not to Answer	*4*	*4.7%*	*0 €*	*0 €*
GLOBAL	**86**	**100.0%**	**-6 710 000 €**	**-13 130 000 €**

industry losses were estimated at 23% for 2020, or more than 8 million euros within the Spanish esports market estimated at 27 million euros (Asociación Española de Videojuegos, 2020). In the next section we will attempt to determine which type of French esports stakeholders were the hardest hit and which fared best economically during the pandemic.

Health Crisis Effects Based on Stakeholders' Characteristics

Given the characteristics of this study's sample, it is possible that the most "robust" or largest stakeholders were impacted the least due to potentially more free cash flow as a result of more sustainable business models. These companies are generally composed of a large number of employees and diversify their activities in order not to be dependent on a single source of revenue. Some large organizations develop a multitude of internal departments that encompass several different esports sectors. For example, the French offices of the multinational corporation Webedia (a media agency that produces activations around esports) includes its own esports player management agency (Bang Bang Management), a tournament management platform (Toornament), its own competition organizer (Electronic Sports World Convention), its own online media (MGG) and television channel (ES1) dedicated to esports, and, finally, its own esports arena for players and spectators. However, in the case of a majority of smaller and thus potentially more fragile stakeholders (i.e., non-profit organizations, smaller companies, self-employed individuals), it is possible that the economic consequences of the pandemic were more significant despite the aid released by the French Government (e.g., funding for employees forced to move from full-time to part-time employment, rescheduling of bank loans, and delays in the payment of social or tax liabilities) (Ministère de l'Économie, des Finances et de la Relance, 2020). Table 29.2 seems to confirm this notion.

In this study we define "micro-companies" as companies with an FTE (Full-time Equivalent) of less than 10. FTE is a rough estimation of the number of employees. For instance, if the average work week is 40 hours, a 0.5 FTE employee would be an employee who works 20 hours per week. As seen in Table 29.2, while small and medium-sized companies (FTE > 10) are proportionally more likely to estimate their losses at between 0 and 29% of their turnover, non-profit organizations, and micro-companies (FTE < 10) are proportionally more likely to have estimated their losses at over 40%. Thus, the latter, which make up 75.6% of the survey respondents (n = 65), represent respectively 100% and 89.3% of the stakeholders who estimate their losses at between 40 and 49% and more than 50% of their revenues. In other words, the most impacted sampled French esports stakeholders by the pandemic were micro-companies with an FTE less than 10.

Conversely, small and medium-sized companies (SMC), which make up only 18.6% of the survey sample (n = 16), represent between 20 and 28.6% of the stakeholders who experienced a decrease of between 0 and

Table 29.2 Estimated percentage of lost revenue for each respondent based on the number of FTEs

	NUMBER OF FULL-TIME EQUIVALENT (FTE) POSITIONS													
	0	**1-5**	**6-10**	**TOTAL**	**%**	**11-20**	**21-50**	**50+**	**TOTAL**	**%**	**Prefer not to Answer**	**TOTAL**	**%**	
Decrease of more than 50%	12	8	5	25	**89.3%**	2			2	7.1%	1	28	32.6%	**89.6 %**
Decrease between 40 and 49%	2	2	2	6	**100.0%**				0	0.0%		6	7.0%	
Decrease between 30 and 39%	1	4		5	71.4%		1		1	14.3%	1	7	8.1%	
Decrease between 20 and 29%	4	6	2	12	63.2%	3	2		5	**26.3%**	2	19	22.1%	
Decrease between 10 and 19%	4	3	1	8	80.0%	2			2	**20.0%**		10	11.6%	
Decrease of less than 10%	3	1	1	5	71.4%	1	1		2	**28.6%**		7	8.1%	
No decrease or increase				0	0.0%		1	1	2	100.0%		2	2.3%	**2.3 %**
Increase of less than 10%				0	0.0%				0	0.0%		0	0	**4.7 %**
Increase between 10 and 19%	1			1	50.0%	1			1	50.0%		2	2.3%	
Increase between 20 and 29%				0	0.0%				0	0.0%	1	1	1.2%	
Increase between 30 and 39%				0	0.0%				0	0.0%		0	0.0%	
Increase between 40 and 49%				0	0.0%				0	0.0%		0	0.0%	
Increase of more than 50%	1			1	100.0%				0	0.0%		1	1.2%	
Prefer not to answer	*1*	*1*		*2*	*66.7%*		*1*		*1*	*33.3%*		*3*	*3.5%*	***3.5 %***
TOTAL	**29**	**25**	**11**	**65**	**75.6%**	**9**	**6**	**1**	**16**	**18.6%**	**5**	**86**	**100.0%**	**100 %**
	MICRO-COMPANIES					**SMALL & MEDIUM COMPANIES (SMC)**								

Note: NPO = non-profit organization.

29%. When aggregated, the estimated losses of micro-companies are estimated to be between 4.76 million and 7.88 million euros, while they are between 1.9 million and 5.11 million euros for small and medium-sized companies.

These results appear to mirror findings by Scerbakov et al. (2022) who investigated the impact of the COVID-19 pandemic on live-stream broadcasters on Twitch. Twitch is a massively popular live-streaming platform that centers on live-streaming video game content, including esports competitions. A longitudinal time-series design analysis of Twitch broadcasters (n = 23,019) revealed that while Twitch benefited from a substantial boost in broadcasters joining, increased content posted, and improved overall views in Twitch during the pandemic, the "established streamers" benefited more strongly than did the newcomer streamers. In other words, while the newcomers (i.e., smaller "companies") may have facilitated outward growth of Twitch through increased Broadcast participation, the increased viewership numbers (which translates to increased revenue for broadcasters) primarily came from already established pre-pandemic broadcasters (i.e., larger "companies").

Finally, results indicated that the most severely impacted esports stakeholders by this health crisis were undoubtedly esports event organizers. Respondents who indicated that they were involved in event organizing (n = 49), of which only 16.3% (n = 8) had "event cancellation" or "business interruption" insurance, accumulated losses estimated at between 4.7 and 8.65 million euros—i.e. approximately two-thirds (between 65.9 and 70%) of the overall losses estimated for all survey respondents.

The effects of the pandemic on esports events are also reflected by the total amounts of cash prizes distributed to esports players. Consequently, numerous tournament cancellations in 2020 led to a decrease in players' winnings and net income. This had less of an impact on esports professional players who were under an organizational contract (e.g., typically professional *League of Legends* or *Counter-Strike: Global Offensive players*), but was a major blow to the vast majority of esports players qualified as amateurs. These players do not have regular income and are highly dependent on the financial gains they earn when they win an esports tournament. Figure 29.5 displays the cumulative amount of cash prizes in 2020, which dropped drastically due to the COVID-19 pandemic.

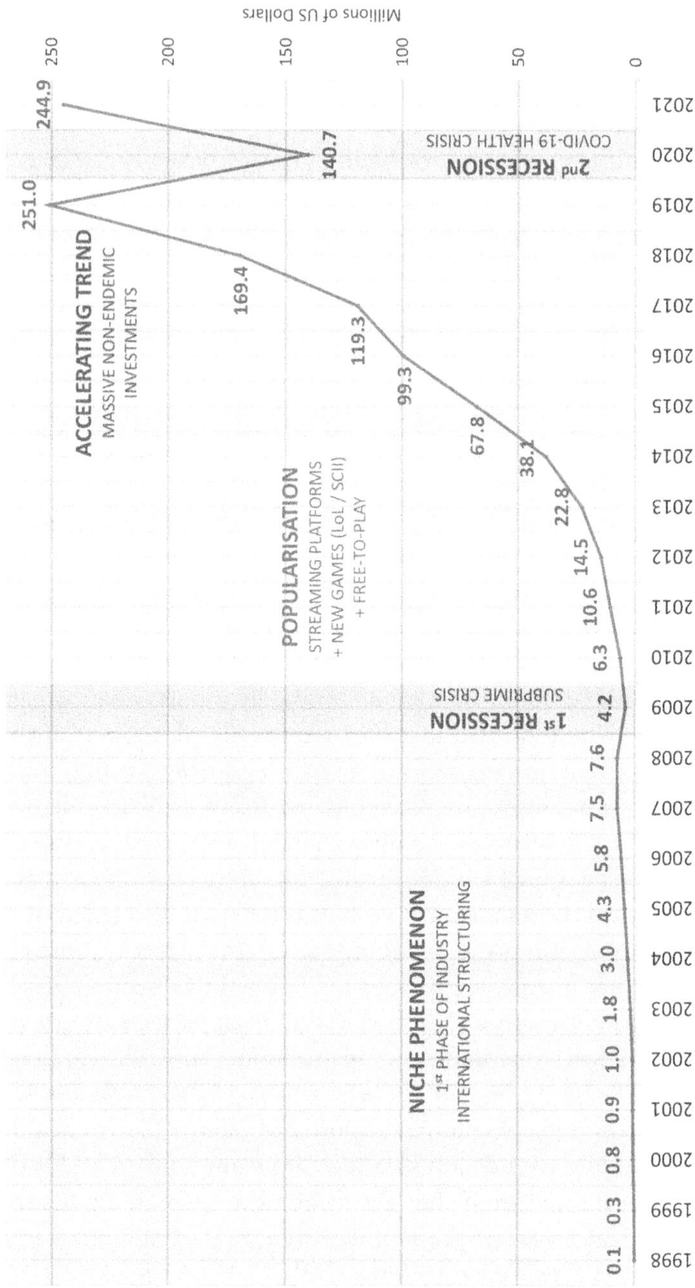

Fig. 29.5 Total prize money distributed in esports per year between 1998 and 2021 per Esports Earnings (2022)

Overall, this study's results confirm, to some extent, those of the annual report of the market research institute Newzoo (October 2020 Update). For the first time since the banking and financial crisis of 2008, the global esports market experienced a regression (i.e., -1.1% in 2020 compared to 2019). After more than ten years of growth, the pandemic retarded the constant worldwide growth of the esports industry, stagnating in 2020 below the symbolic billion-dollar mark for two consecutive years ($947.1 million) (Newzoo, October 2020 Update). Among the most impacted revenue sources, according to Newzoo, were merchandising and ticketing (-50.8% compared to 2019), confirming once again that the event sector of the esports industry may have suffered the most. At the same time, as a direct result of multiple esports competition cancellations, the cumulative annual prize money dropped 43.9%, from $251M in 2019 to $140.7M in 2020 (Esports Earnings, 2022).

Moreover, a joint report by ISFE and EGDF (2021) noted that "the pandemic was still especially hard on smaller and medium-sized companies. To remedy this, EGDF, for example, held the *European Games BizDev Gathering* event for companies to pitch online during the pandemic" (p. 3). While hard economic data was not shared in this report, this sentiment is consistent with our results that the pandemic negatively hurt European smaller companies within the European games industry.

In the specific case of France, an additional hurdle has been highlighted by the pandemic. Since 2016 and Article 101 of the Law for a Digital Republic, only in-person events are excluded from the lottery regulation and therefore can collect registration fees from competitors. In other words, online competitions in France can only be offered free of charge. Indeed, there are many non-profit organizations (i.e., associations) which organize small weekly or monthly in-person tournaments bringing together a few dozen players. In these cases, the registration fees are mainly used to amortize the expenses related to the organization of the event and constitute modest cash prizes for the winners, which make it possible to attract competitors. However, the French law prohibiting fees for online tournaments has prevented these stakeholders from continuing their activity during pandemic lockdown and forced many to cease operations because online competitions cannot charge fees under penalty. In this context, the French regulation of online video game competitions is a particularly urgent issue for the event-based part of the sector, especially for non-profit organizations and micro-companies that are already particularly vulnerable.

Limitations

Despite the methodological precautions taken, limitations of this study must be considered. First, survey data was self-reported by respondents. Next, the study's sample may not be considered representative of the entire French esports ecosystem, thus potentially limiting generalizability of results. For example, French video game publishers were not included in the sample as esports revenues could not be separated from recreational video gaming revenues. The results must therefore be interpreted with caution and are, as such, only indicators of trends within this sample.

Conclusion

Contrary to appearances, the organization of exclusively online competitions, although particularly beneficial for the visibility of the esports sector, does not appear to be a sustainable solution. Despite the maintenance of some major online-streamed competitions without in-person audiences, and the increase in interest in certain tournaments utilizing specific game genres (e.g., simracing, sports video games), the esports sector experienced a regression in its global market revenue due to the COVID-19 pandemic. In the case of France, the results of this study demonstrated a loss of revenue between 13% and 26% compared to the previous year. It appears that online events are only a temporary substitute that may not permit emotions shared on site by competitors and spectators, whether in an international sports arena or in a local festival hall. On the other hand, these physical gatherings are often exhibition spaces for the economic partners and sponsors of the organizers and the teams. In-person events are many times investors' showcases for the last twenty years, and historically could be linked to the greater emergence of esports in the late 1990s as to its further popularization at the turn of the 2010s.

The uncertainty regarding the possibility of resuming in-person competitions that can host spectators currently represented a real threat to the sector. Indeed, the transfer of physical events to online competitions has highlighted the precariousness of the economic models of exclusively online events. Certainly, the pandemic has illuminated esports companies who rely primarily on in-person revenue streams. Conversely, the pandemic may have also showed how successful esports companies must be able to pivot quickly and generate revenues from varying sources. In addition to the lack of ticketing revenue from physical spectators, the difficulty of finding economic partners due to the multiplication of this type of online event over the past year is added.

In sum, the results of this study contradict the idea that the increased general media exposure of esports due to the global health situation adequately "benefited" esports overall economically. While esports has been able to take advantage of its inherent digital nature and continue some of its activities through offering online content (at a time when the cultural and sports industries were at a complete standstill), paradoxically the esports industry in France still suffered, like many other sectors, from the economic and social crisis that the pandemic created. While the digital flexibility that esports offers still remains, the basis of its resilience may reside within in-person competition.

References

Ahn, J., Collis, W., & Jenny, S. (2020). The one billion dollar myth: Methods for sizing the massively undervalued esports revenue landscape. *International Journal of Esports, 1*(1), 1–19. https://www.ijesports.org/article/15/html

Asociación Española de Videojuegos. (2020, May). *Anuario 2020 de la industria del videojuego en España*. http://www.aevi.org.es/web/wp-content/uploads/2021/04/AEVI_Anuario_2020.pdf

Baker, B. (2020, June 17). Esports gets a lift during pandemic. https://penntoday.upenn.edu/news/esports-gets-lift-during-pandemic

Ballinger, A. (2020, July 11). Zwift Virtual Tour de France 2020: Everything you need to know. https://www.cyclingweekly.com/news/racing/tour-de-france/zwift-announce-first-ever-virtual-tour-de-france-for-both-men-and-women-featuring-chris-froome-egan-bernal-and-marianne-vos-458768

Brambilla Hall, S. P. L. (2020, May 15). COVID-19 is taking gaming and esports to the next level. https://www.weforum.org/agenda/2020/05/covid-19-taking-gaming-and-esports-next-level

Cepheïd. (2021, June). *Analyse du marché et perspectives pour le secteur de l'esport* (Rep.). Direction Générale des Entreprises (DGE). https://www.entreprises.gouv.fr/files/files/etudes-et-statistiques/etude_esport_rapport.pdf

Cranmer, E. E., Han, D. I. D., van Gisbergen, M., & Jung, T. (2021). Esports matrix: Structuring the esports research agenda. *Computers in Human Behavior*. [Online]. 117 (July 2020). p. 106671. https://doi.org/10.1016/j.chb.2020.106671

De Moor, W., Terrien, M., Durand, C., & Besombes, N. (2022). The current situation of the French professional esports industry: Economic models of the clubs and regulation of the leagues. *European Sport Management Quarterly*, 1–22.

Dealessandri, M. (2021). 2020 sees record US games spending at $56.9bn: US annual report. *Gamer Network Limited*. https://www.gamesindustry.biz/articles/2021-01-15-2020-sees-record-us-games-spending-at-usd56-9bn-us-annual-report

Direction générale de la migration et des affaires intérieures. (2020, mai). *Communication de la Commission au Parlement Européen, au Conseil Européen et au Conseil concernant la deuxième évaluation de l'application de la restriction temporaire des déplacements non essentiels vers l'UE*. https://ec.europa.eu/transparency/documents-register/detail?ref=COM(2020)222&lang=fr

Entertainment Software Association. (2021). 2021 essential facts about the video game industry. https://www.theesa.com/resource/2021-essential-facts-about-the-video-game-industry

ESPN. (2020, May 1). Murray, Bertens win Madrid Open Virtual Pro titles. (2020, May 01). https://www.espn.com/tennis/story/_/id/29121994/murray-bertens-win-madrid-open-virtual-pro-titles

ESPN News Service. (2020). NASCAR star Kyle Larson fired for using racial slur in virtual race. *Associated Press*. https://www.espn.com/racing/nascar/story/_/id/29034370/nascar-star-kyle-larson-fired-using-racial-slur-virtual-race

Esports Earnings. (2022). Esports Earnings. https://www.esportsearnings.com

Europe 1. (2020, July 07). La rétro sport—L'E-Sport, grand gagnant du confinement. https://www.europe1.fr/emissions/Le-journal-des-sports/la-retro-sport-le-sport-grand-gagnant-du-confinement-3979665

F1 Esports Series. (2020, April 20). Charles Leclerc Takes Back-to-back Virtual Grand Prix Wins! (2020, April 20). https://f1esports.com/news/charles-leclerc-takes-back-to-back-virtual-grand-prix-wins

Formosa, E., Johnson, D., Türkay, S., & Mandryk, R. L. (2022). Need satisfaction, passion and wellbeing effects of videogame play prior to and during the COVID-19 pandemic. *Computers in Human Behavior, 131*, 107232. https://doi.org/10.1016/j.chb.2022.107232

Furchgott, R. (2021, January 18). Pandemic Paved the Way for Sim Racing, but Will It Last? https://www.nytimes.com/2021/01/18/business/sim-racing-enascar.html

Geyser, W. (2021, July 14). The incredible growth of eSports [+eSports statistics]. *Influencer Marketing Hub.* https://influencermarketinghub.com/esports-stats

Gounel, D. (2020, March 26). Coronavirus : L'e-sport, le grand gagnant de cette crise. https://www.midilibre.fr/2020/03/25/coronavirus-le-sport-le-grand-gagnant-de-cette-crise,8819005.php

Haislop, T. (2020, April 13). What is NASCAR iRacing? How the virtual races work, drivers, full schedule & more. https://www.sportingnews.com/us/nascar/news/nascar-iracing-virtual-races-drivers-schedule/a53c8e5widhd14na1jinsz7rq

Interactive Software Federation of Europe & European Games Developer Federation. (2021). Key facts 2020: The year we played together. https://www.isfe.eu/wp-content/uploads/2021/10/2021-ISFE-EGDF-Key-Facts-European-video-games-sector-FINAL.pdf

International Olympic Committee. (2021, April 22). IOC makes landmark move into virtual sports by announcing first-ever Olympic Virtual Series. *IOC News.* https://olympics.com/ioc/news/international-olympic-committee-makes-landmark-move-into-virtual-sports-by-announcing-first-ever-olympic-virtual-series

Jenny, S. E., Manning, R. D., Keiper, M. C., & Olrich, T. W. (2017). Virtual(ly) athletes: Where eSports fit within the definition of "sport". *Quest, 69*(1), 1–18. https://doi.org/10.1080/00336297.2016.1144517

Karhulahti, V. M. (2017). Reconsidering esport: Economics and executive ownership. *Physical Culture and Sport, Studies and Research, 74*(1), 43–53. https://content.sciendo.com/view/journals/pcssr/74/1/article-p43.xml

Lokhman, N., Karashchuk, O., & Kornilova, O. (2018). Analysis of esports as a commercial activity. *Problems and Perspectives in Management, 16*(1), 207–213. https://doi.org/10.21511/ppm.16

Mangeloja, E. (2019). Economics of Esports. In T. Takala, T. Auvinen, M. Vesa, J. Tienari, P. Sajasalo, S. Heikkinen, J. Helms Mills, & M. Kallinen-Kuisma (Eds.), *Electronic Journal of Business Ethics and Organization Studies. 24*(2). *Special issue: Implications of Digitalization on Organizations and Leadership: Esports, Gamification and Beyond* (pp. 34-42).

Ministère de l'Économie, des Finances et de la Relance. (2020). Coronavirus COVID-19 : Soutien aux entreprises. https://www.economie.gouv.fr/covid19-soutien-entreprises

NewZoo. (2021). NewZoo's games, esports, and mobile trends to watch in 2021. https://newzoo.com/insights/trend-reports/newzoos-2021-trends-to-watch-games-esports-mobile

Newzoo 2020 Global Esports Market Report. (2020, October 07). COVID-19 Continues to Impact the Esports Market: Newzoo Revises Its Esports Revenue Forecast. https://newzoo.com/insights/articles/covid-19-continues-to-impact-the-esports-market-newzoo-revises-its-esports-revenue-forecast

Nilsson, A., Rosendahl, I., & Jayaram-Lindström, N. (2022). Gaming and social media use among adolescents in the midst of the COVID-19 pandemic. *Nordic Studies on Alcohol and Drugs, 1-15*, 1. https://doi.org/10.1177/14550725221074997

Nyström, A.-G., McCauley, B., Macey, J., Scholz, T. M., Besombes, N., Cestino, J., Hiltscher, J., Orme, S., Rumble, R., & Törhönen, M. (2022). Current issues of sustainability in esports. *International Journal of Esports, 1*(1), 1. https://www.ijesports.org/article/94/html

Peng, Q., Dickson, G., Scelles, N., Grix, J., & Brannagan, P. M. (2020). Esports Governance: Exploring Stakeholder Dynamics. *Sustainability, 12*(19), 1. https://www.mdpi.com/2071-1050/12/19/8270

Postell, C. & Narayan, K. (2021). Trends in collegiate esports: 2021 report. *Esports Foundry*. https://esportsfoundry.com/Trends-in-Collegiate-Esports.html

Scerbakov, A., Pirker, J., & Kappe, F. (2022). When a pandemic enters the game: The initial and prolonged impact of the COVID-19 pandemic on live-stream broadcasters on Twitch. *Proceedings of the 55th Hawaii International Conference on System Sciences*. Honolulu, Hawaii, USA.

Schary, D. P., Jenny, S. E., & Koshy, A. (2022). Leveling up esports health: Current status and call to action. *International Journal of Esports, 1*(1), 1–16. https://www.ijesports.org/article/70/html

Scholz, T. M. (2020). Deciphering the World of eSports. *International Journal on Media Management, 22*(1), 1–12. https://www.tandfonline.com/action/journalInformation?journalCode=hijm20

SELL. (2021, March). *L'essentiel du jeu vidéo—Le bilan du marché français 2020* (Rep.). https://www.sell.fr/sites/default/files/essentiel-jeu-video/ejv_mars_21_web.pdf

Vansyngel, S., Velpry, A., & Besombes, N. (2018). French esports institutionalization. In *GamiFIN Proceedings*, 123-130.

Wijman, T. (2020, November 24). Global game revenues up an extra $15 billion this year as engagement skyrockets. https://newzoo.com/insights/articles/game-engagement-during-covid-pandemic-adds-15-billion-to-global-games-market-revenue-forecast

Witkowski, E., Midgley, G., Stein, A., Miller, G., & Diamond, J. (2021). Racing with the industry: An interview on motorsports, esports, livestreaming and the COVID-19 pandemic. *Sport in Society*. https://doi.org/10.1080/17430437.2021.1997989

Zalamea, N. (2020, June 1). Every esports event disrupted by the COVID-19 coronavirus outbreak (updated). *One Esports*. https://www.oneesports.gg/gaming/every-esports-event-disrupted-by-the-covid-19-coronavirus-outbreak

30

Disaster Football: Billionaire Owners, Shock Therapy, and the Exploitation of the COVID-19 Pandemic in European Football

Adam Beissel and David L. Andrews

"*Only a crisis—actual or perceived—produces real change*"
Milton Friedman, 1962
"*Never let a good crisis go to waste*"
Attributed to Winston Churchill, mid-1940s

Professional football's universal presence and popularity (Giulianotti, 1999) means it is, arguably, spread more invasively than any other sport through the cultural, social, economic, political, and technological fabrics of myriad national formations. As such, the game provides a revealing site for explicating the extensity and intensity of COVID-19's impact upon elite sport. Among other reverberations to the global game, the pandemic led to: numerous leagues, competitions, and major

A. Beissel (✉)
Miami University, Oxford, OH, USA
e-mail: abeissel@miamioh.edu

D. L. Andrews
Physical Cultural Studies Research Group, Department of Kinesiology, University of Maryland, College Park, MD, USA

D. L. Andrews et al. (eds.), *Sport and Physical Culture in Global Pandemic Times*, Global Culture and Sport Series, https://doi.org/10.1007/978-3-031-14387-8_30

tournaments being cancelled and/or postponed; players being forced to train in solitude or via video conferencing; and, fans being prohibited from attending live matches, in some cases for more than a year. However, the economic implications of COVID-19 strictures encompassed the pandemic's most pronounced effects on the "global football ecosystem" (Parnell et al., 2021), leading some to describe this as an existential "crisis" for the game (Maguire, 2021). Following more than a year of restricted numbers of fans in stadia, reduced television audiences, and numerous leagues confronting rights payment deferrals and grant rebates to international broadcasters, the result were estimated losses of €5bn on aggregate operating revenues in European top divisions in 2019/20 directly attributed to the financial effects of COVID (UEFA Benchmarking Report, 2020). A study by market analyst KPMG estimated that twenty of Europe's biggest clubs lost more than €1bn in revenue in 2020, while almost 10% has been reduced off players' average values (European Champions Report, 2021). In terms of domestic competitions, Premier League clubs in England lost an aggregate sum of £1.4 billion over the two seasons affected by the COVID-19 pandemic, including six (6) clubs losing more than £120m in commercial, matchday, and broadcast revenue (SWISS RAMBLE, 2021). An array of football's most powerful stakeholders (e.g., club owners, financial investors, broadcast partners, multinational advertisers) forced to reconcile the downstream impact of event cancellations, decreasing revenues, and increasing costs with little to no advanced notice nor roadmap for the future. In summation, the professional football industry faced unprecedented times due to the financial impact of the COVID-19 pandemic.

COVID-19 thrust the global football ecosystem–a delicate series of diffuse, interconnected, and mutually dependent networks and flows of capital, labor, and consumption (Parnell et al., 2021)–into a state of profound economic shock across its different spatial, temporal, and social settings. Indeed, disruptions to established ways of operating and producing sustainable football economies revealed the extent to which football is the archetypal postmodern sport, in that it is "unusually dependent on commercial media-financed, impossible-to-repeat live events performed before large co-present crowds that form a key part of the spectacle for the many times larger distant audiences using an expanding range of screens" (Rowe, 2020, p. 706). The inability to realize parts, or at times the entirety, of live football spectacles as the primary economic motors of the football ecosystem resulted in professional sport teams and competitive leagues depleting their financial resources, since most football clubs generate little or no positive cash flows, and leagues distribute the vast majority of centrally collected revenue. Interestingly, the financial impact(s) of the COVID-19 pandemic on football overlapped with already–and in some cases accented–the multiple crises and contradictions that had long beset international football: underlying governance issues; growing inequalities within the game; financial, human rights, and corruption scandals; and, a fragile set of geopolitical relations and agreements (Parnell et al., 2021). While the global football ecosystem has been, at times, considered to have 'recession proof' sustainability (Bond et al., 2022), the ecosystem's economic vulnerabilities and organizational fragilities and effectively were laid bare by the impacts and effects of the COVID-19 pandemic.

In response to the financial crisis, football's leadership concerned itself with at once its own short-term economic survival and unabashed self-interest. However, and equally cynically, the denizens of the sport also saw the pandemic as an opportunity to refine the conditions for more efficiently generating and sharing wealth: To completely re-/un-make the global football ecosystem for their own pecuniary advantage. In this manner, the twin dynamics of crisis exploitation and blatant opportunism would come to characterize football's leadership, and strategic decision-making, in response to the economic disruptions of the COVID-19 pandemic. The COVID-19 pandemic rendered the perfect set of conditions for football's hedge-fund billionaire owners, financial oligarchs, petrostate plutocrats, and the cabal of football's ruling elite, to leverage the pandemic as a mechanism for advancing economic and political agendas that would otherwise be met with great opposition were the global community not already embroiled within multiple crises. Crisis-based opportunism is by no means unique to the COVID-19 pandemic, nor is it solely reserved to sport. Widely referred to as the "shock doctrine" (Klein, 2007), it is the tactic used by political and economic leaders to exploit the aftermath of large-scale natural, political, and/or economic crises, by pushing through theretofore questioned policies, programs, and power grabs or resource grabs. Such “shock doctrine” stratagems are, more broadly, characterized as a “disaster capitalism” typified by free-market legitimated “orchestrated raids on the public sphere in the wake of catastrophic events, combined with the treatment of disasters as exciting market opportunities” (Klein, 2007, p. 6). Thus, “disaster capitalism” mobilizes policies that generate profit for select private industries, consolidate power in the hands of a ruling elite, and exploit and exacerbate systemic inequalities. Long subject to the avaricious impulses of corporate and finance capitalism (Karak, 2017; Millward, 2013; Nauright & Ramfjord, 2010; Rookwood & Hughson, 2017), the economic fallout of the COVID-19 pandemic crisis exposed the entire football ecosystem to its own “shock doctrine”. Mirroring Klein’s insights, Football’s “disaster capitalism” was not about fomenting a crisis; it keyed on strategic and immediate responses to events driven, above all else, by securing profit motive advantages. While disaster profiteering is by no means a new concept to sport (see: Boykoff, 2021; Hall & Amore, 2019; Thorpe, 2016; Zirin, 2007), a close examination demonstrates how European football leaders attempted to use the COVID-19 pandemic to expedite what was tantamount to a disaster capitalist power grab.

The purpose of this chapter is to explore the economic and social impact of the COVID-19 pandemic on European professional football. This is achieved by critically examining how European football’s ruling elite employed the principles and practices of *disaster capitalism,* to exploit the pandemic for economic and political gain, and disrupt the already fragile and contradictory networks that comprise the global football ecosystem. Granted, a comprehensive analysis of disaster capitalism in pandemic football would involve a thorough examination of the multiple actors (e.g., glocal clubs, domestic leagues, continental competitions, and international sport mega-events) operating within the networks of the global football ecosystem across various spatial contexts. However, this chapter will focus solely on two of the most prominent manifestations of disaster capitalism in recent sporting history that occurred in domestic leagues (English Premier League), and continental competitions (European football). This chapter examines how the COVID-19 pandemic—the conditions of which created what we refer to as *disaster football*–served as an opportunity for the activation of football’s shock therapy. An analysis of disaster football informs us about the impact of, and recovery from, the COVID-19 pandemic and how a select group of football owners and investor capitalists exploited this broad-ranging crisis to advance neoliberal capitalist diktats through the enmeshed processes of: (1) market and capital accumulation (*privatization*); (2) consolidation of power and control (*dedemocratization*); and (3) anti-competitive cooperative behavior (*monopolization*). Specifically, the "Project Big Picture" and the European Super League initiatives elucidated: the failures of neoliberal capitalism to adequately address football's growing inequalities; the diminishing authority of the sport's governance structures; and, the struggle between community and capital in the pandemic (sport) economy. More broadly, the spectre of disaster football provides an opportunity to consider the ways disaster capitalist "shock doctrine" are operationalized in generating wealth and power for the world's most powerful.

Project Big Picture: An American Hustle

In October 2020, with stadiums emptied by the COVID-19 pandemic, and revenues plunging for sports leagues the world over, news broke of a radical new proposal, characteristic of the principles and practices of disaster capitalism, that would have resulted in the biggest transformation and restructuring of the English professional game in a generation. Sam Wallace, chief football correspondent for the Daily Telegraph, published a world exclusive story that broke the news of leading clubs' plan to reshape the game, what was referred to as "Project Big Picture" (PBP) (Wallace, 2020). The PBP plan was proposed by leading Premier League clubs Manchester United and Liverpool F.C., and their principal American owners Joel Glazer and John W. Henry, to radically overhaul the power structure of the league, with the aim of financially safeguarding teams in the four divisions that comprise professional football in England. Those behind PBP saw it as an opportunity to address what they considered to be the fundamental flaws in England's professional league system. The English football league structure, known colloquially as the football pyramid, is a series of interconnected leagues for men's association football in England and Wales. As an open-system of sport organization (Fort, 2000), the football league operates a hierarchical format with promotion and relegation between leagues at different levels (or tiers), allowing even the smallest club the theoretical possibility of ultimately rising to the top of the system (the English Premier League). Within the English football league system, there are more than 140 individual leagues, containing more than 480 divisions, of which the top four (4) divisions consist of, at the top, the Premier League (20 teams) and, just beneath it, the EFL (divided into three divisions of 24 clubs each). The 20 clubs in the Premier League and the 72 clubs in the EFL are all full-time professional clubs, with some clubs in the tiers immediately below the EFL operating on a professional or semi-professional level. The COVID-19 pandemic, and the financial impact of fans not being allowed into grounds, led to clubs across England feeling the pressures of collapsing revenues, with a number in the EFL confronting the possibility of insolvency. Premier League clubs remained partially insulated from the full financial fallout of the COVID-19 pandemic. Unlike football clubs in the Premier League, whose majority of revenue comes from lucrative domestic and international broadcast revenue, EFL clubs are wholly reliant on matchday income consisting of gate revenue, merchandise income, and concession sale—all of which were not possible during the prolonged period in which UK government rules prohibited fans from attending matches at stadiums. The loss of matchday income due to the COVID-19 pandemic was estimated at £236m (Maguire, 2020). Thus, with inequality rife through the football pyramid, and a number of EFL clubs facing financial disaster, and even the possibility of going into receivership, the EFL was in dire need of financial assistance. As a result, Premier League clubs offered a one-time financial bail-out, which was designed to save the football pyramid and finally redress the growing inequalities within the English game.

Discussions over ideas similar to those revealed in PBP had been going on for some time between the Premier League's top clubs, in particular Henry and Glazer, and Rick Parry, Chairman of the EFL. What began as an attempt to find a solution to the perennial funding problem throughout England's highest leagues became an urgent matter due to the COVID-19 pandemic's accentuating of the EFL's barely veiled yet enduring financial crisis. The PBP proposal was based on two fundamental compromises: a significant increase in financial support directed from the top flight to the lower leagues; and, in return, a substantial reform of governance in the Premier League. More specifically, the PBP was a Faustian bargain: The Premier League was offering a £250m rescue fund payment up front for EFL clubs, a £100m payment to the Football Association' and 25% of Premier League annual broadcast revenue (up from just 4%) in exchange for reducing the size of the Premier League from 20 to 18 clubs and eliminating the League Cup competition. With fewer domestic fixtures required for Premier League teams each season, there would be more opportunities to pursue more attractive, and commercially lucrative, expanded European competition and highly-profitable overseas tours. To ensure the interests of the largest Premier League clubs were served, the league's one-club one-vote principle would be abolished with nine Premier League clubs (Arsenal, Chelsea, Everton, Liverpool, Manchester United, Manchester City, Southampton, Tottenham, and West Ham) granted special power over rule changes, broadcasting rights, and club ownership approvals, with a majority of six (6) needed to push through any proposed changes (Slater, 2020).

The central principle behind PBP was that by helping fund clubs in the EFL, the top clubs would be both financially supporting and, crucially, securing greater power to shape, the future direction of the English football pyramid. PBP would reserve boardroom voting rights for the nine longest-serving clubs (conveniently encompassing all the current "Big Six" [Arsenal, Chelsea, Liverpool, Manchester United, Manchester City, and Tottenham: three of which are owned by American investors] who would later plan to break away to the European Super League [see below]), with just six teams needed to pass changes in regulations (Maguire, 2020). With this added voting power, the largest clubs would have the power to reduce the league in size, eliminate domestic competitions, and approve changes in the approval process for club ownership changes and takeovers. In other words, English football's biggest clubs would centralize (and effectively cartelize) control over the league's voting structure, in return for greater revenue redistribution further down the football pyramid. Importantly, this reorganization would furnish the largest Premier League clubs greater power and flexibility to pursue further capital accumulation and profit maximization. By reducing the size of the Premier League, and the number of domestic cup competitions, PBP would free up fixture dates for Premier League clubs that could be filled with more lucrative matches in an expanded European competition (which, we would later learn, was to be the European Super League), and more opportunities for international tours and pre-season friendlies. In recompense for divesting themselves of the little power over the football pyramid they possessed, EFL clubs would get a bailout that was vital to cover COVID-19 pandemic losses. In doing so, the price of salvation for those clubs surviving via a hand-to-mouth existence is for them to surrender any realistic hope or ambition of gate-crashing the *de facto* Premier League cartel. With enough voting power to shape the entire Premier League's future, the Big Six could leverage their newly acquired power to enrich their own self-interests and wealth accumulating objectives (e.g., rule changes; schedule adjustments; broadcast rights renegotiation) that would further economic disparities in the league and would also extinguish any realistic hopes for non-Big Six clubs to maintain competitiveness. In other words, survival as a functioning and sustainable football club on the other side of the pandemic, would basically necessitate giving "the 'Big Six' the green light to run the game as they see fit" (Ogden, 2020, para. 6). This grand bargain was, quite simply, an exchange of money for power.

The leaked document outlining details of the PBP proposal to reimagine and reset football divided opinion and sparked a frenzied debate (Crafton, 2020). Upon its revelation, Slater (2020) described the disputed authorship of PBP as duplicitous tale of good and evil, a proposal that was simultaneously "a secretive back-room deal, the reset football has been crying out for, the death of ambition, rare leadership, an American coup, the pyramid's saviour" (para. 3). As news of PBP proposal echoed through the English football media landscape, EFL chairman Rick Parry was quick to defend his involvement in, and contribution to, PBP, pointing out that the existing football pyramid was in need of urgent reform: "it's a broken system, it was broken before COVID. From our perspective, what big picture does is address every single one of those equalities" (quoted in Lane, 2020, para. 12). As Parry continued, "at its heart, it is very simple: it's about taking a major chunk of the media revenues, funnelling them downwards through the game and recognising the relevance of the importance of keeping the pyramid strong, not just in the short term but in the long term" (quoted in Brands & Grounds, 2020, para. 17). For their part, Henry and Glazer remained tight-lipped about their involvement and agenda, though they stood behind the proposal "100 percent" (Buckingham & Slater, 2020, para. 15). Yet, the overwhelming majority of clubs and football fans condemned PBP as nothing more than an elitist power grab for England's biggest clubs. Shortly after news of PBP broke, *The Athletic* reported that those at EFL clubs described it as "unthinkable", a "power and money grab" and a "screen to allow the top six to waltz off into Europe" (Crafton, 2020, para. 8). Premier League clubs below the Big Six were said to have considered this plan a "hostile takeover", rather than a proposal and it should be seen as a "coup or a revolution" (Slater & Ornstein, 2020, para.12). Despite successive Conservative governments' passive encouragement of disaster capitalism flourished (and indeed, their own austerity policies in the aftermath 2007-2009 "Great Recession", engaged in a form of disaster governance), the Johnson administration castigated the ESL for being an example of collusive disaster capitalist opportunism. Outright condemnation came from the UK government's Department for Digital, Culture, Media and Sport, whose representative called the ESL a "backroom deal" (quoted in Lane, 2020, para. 22). Furthermore, through a spokesperson, the United Kingdom Prime Minister, Boris Johnson, communicated his disapproval of the plan: "It is clear that this proposal does not command support throughout the Premier League, and it is exactly this type of backroom dealing that undermines trust in football governance" (quoted in de Menzes, 2020, para. 3).

If at first glance, the deal to 'save' the English game looked too good to be true; indeed, it was. Kieran Maguire's (2020) thorough analysis of the PBP proposal reveals the extent to which the asymmetrical and unequal impact that PBP would have on football clubs throughout the EFL pyramid. As he succinctly observed, "an analysis of the PBP proposal reveals that the (red) devil is in the details" (p. 136). Maguire's analysis reveals: the £250m was not a donation, but rather a loan which would be repaid from future share of broadcast revenues; the proposal included a provision for Premier League clubs to sell their own broadcast rights for up to eight games a season internationally; and the proposal would likely accelerate substantial wealth inequality among the three primary sources of club revenues: broadcast, commercial, and matchday. As Maguire points out, *broadcast revenue* would likely diminish over time, the Big Six would gain disproportional financial benefits from *commercial revenue* deals, and the best players would likely be rested during Premier League matches reducing potential *matchday revenue*. In offering immediate bailout funding to the EFL, the Premier League largest clubs were, according to Smith (2020), 'bribing' EFL clubs facing financial catastrophe to bolster their own power and self-interest. As one Premier League executive put it, "the detail is still missing but the timing is classic exploitation of the short-term crisis with a few dog bones to smooth the transition" (quoted in Crafton, 2020, para. 43). In granting the Big Six expanded power, the ensuing restructuring and rule changes would consolidate money and power among what are already the wealthiest and largest clubs in England. Although at present 58 percent of total revenues are shared by 30 percent of clubs, these figures promised to get more extreme as a result of PBP (Maguire, 2020). The PBP would thus cement the power of the Big Six in perpetuity, with a seemingly permanent financial barrier established between them, the rest of the Premier League, and the entirety of the EFL.

No sooner was it presented to a divided industry–stressed under the financial pressures of COVID-19 pandemic, and desperately in need of meaningful reform–PBP perished under the weight of strong and widespread objection. Indeed, the "whispered plans for the radical restructuring of English football vanished as soon as they were exposed to sunlight" (Smith, 2020, para. 1). In an emergency virtual meeting on 14 October 2020, all 20 Premier League clubs rejected the proposal, but agreed to further financial assistance for League One and League Two Clubs (Buckingham, Slater, & Crafton, 2020). Indeed, such was the pushback from within the game in general, and the Premier League in particular, that even the two clubs which proposed PBP (Liverpool and Manchester United) voted against it in a unanimous Premier League rejection. Despite widespread consensus of deep structural flaws in the game, and acknowledgement that perhaps some PBP ideas were worth considering, defeating PBP was heralded as "a victory for all that was just and right and fair, inasmuch as English soccer's current rapacious capitalism is just and right and fair" (Smith, 2020, para. 10). It would appear that everything is relative, even levels of capitalist exploitation across the English football pyramid.

Despite ultimately failing to gain enough support for approval, the radical nature of PBP rendered it potentially "the greatest sporting heist of the 21st-century" (Calladine, 2020, para. 1). Lest we forget, despite being purportedly guided by self-interest and the promise of re-constituting/re-structuring an influential element of the global football ecosystem, PBP was fundamentally aimed at seizing even more for power for a small group of the world's richest owners and investors –principally, if not exclusively, American–, by overhauling the domestic league's voting structure and systems of control. PBP was an opportunistic power-seizing plan aimed at exploiting the financial crisis caused by COVID-19 pandemic to institute football's own version of economic shock therapy; creating a blank slate for reshaping England's football economy resulting in greater inequality. It was, by "common consent, a 'naked power grab' by English soccer's moneyed elite... cynical and opportunistic...and the people behind it were 'plotters,' absorbed by their own rampant self-interest" (Smith, 2020, para. 9). Furthermore, given the deceptive nature of the repayment plan, and the fact that the terms of the agreement greatly benefit the lender at the expense of the borrower, PBP was in some ways analogous to *a predatory lending scheme*; a £250m loan and an increased revenue share from a source that they intend, eventually, to phase out over time. In exchange for a lifeline, a group of unscrupulous football owners and investors planned to extract more value than the borrower can ever repay, and require clubs' most valuable asset, their vote, as collateral. In other words, PBP was more a buyout than a bailout.

Central to Klein's disaster capitalism thesis is the notion that democracy and neoliberalism are antithetical. As Klein (2007) argues, crises serve as "democracy-free zones—gaps in politics as usual when the need for consent and consensus do not seem to apply" (p. 175). PBP illustrates the ways in which power is accumulated and concentrated through *shock therapy* in disaster capitalism. In the end, PBP was an old-fashioned *American hustle*, the exploitation of the COVID-19 pandemic to institute a form of 'shock therapy', the corollary of which was the accumulation of more power within neoliberal football economies and markets. As such, the PBP saga demonstrates that disaster capitalism is not solely concerned with capital accumulation and wealth consolidation. It was about exploiting crises for the transference of power and seizing of control characteristic of neoliberal capitalism. These pursuits are representative of a corporate capitalist order centralizes for-profit corporations and institutions, transfers power and influence to large corporations and business interest groups, and turns citizens into consumers. In Western societies today, neoliberalism is "the ideology that dominates our lives" Monbiot (2016)— a belief system hat defends, bolsters, and justifies social and economic disparities under capitalism. Hence, the effects of this proto-corporate, process would lead to the acceleration of economic inequality and the *dedemocratization of the English football economy*. Yet, this would not be the only attempt by corporate elite to accumulate wealth and power within the global football ecosystem as a separate, but related, market shock—the European Super League—would come to the fore in a matter of months.

The European Super League: American Splendor

In retrospect it has become evident that PBP was only the opening gambit in English football's COVID-19-propelled turn to disaster football. Although PBP was "unanimously rejected" following its leak to the press, many of its ideas would resurface months later with the European Super League (ESL) proposal, as those at the top try to increase their share of the finances of English football and grow their control over the game. It was later acknowledged that Project Big Picture was floated in preparation for talks on a new deal between the European Club Association (ECA) and the Union of European Football Associations (UEFA), over the Champions League. In actuality, PBP was a precursor to the plans for a European Super League (see below). In other words, PBP was not an alternative to the ESL, but designed to work in parallel whilst dealing with the control of England's domestic game. Simultaneously, the ESL proposal was designed to realise similarly narrowed competitive structures and, and more predictably economic outcomes, at the continental level.

The ESL was a proposed multibillion-dollar breakaway league orchestrated by the billionaire owners and shareholders of several of Europe's wealthiest football clubs. Were it to have been implement, the ESL, would have: heralded the largest transfer of wealth to a small set of clubs in modern European football history; unmoored clubs from football's traditional merit-based competitive structures; and, threatened to upend the governance structures, economics, and relationships that have united European football for nearly a century. The ESL was backed by more than US$4.8 billion in private financing from JPMorgan Chase, and would funnel hundreds of millions of dollars of annual television and sponsorship revenue to the world's richest clubs (Maguire, 2021). Proponents of the ESL claimed that the wealth generated by football's largest clubs would, as Real Madrid President, and ESL architect, Florentino Perez argued, "provide higher-quality matches and additional financial resources for the overall football pyramid" (quoted in Millar, 2021) In Perez's view, the ESL was designed 'to save football' in part driven by his claims that global audiences and international television rights are decreasing because "young people are no longer interested" (quoted in Railston, 2021). For Perez and the other co-signers of the breakaway league, the ESL was a proposal for the evolution and adaptation of football to modern times, a means of reinvigorating younger, global audiences by staging a greater number of more appealing, high-profile matches between European giants, which would aid football's post-pandemic economic recovery.

The details of the ESL proposal included twelve (12) "founding clubs" (AC Milan, Arsenal, Atletico Madrid, Barcelona, Chelsea, Inter Milan, Juventus, Liverpool, Manchester City, Manchester United, Real Madrid and Tottenham) with three other unnamed clubs all serving as permanent members of a close-league competition, that would resemble an Americanized model of sport (Edelman, 2021). Another five (5) clubs would be allowed access to the ESL through a qualification process on an annual basis, to complete the 20-team competition. The format for the competition would see 197 total matches among 20 teams, split into two groups of ten, playing home-and-away in a double round-robin format leading to 18 group matches per team, with fixtures set to take place midweek to avoid disruption to the clubs' involvement in domestic competitions. At the end of the group matches, the top three of each group would qualify for two-legged knockout competition that would take place in a four-week span at the end of the season. Inclusion in the ESL would mean that member clubs would leave the current elite inter-European competition—the UEFA Champions League—and only play against the other designated and protected European "elite" clubs in a closed-league competition. Football is currently organized in a pyramid-like structure, with FIFA at the summit, then the continental confederations like UEFA, and then national associations and leagues. Teams currently qualify for the Champions League annually, based on their performance in their domestic league competitions, meaning a select few teams across Europe qualify to compete in both domestic competitions and the valuable Champions League, affording these teams access to tens of millions in additional broadcast revenues. The paradox of this governance structure is that all of its actors cooperate, but also compete with, each other to organize competitions. Despite these inherent contradictions and complexities, the pyramid system–developed historically based on the principles of competition and meritocracy–is *incompatible* with the commercialization and financialization of the modern game. As Carrington (2021) argues, "the pyramid system of European football makes good sporting sense—but it's a bad financial sense, especially for billionaire owners, who have invested millions into teams and who seek a secure profit from the world's most popular sport" (para. 12). Thus, despite the claims from elite clubs that the ESL would provide a sustainable and competitive environment for the entirety of the football pyramid, the proposed ESL structure would, for the most part, completely remove uncertainty of qualification from the equation. In guaranteeing the best teams in Europe annual membership into the ESL regardless of past performance, the proposed league would contradict embedded principles of competition and meritocracy. Alternatively, the ESL would ensure the stability and predictability of revenues streams, and associated club values for its members, thereby creating a permanent and financially impenetrable zenith to what remained of football's pyramid structure.

The ESL was developed in large part by the billionaire class of football owners and investors—many of whom were American-based sports owners and investors, and hence expectantly attuned to the closed-league franchised nature of the US elite professional sport model—to transform European football into a "hypercapitalistic cartel-based pro sports system" (Baumann, 2021, para. 11). The underlying philosophy behind the proposal was that more revenue could be generated through staging a greater number, and indeed a higher concentration–of high-profile, matches between Europe's elite teams. It was clear that the American-style financialization and cartelization at the root of the ESL, was driven by an economic opportunism to re-make the European football so club owners could simultaneously: (1) enhance capital accumulation and consolidation in the hands of the football elite; and, (2) increase gains on equity and club valuations by mitigating, or in some cases eliminating, financial risks. Regarding the former, each team would likely receive up to €350m as a 'welcome bonuses' for simply joining the league, as well as an annual broadcast and sponsorship deal upwards of €4 billion per annum split disproportionately among the 20 clubs (Neate et al., 2021). With the prospect of more fixtures between European giants like Liverpool, Manchester United, Bayern Munich, Barcelona, and Real Madrid, generating more guaranteed income divided between fewer clubs, the ESL certainly represented a massive financial windfall for Europe's elite clubs still reeling from the financial hardships of the COVID-19 pandemic. Second, the prospect of a closed-league competition would resemble the monopoly-like structures of North American professional sport leagues, which ensure revenues are evenly distributed among a self-selected group, and teams retain membership within the competition, regardless of how poorly they perform. In an industry characterized by ever spiraling operating costs (i.e. player wages), and the prospect of depreciating club valuations owed to COVID-19 related declines in revenue generation, by altering the previously meritocratic football pyramid system, clubs would be provided with the degree of financial security and risk mitigation many were desperate to realise. By ensuring wealth accumulation is no longer tied to sporting success, the ESL would raise the value of assets often considered by some owners to be under-monetized, and overly risky. Thereby, for the chosen few, the

ESL would refashion the upper echelons of the European game to serve the singular purpose of equity finance; the generation of, as near as can be guaranteed, returns on investment for owners and shareholders.

Almost immediately after news of the ESL circulated across the sport media landscape, the proposal elicited a torrent of indignation. Opposition was ferocious, unified, and instantaneous, coming from fans, players, managers, politicians, and soccer's governing bodies alike. Much of the criticism centered on the exclusive nature of the ESL–including notably comments from French President Emmanuel Macron and United Kingdom Prime Minister Boris Johnson–because it seemingly signaled the end of sport's competitive meritocracy, and specifically an abrogation of the principle that clubs should qualify for competitions on the basis of performance alone (Buckingham, 2022). Manchester City manager Josep "Pep" Guardiola criticized the closed-league nature of the league, asserting that football "is not sport if success is guaranteed" (quoted in Gonzalez, 2021, para. 2). He was joined by several notable Premier League rival managers, including Jurgen Klopp of Liverpool, Thomas Tuchel of Chelsea, and Ole Gunnar Solskjaer of Manchester United in voicing strong public opposition to the ESL (Beasley, 2021). In the immediate aftermath of the ESL announcement, there were veiled threats by domestic leagues to expel ESL members from domestic league competitions, or strip them of places in FIFA. UEFA even responded by stating that any players in a breakaway league would forfeit their right to represent their countries internationally (Mendola, 2021). Broadcast partners joined the cacophony of criticism as SKY Sport–the lead domestic broadcaster of the English Premier League–offered its platform to a range of football pundits, including former players Gary Neville and Jamie Carragher, to offer blistering denouncements of the ESL plan. Many of football's major commercial sponsors opposed plans for the European Super League, with some even going as far as ending their contractual agreements with clubs involved; including notably Swiss watch manufacturer Tibus, which ended a multi-million-dollar partnership with Liverpool Football Club. Yet, the most seemingly vociferous objections to the ESL came from football supporters themselves, who, in an unusual act of fan solidarity, united in a groundswell of opposition to halt the ESL. English football supporters took to the streets, neighborhoods, city centers, and stadiums to unite in protest: Chelsea supporters blocked the team bus to the stadium entrance (Johnson, 2021); Liverpool supporters adorned the Anfield gates in black banners condemning club ownership (Pearce, 2021); and, Manchester United supporters protested outside the stadium grounds to demand the resignation of ESL acolyte, and Manchester United Chief Executive, Ed Woodward (Whitwell & Anka, 2021). Soon after the immediate rejection by football fans around the world—some of whom even took to the streets in protest –ESL club leaders and owners seemed to recognize a boundary of their appetites. The covenant that bound this disparate assemblage of investor capitalists, financial oligarchs, and heads of state began to unravel. Manchester City was the first to withdraw, then Manchester United, followed in short succession by the remaining Premier League clubs (Liverpool, Tottenham, Arsenal, and Chelsea). Others soon followed with just Barcelona, Real Madrid, and Juventus committed to the project. Despite being three years in the making, ESL collapsed spectacularly a mere 48 hours on from being launched.

After so many years where UEFA's Champions League competition, and indeed the Premier League itself, willfully succumbed to commercial imperatives and market forces, why was the ESL met with such fierce and overwhelming rejection? Perhaps it was the resigned acknowledgement that football had truly become a global televisual spectacle: one in which the future of football would be shaped by conjoined commercial and televisual impulses–as opposed to the rituals and commitments of the *authentic* football supporter (Giulianotti, 2002)– and thus it was an *experiential change* to football's spectacle hierarchy. The COVID-19 pandemic highlighted the centrality of live spectators to the football spectacle–that "impossible-to-repeat live event performed before large co-present crowds" (Rowe, 2020, p. 706). However, and somewhat counter-intuitively, the football ecosystem's response to the lack of "large co-present crowds" (i.e., the use of simulated crowd visuals and noises) foretold a potential post-COVID future within which the live spectator is, to all intents and purposes, obsolescent. Or perhaps the backlash stemmed from the absence of relegation, the lament over the last vestiges of sporting meritocracy (however fleeting and irregular it might be). Certainly, as a closed-league competition in which a select few of Europe's wealthiest and globalized clubs were guaranteed annual inclusion regardless of on-field performance, the ESL at once reflected a *practical restructuring* to the organizational hierarchies and the competitive meritocracy of the football pyramid.

The ESL represented the desire of a few billionaire owners and shareholders to redefine the conditions for generating and circulating wealth with the global (football) economy. Yet, the ESL was not an entirely new proposal, rather it was the logical continuation of the commercializing, financializing, and globalizing trajectories that European football has been traveling for some time. UEFA–the governing body of Europe's most-prized continental competition, the Champions League–reformed the competition's structure to increase the number of teams involved, the number of games played, and that team qualification is at least partially based on past performance, or what UEFA refers to as "historical coefficients," for a large club who had not qualified through their domestic league. All of these changes have meant an increase in advertising and broadcast revenues to the coffers of European clubs.

Although the experiential transformation and practical restructuring within the ESL plan were certainly part of the public's widespread objections, the fierce backlash was arguably driven far more by the *symbolic transformations* that the ESL represented. As Carrington argues, the ESL "represented a shift from the nostalgic idea of the 'people's game' being organized for the pleasure of fans toward a profit-maximizing approach, in which clubs are viewed more like franchises and fans seen as consumers" (Carrington, 2021, para. 12). Indeed, there was, at times, a visceral popular response to the ESL's particular version of 'shock therapy': a calculated exploitation of the COVID-19 pandemic to institute European football's own version of disaster capitalism, that would transform civic institutions into unapologetic and unfettered corporate engines of profit-maximization. Consequently, as Carrington (2021) writes, "strong local identities and attachments to place are reduced to mere marketing 'narratives' to position competing brands in a global marketplace of team logos and colors" (para. 12). As such, the ESL represented another way in which shock therapy was used during the COVID-19 pandemic to institute market-based reforms and the private accumulation of wealth within the global football ecosystem. Granted, the ESL represented the inevitable conclusion of a pathway the game has been following for a long time: a small number of globally visible and commercially dominant clubs concerned more with producing an entertainment product than the historical commitments of sport performance, and allied communal identification. Yet, these changes were not enough for the owners as there remained untapped wealth to be accumulated and transferred to them. As such, the ESL represented a prophetic window into the late-stage *privatization of the European football economy*—a logical continuation of the steady encroachment of commercialization and marketization of the game orchestrated by a select powerful few. While civic control over European football has steadily succumbed to the financial imperatives of football's investor capitalism, the announcement of the ESL proposal forced a public reflection and recognition of what many football fans had long refused to acknowledge—the decades long process of rampant and unfettered neoliberal capitalism displacing commonly held values of community, collectivism, and solidarity at the foundation of their civic institutions. It was an attempt by football's corporate and technocratic elite to advance the *American splendor* of commercialism, consumption, and capitalism that has long been identified with, and acknowledged to be the generative core, of North American sport leagues (Andrews, 2006; Chen, 2022; Newman, 2014).

Football's Endgame

"made by the poor, stolen by the rich"—anonymous

In this chapter, the PBP and ESL proposals are used to demonstrate how the global football ecosystem was, and continues to be, (re-)shaped by the conjunctural conditions and politics of the COVID-19 pandemic. Taking a structural view of the global football ecosystem through this crisis allows us to better observe, and understand, the networked and interrelated aspects of the various actants constituting football's global organization. Such a framework, which views football as an interconnected system, allows us to explore how "football is vulnerable to the exogenous market shocks, and its inherent fragility has been laid bare by the effects of the COVID-19 pandemic" (p. Parnell et al., 2021, p. 19). More specifically, this analysis offers insights into how the COVID-19 pandemic crisis created an opportunity for a select cadre of football's billionaire owners and commercial investors to institute long-desired changes to the global football ecosystem. These motivations and logics can be understood through the theoretical and practical application of Klein's notion of disaster capitalism, the central premise of which is that wealthy nations, corporations, and individuals exploit the aftermath of natural, political, or economic disaster through a series of market shocks. These are designed to implement radical and transformative neoliberal capitalist proposals, with the intent of generating profit for a select elite. As Klein argues, the reason shocks have been essential for neoliberalization is because many neoliberal policies are so unpopular, and thereby can only be effectively forced through during times of severe and civically disempowering crisis. Drawing upon Klein, both the PBP and ESL serve as archetypal examples of the ways in which complicated, interrelated, and subsequent attempts at 'shock therapy' were experienced and exploited during crises to advance neoliberal capitalism within the global football ecosystem. The series of shock therapies intended to re-structure the global football ecosystem in the interests of markets, capital, and, in particular, a cadre of billionaire football owners and investors, would come to define the conditions and characteristics of disaster football.

An analysis of PBP demonstrates how billionaire owners and commercial investors exploited the financial crises of the COVID-19 pandemic into seizing more power to re-shape domestic football competitions, buying out market competition to increase market share, and establishing the conditions for subsequent attempts at shock therapy. The effects of the PBP proposal would have led to a further dedemocratization of the global football ecosystem. A few months later, those same high-powered individuals attempted to leverage the COVID-19 pandemic as another attempt at shock therapy. The ESL proposal figured to accelerate the commercialization and marketization of European football through instituted experiential, practical, and symbolic changes to the global football ecosystem. The impact of the ESL proposal would be the privatization of civic institutions and the full recognition of clubs as commercial enterprises. Taken in conjunction, PBP and ESL were developed as interrelated and interdependent shock therapies intended to bring about football's endgame: the *monopolization of football*. They were a two-fold strategy devised by a select group of football club owners—many of whom are American investor capitalists—to institute the monopoly-like structure of North American professional sport league; one that would ensure a self-selected and tightly controlled group would work in cooperation with one another to: accumulate capital by maximizing profits; control costs to reduce financial risk; and increase brand value and shareholder equity. More practically, it was about removing the financial risk that jeopardizes commercial values, and providing financial and political guarantees each season without having to go through an annual merit-based qualification process. This model would see a self-controlled and cooperative cartel of restricted competition that would allow the world's wealthiest football clubs to gain market power and accumulate capital without having it trickle-down the football pyramid or circulate through the global football ecosystem.

More importantly, it would allow owners and investors to exert their monopoly power through a coordinated effort to price-fix the cost of labor and transfer further wealth to the capitalist owners of the means of football production. It would have allowed owners to impose a long-desired and oft-discussed salary cap on player wages and transfer fees. Although the monopolistic aspects of this cartelized model have been argued to go against European Union (EU) competition law (Slater, 2021)—a matter that, as of this writing, has yet to be adjudicated by EU courts—the intent to consolidate an industry into conditions where a few firms dominate and cooperate to maximize profit and exploitation of labor was clear. That financial capitalists with profound influence over an inherently profit-driven and commercialized industry desire cooperative market conditions and limited competition should not surprise us. Indeed, as Marx (1977) presaged, the end of capitalism is characterized by two defining features: the accumulation of wealth at the poles, and the centralization of industries through economies of scale. Not unlike other capitalist industries—many of which were the initial source of wealth for football's investment capitalists—football is unequivocally and unabashedly on a political economic trajectory reflective of these two outcomes. In this vein, both proposals were shock therapies aimed at catalyzing football's monopoly conditions which has long been, and will continue to be, the *end of football capitalism*. Crucially, it was the COVID-19 pandemic that provided the contexts and conditions for football's monopoly capitalism to very nearly become a reality. Thus, the conditions of disaster football are characterized by the exploitation of the economic and political crises related to the COVID-19 pandemic, in order to accelerate the already encroaching and advancing privatization, dedemocratization, and monopolization of the global football ecosystem.

The backlash to the PBP and ESL shock therapies was immediate and intense. The fans won, an indication of "how their sense of ownership over clubs and their traditions can be mobilized in ways that might seem quant and provincial in the American context" (Hsu, 2021, para. 15). It has been presented as a great victory for collectivism (Robson, 2021), a case study for examining how to global citizens can rejected the assault of disaster capitalism. The football world's collective response to PBP and the ESL was driven by the recognition of such intersecting inequalities and monopoly power emblematic and inherent to neoliberal global capitalism. And the opportunism of these initiatives, being introduced during the COVID-19 pandemic, was, at once, bound by these conditions. People's experiences of pandemic disaster capitalism, in which billionaires and private corporations accumulate vast sources of wealth and power, informed the ways in which citizens responded to further market shocks to their sacred civic institutions. In this way, perhaps the rejection of these twin proposals suggests there are indeed *limits to capital* (Harvey, 1982) when it comes to certain symbolically-owned civic institutions during crises. Accordingly, disaster football tells us about the capacity for citizens to reject the advances of neoliberal capitalism and, more broadly, how to negotiate to the pandemic shock doctrine that figures to re-shape the global economy as it emerges from the COVID-19 pandemic. While the limited scope of this analysis focused solely on two aspects of the global football ecosystem—domestic leagues (Premier League) and continental competitions (European football)—market shocks were experienced elsewhere within the global football ecosystem (e.g., individual clubs, domestic leagues, continental competitions, and international mega-events). Thus, future research must consider how disaster capitalism continues to shape, and be shaped by, forces and relations of pandemic football. Ultimately, it is important to acknowledge and explicate how the conditions and characteristics of disaster football can serve as a paradigm for understanding the complicated relations of global neoliberal capitalism.

References

Andrews, D. L. (2006). *Sport--commerce--culture: Essays on sport in late capitalist America (Vol. 11).* Peter Lang.

Baumann, M. (2021, April 21). The European Super League never stood a chance. *The Ringer*. Available at: https://www.theringer.com/2021/4/21/22395654/european-super-league-withdrawal-debacle.

Beasley, A. (2021, April 20). Everything Premier League managers have said about the European Super League. *Manchester Evening News*. Available at: https://www.manchestereveningnews.co.uk/sport/football/football-news/everything-managers-said-about-esl-20427683.

Bond, A. J., Cockayne, D., Ludvigsen, J. A. L., Maguire, K., Parnell, D., Plumley, D., et al. (2022). COVID-19: The return of football fans. *Managing Sport and Leisure, 27*(1-2), 108–118.

Boykoff, J. (2021). Celebration Capitalism, Sports Mega-Events, and the Tokyo 2020 Olympics. *Journal of Sport and Gender Studies, 19*, 50–66.

Brands, G. & Grounds, B. (2020, October 14). Project Big Picture Q&A: All you need to know about Premier League shake-up proposal. SkySports.com. Available at: https://www.skysports.com/football/news/11096/12102347/project-big-picture-q-a-all-you-need-to-know-about-premier-league-shake-up-proposal.

Buckingham, P. (2022, April 18). Explained: The binding contract that means all six English clubs are still part of the Super League. *The Athletic*. Available at: https://theathletic.com/3253386/2022/04/18/explained-the-binding-contract-that-means-all-six-english-clubs-are-still-part-of-the-super-league/

Buckingham, P., & Slater, M. (2020, October 15). Explained: 'Project Big Picture is dead'—so what happens now? *The Athletic*. Available at: https://theathletic.com/2138438/2020/10/15/premier-league-project-big-picture-efl/.

Calladine, M. (2020). American Hustle: The Moscow connection—Project Big Picture and the end of football as we know it. *The Ugly Game Wordpress. Available at: https://theuglygame.wordpress.com/2020/10/12/american-hustle-the-moscow-connection-project-big-picture-and-the-end-of-football-as-we-know-it/.*

Carrington, B. (2021, April 23). The Super League lived and died for the same reason: Because money rules soccer. *The Washington Post*. Available at: https://www.washingtonpost.com/outlook/2021/04/23/super-league-americanization-soccer/.

Chen, C. (2022). Naming the ghost of capitalism in sport management. *European Sport Management Quarterly, 1*, 1–22.

Collins, C. (2021, October 18). Updates: Billionaire wealth, U.S. job losses and pandemic profiteers. *Inequality.org*. Available at: https://inequality.org/great-divide/updates-billionaire-pandemic/.

Crafton, A. (2020, October 12). Explained: United, Liverpool and Parry spark 'nuclear war' in English football. *The Athletic*. Available at: https://theathletic.com/2130676/2020/10/12/nuclear-war-liverpool-manchester-united-rick-parry-premier-league-project-big-picture/.

Edelman, M. (2021, April 19). European Super League will bring lucrative U.S. sports model overseas. *Forbes.com*. Available at: https://www.forbes.com/sites/marcedelman/2021/04/19/european-super-league-brings-lucrative-us-sports-model-overseas/?sh=2b1d3d9950b1.

European Champions Report (2021). KPMG Sports Advisory Practice. Available at: https://www.footballbenchmark.com/library/the_european_champions_report_2021

Fort, R. (2000). European and North American sports differences (?). *Scottish Journal of Political Economy, 47*(4), 431–455.

Giulianotti, R. (1999). *Football: A sociology of the global game*. Polity Press.

Giulianotti, R. (2002). Supporters, followers, fans, and flaneurs: A taxonomy of spectator identities in football. *Journal of Sport & Social Issues, 26*(1), 25–46.

Gonzalez, R. (2021, April 20). Pep Guardiola on European Super League: 'It is not a sport if success is guaranteed'. *CBSSports.com*. Available at: https://www.cbssports.com/soccer/news/pep-guardiola-on-european-super-league-it-is-not-a-sport-if-success-is-guaranteed/.

Hall, C. M., & Amore, A. (2019). The 2015 Cricket World Cup in Christchurch: Using an event for post-disaster reimagine and regeneration. *Journal of Place Management and Development*.

Harvey, D. (1982). *The limits to capital*. Verso books.

Hsu, Hua (2021, April 21). The audacity and greed of the Super League. The New Yorker. Available at: https://www.newyorker.com/sports/sporting-scene/the-audacity-and-greed-of-the-super-league.

Johnson, S. (2021, April 20). Petr Chec speaks to Chelsea protestors: 'I know, give everybody time!'. *The Athletic*. Available at: https://theathletic.com/news/european-super-league-chelsea/vd5KDCzFzALB/.

Karak, A. (2017). Accumulation by dispossession: A Marxist history of the formation of the English Premier League. *Review of Radical Political Economics, 49*(4), 615–632.

Klein, N. (2007). *The shock doctrine: The rise of disaster capitalism*. Macmillan.

Lane, B. (2020, October 13). 'Project Big Picture' would see the English Premier League reduced in size, domestic competitions scrapped, and the biggest clubs in the division hold all the power. Business Insider. Available at: https://www.insider.com/project-big-picture-what-is-it-english-premier-league-2020-10.

Maguire, K. (2020). *The Price of Football: Understanding Football Club Finance*. Agenda Publishing.

Maguire, K. (2021). Covid-19 and Football: Crisis Creates Opportunity. *The Political Quarterly, 92*(1), 132–138.

Marx, K. (1977). *Capital: A critique of political economy, volume one*. Vintage Books.

Mendola, N. (2021, April 18). UEFA confirms Super League clubs, players could be banned internationally. NBCSports.com. Available at: https://soccer.nbcsports.com/2021/04/18/uefa-statement-european-super-league-threatens-bans-clubs-players-update/

de Menzes, J. (2020, October 13). Project Big Picture 'exactly the type of backroom dealing that undermines trust in football's governance', says No 10. *The Independent*. Available at: https://www.independent.co.uk/sport/football/premier-league/premier-league-project-big-picture-boris-johnson-backroom-dealing-epl-b990691.html.

Millar, C. (2021, April 19). European Super League debunked: Studying the claims of football's 12 rebel clubs. *The Mirror*. Available at: https://www.mirror.co.uk/sport/football/news/european-super-league-debunked-studying-23941460.

Millward, P. (2013). New football directors in the twenty-first century: Profit and revenue in the English Premier League's transnational age. *Leisure Studies, 32*(4), 399–414.

Monbiot, G. (2016, April 15). Neoliberalism—the ideology at the root of all our problesm. The Guardian. Available at: https://www.theguardian.com/books/2016/apr/15/neoliberalism-ideology-problem-george-monbiot.

Nauright, J., & Ramfjord, J. (2010). Who owns England's game? American professional sporting influences and foreign ownership in the Premier League. *Soccer & Society, 11*(4), 428–441.

Neate, R., Sweney, M., & Wearden, G. (2021, April 19). European Super League clubs promised €200-300m 'welcome bonus'. *The Guardian*. Available at: https://www.theguardian.com/business/2021/apr/19/jp-morgan-european-super-league.

Newman, J. I. (2014). Sport without management. *Journal of Sport Management, 28*(6), 603–615.

Ogden, M. (2020, September 3). Football must face up to stark realities of financial future after COVID-19 crisis. *ESPN.com*. Available at: https://www.espn.com/soccer/english-premier-league/story/4170092/football-must-face-up-to-stark-realities-of-financial-future-after-covid-19-crisis.

Parnell, D., Bond, A. J., Widdop, P., & Cockayne, D. (2021). Football worlds: Business and networks during COVID-19. *Soccer & Society, 22*(1-2), 19–26.

Pearce, J. (2021). Eurpoean Super League: Liverpool fan groups to remove all flags from Kop. The Athletic. Available at: https://theathletic.com/news/european-super-league-liverpool-flags-kop/76eyQ0evqaS1/.

Railston, S. (2021, April 22). Florentino Perez tried to justify Super League by targeting the people that helped to destroy it. *Manchester Evening News*. Available at: https://www.manchestereveningnews.co.uk/sport/football/florentino-perez-tried-justify-super-20434736.

Robson, J. (2021, April 21). European Super League collapse a victor for football fans on game-changing night. *The Evening Standard*. Available at: https://www.standard.co.uk/sport/football/european-super-league-collapse-victory-football-fans-game-changing-night-b930925.html

Rookwood, J., & Hughson, J. (2017). A history of the English Premier League: Cultures, consumption and commerce. In *The English Premier League* (pp. 13-32). Routledge.

Rowe, D. (2020). Subjecting pandemic sport to a sociological procedure. *Journal of Sociology, 56*(4), 704–713.

Slater, M (2020). Explained. Project Big Picture—the winners and losters. The Athletics. Available at: https://theathletic.com/2132829/2020/10/13/project-big-picture-premier-league-efl/.

Slater, M. (2021, September 29). Was the Super League illegal? Why UEFA is in court with Barcelona, Juventus and Real Madrid. The Athletic. Available at: https://theathletic.com/2832247/2021/09/29/was-the-super-league-illegal-why-uefa-is-in-court-with-barcelona-juventus-and-real-madrid/

Smith, R. (2020, October 16). Suggestion for a better big picture for English soccer. *The New York Times*. Available at: https://www.nytimes.com/2020/10/16/sports/soccer/project-big-picture-england-soccer.html.

Swiss Ramble [@swissramble]. (2021, October 23). The COVID-19 pandemic has had a significant adverse impact on football clubs...[Tweet]. Twitter.com. Available at: https://twitter.com/swissramble/status/1429685285755949056?lang=en

UEFA Benchmarking Report. (2020). Benchmarking report highlights profits and polarization. *UEFA.com*. Available at: https://www.uefa.com/insideuefa/protecting-the-game/news/025f-0fe85ed2acf8-db382645ca21-1000%2D%2Dbenchmarking-report-highlights-profits-and-polarisation/.

Wallace, S. (2020, October 11). World exclusive: Man Utd and Liverpool driving 'Project Big Picture'—football's biggest shake-up in a generation. *The Telegraph*. Available at: https://www.telegraph.co.uk/football/2020/10/11/world-exclusive-man-utd-liverpool-driving-project-big-picture/.

Zirin, D. (2007). *Welcome to the terrordome: The pain, politics and promise of sports*. Haymarket Books.

31

Interview(s) with the Vampire: Research Opportunism During a Global Catastrophe

Michael Atkinson

But, We Were on a Break

Arthur Frank's (1997), *The Wounded Storyteller*, documents the ubiquity and power of the restitution narrative. When the anticipated teleology of one's life is disrupted by a sudden disease the reflex for most patients, according to Frank (1997), is to prostrate themselves before the clinician and acquiesce to medical intervention in order to conquer their corporeal calamities and become whole again; in Frank's (1997) terms, patients desperately pine for their pre-illness stories. Frank's (1997) use of the term restitution, given its legal connotations, is particularly compelling as it implies how medicine is an assumed vehicle for restoring the body's expected contractual obligation to function normally. Such a profound myth of corporeal normality is indeed intextuated into the fabric of

M. Atkinson (✉)
University of Toronto, Toronto, ON, Canada
e-mail: michael.atkinson@utoronto.ca

D. L. Andrews et al. (eds.), *Sport and Physical Culture in Global Pandemic Times*, Global Culture and Sport Series, https://doi.org/10.1007/978-3-031-14387-8_31

human existence. But as life instructs, in both radically absurd and deeply traumatizing ways, our narrative fantasies fracture all the time. All the time. Restoration of one's health and accompanying life narrative is possible in many instances, but in others, restitution is either improbable, flatly impossible, or undesirable. Craving restitution is nearly universal, however, and the wide-ranging implications of chasing personal restitution through illness are undeniable. Among such consequences are self-alienation via bio-medicalization, the loss of agency and personal meaning making through illness, and existential inauthenticity in becoming the docile patient waiting for (narrative) salvation.

The global Covid-19 pandemic disrupted, altered, and shattered a great deal of taken-for-granted narrative normalities: from daily timelines to global trade economies, entrenched cultural pastimes, political careers, educational rhythms, collective identities, and most tragically, entire lives. The Covid-19 global illness, as my friend Arthur Frank might instruct (1997), inserted itself as a *narrative break* in immense proportions. Covid-19, as Western news broadcasters were quick to quip during the pandemic's first wave, would be this generation's Second World War. For the first time in twenty-one years, I stopped teaching in-person at a university. My ethnographic research on persons living with invisible disabilities terminated. Up until this point, I'd never spent more than six months away from an ethnographic field in my entire academic career. Meetings shifted to online 'Zoom' space, and I no longer commuted to work as our offices were locked and buildings shuttered. My three children scurried home to experiment with online learning, and I became a school teacher-father to them. Their sports participation ended, their friendships strained. The cruel Canadian winter settled in with full force. One of us nervously ventured out for groceries and sundry items once weekly. I saved money on petrol for my car, I lived in tracksuits, and our house became a congested multi-purpose workspace. An eerie hush fell over my suburban neighbourhood, with residents timid of even coming within 10 metres of one another. I felt lucky to be able to bunker down at home with loved ones. I could work from home 'virtually,' my children had high-speed online access to learning, and none of us would needlessly be exposed to the virus. Within three weeks, however, we had already begun to suffer greatly in the adjustment process and craved restitution.

The meticulously patterned ebbs and flows of my family's collective stories (i.e., going to school, working, dining out, seeing friends, etc.) required immediate revision. Still, I wanted to *behave* like an academic again; drinking my morning coffee, boarding my morning train, interacting with colleagues and students in my office, standing present in the classroom, co-mingling with research participants in the field, and performing the embodied rituals I developed over two decades. Yet in a swift Thanosian snap, my preferred story unravelled and knotted with my partner's and children's frayed stories in twisted, complicated, and frustrating manners. Self-isolation for a mere minute of private thought or quiet contemplation proved impossible. I felt melancholic. At the same time, single friends of mine expressed the crushing weight of solitude and their wish to share co-presence with absolutely anyone. My two dogs incessantly barked during my online lectures and my children constantly bellowed for help with any number of minor tasks around the house. We bickered, the house itself perceptively shrunk to no grander than a matchbox, and we collectively lamented about the numbing effects of physical immobility in our lives. There were narrative shards or memories of our previous normality strewn throughout our house, like my work briefcase and the children's ice hockey sticks. A mood of abandonment and ennui pervaded in our household as we became detached from our imagined life stories.

By mid-April 2020, my daily work tasks were systematic efforts in narrative bridge maintenance, repair, building, and demolition across the interactional chasms created by Covid-19. Perhaps foolishly, I had recently accepted two cumbersome administrative roles within the university: one, the Director of Graduate Studies for my Faculty; and two, the Chair of the University Research Ethics Board. As the Covid-19 work disruption derailed graduate student coursework and research progress, challenged program development we initiated in our Faculty, and through a spanner into the works of long-term Faculty planning, narrative rupture all surrounded me as we scrambled to forge contingency programming. On a broader scale, I became part of a special research ethics task group in the university charged with, for all intents and purposes, halting research at Canada's largest university (and veritably, policing the stoppage). We interpreted and re-wrote standard operating ethical practices for university researchers during the pandemic and helped design a (eventual) research re-start plan. Colleagues at the university routinely bombarded us with hate (e)mail as they opposed the research pause, on grounds ranging from intellectual freedom, tenure and promotion considerations, graduate student allyship, and rights against 'unlawful detention'. At times, I would sit at my computer perusing the daily vitriol from enraged colleagues whilst listening to news accounts of bankrupted shopkeepers or families who recently lost elderly parents to Covid-19 in understaffed long-term care facilities. Complaints rained in whilst I simultaneously received text messages from friends whose businesses teetering on the brink of insolvency, and from nurse friends expressing their shared terror about dying from Covid-19. In Canada like elsewhere, death tolls mounted, depression soared, and precarious labourers were forced into dangerous work conditions as academics around the world took to Twitter to bemoan the oppressive nature of Zoom meetings and the unbearably devastating tolls of online teaching from one's home office. I felt deep antipathy for colleagues during this period but nevertheless reflexively wondered, are they not expressing a learned need for restitution like so many others?

Attempted restitution for academics, including physical cultural studies scholars, through the pandemic generally entailed one of two strategies: in the first instance, lobbying for a return to pre-Covid normal (i.e., denying the realities of Covid-19, decrying mask and health mandates, scoffing at social distancing initiatives, and pressing for research to continue unfettered); and in the second instance, getting on with the business of academia/sport and culture research in innovative, and I would argue cleverly self-productive, manners (i.e., working with and around health rules and regulations by moving research efforts online, pivoting to research agendas focussed on sport and the pandemic, attending virtual conferences, and/or taking to social media to become a public/celebrity/academic voice on the importance of sport, exercise, and leisure are during the pandemic). Rife within both approaches for restitution were narrative undertones and practices of the neo-liberal, hyper-production cultures critical scholars vehemently decry. Quite simply, the academic show, in all of its excess, had to go on at its exponentially pathological rate of production. If one was smart and adaptive, one's research agenda and career progress need not be narratively shattered; it could be resuscitated deftly if one could discover how to produce through, and more depressingly on, Covid-19.

Sitting at home on my computer one day in late June of 2020, I pondered the cognitive bifurcation of throngs of academics during the Covid-19 pandemic. Whilst food shortages, job shortages, familial interaction shortages, money shortages, health care shortages, and any number of other shortages were documented, academics at my home institution and abroad clamoured for *more* publications, *more* conferences, *more* journal special issues, *more* social media attention, and *more* relevance *because* of the pandemic. After all, as Petyr (Littlefinger) Baelish instructed, "chaos is a ladder" and an opportunity to improve one's lot in the stew of collective (Covid-19) suffering and existential angst. As such a deeply privileged group, academics secure in their collective careers and far away from the pandemic's front lines, should have been able to pause and reflect upon the vulnerability of the social fabric—a social fabric that, shockingly, might not need umpteen million studies of sport physical culture at this precise historical conjuncture. Yet early career researchers and graduate students (the most vulnerable during Covid-19 for falling from, or entirely off, the academic production ladder) were appropriately scared. But for tenured, mid- or senior-stage academics, what pressing need for rapid restitution? What impacts would this unmitigated desire and the *depeche mode* of sport-related research on Covid-19 create in the short and long-terms? To be sure, Covid-19 is an historical event worth documenting through empirical research. But were most social scientists (of sport) collectively missing an opportunity to put, as Baudrillard's (1990) expressed in *Fatal Strategies*, sociological research on sport and physical culture on a much-needed 'diet' in the global 'all you can eat' research production culture? I would argue yes, we collectively missed a 'great reset' moment of our own which could have potentially eased the vocational burden of the most vulnerable inside and outside of the academy.

For the remainder of this chapter, I consider whether sport and physical culture researchers have bitten, vampiristically, into endless necks during the Covid-19 global pandemic. From students to fellow colleagues, to administrators, and to vulnerable research participants, the metaphorical blood of many continued to provide ample sustenance for an insatiable research horde desperate to validate the role of critical sociological work on sport. Although my account is undoubtedly partial, biased, incomplete, flawed and wholly perspectival given my multiple roles in academia, my observations on several front lines (as a teacher, researcher, graduate program steward, ethics officer, national grant reviewer, journal co-editor, and human) lead me to question the potential ethical/moral shortcomings of the collective academic appetite for restitution during Covid-19. In no way do I suggest the (literal) business of academia should have stopped outright; but rather the undeterred clamour for restitution amid global suffering requires contemplation and critique (after all, are we not *critical* theorists?). In the next section of this chapter, I discuss the restitution framework, followed immediately by a section articulating how the nascent 'exercise is/as medicine' paradigm attained global credibility even in sociological circles during Covid-19. From there, core ethical questions are presented regarding the practice of research during a pandemic, and interdisciplinary lane-hopping. The final section begs for a consideration of how the pandemic might provide a context for realizing a more slow, thoughtful, committed, and empathetic global research process on sport and physical cultures.

Restitution: Salvation Through a Robust Global Supply Chain

In excess of 240,000 research publications on Covid-19 were disseminated between late August 2019 and December 2020 in Western journals: a staggering 16,000 a month average. Nearly 18,000 of those publications related to social scientific analyses of Covid-19 and the meaning or interpersonal impact of the pandemic on people. At the journal I co-edit, *Qualitative Research in Sport, Exercise and Health*, manuscripts on Covid-19 trickled in as early as April 2020. We decided to desk reject them outright (at least for the first half of 2020), especially the self-indulgent auto-ethnographic pieces, because scholarship rarely manifests in two months of scattergun work. By June of 2020, several sport-related social scientific (virtual) conferences had been organized on Covid-19, calls for papers in special issues on Covid-19 littered social media, and anticipatory anthologies announced. Whilst social sectors frantically scrambled to stay afloat, academics interested in Covid-19 (or merely referencing 'Covid times' in their studies) experienced a modern-day gold rush. Most of us who have instructed students regarding research methods at even the most introductory level found the academic blitzkrieg to be, in a word, outrageous. The long haul of reading about a subject, cautiously considering important research problems related to the subject, contemplating methodologies and design, implementing the study in real time, wading through it meticulously, piecing together analyses (of more than merely 'themes'), painstakingly writing drafts, nervously submitting to an outlet, receiving (frustrating) feedback, revising, resubmitting, and eventually publishing transformed into a 100m sprint. Despite a decade of calls by researchers to find healthier work-life balances (Johnson et al., 2019), to combat the crisis of academic over production and capitalistic commodification (Giroux, 2007), and to advocate for slow methodologies (Honoré, 2004), Covid-19 provided too alluring of an opportunity for critical scholars to stake intellectual claims. Even within the physical cultural studies community, Silk et al. (2014) had made convincing arguments for a slow PCS. Yet in excess of 35,000 publications on the relationship between sport (not sport *and* physical culture) and Covid-19 were produced between December 2019 and May 2022—notably, at a time wherein research was stunted through public health lockdowns and university closures. I wonder how many tens of thousands will follow now that most institutions are fully operational.

Even more personally disappointing, for two and a half decades I have listened to critical sport scholars denounce the dehumanizing nature of market capitalism, its associated systems of structural inequality and resulting cultural hegemony, its colonial foundations, its inherent hyper production and consumption logics, and its institutionally disseminated neo-liberalistic/me-first (bio)ethics. The veracity of such biting criticism is incongruous, on occasion, with academics' collective participation in and personal benefit from these very systems (often in the name of empowering others via some imaginary resistance or social justice work coded as allyship). Guy Debord, an academic hero of mine, might be spinning in his grave from the nascent spectacle of academic production during Covid-19. Early efforts to underline the importance of, or need for, sport, play, and exercise during the pandemic's first waves reeked of uncritical sports evangelism. For instance, review the extant commentaries for the sake of commentary on how Covid might impact sports worlds, implications for sport and exercise during the pandemic, and future considerations for sports researchers The pornographically excessive reflex to academically weigh in on capitalize on Covid-19 without really knowing Covid-19 through *meticulous* study and inquiry (most of us with no previous interest or disciplinary expertise in infectious disease, work/occupation disruption, or public health research) during Covid times, invariably mars the sanctimonious image of the critical, reflexive, and socially conscious scholar. It simultaneously underlines the oppressive production norms so rife and rotten within academia's hallowed halls and to which critical scholars ostensibly consent and reproduce; norms so often 'unpacked' by critical scholars as tyrannically inequitable. The norms include, of course, the excessive publishing through Fordist techniques (cut and paste theory to any emergent substantive issue), the unfettered academic use of public and private money to ostensibly solve others' social problems, the development of shallow expertise on any range of subjects, the ability to pivot one's research agenda to continue production and chase new funding opportunities, and the use of an expanding (and generally poorly paid) cabal of undergraduate and graduate students to maintain the cycle of research production.

Restitution is, then, a powerful metanarrative for an academic inconvenienced by Covid-19. I cannot pause, I cannot stop submitting articles (whilst ironically posting online through social media about the burdens of reviewing articles), I cannot stop chasing external funding (where are the new opportunities?), I cannot stop attending conferences (let's all go online, and my colleagues even get to peer voyeuristically into my home—wait, I better meticulously arrange my bookshelves to impress!), and I simply cannot stop CV building.

True to sociological form, it must be acknowledged, neither did all academics suffer (initial) production delays equally nor were they able to similarly keep calm and carry on. Deryugina et al. (2021) drew attention to the relative gender effects related to productivity through the pandemic. Female, early career researchers with young children, and precariously employed sessional/temporary lecturers, experienced the most significant strains. Carr et al. (2021) argued that academic trainees (a term I personally detest) from marginalized/minority communities (social communities most likely to be exposed to and die from Covid-19 through the first three waves) were also likely to experience the blunt force of research stoppages on their career telemetries. Perhaps unsurprising, then, calls for papers in special issues of journals and edited anthologies on sports and Covid-19 most frequently (that is, almost entirely) were led by mid- to senior-career, White scholars from Western nations; White scholars who are keenly aware of their social/institutional privilege. Such are the outcroppings of embedded structural inequality within academia. Rarely (well, by that I mean never) have I heard senior career scholars in sport and physical cultural studies acknowledge, let alone actionably address, the downward (and inequitable) performance pressures we place on early career researchers through Covid-19 and other times. Anecdotally, similar trends were observable at the journal, *QRSEH*, I co-edit with Kerry McGannon. Drop-offs in submitted articles from BIPOC colleagues and early career researchers (especially women) were noticeable. In my home institution, graduate and postdoctoral students fretted over whether their funding would disappear, whether they could collect data and complete a thesis, where they would live, if their Faculty supervisors would abandon them owing to lack of measurable progress, and whether their research team leaders would request they engage in risky, face-to-face research 'for the sake of the lab'. At the university Research Ethics Board that I Chair, graduate students from across campus (and sadly, from my own Faculty) expressed how they felt both overt and subtle pressure to return to labs. Early career researchers (ECRs) penned letters to Deans, Heads of Schools, and University Presidents inquiring whether unrealistic metrics for assessing tenure or contract renewal (i.e., papers published, grants received, students supervised, etc.) would be altered on both pragmatic and equitable grounds. The most vulnerable among us sought not restitution as much as basic compassion and consideration.

In a spirited debate during a session at the 2018 Qualitative Research in Sport and Exercise conference in Vancouver regarding the need for taking creative methodological risks, my dear friend Kass Gibson pointed out that the road to a culture of innovation/change is best paved by senior colleagues, fully sec(ten)ured in their academic positions. He is correct of course. Through Covid-19, senior colleagues in physical cultural like me (who are, often, working in administrative positions and possess some modicum of institutional authority) had an opportunity to pave a road toward an improved work-life balance for all inside academia by promoting how hyper-productivity is a fatal academic strategy; with its poison fully and finally withdrawn from academic culture during the Covid-19 pandemic. We failed. Restitution fantasies are far too seductive. Twitter became awash with senior colleagues lamenting about how many online classes they have taught, papers graded, whilst boasting about online conferences papers delivered, panels hosted, awards won, and articles published. We normalized research adaptation and churning out papers from home whilst heroically performing childcare and other domestic work, as a means of promoting both our own personal resilience and restitution (with a dash of personal brand promotion). We endlessly highlighted new collaborations and grants received (including funds to study people's Covid-19 sport-related misery). From 2019–2021, I sat on five granting committees for national research funding schemes in Canada. One specifically formed through a unique call for social research on/during Covid-19. Senior academics working as Principal Investigators in collaboration with other mid-career/senior career researchers seized over 85% of the grants across all competitions. Such a brilliant group of global intellectuals could not read the academic room. Gaps between the tiered academic haves and have nots widened during Covid-19, further amplifying pressures on young colleagues to engage more to catch up. Less than one full year into the pandemic, Hunt (2020) painted a dire picture of the academic landscape for ECRs and chastised senior colleagues for their lack of support. Harrop et al. (2021) referred to ECRs as a 'lost generation' of researchers potentially unable to academically draw level with their senior peers. Dozens of articles across the life/social sciences underlined the grim outlook for ECRs as fallout from an unyielding and enduring publish or perish culture. But here's a picture of me for your social media viewing, sat at home, opening the Amazon box which has delivered a first copy of my new book. I'll add text to the top of the media post expressing, "I couldn't have done this without all your help. Thoughts and prayers to everyone struggling right now." Statements from sociologists of sport and physical culture analysing the terrain for ECRs? Relative silence save for quasi-supportive platitudes on social media. Yet submissions from senior colleagues working collaboratively, or leading a team of graduate students, at my journal were stable and then skyrocketed during Covid-19—and yet, requests sent to them to review for our journal were the most frequently rejected week in and week out. They were, as disclosed to me privately, simply 'too busy' or 'too burnt out' to review. Reviewing stood in the way of restitution. Who reviewed most frequently? ECRs of course. After all, someone had to ensure senior colleagues' progress would not be impeded. I decided to stop disproportionately asking ECRs for reviews. It felt exploitive. Turnaround times at the journal have now risen and senior colleagues petulantly complain.

Senior academics not only failed our junior colleagues through a collective zeitgeist and privileged for restitution, but we also failed ourselves as a broader scholarly community through Covid-19. A little over a year prior to the pandemic, the Canadian Association of University Teachers (CAUT) Bulletin published an article (May 2018) articulating the psycho-emotional costs of living within highly competitive and (quantified) results driven academic cultures. These CAUT (2018) findings hardly shocked anyone attentive to the dehumanizing impacts of corporate audit cultures in universities. Cries of burnout, depression, overload, and exasperation have filled academic corridors for my twenty-two years as a professor, and I assume they echoed long before those corridors contoured my shadow. But by December 2021, yet another sociological study of academics' experiences during Covid-19 featured in the CAUT Bulletin, discussing how the ever so brief productivity dip through Covid-19 among senior colleagues produced significant anxiety among them. Not in the sense that senior, tenured colleagues feared institutional reprisal for decreased productivity, no. Rather, in the sense that senior colleagues were initially perturbed by being prevented from collecting data (or, perhaps more accurately, sending out legions of students to collect said data) as typically accustomed (CAUT, 2021). Instead of embracing an opportunity to publish less frequently, think more deeply, and collaborate more intentionally (desires expressed to me by hundreds of colleagues over the years), restitution is the almost always preferred occupational drug. Chaos, it seems, isn't much of a ladder after all, except for the privileged few.

At the outset of the pandemic, I foolishly worried that the flow of original research to our journal, QRSEH, would dry out by mid 2020. Surely, no one was doing research, I told myself. Sport and physical cultural spaces shut down, close interpersonal/moving/contact became athletes prohibited, and social gatherings in countries like Canada were either banned outright or limited to a select few within one's family. Lacking the sociological imagination to consider how academics would adapt, I became gobsmacked the flow did not thin but rather swelled. People switched gears and hastily researched the effects of lockdowns, closures, and corporeal fear among people in sport. Logical. Do not read decades of research on pandemics and their social effects, scour the literature on the subjective experiences of fear/trauma during social or environmental catastrophes, tap the collective lexicon of sociological, psychological, or theological thought on human suffering, or even assess whether extant critical theories are even prepared to account for Covid-19 conditions and events. No need. Not at all. Covid-19 is a novel case study, and I must plant the first flag in my substantive area. There is no shortage of case studies, in fact there is a global supply chain of them. A base of critical theory, a pinch of new materialism, a healthy measure of online methods, heated in [x] community of sport participants, and a new research cake is ready in under thirty minutes.

While collective expression from academics through 2020 in Canada and abroad would almost (self)portray them as characters from Steinbeck's (1939), *Grapes of Wrath*—forced from their craft/graft in local communities during dust bowl research times—a significant portion transformed into those featured in Rice's (1976), *Interview with the Vampire*. As a researcher who has spent nearly thirty years studying people's suffering in one context or another, the rapid turn to study deeply vulnerable people during Covid-19 felt unsavoury and vampiristic at first—even to someone like me who anticipates pangs of guilt when researching other people's horribly arduous lived experiences. Personal tragedy, loss, depression, and fear are all standard research fare among academics, to be sure, but studying such during a period of intense, and *en masse*, corporeal fear and anxiety is relatively unprecedented. It felt too soon, it felt too forced, and it felt too insensitive as people were reeling with deep existential uncertainty. And yes, researching the impacts of closing the community pool down at the local leisure centre or children's experiences wearing cloth masks whilst swinging a baseball bat, felt proportionately inconsequential in communities besieged with so many other health, economic, psychological, spiritual, and emotional concerns. Further still, the use of others' ongoing pain, uncertainty, anxiety, frustration, loss, dislocation, and angst through online surveys and virtual interviews to secure and reinforce our version of a vampire's eternal life (promotion and tenure) felt wholly unethical. But then again, maybe it was entirely ethical and to be expected as this current historical conjuncture in critical sport studies.

Exercise as (Personal and Social) Medicine: The Birth of the (Not So) Critical Clinic

In Andrews' (2008) now seminal critique of kinesiology and its scientific hegemony, he warned about the loss of the *critical* focus of qualitative analyses of sport and physical culture within a diffuse trend of privileging sport research with an instrumental/applied focus. At the time of writing, a wave of what is called 'translational' or 'knowledge exchange' philosophies swept through academia. In simpler terms, not only did one's research need to be manifestly scientific (hence the contemporary obsession with scientific 'rigour' in qualitative sports studies), but research should also move goal posts forward in measurable, defined, immediate, and problem-solving manners. During the period, and I argue uncoincidentally, the field of critical scholarship resolutely turned to intersectional analyses of sport participation (notably, *barriers* to sport participation), sport for development and peace began to flourish, and early percolations of new materialism (the unholy coupling of biology with sociology) popped up in journals. Furthermore, as physical education, human movement, or recreation departments transformed into proper Kinesiology and Sport Science units around the world, space contracted for focussed *sociology* of sport research on how people simply 'do' sport and physical culture. For a doubly marginalized group of scholars easily derided as academically inconsequential (not quite sociologists, not quite sport scientists), the survival of sociologists of sport and physical culture depended upon demonstrating *functional utility* in applied, translational manners with a critical flavour; now referred to ubiquitously as social justice work.

For the last decade, intersectional studies of sport increasingly attested to how differences in race, class, gender, sexuality and religion reproduce social hierarchies and limit people's potential as citizens with rights to participate (Carter-Francique & Flowers, 2013). Sport for development and peace research instructed how sport programs could not only be used to achieve United Nations Development Goals (Millington & Darnell, 2020), but also how sport programming can functionally 'cure' problems ranging from HIV transmission to violence against girls/women to poverty to educational differences. New materialist studies tipped hats to positivist hierarchies in sport research, perhaps inadvertently admitting that critical scholarship requires the 'hard' sciences for robust understandings of the human condition (rarely, if I might add, is the reverse true in sport sciences). Today, Karen Barad, a PhD in quantum field theory and particle physics, is more likely to be cited in the sociology of sport and physical culture literature than Judith Butler. Together and separately, trends in critical scholarship ignored Andrews' warnings (2008) and Ingham's (1997) much earlier thoughts on the hegemony of scientific/rationalized paradigms in sport and physical culture research. Critical work now has to solve concrete problems to be fundable (in activist terms, 'make a difference' by and curing sexism, racism, homophobia, material disparities, etc.), has to be understandable and palatable to non-critical peers (as evidenced by the enduring arguments to dumb down the esoterically impenetrable language used by critical scholars), and had to illustrate once and for all that on a social basis sport does in fact matter (i.e., as a path to social integration, equity, and inclusion beset against a backdrop of shared social values—namely, justice). It is if Parson's (1937), *The Structure of Social Action*, had been resuscitated and rebranded in a strangely structural functionalist *oeuvre* with critical scholars becoming fully fledged social engineers (sorry, allies). The icing on the *nouveau functionalist* coup d'état in the sociology of sport and physical culture would be spread via the invisible hand of the North American 'exercise is medicine' movement.

In late 2007, Exercise is Medicine (EiM), a non-profit initiative co-launched by the American College of Sports Medicine and the American Medical Association, would unintentionally change (even critical) sport research in North America by providing a conceptual solution to nagging problems of relevance both inside and outside the academy. To grossly reduce the field within a solitary sentence, EiM suggests that exercise is indeed a powerful, preventative cure-all for most human ailments (Williams & Gibson, 2018). Exercise/sport is a magical pill in not only physiological (e.g., disease prevention, ambulatory improvement, life extending) and psychological/emotional manners (e.g., it fights anxiety, depression, improves happiness and sense of self), it also has the power to bring communities together through shared embodied practices and social values (an old functionalist idea). The degree to which the EiM philosophy has been employed as a lever to justify a full spate of sport related research in North America and elsewhere (let alone improve the cultural perception that sport science is merely 'phys ed' for 'jocks') cannot be understated (see Cairney et al., 2018). Sport, exercise, physical activity is at once individually medicinal, a public health intervention, cost effective, equity producing, history producing, and a fundamental human right (unless you are an internationally competitive Russian athlete in the present moment). Encouraging people to participate in order to remedy a broad range of personal/social problems is required, with documenting then removing barriers for all as a fundamental task.

Critical intersectional research, sport for development research, and new materialist research moved quickly to the fore of Kinesiology programs not because senior administrators developed a social conscience about issues related to power and culture or the promise of interdisciplinary thinking, but because critical research has become conservatively Kinesiological and translational along EiM lines. Equity and inclusion through sport are clearly important because they are primary social determinants of health. If racism and sexism are cultural diseases produced through historically pathological social structures, inclusive, tolerant, and diverse sport participation is an allopathic treatment not only for individuals, but entire social 'at risk' groups and indeed social structures. Critical work is a now little more than a sub-branch of epidemiology in public health units. Indeed, White scholars are now highly attentive to race in their research as a means of attending to the social determinants of health for all marginalized people (in Canada, a punctuated trend is for White persons to become experts on First Nations/Indigenous populations and sport—even becoming the thematic structure of academic conferences with very few Indigenous persons in attendance). Social scientists, without relevant psychological training or certification, now promulgate how sport and exercise can broadly help with mental health issues in the population. We used to study how sport produces poor mental health among athletes owing to power imbalances and exploitive socialization processes within unyielding performance sport cultures. Sport for development and peace can be reconciled with functional economic and globalized development. Sport for peace and development and Africa ostensibly erases the scars of colonialism, ongoing resource exploitation, and lack of health provision and aid from the West (like actual vaccines for a range of diseases). New materialism creates collaborative, fundable projects for national granting/health agencies highlight the 'cell to society' mantras in research. To modify Brohm (1978), then, in the collective embrace of highly corporatized, sanitized, and institutionalized EiM ideologies by sport researchers, critical studies have conformed to the ubiquitous trend that all research must exist within a 'prison' of measured function and impact.

None of the critique above is offered as condemnation of the turn in the social scientific study of sport and physical culture toward issues in justice, development, or new theoretical modes of inquiry. All three have long-standing, and highly valued, traditions in the field. The transformation of a huge segment of the field does, however, play a significant role in rationalizing and framing how and why sport and physical culture research had to proceed without pause during the pandemic; it is simply too important to be ignored.

We Ought Not To, Maybe Because We Ought Not To

My disdain for Foucauldian theory is well known by colleagues. But even I reflected on the glaring similarities between researchers engaged with Covid-19 research and Foucault's (2021) account of Christian confession practices in *Confessions of the Flesh: The History of Sexuality Volume IV*. In a disciplinary attempt to reproduce functionalist 'sport for something progressive' discourses through Covid-19, people involved in a spectrum of sport and physical cultural zones have been asked to confess about the effects of Covid-19 on their lives through very predictable tropes. Confess not of your sin, but of your suffering as a sexed, gendered, raced, and classed persons in hyper-discriminatory sports worlds. Investigators were perfectly correct in pointing out how marginalized persons in sport and physical culture are disproportionately affected by Covid-19 hardships. But in review of sociological work on sport and Covid-19, vulnerable communities were the most frequently studied. On the one hand, documenting inequality and inequity is foundational sociology and must be lauded. On the other hand, considering how either research agendas or radically contextual research could not materially improve these persons' sporting experiences or lives during Covid-19, ethical questions pertaining to the process of soliciting confessions about suffering without supplying remedy or relief must be raised. At the least a Catholic priest offers temporary absolution through confession. The researcher, most of the time, only offers collaboration, co-production, allyship, voice, or a compensatory $20 gift card to Starbucks.

Covid-19 researchers might argue that documenting sport and physical culture in the present era is morally good, because, as a consequence of said research interventions, social injustice is further exposed in the slow process of producing a more perfect social union inside and outside of sport. In this sense, critical researchers *ought to* engage in pandemic studies precisely because research is a functional act geared toward social justice critique and realization. Seeking confession from research participants is not only morally warranted (in fact, isn't one's silence complicity in social oppression?), critical researchers are obliged to pursue accounts of Covid-19 experiences in pursuit of the collective good. From another, and deontological (Hooker, 2012) ethical lens, if a researcher's primary *duty* is to engage in research which minimizes harm on those persons studied as a categorical imperative (see the TCPS-2 in Canada, for instance) then asking for painful confessions during times of intense personal and collective suffering may be risky ethical business. Notwithstanding the ostensible benefits of further evidencing how sport worlds are inhumanely replete with oh so many 'isms' (which they are) through Covid-19 research, unless researchers demonstrate the immediate functional benefits of such research in tangible manners for participants, is such research ethical? I argue, maybe, just maybe, sociologists of sport and physical culture ought to have taken the collective foot of the research pedal for two years and let vulnerable alone whilst the latter's lives were in cataclysmic disarray.

As the Alpha (January 2020) and Beta variants of Covid-19 (July 2020) ripped through global populations, research agendas for the sociology of sport were crafted and published even before either the first or second global wave of the virus were fully understood (Evans et al., 2020; Ward, 2020). The period between January and July of 2020 produced the most global fear as hospitalizations and deaths soared exponentially. The abruptness of global lockdowns was astounding. I waited, with bated breath, for someone, anyone, to voice a plea for researchers to resist the urge to plunge into the Covid-19 terrain. As a journal co-Editor, graduate studies director, and Ethics Board Chair, my duties conflicted. I chose to lobby for a research shutdown in my own backyard out of respect for others' social, mental, and emotional safety. My rationalizations were grounded in recognizing the totalizing narrative disruptions in people's lives (like my own) that caused daily suffering and chaos; the need to protect the most vulnerable research participants from unnecessary poking and prodding during a pandemic; and the notion that stories about the pandemic could be confessed to researchers well after the pandemic subsided. Quite simply, I thought we ought not to ask for confessions, because we fundamentally ought not to in fulfilling our duty to care for vulnerable persons. I lobbied with others on behalf of ECRs to have their tenure clocks stopped, for graduate students to receive immediate emergency funding and extensions to their programs, and for colleagues to publish less and self-care more. I could not conceive research as social justice for anyone during the first two years of the pandemic.

For me, the first two years of the pandemic in Canada became a time to reflect on the ethical basis of my own research process and the blanket assumption that all critical research is by definition, purposeful, impactful, and morally justifiable research. First, in reflecting on the bulging corpus of 'life during Covid-19' sport research I cannot help but wonder whether much will have, in academic-speak, and discernable *impact beyond citations and references*. To assert that virtual or survey-based research on athletes who were, for example, unable to compete for their countries in national competitions, amateurs who lost funding, or programs shuttered due to economic collapse could right these wrongs is patently disingenuous. Written testimonials of people's losses, pain, suffering, and life-course disruptions are, at times, pale academic museum displays representing the fundamental unfairness of human existence. My over twenty-five years of involvement in the sport and physical cultural studies academic community instructs that all of the social inequalities demonstrated through Covid-19 were highly predictable: women's sports would suffer first and profoundly (see: feminist theories), people would find physical cultural 'salvation' (to steal from Brian Pronger) in technology by working out at home in their bedrooms on their Peloton bikes or through a freshly minted fitness app, an oligarchy of corporate sport industrialists would profit (see: all cultural studies and political economy theories), people around the world would say 'fuck it' and still gather to play despite lockdowns (see: all critical theories), child and elite athletes would experience anomie (see: all socialization theories), activists would lobby for sport as a human right (see: all sport for development theories), racial disparities in sport would be underlined (see: all critical race and intersectional theories), and class differences in sport (see: basically every social theory) in and through (and beyond) Covid-19 would be documented. In Baudrillard's (2002) phraseology, Covid-19 research has been a conceptual *non-event* in sport and physical culture thinking. The lion's share of what has been written about Covid-19 scarcely advances theory in physical cultural studies because theoretical readings were predominantly pre-populated into research on Covid-19 (see: above). A rich substantive literature now documents the lived events at this historical Covid-19 conjuncture, but whether any conceptual insight developed through the current moment will endure is doubtful. In part this also owes to the fundamental resistance of practitioners in the sociology of sport/physical cultural studies to engage in meaningful theoretical melding with scholars from the medical humanities, the sociology of health and medicine, public health, and epidemiology in order to pursue long-term interdisciplinary work on viruses, sickness, illness, and disease and their complicated intermingling with sport and physical cultural practices.

Second, questions whether Covid-19 research is a long-term project or a temporary opportunity loom large. Stated differently, will there be any discernable substantive interest in viruses, disease, and sport when the Covid-19 circus leaves town? The dearth of social science or critical research on issues connecting illness, disease, population health and sport prior to the Covid-19 pandemic would lead one to predict the research curve on Covid-19 will soon flatten. But long-term, concatenated, and conceptually driven projects could produce considerable theoretical and conceptual fruit as a means of exploring the theoretical, trans-disciplinary, methodologically innovative and boundary crossing exegeses often promised by proponents of the physical cultural studies intellectual project. Hit and run pieces on Covid-19 and sport are far less promising. From a research ethics perspective in Canada, our national policy document outlining ethical research practices (*Tri-Council Policy Statement: Ethical Conduct for Research Involving Humans, Version 2*) indicates studies without solid academic rationale, include researchers with expertise on the subject, and likely lead to demonstrable social benefits are patently unethical and foist undue burden on research participants. In the language of the TCPS-2, such projects are entirely socially unjust and we ought not to conduct them.

Third, and finally, will the body of Covid-19 research be integrated into teaching, graduate student education platforms, academic program development, and conference composition and cross-pollination in meaningful ways beyond 2022? My money is on the answer, no. I certainly struggle to remember enduring or impactful sport research on H1N1 ('swine flu'), Avian influenza, or Ebola either during or after the respective global health scares around them. I, for example, presently teach the only senior undergraduate course in Canadian sport science departments focussed exclusively on social scientific dissections of disease, illness, sport, and physical culture. Further, are there inherent disciplinary risks in coupling even more closely with public health and medicine in the extension of critical sport research's institutional mandate? Public health, education, and medical Faculties are already expanding and diversifying their rosters to include researchers pursuing sport studies from translational/exercise is medicine standpoints. Public Health or Medicine Faculties, often larger than their Kinesiology counterparts within higher educational institutions, might envelope translational sport and culture research in future and render autonomous sport and exercise divisions redundant.

Epilogue: Letting Covid-19 Stories Breathe

At the time of writing this chapter, I have experienced nearly two and a half years of life in a pandemic. I am fatigued, exasperated, and on many days, unmotivated. I cannot fathom a single condition or context in which I would wilfully consent to Covid-19 research as a subject. As Covid-19 raged between early 2020 and late 2021, people were constantly instructed to self-monitor, wash incessantly, receive inoculations, carry vaccine passports, confess their fear and depression, submit to screening, allow others to Zoom into their homes thereby collapsing work/family boundaries, speak to one another behind plastic or glass partitions, and in the most tragic cases, say goodbye to loved ones. I had to acknowledge the relative insignificance of my research agenda during such a physical cultural apocalypse. Yet in this milieu of suffering, I watched colleagues in sport sciences ask people to engage in a 30-minute virtual interviews or surveys to explore what strategies they engage to 'get in their daily steps' during lockdown. At the Research Ethics Board I fielded emails from irate colleagues whose research programs (on non-Covid related subjects) sputtered. Those stories seemed relatively trivial and indifferent to people mired in trauma, and I remember thinking this is precisely why people hate academics.

The funny, beautiful, and maddening thing about stories is that they are seldom recounted only once. People carry with them a suitcase full of stories and retell them in context. The race to formulate public first drafts of sport-related Covid-19 stories scarcely made sense because 'lockdown' stories will be (re)told for generations. From my perspective, and in using Frank's (2010) terms, our collective Covid-19 stories needed to 'breathe' whilst still unfolding. Convention in trauma research (generally speaking) is to refrain from soliciting stories of suffering from people in the thick of their trauma. Relevant stories about the long-term impact of Covid-19 on people in sport and physical cultural worlds will be around for years. Linking back to the previous section in this chapter, there are times when we categorically *ought not* to inquire. Covid-19 'cause' research was desperately required, whilst Covid-19 'effect' research could wait. Further, the odds of another viral pandemic occurring within the next few years, for which Covid-19 research on sport and physical culture could prove instructive, are exceptionally small. In review of the corpus of literature now available in the sociology of sport and physical cultural studies during Covid-times, are the vast majority of findings especially novel, surprising, telling, or conceptually game changing in the field?

Still, there can be no denying how important sport and physical cultural stories are in social restitution processes. In Canada, cases where people were able to 'return to play' signalled small victories in the broad public battle against Covid-19. Public parks re-opened, and children could play with one another again. Amateur sports re-commenced with modified rules. Professional sports followed, allowing social distanced people to symbolically reconnect once again. Sport around the world slowly returned to a modified normal, true to cherished and dominant restitution narrative nestled in our collective consciousness(es). The public goal has never been to adapt, recalibrate, reorganize, create new possibilities through, or fundamentally alter local or national sport/physical cultures beyond Covid-19, only to restore sport normality pre-2020. Important is how, as attested to by many chapters in this book, publics have 'run' to sport as a vehicle for escaping the processual abnormality produced via the pandemic. If sport's social assemblages returned triumphantly and defiantly, surely the war against Covid-19 drew to a close. Sport/physical culture is a restitutive dreamland. One example of sporting restitution stands out for me. In late spring of 2021 in Canada, fans were finally allowed back into areas to watch the National Hockey League ice hockey playoffs in Montréal. Roughly one-quarter of the Bell Centre was filled with spectators. Coldplay's song "Fix You" played over the music system as players were ushered onto the ice surface to start the game. People stood in ovation at the arena and cried, thousands gathered outside the Bell Centre in defiance of public health orders, and viewers at home across homes in Canada hugged each other in collective, restitutional relief. These stories matter, of course. But they did not require intervention by a researcher to co-produce or witness them. They were stories exhaled naturally as a sport and a nation collectivity breathed.

Writing this chapter has neither been straightforward nor pleasing. As a physical cultural studies researcher with an unyielding penchant for gritty ethnographies, reflecting on how I refrained my plying my trade while remaining at a physical distance from others was discomforting. I want restitution because embodied ethnographic acts matter to me. I want to breathe again with people who run, jump, bend, and twist. I also understand the salience of sport and physical culture in people's lives, and the thousands of manners by which Covid-19 disruptions, dislocations, dissociations, and disenfranchisement from sport has damaged lives. It's important to document them. Indeed, my entire adult life has been devoted to defending the cultural relevance of sport as a serious academic subject. Critiquing sport research during the pandemic ranks, singularly, as the most unsatisfying task I have accepted as a sociologist. But the promise of physical cultural studies is rooted in its potential to push academics to reconsider dominant sport, let alone sport research, narratives. In the case of this chapter, I push each of us to consider whether a more ethically informed and less vampiristic physical cultural studies is achieved by learning lessons from the pandemic regarding Western culture's inability to decelerate, to produce and consume less, and attend to the vulnerable in empathic manners. Just as physical cultural studies researchers seek to instruct sociologists of sport that embodied research includes the widest range of human movement as meaningful cultural expression, physical cultural studies proponents must pursue unapologetically theoretical, artistic, expressive, thought-provoking, conceptually unsafe, philosophical, and experimental research that ventures beyond the conservatively rational and translational now dominant in the sub-discipline. I wrote this chapter because as critical sport research has attained disciplinary power, it is important to speak truth to such power.

References

Andrews, D. (2008). Kinesiology's inconvenient truth: The physical cultural studies imperative. *Quest, 60*(1), 46–63.

Baudrillard, J. (1990). *Fatal strategies*. Semiotexte.

Baudrillard, J. (2002). L'esprit du terrorisme. *Harper's Magazine*, February: 13–18.

Brohm, J.-M. (1978). *Sport: A prison of measured time*. Pluto Press.

Cairney, J., McGannon, K., & Atkinson, M. (2018). Exercise is medicine: Critical considerations in the qualitative research landscape. *Qualitative Research in Sport, Exercise and Health, 10*(4), 391–399.

Carr, E., Davis, K., Bergin-Cartwright, G., Lavelle, G., Leightley, D., Oetzmann, C., Polling, C., Stevelink, S., Wickersham, A., Razavi, R., & Hotopf, M. (2021). Mental health among UK university staff and postgraduate students in the early stages of the COVID-19 pandemic. *Occupational and Environmental Medicine, 79*(4), 259–267.

Carter-Francique, A., & Flowers, C. (2013). Intersections of race, ethnicity, and gender in sport. In E. Roper (Ed.), *Gender relations in sport: Teaching gender* (pp. 73–94). Rotterdam Sense Publishers.

CAUT Bulletin. (2018) Academic anxiety. May, 13–18.

CAUT Bulletin. (2021). The psychological toll for academic staff. December, 16–21.

Deryugina, T., Shurchkov, O., & Stearns, J. (2021). COVID-19 disruptions disproportionately affect female academics. *AEA Papers and Proceedings, 111*, 164–168.

Evans, A., Blackwell, J., Dolan, P., Fahlén, J., Hoekman, R., Lenneis, V., McNarry, G., Smith, M., & Wilcock, L. (2020). Sport in the face of the COVID-19 pandemic: Towards an agenda for research in the sociology of sport. *European Journal for Sport and Society, 17*(2), 85–95.

Foucault, M. (2021). *Confessions of the flesh: The history of sexuality, volume IV*. Pantheon.

Frank, A. (1997). *The wounded storyteller: Body, illness, and ethics*. The University of Chicago Press.

Frank, A. (2010). *Letting stories breathe: A socio-narratology*. The University of Chicago Press.
Giroux, H. (2007). *University in chains: Confronting the military-industrial-academic complex*. Routledge.
Harrop, C., Bfal, V., Carpenter, K., & Halladay, A. (2021). A lost generation? The impact of the COVID-19 pandemic on early career ASD researchers. *Autism Research, 14*, 1078–1087.
Honoré, C. (2004). *In praise of slowness: Challenging the cult of speed*. Harper Collins.
Hooker, B. (2012). *Developing deontology: New essays in ethical theory*. Wiley.
Hunt, J. (2020). Being vulnerable: Early-career researchers feel discouraged from exposing vulnerability even during a global crisis. *eLife*. https://doi.org/10.7554/eLife.59285
Ingham, A. (1997). Toward a department of physical cultural studies and an end to tribal warfare. In J. Fernandez-Balboa (Ed.), *Critical postmoderism in human movement, physical education, and sport* (pp. 157–182). State University of New York Press.
Johnson, S., Willis, S., & Evans, J. (2019). An examination of stressors, strain and resilience in academic and non-academic UK university job roles. *International Journal of Stress Management, 26*(2), 162–172.
Millington, R., & Darnell, S. (2020). *Sport, development and environmental sustainability*. Routledge.
Parsons, T. (1937). *The structure of social action*. The Free Press.
Rice, A. (1976). *Interview with the vampire*. Ballantine Books.
Silk, M., Francombe, J., & Andrews, D. (2014). Slowing the social sciences of sport: On the possibilities of physical culture. *Sport in Society, 17*(10), 1266–1289.
Steinbeck, J. (1939). *The grapes of wrath*. Viking Press.
Ward, P. (2020). A sociology of the Covid-19 pandemic: A commentary and research agenda for sociologists. *Journal of Sociology, 56*(4), 726–735.
Williams, O., & Gibson, K. (2018). Exercise as a poisoned elixir: Inactivity, inequality and intervention. *Qualitative Research in Sport Exercise and Health, 10*, 412–428.

Index[1]

A

Ableism, 270–274, 277, 283, 287–288, 563
Actor-network theory (ANT), 355, 356, 373–378, 381
Acquired Immune Deficiency Syndrome (AIDS), 297–306, 308–311, 313, 420, 575
Adolescents, 146–149, 151, 157–160, 721
Affect, 8, 12, 14, 17, 18, 121, 148, 157, 226, 242, 243, 249, 253, 254, 259, 261–263, 270, 309, 349, 351, 355, 359, 360, 363–366, 532, 581, 598, 604, 606, 626, 639, 656, 699, 710
Affective contagion, 11–12
Agential realism, 121, 145–161
Amateurism, 628, 629, 631
Anthropocene, 105, 109, 356, 545–564
Anti-Blackness, 625, 639, 640
Antiracism, 336
Aotearoa New Zealand, 19, 118–120, 124, 138, 171, 172, 173n4, 471–492, 602
Assemblage, 1–29, 39, 40, 47, 66, 68, 70, 73, 94, 106, 122, 134, 150, 242, 246, 248, 249, 334, 338, 348, 351, 353–356, 359, 360, 362–367, 430, 657, 759, 792
Association of football, 378, 379, 381, 387, 749

[1] Note: Page numbers followed by 'n' refer to notes.

D. L. Andrews et al. (eds.), *Sport and Physical Culture in Global Pandemic Times*, Global Culture and Sport Series, https://doi.org/10.1007/978-3-031-14387-8

Athlete activism, 73, 82, 335
Atmospheres, 91–111, 137, 156, 426, 438, 550, 602, 609, 610, 667, 669
Austerity, 497, 501, 535, 751
Autonomy, 92, 94, 99, 170, 474, 487, 500, 534, 561, 587, 791

B
Beach, 9, 161, 165–183, 202, 214, 610, 611, 650
Becoming, 16, 20, 106, 117–139, 145–161, 245, 283, 332, 348, 351, 353, 357, 364, 385, 439, 498, 505, 523, 602, 656, 702, 772, 785, 786
Biopolitics, 6, 18, 37, 39, 453, 455, 463
Blue space, 174, 202, 224, 600, 611, 616
Board of Control for Cricket in India (BCCI), 395–412
Bodily boundaries, 8–11, 132
Body of sport, 373–375, 378–382, 387
Bourdieu, Pierre, 108n5, 327, 696–698, 703, 708–710
Brazil, 2, 4, 19, 38, 172, 419–440, 533
Bubbles, 13, 53, 77, 78, 80, 125, 126, 133, 244, 299, 308, 312, 383, 384, 404–407, 409, 410, 445, 547, 571, 572, 651–655, 663
Business, 38, 43–46, 46n3, 50, 79, 99, 125, 126, 129, 137, 138, 192n1, 287, 303, 312, 321, 397–399, 404, 407, 408, 411, 412, 497, 507, 525, 546, 547, 583, 632, 634, 645, 649–651, 726, 727, 729, 730, 754, 774, 788

C
Capitalism, 16, 206, 328, 447, 518, 545, 549, 551–555, 561, 616, 667–684, 746, 747, 751–754, 760–765, 777
Cardiac rehabilitation, 692–696, 700–702, 706
Care, 2, 9, 17, 19, 55, 95, 98, 117–119, 121, 122, 124–132, 135, 137–139, 201, 208, 244, 253, 256, 272, 276, 288, 298, 307, 309, 359, 365, 380, 396, 406, 426, 447–449, 451, 454, 461, 464, 480, 502, 506, 527, 533, 535, 579, 585–588, 597, 603, 611, 616, 617, 623–640, 661, 692, 694, 695, 697, 698, 706, 707, 774, 775, 788
Cartography, 91–111, 373–388
Celebration capitalism, 667–684
China, 2–4, 19, 37–59, 95, 171, 175, 295, 305, 683
Chinese Communist Party (CCP), 38, 39, 41, 42, 44, 44n1, 46, 48–52, 54, 57
Climate change, 48, 191, 261, 508, 554, 570, 616
Coaching practice, 40, 374, 375, 382–384, 386, 388
Colonization, 487, 552
Colorblindness, 323, 334
College athletes, 569, 570, 573, 574, 576, 581, 583, 585–587, 628, 636–638

College football, 74, 571, 572, 584, 625–634, 636, 638–640
Community, 1, 4, 6, 7, 10, 11, 13, 15–18, 20–22, 51, 56, 80, 96, 98, 100, 104, 117–139, 159, 160, 171, 172, 176–178, 180, 183, 193, 202, 206, 214, 216, 219, 227, 229, 230, 241–243, 245–247, 255, 256, 272, 274, 275, 277–282, 285, 287–289, 295–314, 322, 329, 334, 338, 354, 355, 359, 361, 364, 374, 409, 421, 423, 424, 438, 439, 446, 449, 450, 453–455, 461–463, 471–473, 475, 476, 481, 484–488, 490–492, 502, 526–529, 531, 532, 558, 572, 575, 577, 581, 582, 597, 599, 610, 629, 637, 646, 651, 652, 675, 679, 680, 682, 718, 745, 747, 761, 777, 779, 781–783, 785, 787, 789
Connection and convergence, 16–18
Coronapolitics, 65–84
Coronavirus, 6, 12, 17, 66, 68, 70, 71, 73, 76–80, 83, 121, 148, 152, 165, 167, 178, 241, 256, 295, 302, 304, 311, 348, 439, 448, 521, 523, 525, 527, 528, 535, 563, 576, 578, 580, 624, 632, 634, 646, 647, 652, 661, 668, 676, 678–684
Cosmopolitics, 105–111
COVID-19, 1–6, 8–14, 16, 18–20, 37, 39, 40, 47–49, 51, 53, 54, 56, 71, 76, 91, 95, 98, 117–123, 125, 126, 132–134, 137–139, 145–148, 152, 156, 158–161, 165–184, 191–208, 214, 226, 227, 229–231, 242–250, 256, 259, 261, 263, 270, 272, 274–282, 284, 287, 288, 295–314, 321–341, 347–367, 373, 378–381, 383, 387, 395–397, 406, 408, 420, 421, 425, 427–429, 431, 438, 439, 446–451, 453, 454n3, 459–462, 471–492, 495–510, 517–536, 545–564, 569–588, 597–599, 601, 604, 608, 613, 616, 633, 645–663, 667–684, 691–710, 715, 716, 721, 724, 725, 728, 729, 733, 736, 738, 743–765, 772–782, 787–794
COVID-19 syndemic, 420, 431, 438
Cricket, 45, 181, 395–412, 527
Critical pedagogy, 204, 326
Critical race theory (CRT), 75, 322, 323, 335–337, 340
Cultural pedagogies, 203, 419–440
Cultural politics, 43, 45, 66, 80, 165–184, 336

D

Debt, 57, 192, 218, 496–505, 507–510
Decorum/decay, 94, 102–105
Delivery workers, 420, 428–431, 435–438
Differential vulnerability, 100–102, 105, 109, 110
Diffraction, 40, 41, 52–59, 157, 194, 208, 420
Digital technologies, 16, 17, 118, 123, 124, 127–132, 136, 138, 139, 150, 357, 364, 604
Digital photo diaries, 597–617

Disability, social model of, 270, 275–277
Disaster capitalism, 670–672, 678, 683, 746, 747, 751, 753, 754, 760, 762, 764

E

Ecological feelings, 107, 108
Economic, 7, 8, 16, 21, 37, 56, 57, 59, 66, 83, 97, 99, 100, 103, 109, 119, 120, 125, 167, 168, 173, 178, 216, 220, 244, 272, 288, 296, 299, 301, 302, 313, 321, 323, 325, 333, 334, 336, 348, 399, 407, 411, 427, 432, 436, 437, 461, 463, 475, 476, 487, 488, 496, 497, 499, 500, 507, 518, 519, 546, 553, 554, 557, 561, 563, 575, 579, 582, 600, 611, 613, 616, 625, 636, 669, 670, 674, 680, 697, 715, 718, 722, 724–726, 729, 731, 735–737, 743–746, 750, 753–755, 757, 762–764, 783, 786, 789
Embodiment, 8, 39, 50, 128, 203, 242, 353, 358, 562, 597–617, 662, 701
English Premier League (EPL), 518, 523–527, 531, 746, 748, 758
Environment, 17, 99, 106, 110, 118, 123, 128, 129, 132, 134, 136, 178, 192n1, 200, 202, 214, 215, 224, 228, 246, 253, 272, 273, 275, 277, 281, 282, 286, 287, 337, 338, 340, 349, 353–357, 359, 361, 409, 421, 424, 436, 472, 489, 509, 510, 518, 523, 546, 547, 550, 555, 562, 563, 575, 586, 598, 600, 603, 611, 639, 648, 649, 660, 673, 701, 707, 724, 756
Equity, 208, 221, 243, 324, 341, 490, 500, 501, 582, 757, 758, 763, 784, 785
Esports, 553, 648, 715–737
Ethics, 12, 19, 117–139, 169, 191, 251, 326, 585–588, 773, 776, 777, 790
Ethnography, 374, 793
European Super League, 747, 749–751, 754–762, 764
Exercise, 9, 10, 43, 48, 169, 174, 175, 177–179, 181–183, 245, 284, 327, 336, 339, 522, 597–599, 602, 606, 610, 660, 692, 694, 695, 698, 700, 701, 703, 706, 707, 722, 724, 776, 778, 783–786, 791
Exploitation, 109, 206, 215, 216, 549, 552, 556, 581, 585–586, 588, 628–630, 633, 636, 637, 639, 647, 743–765, 786

F

Fascism, 67–71, 77, 82, 84, 427
Fatherhood, 447
Feminist materialisms, 7, 13, 17, 138, 242, 248, 261
Feminist new materialism
  innovation, 358, 363, 366
  virtual programs, 353, 354, 358, 366
Field hockey, 243, 254
Fight Island, 646, 648, 650, 654–663

Fitness professionals, 117–139, 274, 278, 281
Food banks, 517–536
Football (American), 571, 626, 632, 638, 639
Football fans, 40, 42, 420, 423, 425, 427, 517, 524–527, 751, 759, 761
Football, 37–53, 57–59, 74, 75, 79, 123, 126, 128, 134, 243, 254, 260, 261, 307, 333, 334, 362, 374, 378–381, 385, 387, 398, 419–440, 460, 517, 518, 522–531, 533, 534, 547, 569, 571–574, 577, 578, 580–581, 584, 588, 623–640, 662, 743–765
  See also Soccer
France, 38, 171, 173n4, 376, 398, 716, 724–726, 729, 735–737
Furlough, 499, 517–536, 704

G

Gendered pandemic, 119–120
Gendered performances, 199, 250
Gender equity, 243
Geography, 19, 217, 241, 445–464, 601, 645–663, 670, 704
Gig economy, 420, 428–431, 434–436, 438–440
Girls, 128, 241–264, 350, 354, 363–365, 459, 484, 486, 784
Global football ecosystem, 744–746, 753, 754, 760–764
Governance, 38, 58, 102, 137, 178, 287, 407–410, 478, 483, 508, 745, 747, 749, 751, 755, 756
Governing, 43, 44, 100, 167, 350, 360, 373–375, 378, 378n2, 379, 381, 382, 387, 411, 517, 523, 533, 535, 723, 758, 760
Government, 2–5, 9, 10, 38, 43, 48–51, 51n5, 52–59, 91, 93, 95, 100, 101, 119, 120, 125, 168, 170, 172–177, 179–182, 221, 224, 256, 273, 296, 298, 301–303, 311–313, 330, 349, 361, 374, 378, 379, 399, 400, 403–412, 419, 420, 424, 426–428, 433, 434, 439, 472–475, 488, 491, 492, 495–510, 517, 519–521, 523–525, 527–530, 532, 535, 536, 563, 650, 668, 670–672, 674, 676, 681, 700, 725, 726, 748, 751
Graduate students, 192–196, 201, 206–208, 337, 554, 773–775, 778, 779, 781, 788, 790
Great Migration, 220
Green space, 202, 213–231, 273, 279, 600, 614–616

H

Health, 2, 47, 92, 117, 174, 202, 214, 227–230, 241, 272, 296, 322, 350, 373, 396, 420, 447–451, 483, 496, 520, 555, 569, 597, 625, 646, 675, 692, 705–708, 715–737, 772
Health inequalities/inequity, 97, 577, 581, 582, 586, 601, 616
HIV, 297, 298, 301, 307, 309, 310, 313, 784

I

Identity, 19, 40–42, 69, 169, 170, 183, 204, 224, 231, 245, 261–263, 270, 328–331, 374, 386, 401, 423, 491, 548, 554, 556, 559, 630, 631, 656, 760, 772
Idleness, 555, 561–564
Indian Premier League (IPL), 395–412
Indigenous, 15, 46n4, 425, 461, 473, 477–480, 487, 488, 558, 560, 624, 786
Industry, 2, 46, 50, 111, 118, 120, 123, 126, 139, 166, 322, 401, 446, 449, 454n3, 460, 463, 491, 506, 527, 533, 546–549, 553–555, 564, 653, 669, 671, 676, 695, 715–737, 744, 746, 752, 757, 763
Innovation, 19, 56, 281, 350, 358, 359, 362, 363, 780
International Olympic Committee (IOC), 547, 667–671, 676, 678–683, 723, 724
Interviewing, 39, 693
Intra-action/intra-acting, 11, 13, 14, 41, 109, 121, 132, 135, 137, 150, 151, 160, 161, 192, 242, 249, 250
Intrusion of Gaia, 92, 94, 105–108, 110

J

January 6th, 2021, 65, 522

K

Kaupapa Māori, 473, 474, 476–481, 486, 487, 490, 491
Kholi, Virat, 398–400, 411

L

Labor, 42, 43, 72, 82, 83, 117, 132, 201, 215, 217, 218, 426, 428, 429, 436, 450, 503, 506, 552, 571, 581, 583, 585–586, 588, 626, 627, 630, 631, 633–640, 654, 668, 744, 763
Latour, Bruno, 102, 106, 110, 374, 374n1, 375–378, 381, 383, 387, 388, 549
Leisure time physical activity (LTPA), 271–274, 278–281, 286
Lifestyle sport, 169, 548, 557, 558
Lockdown, 2–4, 6, 9, 40–42, 52n6, 57, 66, 91–111, 118, 119, 124–128, 132, 133, 135–137, 147, 152–155, 159, 160, 165–184, 242, 243, 245, 247, 253, 254, 256–259, 263, 278, 321, 322, 329, 349, 364, 373–375, 378, 379, 381–387, 404, 407–409, 425, 426, 438, 446, 453, 471, 517, 518, 520, 522, 523, 525–527, 563, 597–617, 691, 693, 696, 698, 699, 702–705, 716, 721, 722, 724, 735, 777, 782, 788, 789, 791, 792
Longing, 137, 139, 196, 201, 387, 597–617

M

Methods, 16, 17, 70–72, 118, 123–124, 151, 205, 242, 243, 246–251, 253–264, 354, 449, 452, 605, 607, 693, 726, 777, 782
More-than-human, 6, 8, 11–13, 15, 16, 94, 108, 121, 122, 124, 130, 137–139, 160, 248, 261, 263, 352–354, 356, 359, 366, 547, 548, 550, 553, 559, 560, 562, 563, 598, 604–606, 610, 615, 616

N

National Collegiate Athletic Association (NCAA), 74, 296, 446, 456, 547, 569–588, 630, 631, 633, 636, 638, 640
Nationalism, 46, 65–84, 302, 335, 505, 613, 672
National Park Service (NPS), 215, 222
Nature inequities, 224
Nature privilege, 231
Neoliberalism, 18, 66, 67, 298, 302, 305, 411, 447–451, 464, 495, 496, 507, 510, 587, 670, 753, 754
Nonhumans, 7, 8, 12–16, 19, 102, 103, 105, 109, 121, 122, 124, 130, 131, 135, 137, 149, 248, 253, 259, 348, 351–360, 362–367, 376, 377, 383, 551, 552, 559, 560, 604

O

Olympics/Olympic Games, 16, 65, 71, 409, 472, 496, 497, 504–505, 508, 509, 553, 648, 667–684
Online activity, 130, 285, 288, 349, 362, 364, 737

P

Pandemic, 1–22, 29, 37–59, 65–84, 91–111, 117–139, 145–149, 152, 158–160, 165–183, 191–208, 213–231, 241–264, 270, 272, 274–281, 284, 286–289, 295–314, 321, 322, 335, 339, 341, 347–352, 358, 359, 362–367, 373–388, 395–412, 425, 431, 439, 445–464, 472, 473, 491, 495–510, 517–536, 545–547, 549, 551, 563, 564, 569–574, 576–578, 581, 584–588, 597–602, 604–611, 613, 615, 616, 623–640, 645–652, 654–656, 658–663, 669, 672, 680, 691–694, 696–710, 715, 716, 721–726, 728–731, 733, 735–737, 743–765, 772, 774–776, 778–782, 786–793
Pandemic atmospheres, 91–111
Parenting, 445–464
Pariah, 295–314
Participation in sport, 354, 373, 374, 387, 388
Pay-Per-View (PPV), 517, 525, 526, 663

Pedagogy(ies), 21, 29, 193, 201–206, 208, 321–341, 419–440, 554, 658
People, 1, 2, 6, 8–10, 19, 20, 39, 41, 43, 46, 46n3, 48–52, 54, 55, 57–59, 68, 79, 92, 93, 95, 96, 99, 100, 100n2, 108, 109, 123, 126, 128–131, 133–138, 153, 155, 168, 169, 173, 174, 176, 177, 193–198, 200, 204, 208, 216–218, 220, 222, 225, 229, 231, 242, 243, 245, 248, 253, 256, 259, 270–284, 286–288, 296, 298, 307, 309, 310, 324, 325, 327, 329–333, 335, 336, 339, 340, 348, 361–363, 365, 373–375, 378, 382, 395, 396, 401, 404–407, 409, 411, 412, 419, 421, 423, 427, 431, 432, 439, 440, 448, 449, 453, 461, 463, 474, 474n1, 474n2, 481, 483, 484, 487, 489, 492, 499, 500, 502, 503, 506, 518–520, 522, 527, 529, 534–536, 550, 563, 571, 572, 597, 598, 600–603, 605–610, 614, 616, 624, 626n1, 632, 648, 658, 668, 674, 675, 681–683, 691–693, 697, 704–707, 753, 755, 760, 764, 776, 780, 782–789, 791–793
Physical activity, 7, 9, 10, 91, 93, 97, 109, 120, 123, 124, 127, 130, 134, 136, 146–148, 150, 203, 204, 225, 228, 244, 245, 269–289, 349, 350, 353, 361, 362, 364, 365, 449–451, 453, 456, 457, 460, 464, 475, 476, 486, 496, 502, 509, 510, 547, 556, 559–561, 597–602, 605, 606, 611, 615, 616, 691, 694, 697, 698, 700–704, 706, 708, 709, 785
Physical cultural studies (PCS), 21, 22, 29, 191–208, 326, 327, 461, 495, 498, 502, 507, 510, 561, 605, 774, 777, 779, 789, 790, 792, 793
Physical culture, 6, 7, 18–22, 37, 40, 41, 69, 97, 108–111, 128, 168, 170, 171, 193, 202, 203, 248, 271–274, 279–282, 348, 352, 354–358, 447, 452, 462, 495–510, 548, 552, 555–564, 574, 662, 698, 775–777, 781, 783–789, 791–793
Place, 3, 9, 41, 44, 45, 49, 53, 91–94, 98, 100, 108, 123, 137, 148, 150, 154, 161, 173, 173n4, 174, 175, 177, 179, 181–183, 192, 193, 201, 208, 213, 214, 216, 217, 221, 224, 225, 228, 242, 248–251, 253, 256, 259, 273, 286, 308, 333, 336, 347, 351, 353, 354, 356, 358–360, 363–366, 374, 376, 379, 381, 382, 384, 385, 387, 404, 429, 432, 449, 454n4, 456, 459, 462, 471, 482, 484, 518, 519, 521–523, 550, 551, 562, 583, 602, 609, 629, 633, 634, 646, 648, 650, 659, 661, 669, 681, 691–693, 696, 698, 701–705, 708, 709, 726, 756, 758, 760, 779

Policy, 4, 11, 13, 16, 53, 54, 56, 57, 75, 76, 94, 103, 120, 121, 125, 139, 175, 221, 223, 224, 226, 230, 244, 263, 271, 273, 277, 279, 281, 289, 296, 302, 307, 313, 322–324, 329, 330, 351, 359, 360, 363, 365, 374, 379, 381, 421, 437, 446, 447, 473, 475, 478, 479, 484–485, 488, 491, 496, 498, 499, 501–503, 506–510, 574, 578, 613, 646, 653, 663, 670, 671, 680, 745, 746, 751, 762, 790
Political economy, 45, 496, 498, 518, 789
Political economy of sport, 498
Politics, 2, 5, 6, 12, 14, 17–19, 21, 29, 40, 41, 43, 45, 48, 50, 51, 53, 65–84, 97, 100–104, 108–111, 165–183, 204, 206, 220, 247, 261, 301, 323, 325–327, 332, 335–339, 341, 348, 352, 357, 358, 398, 399, 423, 426, 433, 436, 437, 447, 449, 455, 464, 486, 496, 499, 501–503, 505, 507, 597–617, 646–648, 651–656, 669, 671, 753, 761
Popular resistance, 420, 430, 437
Post-sport, 545–564
Praxis, 4, 40, 94, 192, 202, 206, 283, 326, 327
Precarity, 2, 191–208, 436, 631, 696
Processes of becoming, 122, 130, 131, 148, 602
Professional sport, 81, 118, 244, 272, 296–298, 307, 308, 313, 379, 380, 449, 450, 517, 533, 553, 572, 631, 650, 652, 658, 745, 757, 763, 792
Project Big Picture (PBP), 747–754, 761, 762, 764
Propaganda, 54, 67, 70, 72, 76, 305, 322, 336, 679
Protest, 4, 11, 99, 166–168, 168n1, 170–183, 310, 322, 335–337, 419–440, 533, 536, 676, 680, 759
Proximity, 95n1, 137, 191–208, 220, 228–231, 278, 349, 378, 398, 599, 648, 650

Q

Qualitative research, 355
Quasi-governmental institution, 397, 411–412

R

Race, 48, 75, 83, 84, 171, 198, 214, 216, 220, 226, 227, 231, 241, 270, 321–341, 434, 490, 518, 522, 557, 563, 577, 626, 658, 724, 784, 786, 789, 792
Reconciliation, 218, 222, 489
Reflexivity, 331, 358, 451, 696, 698, 709
Relationships, 6, 7, 9, 12, 40, 44n1, 68, 69, 71, 80, 81, 101, 131, 137, 158, 193, 202, 208, 213, 215, 230, 231, 246, 248, 258, 276, 299, 300, 310, 313, 326, 351, 362, 396, 400, 449, 464, 473–477, 479–486, 488, 489, 491, 492, 497, 502, 503, 509, 517, 518, 532, 533, 547, 555, 580, 600, 606–608, 638, 646, 647, 660–662, 692, 695, 703, 755, 777

Reorienting, 373–388
Resilience, 11, 107, 487–488, 491, 737, 780
Re-turning, 10, 12, 14, 18–29, 74, 118, 120–122, 132–139, 199, 244, 245, 254–261, 307, 308, 340, 380, 383, 462, 487, 563, 578, 632, 703
Risk, 8, 10, 11, 13, 14, 16, 20, 21, 55, 97, 99, 134, 139, 147, 159, 167, 169, 172, 174, 175, 204, 207, 208, 221, 225, 227, 228, 243, 246, 254, 261, 270, 275–277, 304, 307, 309, 328, 373, 379, 383, 385, 388, 405, 406, 420, 425, 427, 431, 448, 523, 530, 534, 545, 571–574, 576–581, 584–586, 599, 601, 615, 625, 628, 631, 632, 634, 635, 646, 661, 671, 681, 692, 694, 704, 707, 757, 763, 780, 786, 791
Ruination, 110

S

Self-reflexivity, 324–328
Sexuality, 297, 328, 339, 675, 784
Shock therapy, 743–765
Soccer, 37, 43, 45, 181, 243, 254, 255, 260, 262, 322, 350, 446, 450, 452–455, 455n4, 456, 459–461, 518, 752, 753, 758
  See also Football
Social class, 309, 328, 424, 434, 463, 531, 695, 697, 704
Social determinants of health, 221, 226, 283, 785, 786
Society, 42, 52, 53, 58, 84, 98, 106, 119, 132, 147, 148, 167–170, 180, 182, 183, 193, 208, 215, 217, 223, 226, 296, 303, 304, 308, 326–330, 332, 335, 339–341, 351, 355, 362, 376, 377, 381, 396, 420, 427, 429, 433, 434, 447, 477, 480, 496, 502, 508–510, 519, 535, 545, 547, 549, 551, 555, 558, 561, 588, 652, 656, 671, 683, 754, 786
Sociology of sport/sport sociology, 7, 18–29, 207, 348, 352–356, 507, 510, 554, 574, 577, 784, 785, 788, 790, 792
South Africa, 19, 165–184, 398
Spacetimemattering, 12–14, 194, 208, 242, 255, 259, 261
Sport, 6, 12–14, 18–29, 38, 66–69, 72–83, 93, 117–139, 147, 169, 203, 241–264, 270, 296, 321–341, 348, 373, 378–381, 396, 420, 445–464, 471–492, 495–510, 517–536, 546, 569–588, 626, 645–663, 671, 716, 743, 774
Sport for Development (SFD), 347–367, 783–786, 789
Sport-for-development and peace, 347–367, 783, 784, 786
Sport management, 554, 555
Sports-media complex, 397, 398, 400–402, 410
Sport sociology as discipline, 554
Stigma, 284, 298, 299, 305–308, 310, 312, 434
Surfing, 10, 123, 165–184, 557, 600, 610, 616

Surveillance, 3, 4, 37, 51, 55, 56, 58, 59, 92, 93, 97, 101, 103, 104, 107, 109, 276, 284, 297, 299, 302, 308, 333, 495, 629, 676
Sustainability, 547, 548, 555, 671, 673, 674, 678, 725, 745
Syndemics, 419–440, 569–588

T

Technologies, 3–5, 7, 14, 16, 17, 28, 39, 43, 51, 54–56, 67, 118, 123, 124, 127–132, 134–136, 138, 139, 149, 150, 152, 153, 156, 159, 199, 259, 281, 282, 299, 347–367, 384, 428, 436, 460n8, 545, 604, 605, 615, 676, 723, 789
Time capsule, 241–264
Tokyo 2020, 471, 667–684
Tokyo 2021, 71
Trump, Donald, 4, 65, 66, 69, 72–74, 77–80, 82, 298, 300–306, 310, 311, 313, 335, 336, 341, 571, 572, 645–647, 651–657, 661, 662, 679

U

Uber-sport, 15, 66, 68, 69, 71, 72, 77, 79–82, 84, 333, 547, 656, 657, 662
Ultimate Fighting Championship (UFC), 547, 633, 645–663
United Kingdom (UK), 2–4, 19, 38, 46n4, 118, 229, 249, 280, 360, 361, 381, 496, 499, 517–520, 522, 523, 527, 528, 531, 533–536, 683, 696, 751, 758
United Kingdom government, 378, 379, 387, 517, 519, 520, 523–525, 527, 529, 703, 709, 748, 751

V

Vaccine hesitancy, 517–536
Video game, 718, 720–722, 724, 725, 733, 735, 736
Violence, 13, 15, 16, 102, 109, 218, 219, 244, 246, 322, 323, 328, 335, 341, 365, 423, 434, 437, 461, 555, 575, 577, 583, 623–640, 659, 663, 670, 684, 708, 784
Virtual programs, 350, 353
Vital matter, 14–16
Vulnerabilities, 8, 11, 100–102, 105, 109, 110, 130, 131, 205, 439, 602, 631, 709, 745, 775

W

Women, 10, 44, 72, 117–139, 215–217, 219, 223, 244–248, 263, 273, 281, 310, 322, 336, 350, 354, 363–365, 451, 456, 461, 486, 535, 579, 602, 606, 634, 675, 779, 784, 789
Wuhan, 2, 3, 5, 47, 52, 57, 175, 295, 304, 521

Y

Youth sport, 246, 349, 445–464

Printed by Printforce, the Netherlands